ARDENT MEDIA INC
is pleased to announce the birth of:
CONTRACEPTIVE TECHNOLOGY

In PDF format on CDROM

For the first time, some *Contraceptive Technology* (CT) books also include a CD-ROM with the complete text of CT in direct electronic conversion. Jump links are included so that you can go directly from the table of contents to any chapter or any topic listed in the subheads in the contents. Electronic links are also included to the 300 Web sites recommended by the authors in CT so that you can go online with your CD-ROM and access instantly a wealth of helpful information to complement CT. As well, you will be able to quickly print out patient instructions for those you counsel, or other content for your own use.

Please read this overview BEFORE opening your CD-ROM.

If your copy of CT does not include a CD-ROM, you will find ordering instructions in the back of this book. Please save your receipt if you have purchased or when you do purchase the CD-ROM or book/CD combo to mail with the CD (or PDA) Registration Form in the back of this book. This will enable us to email you a password to activate your CD-ROM. Please print out and save this email and keep it in a safe place.

If you are considering the purchase of a CD-ROM or PDA format but are not sure if it is right for your needs or the needs of your organization, we ask that you fill out and mail the New Media Survey in the back of this book, including your specific needs and we will help you meet those needs.

Each CD-ROM is for a single-user only unless you purchase a network license. Your password will work only on one computer. If you purchase a new computer there is no additional charge to issue you a new password (your old password will be disabled). If you want a CD-ROM for two of your own computers, you may purchase a second CD-ROM at half the current list price.

For organizations with multiple computer users, we can provide either bulk quantity CD-ROMs at a discount, or you can purchase a network license if your computers are networked. Please fill out the New Media Survey in the back of this book, describe your needs and send it to us so that we can provide a solution. If your organization desires the ability to cut and paste for use within the network, a network license must be purchased as this function is not supported on single-user CD-ROMs.

We encourage you to make one backup copy of your CD-ROM. You may use the CD-ROM on a computer or workstation but may not copy or reproduce it through a LAN or other network. Please do not risk the disabling of your access password.

If you or your organization wish to print out, reproduce or distribute any of the content on the CD for a purpose other than individual counseling or use (for example, for a class, workshop or seminar with multiple participants) please mail us the New Media Survey or Registration Form in the back of this book describing your permissions request and we will contact you with a solution to obtain the written permission you need for a network license, other license, or provide you bulk CDs at a discount.

Hardware requirements:
PC or Mac with CD-ROM Drive

Software requirements:
PC; Win 95 or greater
Mac; OS 7 or greater
Adobe Acrobat Reader 4 or better
Download free Reader at www.adobe.com

Accessing the CD:
Place the CD in the CD Drive. The Single-User Purchaser Agreement should open automatically. Click on "I Agree" and the table of contents will open. If the Single-User Purchaser Agreement does not open, then browse the CD and double click on the file "Single User Purchaser Agreement.pdf".

If you do not yet have a password, print out, complete and mail the registration form to Ardent Media. The registration form is also located at the end of the table of contents on the CD.

You will find the complete Single-User Purchaser Agreement on the CD-ROM. Please read it carefully. By clicking on "I Agree" you are agreeing to be bound by its terms.

Thank you for helping *Contraceptive Technology* enter the electronic era.

Please complete the
CD-ROM/PDA REGISTRATION FORM
located at the end of this book

To register your CD-ROM or PDA format and receive an access password, enclose with the Registration Form:

- For Laptop or Desktop, specify PC or Mac
- For PDA, specify Palm or Pocket PC
- Enclose a copy of your receipt or proof of purchase for *Contraceptive Technology* in CD, PDA, or CD/book format. If purchased for you, enclose that proof of purchase.

ARDENT MEDIA INC

is pleased to announce that its expecting the birth in November 2004 of CONTRACEPTIVE TECHNOLOGY

In PDF format for
PDA (Personal Digital Assistant)

This single-user version now being completed will be a direct electronic conversion to PDA format, sent to you on CD-ROM or we will email to you instructions to download from the Web. It will download to either a Palm or Pocket PC PDA. You will be able to create your own custom version of *Contraceptive Technology* by downloading the chapters or sections that you refer to the most. The security features described for the CD-ROM will also apply to the PDA. The single-user PDA will not provide for printing out of any content as the CD-ROM will. The single-user PDA will only be for on screen viewing and will not run on a network.

Because the PDA is still in completion, we welcome your suggestions. If you need to be able to print from the PDA format or have other special requirements, please include that in the New Media Survey, located at the end of this book. Please include your email address so we can notifty you of pre-publication offers, such as a sample chapter in PDA format that we hope to make available for download or on CD-ROM. Please specify Palm or Pocket PC format.

If you are ordering the PDA format by credit card, your card will not be charged until it is sent to you either on CD or instructions are emailed to you to download from the Web. If you are sending a check in payment for the PDA format along with any other materials on the order form in the back of this book, please make a separate check for the PDA. We will deposit it only when the PDA format is sent to you.

Thank you for your interest in this exciting new way to access *Contraceptive Technology*.

Contraceptive Technology

Eighteenth Revised Edition

Robert A. Hatcher, MD, MPH

James Trussell, PhD

Felicia H. Stewart, MD

Anita L. Nelson, MD

Willard Cates Jr., MD, MPH

Felicia Guest, MPH, CHES

Deborah Kowal, MA, PA

ARDENT MEDIA, INC.

NEW YORK

Bulk Purchase Discounts: For discounts on orders of 25 copies or more, please fax the number above, write the address above or call (212) 861-1501. Please state if you are a non-profit organization and the number of copies you are interested in purchasing. Bulk discount orders are nonreturnable.

Note to Book Sellers: All returns require written permission and label from the publisher. CD-ROMs returnable only if packaging unopened. Write to the address above or fax the number above for permission.

ISSN 0091-9721

ISBN 0-9664902-2-3 (Paperback with CD-ROM)
ISBN 0-9664902-3-1 (Hardcover Reference with CD-ROM)
ISBN 0-9664902-5-8 (Hardcover Reference)
ISBN 0-9664902-6-6 (Paperback)

TRADEMARKS: All brand and product names are trademarks or registered trademarks of their respective companies. It has been attempted throughout this text to distinguish proprietary trademarks from generic or descriptive terms by following the capitalization style used by the manufacturer; however, the publisher cannot attest to the accuracy of this information. Use of a term in this text should not be regarded as affecting the validity of any trademark or service mark.

1 3 5 7 9 10 6 4 2

Printed in the United States of America.

The paper used in this publication meets the minimum requirements of American National Standard for Information Sciences — Permanence of Paper for Printed Library Materials, ANSI Z39.48-1984.

DISCLAIMER

The information contained herein is intended to be used by physicians and other qualified healthcare professionals. The information is not intended to be used for medical diagnosis or treatment by persons who are not qualified healthcare professionals. Such persons should not rely upon or use the information contained herein in place of a visit, call, or consultation with, or the advice of their personal physician or other qualified healthcare provider.

Physicians and other qualified healthcare professionals should recognize that this book is to be used only as a reference aid, and that this book is not intended to be a substitute for their exercise of professional judgment. Since medical science is always changing, physicians and other qualified healthcare professionals users are advised to confirm the information contained herein with an independent source. The authors and contributors are not liable for errors and omissions.

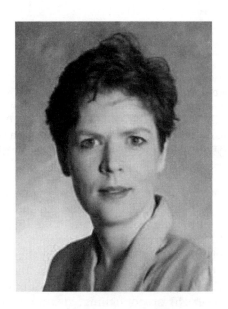

In memory of

Charlotte Ehrengard Ellertson, MPA, PhD

March 2, 1966 – March 21, 2004

Beloved friend, inspiring colleague, visionary scholar, effective activist

Dedication

Blessed is she who is flexible, for she shall not be 'bent out of shape.'
—Maxine Keel

We dedicate this edition of *Contraceptive Technology* to Maxine Keel.

Maxine has been the administrative assistant to founding author Bob Hatcher for 20 years, gracefully managing a hub office and welcoming a steady stream of visitors, medical students and residents, phone callers, and electronic messengers.

A fundraising and organizing genius and family planning advocate of the highest order, she recruited and shepherded the many students who participated in the seminal summer program in family planning at Grady Memorial Hospital/Emory University. She communicates with staff, faculty, and donors with candor and passion about the importance of our field. And even in these perilous economic times, they usually respond with support! We think her glorious Boston accent has something to do with it, along with her gift of storytelling, creating a vivid and moving rationale for family planning care and professional education.

Maxine generates a great deal of the energy for our *Contraceptive Technology* publications and conferences, especially our annual Atlanta conference that sometimes seems to exist as an act of her will.

Maxine, we send you our deep gratitude and boundless affection.

Foreword

In 1967, Beach Conger, MD, an Epidemic Intelligence Service (EIS) officer with the Centers for Disease Control working with me in family planning at Grady Memorial Hospital in Atlanta, asked in his usual straightforward style, "Hatcher, if you believe so much in the importance of birth control services, why don't you prepare an outline on it for medical students? " His prodding changed my life and led to 18 editions of *Contraceptive Technology*.

The first edition contained 32 pages and, thanks to Rockefeller Foundation support, went to third-year medical students at Chicago, Columbia, Emory, Johns Hopkins, Meharry, Mississippi, New York Medical College, Pennsylvania, Temple, and Yale.

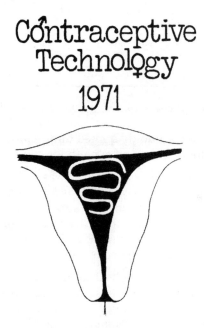

Prepared for Third Year Medical Students,
Physicians, Students, and others interested
in Contraceptive Technology.

Supported by a grant from The Rockefeller Foundation, 1971

THE EMORY UNIVERSITY FAMILY PLANNING PROGRAM
DEPARTMENT OF GYNECOLOGY AND OBSTETRICS
EMORY UNIVERSITY SCHOOL OF MEDICINE
ATLANTA, GEORGIA

Figure F-1   First bound edition of *Contraceptive Technology*, 1971

More than 30 years later, the fundamental things continue to apply, as the song says. Look, for example, at how closely the failure rates we published in 1971 compare with some of the 2004 failure rates. For other methods, failure rates have decreased as methods have improved:

CONTRACEPTIVE FAILURE RATES

	1971 Constant Users	2004 Perfect Use	1971 Actual Users	2004 Typical Use
Chance (sexually active)	80	85	80	85
Coitus Interruptus	15.6	4	22.5	27
Condom (male) .	2.6	2	11.1–28.3	15
Diaphragm	2–3	6	8.8–33.6	16
IUD	1.0–2.7	0.1–1.5	6.1	0.1–2.0
Oral Contraceptive	0.1–1.0	0.3	16.5	8
I.M. Long-Acting Progestin	0.23	0.3	5–10	3
Rhythm (calendar)	14	9	38.5–40	25
Spermicidal Foam	3.05–3.14	8	29	29
Vasectomy	<0.15	0.10	0.15	0.15
Tubal Ligation	0.04	0.5	0.04	0.5

James Trussell, PhD, has calculated the failure rates in the past dozen editions. His work is respected worldwide, and his table on contraceptive failure rates is the most commonly quoted information in this book. The package inserts for most contraceptive methods contain this table.

Jack Lippes, MD, whose Lippes Loop IUD was featured on the cover of the first bound edition of *Contraceptive Technology*, once said, "My curiosity and a little plastic coil have opened up amazing vistas to me. I've been all over the world because of this simple device I designed on my kitchen table." In a similar manner, *Contraceptive Technology* has opened up amazing vistas for me. I've been to every state and to several foreign countries.

Contraceptive Technology has evolved from that 32-page booklet to an 850-page reference text, as the body of scientific knowledge on contraception other reproductive health issues has grown enormously. International editions include *Family Planning Methods and Practice: AFRICA* (available free through the CDC) and *Contraceptive Technology: International Edition*. These various editions have been translated into Russian, Turkish, Arabic, French, and Spanish.

I reflect on the history of this book as I finish my tenure as a chapter author and begin a new role as founding author and advisor. For me, one of the best parts of writing this book has been working with my co-authors: the brilliant and irrepressible James Trussell; the optimistic and indefatigable Ward Cates and his entire family; the wordsmith and lover of the Atlanta Braves, Fifi Guest; the creative and insightful Felicia Stewart;

our editor and patient negotiator on countless details, Debbie Kowal; our deceased beloved friend, Gary Stewart; and the newest member of this writing team, the gentle, gifted teacher Anita Nelson.

For the last 13 years, the authors have held Contraceptive Technology conferences three times a year—on each coast and in Atlanta. We have shared the podium with many devoted and brilliant family planning experts. Sharon Schnare and Michael Policar deserve special recognition.

I use material from *Contraceptive Technology* with medical students rotating through the Department of Gynecology and Obstetrics at Emory. I always try to impart this foundational truth to these new clinicians:

> "The most important reproductive health problems facing the world today—everything from unintended births, maternal and infant mortalities, abortion deaths, rape and the physical abuse of women, and teenage pregnancy—cannot and will not be solved unless and until the status of women improves."

It is the fervent hope of the authors of *Contraceptive Technology* that accurate information about the current contraceptive options—which have changed over the course of the 18 editions—will improve the status of women by offering each woman the opportunity to choose if and when she will bear children. Margaret Sanger said that no woman could be completely free unless she had control over her own reproductive destiny. Even now, in the 21st century, too many women still lack this freedom. Our book advocates for the medical, economic, social, and political changes necessary for women to gain control of their own reproductive destiny.

What a joy it has been for me to spend a lifetime working on this endeavor.

Robert A. Hatcher MD, MPH
Professor of Gynecology and Obstetrics
Emory University School of Medicine

Preface

This 18th edition of Contraceptive Technology includes an outpouring of new scientific and medical developments that have emerged in just the past five years. While we are eager to share with you the latest, exciting scientific and medical developments, it is equally important to take a moment to talk about why researching, teaching, and providing reproductive health care remains so satisfying and rewarding to each of us.

The first edition of *Contraceptive Technology* was published over thirty years ago when hormonal contraceptives had only recently become commonplace. Since then, an entire generation has grown up with the potential benefits of a variety of safe and effective contraceptive methods. These technologies have enabled men and women to decide when and whether to become parents, a profound advance that has indelibly shaped modern life.

When we talk with patients about their sexual and reproductive health, counsel patients about their contraceptive options, provide abortion care to patients who have decided to terminate an unintended pregnancy, work to shape public policy, or contribute to reproductive health research, we are engaged in a critically important and deeply moral undertaking. Reproductive health care enables individuals and couples to make and implement some of the most important decisions that shape their lives, and thus also shape society. Reproductive health care reflects a deep commitment to the moral importance of parenthood and children. Our work helps ensure that every pregnancy is intended and as safe as possible, and that children are born when their parents are best able to provide the love and support they need to thrive. In sum, reproductive health care makes an essential contribution to the human infrastructure we count on for our society's well-being, opportunity, security, freedom. Our participation in strengthening individuals, families, and the community provides each of us with a foundation for our own unique moral code, which brings meaning to our lives.

As scientists, clinicians, and educators, we may not be accustomed to talking about values and the spiritual aspects of what we do. But despite our shyness, we need to do a better job of explaining our own moral values as we work with colleagues and patients—we need to teach the *why* as well as the *what, when, how* and science of reproductive health. Otherwise, it is easy to understand how the moral high ground has increasingly seemed to belong to those who oppose efforts to provide reproductive health care. For many of us, the moral importance of our work is its most compelling appeal, and it helps sustain us in the face of political and economic challenges. As one abortion provider interviewed in the mid-1990s said, "There is nothing else I do in my medical practice where people look me in the eye, in quite the same way, and say 'thank you.' I feel I am empowering women." [1]

It is not only abortion that is under attack. Emergency contraception, IUDs, and OCs are challenged by arguments based on hypothetical grounds that are sustained despite compelling scientific evidence to the contrary. Failure to provide insurance coverage for contraception stands as *prima facie* evidence of the second-class status of women in this country. In the face of overpopulation, spreading poverty, and challenges to individual freedoms, we need to rededicate ourselves to the goal that women do have the right to control their own fertility and that they need access to information, service and psychological support for their decisions. And we need to remember how important fertility control is to helping improve pregnancy outcomes.

As authors, we are inspired by the commitment and courage—and the moral example—we see in the work of so many colleagues. We appreciate deeply your help. This volume would not have been possible without the dedicated efforts and great talents of scores of people: invited chapter authors, contributors, editors, our formal and informal advisors and reviewers, and our thoughtful readers. We invite you to join our contributors. Tell us what is helpful, what is missing, and what needs to be improved.

In this time of great challenges in reproductive health, we need to work together to ensure the best possible reproductive health care for our patients and our society. We thank you for your interest in reproductive health, and hope that this book will be helpful to you.

Felicia H. Stewart, MD,
writing for the authors
of the eighteenth edition

---

[1] Joffe C. Doctors of Conscience: The Struggle to Provide Abortion Before and After Roe v. Wade. Boston: Beacon Press, 1995. 210.

The Authors

Robert A. Hatcher, MD, MPH
Professor of Gynecology and Obstetrics
Emory University School of Medicine

James Trussell, PhD
Professor of Economics and Public Affairs
Director, Office of Population Research
Princeton University

Felicia H. Stewart, MD
Adjunct Professor, Department of Obstetrics, Gynecology
  and Reproductive Sciences
Co-Director, UCSF Center for Reproductive Health Research & Policy
University of California, San Francisco

Anita L. Nelson, MD
Professor, Obstetrics and Gynecology
David Geffen School of Medicine at UCLA
Medical Director, Women's Health Care Programs
Harbor-UCLA Medical Center

Willard Cates, Jr., MD, MPH
President and CEO, Institute for Family Health
Family Health International

Felicia Guest, MPH, CHES
Director of Training, Southeast AIDS Training and Education Center
Emory University School of Medicine

Deborah Kowal, MA, PA
President and CEO, Contraceptive Technology Communications, Inc.
Adjunct Assistant Professor, Department of International Health
Rollins School of Public Health, Emory University

Invited Chapter Authors

Marcos Arevalo, MD, MPH
Director of Biomedical Research, Institute for Reproductive Health
Assistant Professor, Department of Obstetrics and Gynecology
Georgetown University Medical Center

Sarah S. Brown, MSPH
Director, The National Campaign to Prevent Teen Pregnancy

Charles S. Carignan, MD
Vice President, Clinical Affairs and Medical Director,
    Boston Scientific Corporation

Charlotte Ellertson, MPA, PhD*
President, Ibis Reproductive Health

Henry L. Gabelnick, PhD
Director, CONRAD
Professor of Obstetrics and Gynecology, Eastern Virginia Medical School

David A. Grimes, MD
Vice President of Biomedical Affairs, Family Health International
Clinical Professor, Department of Obstetrics and Gynecology,
    University of North Carolina School of Medicine

Debra W. Haffner, MDiv, MPH
Director, Religious Institute on Sexual Morality, Justice, and Healing
Community Minister, Unitarian Church of Westport

Carol J. Rowland Hogue, PhD, MPH
Terry Professor of Maternal and Child Health
Professor of Epidemiology, The Rollins School of Public Health
Senior Fellow, Center for Interdisciplinary Study of Religion
Emory University

Roy Jacobstein, MD, MPH
Medical Director, EngenderHealth

Victoria Jennings, PhD
Professor of Obstetrics and Gynecology,
Georgetown University Medical Center
Director, Institute for Reproductive Health, Georgetown University

Kathy Irene Kennedy, DrPH
Associate Clinical Professor of Preventive Medicine, University
    of Colorado Health Sciences Center
Director, Regional Institute for Health and Environmental Leadership

---

* Deceased, March 21, 2004.

Luella Klein, MD
Charles Howard Candler Professor, Department of Gynecology
  and Obstetrics, Emory University School of Medicine
Director, Maternal and Child Health Program, Grady Health System

John R. Marshall, MD
Clinical Professor of Obstetrics and Gynecology, UCLA School of Medicine
Attending Physician, Harbor/UCLA Medical Center

Anne Brawner Namnoum, MD
Atlanta Center for Reproductive Medicine

Michael S. Policar, MD, MPH
Vice President of Medical Affairs, NorthBay Healthcare System
Associate Clinical Professor, Department of Obstetrics, Gynecology and
  Reproductive Services, University of California-San Francisco

Amy E. Pollack, MD, MPH, FACOG
President, EngenderHealth
Adjunct Assistant Professor of Public Health, Mailman School of Public
  Health of Columbia University

Elizabeth Gray Raymond, MD, MPH
Associate Medical Director, Family Health International

Tara Shochet, MPH
Doctoral Student, School of Public Health
Demography Trainee, Population Studies Center
University of Michigan

William R. Stayton, ThD, PhD
Professor and Director, Human Sexuality Program, Widener University

Markus J. Steiner, PhD
Senior Epidemiologist, Family Health International

Paul F.A. Van Look, MD, PhD, FRCOG
Director, Department of Reproductive Health and Research,
  World Health Organization

Lee Warner, PhD, MPH
Epidemiologist, Department of Epidemiology, Rollins School of Public
  Health of Emory University

Production staff
  Managing editor: Deborah Kowal, MA, PA
  Designer/typesetter: Karen Stuart, Command Information Services
  Cover Artist: KC Hatcher
  Proofreader: Kathleen Ditchfield
  Indexer: Barbara Lutkins

Contributors to Contraceptive Technology, Eighteenth Edition

Many individuals contributed to this edition of *Contraceptive Technology*. They helped ensure the completeness, accuracy, timeliness, and usefulness of the information contained herein. The Authors (listed in the first grouping) alone are responsible for errors and opinions.

Authors

Willard Cates Jr., MD, MPH
Felicia Guest, MPH, CHES
Robert A. Hatcher, MD, MPH
Deborah Kowal, MA, PA
Anita L. Nelson, MD
Felicia H. Stewart, MD
James Trussell, PhD

Invited Chapter Authors

Marcos Arevalo, MD, MPH
Sarah S. Brown, MSPH
Charles S. Carignan, MD
Charlotte Ellertson, MPA, PhD*
Henry L. Gabelnick, PhD
David A. Grimes, MD
Debra W. Haffner, MDiv, MPH
Carol J. Rowland Hogue, PhD, MPH
Roy Jacobstein, MD, MPH
Victoria Jennings, PhD
Kathy I. Kennedy, DrPH
Luella Klein, MD
John R. Marshall, MD
Anne Brawner Namnoum, MD
Michael S. Policar, MD, MPH
Amy E. Pollack, MD, MPH, FACOG
Elizabeth G. Raymond, MD, MPH
Tara Shochet, MPH
William R. Stayton, ThD, PhD
Marcus J. Steiner, PhD
Paul F.A. Van Look, MD, PhD
Lee Warner, PhD, MPH

Contributors

Melanie Adams
Nancy Alexander, PhD
Marcia Ann Angle, MD, MPH
Susan Ashford, MN, RNC
Christine Bachrach, PhD
Daniel Bao
Sharon Bell
James Bellinger, PAC
Kelly Blanchard, MSc
Paul Blumenthal, MD, MPH
Lynn Borgatta, MD, MPH
Michael Bracher, PhD
Glenn D. Braunstein, MD
Michael Burnhill, MD
Josefina J. Card, PhD
Eli Carter
Philip D. Darney, MD, MSc
Jacqueline Darroch, PhD
Jennifer Del Medico
Rosalie Dominik, DrPH
Laneta Dorflinger, PhD
Batra Elul, MSc
Thomas J. Espenshade, MAT, PhD
Paul Feldblum, PhD
Monica M. Gaines, MBMA
Joan Mogul Garrity
Vanessa Garver
Vickey Gibbons
David Gittelman
John Guillebaud, MA, FRCSE, FRCOG, MFFP
Polly F. Harrison, PhD
Stanley K. Henshaw, PhD
Douglas Huber, MD, MSc
Ken Hunt
Timothy Johnson, PhD
Kirtly Parker Jones, MD
Mary L. Kamb, MD, MPH
Leslie M. Kantor, MPH
Cynthia Kay
Maxine Keel
Philip Kestelman, MA, MSc
Douglas Kirby, PhD
Ronald L. Kleinman, MD
Lorraine Klerman, DrPH
Jacqueline Koenig, MSB
Miriam H. Labbok, MD, MPH
Virginia Lamprecht, RN, BSN, MSPH
Deanna Lewis, BA
Mark C. Maltzer, MD
Rebecca Maynard, PhD
Jack Moseley, MD
Kathryn Murrell, MA
LeRoy E. Nelson
Colleen O'Donnell
Chloe O'Gara, EdD
David Olive, MD
Maureen Paul
Herbert Peterson, MD
Linda Piccinino, MPS
Susan Pinsky, MD
Linda S. Potter, DrPH
Malcolm Potts, MB, BChir, PhD
Lisa Rarick, MD
Roberto Rivera, MD
Jeffrey Sacks, MD
Gigi Santow, PhD
Karena Sapsis, MPH, CHES
Margaret Scarlett, DDS
George Schmid, MD
Sharon Schnare, FNP, CNM, MSN
James Shelton, MD, MPH
R.V. Short, PhD, ScD
Irving Sivin, MA
Richard Soderstrom, MD
Jeff Spieler, PhD (Hon.)
Karen Stein, MD, MPH
Zena Stein, MD
Gary K. Stewart, MD, MPH
Katherine M. Stone, MD
Philip Stubblefield, MD
Kathleen Toomey, MD, MPH
Amanda Troxler
Abby Norris Turner
Elizabeth Wentzel
Gary West, MPH
Nicole Wilcox, MPH
Beverly Winikoff, MD, MPH
Lisa Wynn, PhD
Miriam Zieman, MD

* Deceased, March 21, 2004.

Table of Contents

Forthcoming Books and Conferences

CD-ROM/PDA Registration Form and New Media Survey

Ordering Information and Order Form

List of Tables

List of Figures

Expanding Perspectives on Reproductive Health

Deborah Kowal, MA, PA

- Evolving market forces and consumer expectations are changing the scope of reproductive health services.
- Many primary care providers are delivering reproductive health services. Conversely, many reproductive health care providers are delivering primary care services.
- Family planning helps not only individuals and families, but also the community at large.

In recent years, reproductive health care in the United States, in parallel with other medical disciplines, has changed to meet the challenges of evolving market forces and broadened consumer expectations. As a result, integrated reproductive health care has expanded in concept. In many cases, shifting management and insurance schemes have placed reproductive health within the domain of primary care. For an increasing number of women, the clinician who provided only family planning now often serves as their health care provider for all primary care. For others, their primary care provider now delivers the family planning services they may previously have received elsewhere.

A broader scope of family planning services includes not only fertility but also infertility, not only sexually transmitted infections (STIs) but also reproductive tract infections (RTIs) overall, not only menstruation and fertilization but also the preconceptual and interconceptual periods and menopause, and finally, not only reproductive tract problems but the wide range of risk factors that influence a woman's health in general. As reproductive health care expands in scope, however, two goals are paramount. First, the planning, or preventive focus, of family planning must remain a central activity. Second, reproductive health must be recognized for its broader public health impact.

PREVENTIVE HEALTH SERVICES

Family planning has always rested on the notion of thoughtful prevention rather than emphasizing the curative orientation practiced in many other medical arenas. This notion of prevention must carry through the entire practice of reproductive health, from providing contraceptives and reducing exposure to STIs to improving a woman's general health so she can conceive and deliver a healthy infant and to minimizing her risk factors for the diseases and injuries that curtail her life or quality of life.

By knowing which conditions commonly afflict your patient's population group, you can make more efficient use of resources and better assess your patient's risk factors. For example, the most common causes of mortality among women in various age groups provide a starting point (Table 1-1). Simply by screening for the risk factors associated with these problems and counseling about prevention, you can provide a high level of care for a substantial proportion of the patient population. In addition, by knowing what other conditions are uncommon or exceedingly rare, you can limit excessive workups and better identify those cases that truly merit extensive and expensive approaches. Health care provision should be based on more than "Can the patient (or the third-party payor) pay for this?"

Table 1-1 Leading causes of mortality among women

15-19 years	20-24 years	25-34 years	35-44 years	45-54 years	55-64 years	65+ years
Accidents	Accidents	Accidents	Cancer	Cancer	Cancer	Heart disease
Assault	Assault	Cancer	Accidents	Heart disease	Heart disease	Cancer
Cancer	Cancer	Heart disease	Heart disease	Accidents	Lung disease	Stroke
Suicide	Suicide	Suicide	HIV disease	Stroke	Stroke	Lung disease
Heart disease	Heart disease	Assault	Suicide	Diabetes	Diabetes	Influenza/ pneumonia

Source: NCHS (2001).[1]

The U.S. Preventive Services Task Force has designed a recommended schedule of periodic health examinations that cover both general and reproductive health care (Table 1-2). The recommended services reflect only those areas reviewed by the Task Force or those interventions that have documented evidence of value.[2,3] While many approaches to periodic health screening have been proposed, the Task Force recommendations are considered the blueprint for screening guidelines. These guidelines were developed using an evidence-based methodology. Above all, the Task Force emphasizes that the most cost-effective approach to health is through primary prevention, and primary prevention is most likely met through focused risk assessment and counseling rather than through periodic "one-size-fits-all" laboratory testing and physical examinations. When and how often the preventive services are performed (or other services added) must be based on an individual patient's medical history, physical findings, and risk factors. The Task Force updates the screening recommendations as more evidence becomes available; consult the website: www.ahcpr.gov/clinic/gcpspu.htm.

Table 1-2 Periodic health screening recommendations, U.S. Preventive Services Task Force

Screening/Intervention	Strength of Recommendation
Gynecologic Cancers	
OCs to prevent ovarian and endometrial cancer	B
Avoid high risk sexual activity; use condoms	A
Cervical cancer	
Pap smears at least every 3 years	A
New technologies to screen	I
Routine HPV testing	I
Breast cancer	
Mammography every 1–2 years for women 40 and older	B
Routine clinical breast exam alone	I
Routine breast self-examination	I
Ovarian cancer	
Routine pelvic exam, ultrasound or serum tumor markers:	
General population	D
High-risk women	C
Colorectal cancer	
Fecal occult blood testing for women over 50	A
Sigmoidoscopy for women over 50	A
Hormone Replacement Therapy	
Use of estrogen and progestin to prevent chronic conditions	D
Use of unopposed estrogen for women with hysterectomy to prevent chronic conditions	I
Osteoporosis	
Routine screen for women 65 and older	B
Routine screen for high-risk women 60 and older	B
Routine screen for women younger than 60	C
Bacterial vaginosis in pregnancy	
Routine screen for high-risk pregnant women	I
Routine screen for average pregnant women	D
Chlamydia infection	
Routine screen for sexually active women 25 and younger	A
Routine screen for asymptomatic low-risk general population	C
Routine screen for asymptomatic pregnant women 25 and younger	B
Routine screen for asymptomatic low-risk pregnant women older than 25	C
Genital herpes simplex	
Routine screen general population	D
Routine screen pregnant women	D
Examination of women in labor	C

(continued)

Table 1-2 Periodic health screening recommendations, U.S. Preventive Services
Task Force—*(cont.)*

Screening/Intervention	Strength of Recommendation
Gonorrhea	
Routine screen or culture of high-risk women	B
Routine screen or culture of high-risk pregnant women	B
Other pregnant women	C
General population	D
Human immunodeficiency virus	
Periodic screen for at-risk adults and adolescents	A
Screen for at-risk pregnant women	A
Universal screen for low-risk pregnant women in low-prevalence areas	C
Asymptomatic bacteriuria	
Routine urine culture	
Pregnant women 12–16 weeks gestation	A
Routine urine dipstick	
Pregnant women	D
Diabetic women	C
School-aged girls	E

Source: U.S. Preventive Services Task Force (1996, 2003).[2, 3]

Strength of recommendations:

A   The USPSTF strongly recommends that clinicians routinely provide [the service] to eligible patients. (The USPSTF found good evidence that [the service] improves important health outcomes and concludes that benefits substantially outweigh harms.)

B   The USPSTF recommends that clinicians routinely provide [the service] to eligible patients. (The USPSTF found at least fair evidence that [the service] improves important health outcomes and concludes that benefits outweigh harms.)

C   The USPSTF makes no recommendation for or against routine provision of [the service]. (The USPSTF found at least fair evidence that [the service] can improve health outcomes but concludes that the balance of the benefits and harms is too close to justify a general recommendation.)

D   The USPSTF recommends against routinely providing [the service] to asymptomatic patients. (The USPSTF found at least fair evidence that [the service] is ineffective or that harms outweigh benefits.)

I   The USPSTF concludes that the evidence is insufficient to recommend for or against routinely providing [the service]. (Evidence that [the service] is effective is lacking, of poor quality, or conflicting and the balance of benefits and harms cannot be determined.)

RISK FACTORS AFFECTING WOMEN'S HEALTH

Unintended pregnancy. Annually, nearly half of the 6.3 million pregnancies in the United States are unintended.[4, 5] About 7.5% of women at risk of pregnancy do not use contraception.[4] Those who do use contraception still face some risk of unintended pregnancy because their use of their chosen method is imperfect. (See Chapter 10 on Essentials of Contraception.) Adequate instruction in how to use a method, provision of a back-up method, and information about emergency contraception could reduce the risk of unintended pregnancy. (See Chapter 12 on Emergency Contraception.)

Exposure to STIs. HIV is fatal, and hepatitis B can be life-threatening; other STIs can cause infertility and pain.[6] The estimated total number of people newly infected each year with curable STIs is 15 million in the United States.[7] Most STIs show a "biologic sexism," meaning that women are more likely than men to acquire an STI from a sexual encounter[8] (see Chapter 8 on Reproductive Tract Infections). They are also more likely to suffer more severe consequences, including PID, infertility, ectopic pregnancy, chronic pelvic pain, and cervical cancer. Younger patients, arguably with the most to lose from a fertility standpoint, account for most STI cases.[9] Abstinence, a mutually faithful relationship, and use of condoms merit discussion during each patient encounter.

Cigarette smoking. Just as for men, tobacco smoke is associated with several types of cancer including lung cancer, other lung diseases, and cardiovascular conditions in women smokers. Women smokers have an increased risk of cervical cancer, premature menopause, and impaired fertility. Women who smoke during pregnancy have an increased risk of having an infant of low birthweight, a miscarriage, a stillbirth, or an infant death.[10,11] The oral contraceptive user who smokes heavily faces an increased risk of myocardial infarction[12] and thrombotic and hemorrhagic stroke. (See Chapter 19 on Combined Hormonal Contraceptive Methods.) About one-fourth of women age 18 and older smoke, with smoking concentrated primarily among younger women.[13] Together, these smoking-related diseases killed 165,000 women in 1999. Lung cancer kills more women (68,000) than does breast cancer (41,000).[13] Counseling about smoking cessation undoubtedly belongs in the reproductive health office visit.

Substance use. Alcohol use is associated with impaired judgment, increased risk of motor vehicle accidents, use of other addictive substances, cirrhosis, stroke, and hypertension. It is also a leading cause of birth defects.[10] Cocaine may cause sinusitis, allergic rhinitis, upper respiratory tract infections, epistaxis, and weight loss. Marijuana causes fatigue, panic attacks, and anxiety. Sedatives may be associated with headaches, nausea, paranoia, and sleep disturbances.

Violence. Violence against women is so common[14] that health care providers overlook a critical aspect of care if they fail to ask about abuse history. One of 6 women has experienced attempted to completed rape. Each year, more than 50% of women are victims of physical assault. About one million women are stalked annually. Violence against women is primarily, though not exclusively, a crime committed against the young. Of women who have been raped, 22% were under age 12 and 32% were 12 to 17 years of age when they were first raped. Among women age 15 to 24 years, homicide is the second most common cause of death.[1] The warnings of "stranger danger" are misleading—76% of women who were raped or physically assaulted report that the perpetrator was a current or former husband, cohabiting partner, or date.[14] Domestic violence is more common than rape or muggings.

Poor nutrition and exercise patterns. Overnutrition leading to obesity is the primary nutritional problem in the United States. The obese are at increased risk of cardiovascular disease, diabetes, gallbladder disease, some forms of arthritis, and some cancers.[10] Although U.S. women can choose from an abundance of foods, many still have a deficit of vitamins and minerals such as calcium, iron, vitamin B, and folic acid. The fact that folic acid deficiency is associated with neural tube defects implies other nutritional factors may also play heavily in conceptual and pregnancy outcomes. A lack of exercise is associated with cardiovascular illnesses, musculoskeletal problems, and respiratory insufficiency. Exercise not only reduces the risk of these health problems, but it may also have a favorable effect on mood, depression, anxiety, and self-esteem.

Poverty. The fastest growing segments of people living in poverty are women and children. Over half the poor families in the United States are headed by women with no spouse present.[15] Poverty is not a lifestyle choice; it generally cannot be remedied by changing a lifestyle behavior. However, being poor is a risk factor that must be addressed by clinicians. Poverty is associated with inadequate health care and nutrition, excess stress, and limited alternatives. Having contraceptive services, including thorough education and counseling, is paramount in helping your patient avoid the emotional and financial toll of unintended pregnancy or STI. In many cases, as a contraceptive provider, you may be the indigent woman's only health care provider.

REFERENCES

1. Anderson RN. Deaths: leading causes for 1999. National vital statistics report 2000;49(11).
2. U.S. Preventive Services Task Force. Guide to clinical preventive services. 2nd edition. Baltimore MD: Williams & Wilkins, 1996.
3. U.S. Preventive Services Task Force. Update, 2002 release. www.ahcpr.gov/clinic/gcpspu.htm. Retrieved December 2003.
4. Abma JC, Chandra A, Mosher WD, Peterson LS, Piccinino LJ. Fertility, family planning and women's health: new data from the 1995 National Survey of Family Growth. Vital Health Stat 1997;Series 23, Number 19.
5. Henshaw SK, Unintended pregnancy in the United States. Fam Plann Perspect 1998;30:24-29, 46.
6. Eng TR, Butler WR (eds). The hidden epidemic: confronting sexually transmitted diseases. Washington D.C.: National Academy Press, 1997.
7. Cates W Jr and the American Social Health Association Panel. Estimates of the incidence and prevalence of sexually transmitted diseases in the United States. Sex Transm Dis 1999; 26(4 Suppl):S2-7.
8. Anderson RM. Transmission dynamics of sexually transmitted infections. In: Holmes KK, et al. Sexually Transmitted Diseases. Third edition. New York: McGraw Hill, 1999: 25-37.

9. Mosure DJ, Berman S, Fine D, DeLisle S, Cates W Jr, Boring JR 3rd. Genital chlamydia infections in sexually active female adolescents: do we really need to screen everyone? J Adolesc Health 1997; 20(1):6-13.

10. Department of Health and Human Services. Healthy people 2010. Conference edition, volume 1. Washington D.C.: U.S. Government Printing Office, January 2000.

11. Stein Z. Smoking and reproductive health. J Am Med Women's Assoc 1996;51:29-30.

12. Tanis BC, van den Bosch MAAJ, Kemmeren JM, et al. Oral contraceptives and the risk of myocardial infarction. N Engl J Med 2001;345:1787-1793.

13. Satcher D. Women and smoking: a report of the surgeon general. Washington DC: Department of Health and Human Services, 2001.

14. Tjaden P, Thoennes N. Prevalence, incidence, and consequences of violence against women: findings from the national violence against women survey. Atlanta, GA: Centers for Disease Control and Prevention, National Center for Injury Prevention and Control. November 1998.

15. Census Bureau. Current population reports, series P60-188. Income, poverty, and valuation of noncash benefits: 1993. Washington D.C.: U.S. Census Bureau, 1994.

Sexuality and Reproductive Health[a]

Debra W. Haffner, MDiv, MPH
William R. Stayton, ThD, PhD

- Sexuality is a natural and healthy part of living.
- Sexuality involves more than sex, and sex involves more than intercourse.
- Sexual feelings and sexual behaviors are integral aspects of reproductive health.
- A client's sexual attitudes, behaviors, and relationships all influence how effective a particular contraceptive method will be.
- Understanding sexual behavior is critical for designing interventions that will reduce unintended pregnancies and sexually transmitted infections (STIs), including infection with the human immunodeficiency virus (HIV).

Sexuality and reproductive health care are interdependent. Reproductive health care providers help people manage their sexual lives. Although contraceptive services have traditionally helped plan the number and spacing of children, most clients seek contraception primarily to separate procreation from the recreational aspects of sexual intercourse.[b]

Sexuality, however, is about much more than sexual intercourse. It encompasses the sexual knowledge, beliefs, attitudes, values, and behaviors of individuals. It includes not only anatomy, physiology, and biochemistry of the sexual response system, but also identity, orientation, roles, personality, thoughts, feelings, and relationships. The expression of sexuality is influenced by ethical, spiritual, cultural, and moral concerns.[1]

---

[a] Portions of this chapter have been adapted with permission from the following sources: Haffner D (ed). Facing facts: sexual health for America's adolescents. New York: SIECUS, 1995. Stayton W. Sexual and gender identity disorders in a relational perspective. In: Kaslow FW (ed). Handbook of relational diagnosis and dysfunctional family patterns. New York: John Wiley & Sons, 1996.

[b] While this chapter is directed primarily to heterosexual couples needing contraception, the authors believe sexuality is an important part of most adults' lives: gay men, lesbians, post-reproductive age women, the physically or mentally challenged, and so on.

Men's and women's sexual attitudes and behaviors influence their choice of contraception and their ability to use the methods effectively. On a very fundamental level, individuals' reproductive health care decisions rest on their ability to make informed and healthy choices about their sexuality. The decision to become sexually involved—whether the relationship is consensual, whether it is monogamous, whether it is protected against unplanned pregnancy and sexually transmitted infections (STIs), or whether sexuality is a pleasurable or painful part of life—is related to the ability to make responsible sexual choices.

Many reproductive health care clinicians have treated an individual's sexuality needs as separate and distinct from contraceptive and other reproductive health needs. Practitioners may not have been trained in addressing sexual health concerns. The pressure to reach the largest number of people in an efficient manner may limit counseling to method instruction and preclude time for helping clients manage their sexual lives in a way consistent with their own values and goals.

The 1994 International Conference on Population and Development directly recognized the relationship of sexuality to reproductive health, acknowledging that sexuality issues must be addressed in reproductive health care settings: "Reproductive health therefore implies that people are able to have a satisfying and safe sex life and that they have the capability to reproduce and the freedom to decide if, when, and how often to do so . . . Reproductive health . . . also includes sexual health, the purpose of which is the enhancement of life and personal relations, and not merely counseling and care related to reproduction and sexually transmitted diseases."[2] The report was endorsed by more than 200 countries.

Practitioners have a unique opportunity to provide information, education, and counseling to clients who might otherwise have no readily available resource for help. As important, addressing sexual concerns directly with clients as they choose their method may improve how effectively they use contraception.

SEXUAL BEHAVIOR IN THE UNITED STATES

Human sexual interaction is surely the least understood, least investigated behavior in daily life, so reproductive health care practitioners are placed at a serious disadvantage. Solid information on contraceptive use during penile-vaginal intercourse yields knowledge about contraceptive failure and pregnancy risk taking. Solid information on heterosexual and same-gender sexual practices (anal, vaginal, and oral intercourse) and partner networks (who does what with whom and when) yields knowledge about the transmission of STIs, including infection with the human immunodeficiency virus (HIV). Understanding the psychological and social reasons for sexual behaviors is necessary for designing effective interventions to reduce risk taking with regard to pregnancy and infection. Understanding and combating STI transmission can be even more difficult than understanding and combating unintended pregnancy—the sexual behaviors that result in an STI are more varied, and the sexual networks extend beyond the present into the past.

Until recently, information about sexual behaviors was limited to questions included in surveys primarily devoted to other topics, such as general social, family, or fertility surveys or non-generalizable surveys of college students or the readers of magazines. In 1994, the National Opinion Research Center (NORC) at the University of Chicago completed the largest, most current study of sexual behaviors in the United States. The study was based on interviews with a national probability household sample of more than 3,400 men and women age 18 to 59 years.[3]

In general, Americans are having less sex than was generally believed. Eighty-three percent of American adults age 18 to 59 had one partner or no partner in the last year of the study, and most people had sexual relations a few times a month. American adults were about equally divided among those who have sexual relations with a partner at least twice a week, a few times a month, a few times a year, or not at all (Table 2-1[3]).

Younger Americans behave significantly differently than older Americans. Younger people begin having intercourse earlier, marry later, and have more lifetime partners. One of the surprises of the study is that marriage is a great leveler. Married adults share remarkably similar patterns of sexual behavior, regardless of attitudes, premarital experience, religious or ethnic background, or geography. The vast majority of married people report that they are monogamous, engage in sex a few times a month, and focus on penile-vaginal intercourse as their primary sexual behavior.

Table 2-1   Survey of sexual behaviors in the United States, 1994

- 83% of Americans had one partner or no partner in the last year.
- Most married couples have sexual intercourse a few times a month.
- The most frequent and most enjoyed sexual behavior for heterosexual adults is penile-vaginal intercourse.
- One-fourth of adults have oral sex regularly.
- 10% of married women and 25% of married men have had an affair.
- More than 4 in 10 adults have had 5 or more sexual partners in their lifetime.
- One in 5 Americans had a new sexual partner in the past 12 months.
- The median number of lifetime sexual partners by age 60 is 2 for women and 6 for men.

Source: Laumann (1994).[3]

Gender differences clearly exist when it comes to sexual attitudes and behaviors. Men are much more likely than women to report recreational sex, a greater number of partners, a greater interest in a variety of sexual activities, and less monogamy. Women are much more likely to say their first intercourse was as a result of peer pressure, they do not consistently have orgasms, and they have never masturbated. Men also reported greater access to sexual partners, particularly as they age; although almost 6 in 10 single men age 45 to 59 had a partner last year, only one-third of women did. In fact, 6 in 10 single women in this age group had no partner during the last 12 months of the study.

ADOLESCENT SEXUAL BEHAVIOR

Historically, young women and young men did not reach physical maturity until their middle adolescent years. Marriage and other adult responsibilities followed puberty closely. Today's adolescents are different from young people of generations ago. They reach puberty earlier, have intercourse earlier, and marry later. Women and men who marry today do so 3 to 4 years later than young people did in the 1950s.

A majority of American adolescents date, 85% have had a boyfriend or girlfriend, 85% to 90% have kissed someone romantically, and 79% have engaged in "deep kissing."[4, 5] Almost all American adolescents engage in some type of sexual behavior. Although policy debates have tended to focus on sexual intercourse and its negative consequences, young people explore dating, relationships, and intimacy from a much wider frame-work.[6]

The majority of young people move from kissing to other more intimate sexual behaviors during their adolescent years. More than half of all adolescents have engaged in "petting behaviors." By the age of 14, more than half of all boys have touched a girl's breasts, and a fourth have touched a girl's vulva.[4, 5] By the age of 18, more than three-fourths have engaged in heavy petting.[4, 5] One-fourth to one-half of young people reported experience with fellatio or cunnilingus.[4, 5, 7]

Some data suggest the progression from kissing to noncoital behaviors to intercourse varies among different groups of adolescents. While many adolescents move through a progression of intimate behaviors, lower-income adolescents are less likely to follow this progression, moving more rapidly from kissing directly to sexual intercourse.[8]

In the past two decades, there has been a significant change in the numbers of young people who have had intercourse at young ages. At each age of adolescence, higher proportions of adolescent men and women have had sexual intercourse today than had done so 20 years ago.[9]

More than 80% of Americans first have intercourse as adolescents.[9] More than half of women and almost three-fourths of men age 15 to 19 have had sexual intercourse. However, despite the large numbers of young people who experiment with a variety of sexual behaviors, intercourse is generally less widespread and certainly less frequent than many adolescents and adults believe. In fact, teenage pregnancy and birth declined dramatically in the 1990s.[10]

Despite the public impression to the contrary, most adolescents who have intercourse do so responsibly. The majority of adolescents use contraceptives as consistently and effectively as most adults. In 1979, less than half of adolescents used a contraceptive at first intercourse.[11] By 1990, that proportion had increased to more than 70%.[12] Recent surveys suggest as many as 60% of adolescents now use condoms; these proportions are 2 to 3 times higher than those reported in the 1970s.[13] However, in every survey, less than half of the adolescents who recently used condoms did so all of the time.[14]

SAME-GENDER SEXUAL BEHAVIOR

Reproductive health care practitioners have long understood that presuming heterosexuality can compromise care. Many clinic counselors report they see lesbian clients who prefer the reproductive health care they receive at contraceptive clinics. Many lesbians reluctantly take condoms and foam as a method in exchange for their annual Papanicolaou smears and pelvic exams. However, there are little reliable data on same-gender sexual practices of men and almost none on women who have sex with other women.

In 1948, Alfred Kinsey, in his landmark report on the sexual behaviors of American men, reported that 37% of the total male population had an overt homosexual experience (that did not include orgasm) between adolescence and old age, that 10% of males are more or less exclusively homosexual for at least 3 years between the ages of 16 and 65, and that 4% of white males are exclusively homosexual throughout their lives.[15] Kinsey never published comparable figures for women. These findings about men, which were not based on random samples, led to the widely quoted figure that 10% of American adults are homosexual.

The NORC[3] study used a range of questions to elicit information on same-gender sexual attraction, behavior, and identification. Unfortunately, the small numbers in this study do not reveal a great deal about self-identified gays and lesbians. Respondents were asked, "Do you consider yourself heterosexual, homosexual, bisexual, or something else?" Few women (1.4%) reported themselves as homosexual or bisexual; 2.8% of men did. This finding was very similar to other recent studies in the United States, England, and France that found 2% to 4% of adults self-identified as gay or lesbian. However, in the NORC study, 10% of the men and 9% of the women reported feeling same-gender sexual attraction, having had sex with someone of the same sex, or self-identifying as gay or lesbian. Forty-four percent of these men and 59% of these women reported desire only.[3]

WHAT DO PEOPLE DO?

The media often give the impression that everybody in America is having more sex, hotter sex, and better sex than they really are. In fact, most

Americans are fairly conservative in their sexual practices. When the Kinsey studies were first published, Americans were surprised to find a significant minority of people had visited prostitutes, many people had at least one same-gender sexual experience, and there was a substantial rate of extramarital affairs.[15, 16] These data, with all their limitations, suggest changes in sexual behaviors probably began around the turn of the century, and the so-called sexual revolution of the 1960s and 1970s was really just a continuation, and perhaps an acceleration, of these trends.[17]

Several factors have been offered as explanations for these trends. During the mid-1900s, larger numbers of young Americans began to go to college, and the age of marriage was delayed as a result of this education. More women entered the labor force and became financially independent. Marrying later and divorcing more, adults who were single and sexually available increased in number.

In 1948 and 1953, Kinsey found that by the age of 25, three-fourths of men but only one-third of women had had sexual intercourse.[15, 16] By 1992, 89% of men and 94% of women age 18 to 24 had had vaginal intercourse. Only 5% of American adults were virgins. The vast majority of Americans first have intercourse by their twentieth birthday, and almost all adults, regardless of marital status, are sexually experienced by their mid-twenties.[3]

The NORC[3] study found that the most frequent, and most enjoyed, sexual behavior for heterosexual adults is penile-vaginal intercourse. About two-thirds of men and 60% of women have had oral sex, although only about a fourth do so regularly. Oral sex is more common in short-term relationships and more likely among whites compared with blacks. Older adults (over age 50) are less likely to engage in oral sex. About one-fourth of men and one-fifth of women report having ever had anal sex, and about 10% of single men and women have had heterosexual anal sex. Rates of anal sex are higher among Hispanics.

Frequency of sexual interactions is a factor of age, relationship duration, and marital status. In general, cohabiting couples have more sex than married couples; married people have more sex than singles. Due to increased age of marriage and the high divorce levels, there are now significantly more heterosexual adults who are not married but are nevertheless sexually involved.[17]

Ten percent of women and 25% of men report they have had an extramarital sexual relationship.[3] Since more men are involved in affairs, presumably without their wives' knowledge, more women may be at risk of STIs than they expect. Research is not available on what proportion of men have same-gender relationships outside of marriage. "These findings suggest not only that the clinician would be wise to ask about behavior rather than sexual orientation, but also that some married persons will perceive themselves to be at no (or low) risk of STIs when in fact their spouse's extramarital sexual activities may place them at risk."[17]

Risk of HIV and Other STIs

The authors of the NORC study[3] convincingly argue that the 83% of American adults age 18 to 59 years who had either one partner or no partner last year faced little risk of exposure to HIV, unless one or both partners are exposed by sharing injecting-drug equipment. Indeed, they found most American adults have sexual relationships with people very much like themselves; this fact, coupled with the limited infectivity of HIV, is part of the reason that HIV infection has not exploded among heterosexuals in the United States.

However, both the HIV and STI epidemics have clearly affected large numbers of people attending reproductive health clinics. Many people's behaviors place them at risk of infections, and clinics must now address how clients are protecting themselves against these risks. The NORC[3] study found risky behaviors:

- More than 4 in 10 Americans age 18 to 59 years have had 5 or more partners. An estimated 13 million Americans have had 21 or more partners since the age of 18.
- One in 6 Americans report they have had an STI.
- One in 5 Americans have had a new sexual partner in the past 12 months—25% of the men and 15% of the women. Of these, 8.5% had a one-encounter sexual relationship; 12% had a sexual relationship that lasted less than 2 months. The more partners one has had, the less likely they are to be known well, the less likely they are to be from the same social networks, and the less exclusive the relationships are likely to be.
- Condom use is still very low. Only 20% of people who had 3 or more partners in the past 3 years always used condoms with their primary partner. Although knowledge of AIDS is very high, less than half of those surveyed said using a condom is a very effective way to prevent HIV.

Nonvoluntary Sexual Activity

Not all sexual behavior is voluntary, and a history of sexual abuse and sexual assault may severely compromise one's ability to have safe, satisfying sexual relationships. It is important for clinicians to ask questions about prior sexual assault and abuse. It is not uncommon for young adolescent women to reveal they are being forced into sexual relationships with older men, some of whom live in the same household.

Almost one-fourth of women report they have been forced to have sexual relations during their adult lives, most often by their committed partner. In the NORC study,[3] 22% of women report they had been forced by their partners to have sexual relations, while only 3% of men report they had ever forced a woman. Just under one in 5 men and women report having been sexually abused as children. At least 683,000 adult American women are raped each year.[18] A history of sexual abuse seems to have especially pernicious effects. Women with histories of sexual abuse are more likely than other women to be unhappy, have more than 10 lifetime sex partners, lack interest in sex, be unable to have orgasms, feel sex was not pleasurable in the past year, and report other sexual problems.

Adolescents are particularly vulnerable to sexual abuse, and 6% of boys and 15% of girls are sexually assaulted prior to their sixteenth birthday. In a study of adolescent girls in foster care, 43% reported experiencing some type of sexual abuse. The most prevalent type of abuse was being touched or fondled by an adult against her wishes. One in 6 reported being forced to have intercourse with an adult. One-third of the young women had been sexually abused before their tenth birthday.[19] In fact, nearly one-third of rapes are committed against women 11 to 17 years of age.[18] Nearly three-fourths of young women who had intercourse before age 14 report the experience was involuntary.[9,20]

A disproportionate number of young women who become pregnant during adolescence are victims of childhood sexual abuse. In one study of adolescents who were pregnant or were parents, 70% of whites, 42% of blacks, and 37% of Hispanics had been sexually abused as a child.[21] In another study, 64% of parenting and pregnant adolescents reported they had at least one unwanted sexual experience.[20]

SEXUAL ANATOMY
MALE SEXUAL ANATOMY

Men tend to be conditioned to focus on genital sexual stimulation rather than whole-body touch arousal. Retraining to be comfortable and to accept and enjoy whole-body stimulation may be a desirable sexual goal for some men. Except for those men who do not respond to nipple caresses and those who deny their sensitivity because of the fear of being unmasculine, the remainder of men are likely to be pleased and excited by nipple stimulation. The sexual sensitivity of male genitalia varies strikingly according to anatomic area. The sites of highly pleasurable sensitivity (in order of decreasing response to touch) are as follows:

- Area of frenular attachment on ventral surface of penis, just behind the glans
- Coronal ridge of glans
- Urethral meatus
- Shaft of the penis
- Penile base located within the perineal area between the area of scrotal attachment and the anus
- Scrotum and testicles
- Perianal skin

FEMALE SEXUAL ANATOMY

Virtually any portion of a woman's skin may give pleasurable and exciting sensations when caressed, providing she is willing and not distracted by extraneous thoughts or events. Women tend to be whole-body oriented for sexual touching rather than genitally oriented as men are trained to be. Breast and nipple sensitivity tends to be high in most women, but some women do not find breast caressing particularly arousing.

For most women, the glans and shaft of the clitoris, the inner surfaces of the labia minora, and the first inch and a half of the vagina are the most sexually sensitive areas of all. Indeed, the clitoral head (glans) may be so exceedingly sensitive that direct touch is sometimes or always uncomfortable. Many women enjoy indirect clitoral touch by caressing the clitoral shaft rather than the glans. Women, as well as men, have (or may acquire) high levels of sexual responsiveness to anal penetration.

The frequency, sensation, intensity, and duration of orgasm are highly variable in women. Women also vary greatly in what stimuli induce orgasm for them (dream, fantasy, breast stimulation, masturbation, a partner's hand, a partner's mouth, intercourse, or other stimulation). It is common for healthy, normal women not to be orgasmic through penile-vaginal thrusting alone.

Researchers suggest that women may have three different types of orgasm.[22,23] First is a vulvar, or tenting, orgasm, where the clitoris or some outside stimuli such as fantasy or breast stimulation is the main focus of the orgasmic experience. Second, a uterine or A-frame orgasm is felt deeper inside the abdomen and may be triggered by stimulation of the G-spot, or Grafenberg spot, an area in the anterior vaginal wall that is sensitive to sexual stimulation. Some women report ejaculating a milky-white fluid from the urethra when they reach orgasm through this stimulation. The ejaculate is described as different from urine, differing in color, clarity, and odor, and does not stain. It should be regarded as a normal variant of the female sexual response and not as a symptom of urinary incontinence. The third type of orgasm is a blended orgasm, which is a combination of the first two.

SEXUAL RESPONSE

In the past 40 years, the medical and behavioral sciences have yielded information about healthy sexual functioning. Sexual arousal and response are natural to everyone from birth to death. They are not experiences that begin at adolescence and end with menopause, but rather occur to be enjoyed and experienced throughout the life cycle. Reproductive health care providers can incorporate the information that is now available into clinical practice.

There have been three major contributions to the overall understanding and knowledge of adult sexual response.

FOUR PHASES OF RESPONSE

William Masters and Virginia Johnson can be credited with beginning the modern movement toward our understanding of the sexual response cycle. They divided the sexual response cycle into four phases: excitement (or arousal), plateau, orgasm, and resolution. In their seminal book, Human Sexual Response (1966),[24] they detail these phases of the response cycle for both men and women (Figure 2-1).

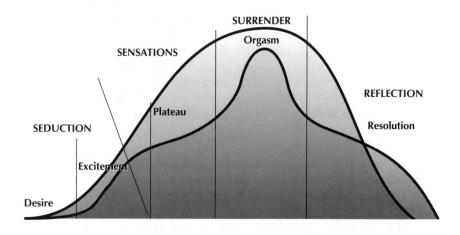

Masters W et al. (1966)[24]; Kaplan HS (1979)[28]; Stayton WR (1989).[29]

Figure 2-1   Sexual response curve

TRIPHASIC MODEL

Another major contribution to our understanding of sexual function comes from Helen Singer Kaplan.[25–27] She described sexual response in a triphasic model consisting of desire, excitement, and orgasm. In discussing her differences with the Masters and Johnson model, she combined their excitement and plateau stages as describing different degrees of the vasodilatory excitement phase. She believed the resolution stage of the Masters and Johnson model merely refers to the absence of sexual arousal.

Kaplan stressed it is natural to have sexual desire.[28] She discussed all the factors that contribute to the inhibition of sexual desire: medication, relational problems, sexual abuse, and the effects of illness and disease. Among the major psychological contributors to sexual desire disorders are childhood sexual abuse, rape, negative attitudes towards sexuality, low self-esteem, religious orthodoxy, and relational problems.

EROTIC STIMULUS PATHWAY

A most important contribution to the knowledge base in clinical sexology comes from the Erotic Stimulus Pathway (ESP) theory of David

M. Reed.[29] The ESP theory enhances our understanding and ability to treat sexual dysfunctions. Reed divides the sexual response cycle into four phases that correspond to those of Kaplan and Masters and Johnson (Figure 2-1). For many people, these phases are learned developmentally.

In the seduction phase a person learns how to get aroused sexually and how to attract someone else sexually. Seduction translates into memories and rituals. For example, adolescents may spend much time on personal appearance, choice of clothes, and mannerisms. These can enhance positive self-esteem if the adolescents like the way they feel. If the adolescents feel good about the way they look and feel, then attracting another person will be much easier. As the adolescents get older, these positive feelings are translated into sexual desire and arousal. These seductive techniques are stored in the memory and can be activated later on in life.

In the sensations phase, the different senses can enhance sexual excitement and ideally prolong the plateau phase. The early experiences of touch (holding hands, putting arms around a loved one) become very important. The sense of vision (staring at a loved one, holding an image of him or her when absent) is a way of maintaining interest and arousal. Hearing the loved one in intimate conversation or over the telephone becomes very important. Hearing the sounds of a partner responding to sexual stimulation can be titillating. The smell of the loved one, either a particular scent he or she wears or the sexual smell, brings additional excitement. Finally, the taste of a food or drink or the taste of the loved one become important to memory and fantasy. All these senses extend the excitement into a plateau phase, which makes one want to continue the pleasurable moment over a longer period of time. These seduction and sensation experiences are the psychological input to the physiology of sexual response. They are the precursors to sexual climax and orgasm.

In the surrender phase, orgasm is a "psycho-physiological surprise." The psychodynamic issues surrounding orgasm are power and control. Persons with orgasmic dysfunction may be in a power struggle with themselves or with their partners or with the messages received about sex. Over-control or under-control can affect orgasmic potential and the ability to allow all of the passion to be expressed.

Finally, the reflection phase is central to the sexual experience, especially for the person having intercourse for the first time. How does the person feel immediately after the experience? If the person feels it was a positive experience, the reflection will create positive feedback that will affect future desire. If it is negative, it will diminish future desire, at least for that specific partner, if not for sex itself. It is important that the first sexual experience not be traumatic, otherwise it can have a negative effect on future sexual encounters. For example, in a case of sexual abuse or rape, it can take years for the victim to be able to experience sex in a positive way. The effects of early negative sexual experiences can manifest in lack of sexual desire, vaginismus or dyspareunia, orgasmic disorders, sexual orientation confusion, gender dysphoria, low self-esteem, and erotophobia.

CONTRACEPTIVE CHOICE AND SEXUALITY

Attitudes about sexuality and the characteristics of sexual relationships influence choice of a contraceptive method, how effectively the method is used, and satisfaction with the method. Ambivalence about sexuality contributes to unintended pregnancies and STIs. For example, a 1996 study of women found "women who think planning ahead for birth control can spoil the fun of sex are no more or less likely to use contraceptives, but they are less likely to be satisfied with their method, and, if they use the pill, less likely to use it consistently."[30]

There is no perfect, 100% effective, 100% easy-to-use, pleasurable contraceptive. Clients can be advised to consider comfort with their body, desire to keep contraception independent of intercourse, degree of cooperation they can expect from their partner, and whether they also need protection against STIs (Table 2-2).

FEAR OF INFECTION

Worry about HIV, genital warts, and other incurable viral STIs often clouds the sexual experience for couples. It can be discouraging to realize that assuring protection from unwanted pregnancy is only half the battle for couples with any possible STI risk. Some people give up on sex altogether, some manage excellent safer sex techniques, but many more give up on safety. The clinician's task is to help at-risk patients in their efforts to keep sex pleasurable and infection-free, tailoring advice to fit an individual patient's sexual patterns.

Table 2-2 Sexuality issues and contraceptive selection

	Used at Time of Coitus	Partner Support Required	Affects Sexual Functioning	Can Be Used in Love-making	Okay for Multiple Partners
Pill	No	No	May	No	Yes? With condoms
Diaphragm	Yes	No	No	Yes	Yes? With condoms
Condom	Yes	Yes	Yes	Yes	Yes
IUD	No	No	No	No	No
Abstinence	NA	Yes	Yes	Yes	Yes
Coitus Interruptus	Yes	Yes	Yes	Yes	Yes? With condoms
Fertility Awareness	Yes	Yes	May	Yes	No
Sterilization	No	No	No	No	Yes? With condoms

FEAR OF PREGNANCY AND INFERTILITY

Fear or hope for pregnancy may powerfully affect sexual desire and performance. For men, the subject of pregnancy may cause concerns, but their level of concern tends to be lower than women's. Even among perimenopausal, postmenopausal, contracepting, or sterilized women, the fantasy, memory, hope, fear, anticipation, dread, joy, or desperation and despondency of pregnancy have an impact on identity that men generally do not feel. A woman who has more children than she wants may feel she literally risks the further destruction of her life every time she has penile-vaginal intercourse. An infertile woman may put her feminine identity on the line every month she tries to conceive and is likely to feel emotionally intimidated by the typical infertility workup.

Instructions to time intercourse around ovulation can be particularly stressful for both partners. Even among well-adjusted couples, such instructions are likely to precipitate performance anxiety as well as power and control conflicts. After couples begin timed intercourse, the man may experience an inability to achieve or maintain erections and the couple may have major conflicts. The spontaneity and romantic parts of lovemaking disappear, and couples often panic. Couples trying timed intercourse often need counseling and a break from the pressure of trying to conceive.

INFLUENCE OF CONTRACEPTIVE CHOICE

Hormonal Contraceptives

The primary sexual advantage of oral contraceptive pills, progestin-only pills, Nuva-Ring, Evra patch, injectables, and implants is that their use is entirely independent of coitus—they do not interrupt lovemaking. Further, women can adopt these methods without the cooperation, or even the knowledge, of their partners. For some couples, assurance of safety from pregnancy leads to increased frequency and satisfaction with sex. There are no timing issues, no stopping to use the method, and virtually no fear of pregnancy. Some women experience increased sexual desire when taking hormones.

Conversely, one of the occasional side effects of some hormonal contraceptives is diminution or loss of sexual desire. A woman whose usual sexual response pattern is well established over time is likely to recognize immediately any loss of desire that closely follows the initiation of a new hormonal method as an undesirable effect of the method. Such patients will usually report their symptom. A different hormonal method may alleviate the problem.

Vaginal Barriers and Spermicides

Diaphragms, cervical caps, films, suppositories, and foam may either increase sexual pleasure or impair sexual functioning. Clients must be comfortable touching and handling their genitals to use these methods successfully. Using these methods often requires women to plan for intercourse in advance or to interrupt lovemaking. Some couples include inserting the method as part of their sexual play. The extra lubrication is a plus for some couples and a messy interference for others.

For some women, inserting a vaginal barrier method before the beginning of a sexual interaction may increase excitement about the upcoming behavior. For others, carrying the equipment when going out for a date may feel uncomfortable and can alter the negotiation between partners. Inserting the method during precoital play carries the risk of interrupting a tender and romantic interlude with a purely mechanical task. One possible negative sexual outcome of diaphragm use for some women is an increased risk of cystitis infections, thereby making intercourse painful if not impossible. This is particularly true for couples having very frequent or particularly rigorous intercourse. (See Chapter 17 on Vaginal Spermicides and Chapter 18 on Vaginal Barriers.)

The female condom offers particular challenges related to sexual functioning. Although some women users report that it increased their pleasure during intercourse, others report it as awkward to place and use. The external ring requires that oral sex take place before insertion or after removal. Couples have reported the method "squeaks" during intercourse. As one sexologist reports, "This is not a method for a couple without a sense of humor."

Condoms

For many couples, condoms are a sexual boon, while for others, their use dampens sexual experience. Condom use requires that the couple communicate about their decision to have intercourse, which is likely to benefit both the sexual interaction and the relationship as a whole. Condoms can help men maintain their erection longer, perhaps increasing the likelihood that women will achieve orgasm during intercourse.

Yet, everyone knows men who feel using a condom is "like taking a shower with a raincoat on." Couples need careful encouragement on how to integrate putting on the condom as part of foreplay prior to intercourse. Men need to be encouraged to practice condom use when they are not with a partner so they increase their condom skills; women can experiment with erotic techniques for putting condoms on their partners. Some men report they lose their erections when faced with an unrolled condom; practice in private should help alleviate this problem. Speak with young women about how to bring up and negotiate condom use with their male partners. Because so many women have older partners, power issues related to condom use are very real. Role play discussing condom use with her partner and help her develop strategies with a resistant partner. Encourage clients to bring their male partners to the clinic for education and counseling.

Some men lose their erection rapidly after ejaculation whereas others maintain a relatively erect penis for some time, perhaps as long as 15 to 20 minutes. Because even a few minutes of rest and relaxation while the penis is still inside the partner may result in spillage of semen, men should hold the rim of the male condom at the base of the penis as they withdraw. Doing so prevents the condom from slipping off. (See Chapter 16 on Male Condoms.)

Coitus Interruptus

Withdrawal requires the man to pull out and move away from his partner when his desire is to push deeper and hold more firmly. For some heterosexual couples, this contraceptive method may leave the woman in a state of high excitement without orgasmic relief. Couples using withdrawal should make a special effort to reinstitute sexual play after withdrawal to make sure both partners have achieved gratification and relief of sexual tension. The method can encourage attention on performance rather than pleasure.

In adult or X-rated productions, the man often withdraws, ejaculates after a few moments of manual stroking, and then rapidly reinserts. It should be noted that this withdrawal is for the purpose of showing the viewer his ejaculation and is not for contraception. Rapid reinsertion when seminal fluid is still in the urethra as well as on the glans and shaft is not a satisfactory technique for contraception. Reinsertion should not take place without cleansing the male genitalia (washcloth and warm water with or without soap) and urinating to flush the urethra. (See Chapter 14 on Coitus Interruptus.)

Abstinence

It is likely all adults will go through periods of abstinence. In some cases, single people choose abstinence because of their conviction that sexual intercourse should occur only in marriage. Some single people remain abstinent because they lack a desirable partner. Some couples experience periods of abstinence because of illness, physical separation, or relationship conflicts.

There is no uniformly accepted definition of abstinence. Some people have defined abstinence as no genital contact of any kind outside of a monogamous marriage. Others have defined abstinence as not engaging in penetrative behaviors.

Young people need support for choosing abstinence until they are physically, emotionally, and cognitively ready for a mature sexual relationship. Adolescents need to know that "not everybody is doing it": although many American adolescents have had sexual intercourse, many have not. Adolescents need to understand that sexual intercourse is not a way to achieve adulthood, that adolescents in romantic relationships can express sexual feelings without engaging in intercourse, and that there are many ways to give and receive sexual pleasure without the risks associated with penetrative behaviors.[31] Spend ample time with adolescent clients addressing their decision to be sexually involved.

Adult couples may achieve satisfaction with sexual abstinence providing both select this alternative as the one that most closely meets their individual needs. A relationship can be almost anything so long as both partners agree on what it is to be. When one partner does not agree to abstinence but does not wish to give up the relationship, then a continuing conflict arises that will have emotional consequences for each individual and for the couple. One or both partner(s) may choose abstinence for contraception, for protection from an STI, as part of sexual aversion, or as a symptom of alcoholism or other addiction, depression, or distraction. The person who feels abandoned because of a partner's decision to abstain may use masturbation as an alternative, may reluctantly accept abstinence also, or may choose to seek another partner outside of the primary relationship. (See Chapter 13 on Abstinence and the Range of Sexual Expression.)

The couple practicing sexual abstinence may lose a major method of nonverbal communication in their relationship and may find it difficult to compensate by communicating in less intimate ways. They must make special efforts to maintain or strengthen other forms of communication.

Fertility Awareness

Couples using fertility awareness methods must carefully assess their impact on their sexual relationship. Both partners must be committed to fertility awareness as the primary contraceptive method for it to be effective. Couples must negotiate in advance what the use of this method will mean during the fertile days: will they abstain from all sexual behaviors, will they abstain only from penile-vaginal intercourse, or will they use a barrier method? How sure are they that they will be able to maintain sexual limits once sexual activity is in progress? It is even possible that abstaining from sexual intercourse may enhance the experience when it does occur.

Intrauterine Devices

The primary advantage of the intrauterine device (IUD) as regards sexual functioning, is that like the pill, its use is completely separate from coitus and it is highly effective. IUD users do not need cooperation from their partner. However, women who experience severe or frequent bleeding with the IUD may find it affects their own and their partner's aesthetic experience during intercourse. (See Chapter 21 on Intrauterine Devices.)

Voluntary Surgical Contraception

Sterilization could improve or hinder sexual functioning. Men considering vasectomy need careful counseling that a vasectomy will not affect or impair their ability to have an erection. As many men are not familiar with their reproductive anatomy, beyond their penis and scrotum, begin with basic anatomy education, including the sexual function of different organs. Help men understand that vasectomy does not affect their erectile or orgasmic potential.

For many women, sterilization removes the fear of pregnancy and leads to an increase in desire and frequency of intercourse. For others, reproductive capacity is intimately connected with sexual desire, and sterilization may have the opposite effect. These issues should be carefully discussed as part of the informed consent process. (See Chapter 22 on Female and Male Sterilization.)

BRIEF INTRODUCTION TO SEXUAL COUNSELING

Few patients who have a sexual problem or dysfunction are beyond help, if they want to change and if the counselor is willing to help. By simply allowing them a place to ventilate or by providing basic information, counselors can often help patients solve their problems. A brief sexual history is a good place to start (Table 2-3).

The PLISSIT counseling model was developed for providers who are not psychiatrists, psychologists, or sexual therapists but who wish to address the sexual needs and concerns of their patients and make appropriate referrals when necessary.[32] PLISSIT is an acronym for four stages of counseling: Permission giving, Limited Information giving, Specific Suggestions, and Intensive Therapy.

Permission giving is not the same as telling the patient what to do. Permission is usually for thoughts, feelings, or behaviors and may be expressed as permission to do or not to do. Permission giving from a knowledgeable professional figure is quite powerful. Counselors are not required to give permission for thoughts, feelings, or behaviors that violate their professional value system; however, they are required by professional honesty to indicate to the patient that such is the case and to be frank about differing beliefs and values among professionals. For example, no qualified professionals approve of rape or child sexual abuse. The law requires reporting of all suspect child abuse to the police. This duty supersedes medical confidentiality. Professionals ought not approve of behaviors that threaten the physical or psychological health of patients and their partners.

Table 2-3 Taking a sexual history

The following questions may be helpful in encouraging clients to talk about their sexual lives or to choose a contraceptive method:

1. Tell me about your earliest sexual experience.
2. Briefly give me a history of your sexual experiences to date.
3. Did you agree to these experiences?
4. How has contraception fit into your sexual behaviors?
5. Are you willing to use a contraceptive method at the time of intercourse?
6. Does your partner actively support your use of contraception?
7. Are you looking for a method you can integrate into lovemaking?
8. How likely is it that you will have more than one sexual partner?
9. Do you have any questions or concerns that you would like to discuss about your present sexual response or your relationship?

Limited information giving usually involves discussing anatomy and physiology as well as dispelling myths about sex. This task is often easy for health care providers because of knowledge about anatomy and physiology. Sexual myths are common, but trained health workers can usually dispel them easily.

Specific suggestions involve skill-building such as changing position for sexual activities, using lubricants (for dyspareunia), considering Viagra for erectile dysfunction, or using a squeeze or stop-start technique (for rapid ejaculation).

Intensive therapy will probably prove too time-consuming and involved for all but those who are specially trained and wish to devote considerable time to such work. Intensive therapy may be necessary for body-image problems, relationship problems, identity issues, depression, personality disorders, or psychoses.

Patients are rarely hesitant to provide sexual information if the clinician is professional, concerned, self-confident, and nonjudgmental. Even though the patient may offer no data on the first visit, the experience demonstrates willingness to deal with these special subjects, and, often on subsequent visits, patients will offer additional significant and useful data.

If the patient has beliefs or practices that may be harmful or dysfunctional (not merely different from the provider), it is important to talk about the consequences of those beliefs and practices and discuss alternatives. If a clinician is unwilling to offer care because of personal values or professional ethics, they can recommend an alternative source of reputable help. Family planning clinicians should have a referral list of certified sex counselors and therapists.

COMMONLY ASKED QUESTIONS

A client's questions about sexuality often indirectly approach personal worries and concerns:

- How often do most couples my age have sex?
- Is it normal to have times in your marriage when you do not want to have sex?
- How often is it okay to masturbate?

The client with these questions is often asking "Am I normal?" Factual information about frequency may help assure the client, but she may also need time to process her own feelings about sexual behavior. Clients can be reassured there is no "right" answer to these questions; people must decide, alone or with their partner, what frequency is acceptable. Assure married clients that sexual drives fluctuate during different periods of life, so communication is essential. The questioner on masturbation needs to know that "once is too much if you don't like it," and that too much is when it interferes with your life, relationship, and work.

- My partner wants to (fill in behavior) and I do not. What can I do?
- My partner wants less sex than I do. What can I do?
- What can I do to improve my sex life?

These clients are seeking assistance with couple issues. For example, they may need permission to discuss this issue with their partner. They may need encouragement to say "no" to sexual behaviors or to ask for more control and input over sexual encounters. These clients and partners may need to be referred for counseling.

- Intercourse is painful for me.
- My partner cannot maintain an erection.
- I have never had an orgasm.

These clients may be helped by simple information. The clinician needs to elicit additional information from the client: how often does this happen? Under what conditions does it happen? The information given in the next section may be helpful.

- How can I tell if my partner has an STI?
- How do I know if my partner is being honest with me?

The reality is that no one can ever know for sure if a partner is being completely honest about past or current sexual history. Unfortunately, some people do lie to their partners, and in some cases, some people may not be aware themselves of their past exposure to STIs and even HIV. To eliminate transmission risk, condoms must be used with each and every act of vaginal, oral, and anal intercourse when a partner's health history is unknown. Of course, if the partner has obvious genital sores, lesions, or secretions, all sexual contact is best avoided until medical advice has been sought and the condition diagnosed and treated.

INTRODUCTION TO COMMON SEXUAL DYSFUNCTIONS

Sexual dysfunctions are indeed common. Among the 3400 National Health and Social Life Survey respondents age 18-59, 43% of women and 31% of men confronted such problems in the past year.[33]

Sex therapy in its beginnings was framed in relational terms. In their book, *Human Sexual Inadequacy*, Masters and Johnson said "there is no such thing as an uninvolved partner in any marriage in which there is some form of sexual inadequacy."[34] Even though some sexual dysfunctions, such as female orgasmic disorder, can be treated on an individual basis, it is still important to offer to include her partner so she can become orgasmic with her partner as well as alone.

The effects of a sexual dysfunction on a relationship cannot be overstated. Performance fears, anxiety, and low self-esteem often are direct results of a person feeling like a failure in the bedroom. Depression is common in either or both partners if they cannot get aroused or feel they cannot satisfy their partner. On the other hand, improving sexual functioning can help the entire relationship blossom, just as resolving some of the marital discord can promote a more relaxed and satisfying sexual interaction.

Since 1970, not only has much more been learned about sexual function and dysfunction, but the field of sex therapy has expanded to include a wider range of sexual issues such as sex therapy with persons with a disability, both physical and mental, and gender identity issues.

Most people were not taught to be good lovers. While we are all born sexual and with the capacity for sexual response, we are not born lovers. In America's sexually repressive and sex-negative culture, being a good lover is a matter of learning new attitudes and skills; sex instruction with adults can provide the "how to" of being a lover. Overcoming a sexual dysfunction can be a by-product of learning and practicing the techniques of being a considerate and passionate lover.

While most clinics do not provide sex therapy, it is important to know when to refer a client to a competent sex therapist. Refer clients who require more than information and education to a qualified gynecologist, sex counselor, or therapist. Develop a list of certified practitioners in your area for referrals to a certified sex counselor or therapist. Contact the American Association of Sex Educators, Counselors and Therapists (AASECT), PO Box 5488, Richmond, VA, 23220 or via the website at www. aasect.org. In this section are simple suggestions for assessing when to refer a client for sex or relationship therapy.

ETIOLOGY OF SEXUAL DYSFUNCTION

Human sexual response consists of a complex orchestration of emotional and hormonal influences, via the autonomic nervous system, to trigger basic reflexes. Any agent that alters metabolism, stimulates or depresses the central nervous system, or locally influences anatomy or physiology is likely to affect sexual functioning.[35] Stress, emotional well-being, relational issues, and general health affect sexual intimacy and functioning.

Organic factors. Any possibility of organic, physiological, or chemical factors in the sexual dysfunction should be ruled out. Emotional and physiological illness, neurological disorders, use of illicit drugs or medications, or psychotropic drugs can raise or lower sexual desire or function. Couples need a complete physical examination when beginning treatment. (See Chapter 6 on Menstrual Problems and Common Gynecologic Concerns.)

Individual psychodynamics. When Masters and Johnson[34] first presented their material on sexual inadequacy, it was believed that more than 90% of sexual dysfunction was psychologically caused. Performance anxiety was believed to be the chief culprit. Classically trained analysts believed most sexual dysfunctions were the result of psychological issues such as unresolved Oedipal wishes. Other causes of sexual dysfunction were thought to be borderline personality disorder, obsessive-compulsive personality disorders, anxiety disorders, and depression. While it is true that all of these can affect sexual function, they are not the only factors to be evaluated.

Relationship. It is common for therapists to believe from their own clinical experience and from familiarity with the sex therapy literature that most sexual problems are due to significant relationship problems. Hostility, battles for power and control, poor communications, and excessive dependency are incompatible with sexual intimacy and good functioning. For sex therapy to be successful, problems with the relationship need to be resolved. Otherwise, the behavioral suggestions recommended later in this section will not work and can even increase marital discord. Many clients will need to be referred for couples counseling.

Sociocultural and religious factors. The United States is one of the most sexually repressive cultures in history when compared with both ancient and other contemporary societies. Kaplan as well as Masters and Johnson held that religious orthodoxy has played a major part in the widespread sexual dysfunction of our day. Guilt, fear, and the denial of sex as pleasure have led to sexual inhibition. In recent decades, widely held gender-role stereotypes (males as aggressive, females as passive, and so on) have been challenged. Cultural imprinting or conditioning (males pressured to perform quickly; females conditioned to not stimulate the male directly) can create sexual dysfunctions.

SEXUAL DESIRE DISORDERS

The desire disorders[28] are associated with Reed's seduction phase. In any given case, it must be determined when seduction takes place: in the present or the past? These disorders must create enough distress and interpersonal difficulty for both partners to be motivated to change.

Lack of desire may be lifelong or acquired; that is, desire may have once been there, but then have diminished for some reason. A lack of desire may be generalized, that is, experienced in every situation; or it may be situational, occurring only in certain situations. For example, one may have desire on vacation but not at home in familiar surroundings. Or one may lack lustful feelings with a long-term partner but feel aroused by others. The dysfunction may be due only to psychological factors or to a combination of psychological and organic disease or chemical factors. Sexual desire disorders should be referred to a trained sex therapist.

In hypoactive sexual desire disorder, there is a lack of desire for sexual activity and often an inability to experience sexual fantasies. In a sexual aversion disorder, there is an aversion or avoidance to kissing, touching, and genital sexual contact. A picture or genital model can be used to discuss the client's feelings about observing or touching the model.

SEXUAL AROUSAL DISORDERS

An arousal disorder has an impact on a couple's emotional well-being, whether the disorder affects a woman or a man, and whether medical intervention is successful or not. Consider whether medical interventions should be linked to psychotherapeutic support for the couple, either in the clinical setting or by referral. For example, it is common for the non-dysfunctional partner to feel he or she is no longer attractive, or to worry that the partner is attracted to someone else. People experiencing a dysfunction may lose self-confidence, and may believe that their desire for the partner is permanently lost. Both may feel powerless and fearful. Even if a medical intervention is technically successful, sexual desire may still be affected if interpersonal issues are not addressed and treated.

Female sexual arousal disorder. Women who have difficulty becoming aroused will have difficulty lubricating and feeling erotic genital sensations. There is little or no genital swelling. It is important to evaluate the couple's foreplay patterns to assess whether there has been enough attention paid to the woman's arousal. If her partner is anxious about his potential loss of erection, he may initiate intercourse before she is physically and/or emotionally prepared.

The first step is a thorough medical evaluation, looking especially for drug therapies such as selective serotonin reuptake inhibitors (SSRIs), neurologic disorders, and chronic conditions such as diabetes that can impair sexual function. Then, interventions to consider are over-the-counter lubricants such as Astroglide, Replens, and K-Y Jelly, and, for perimenopausal women, hormonal creams or other hormonal treatment to diminish vaginal dryness. (See Chapter 5 on Menopause.) A prescription-only mechanical intervention to increase genital blood flow, a clitoral pump known as the Eros-CTD Treatment™ (Clitoral Therapy Device), is available through UroMetrics, Inc. at 877-774-1442 (toll-free) for around $360. A number of testosterone and other hormonal products and vasodilators are under study as treatments for female arousal disorders,[36] but not FDA-approved (or not approved for this indication) as of early 2004, although the results of current studies are promising. These pharmacotherapeutic agents are meant to enhance the desire for sex, increase arousal response, and/or improve blood flow to the genitals.

While product labeling states that Viagra and now Levitra are indicated only for the treatment of erectile dysfunction,[37] these drugs have been used to treat women, and women often ask their reproductive health care providers about Viagra. It has not proven to be effective in treating sexual dysfunction in women as it has in men, with the exception of SSRI-associated dysfunction.[38] The risk is that long-term use has not been tested. Wellbutrin, an antidepressant, may increase sexual interest in women who are not depressed.

Male erectile disorder. If a man has difficulty gaining or maintaining an adequate erection suitable for sexual activity, he suffers from erectile disorder. The first step is a thorough medical evaluation, looking especially for ischemic heart disease, diabetes, prostate cancer treatment, neurological disorders, and use of SSRIs. Then, a mechanical intervention to consider is the vacuum pump to draw blood into the penis. When an erection is attained, a rubber band or similar device is placed over the base of the penis to hold the blood in. The pump is a prescription product from ErecAid System, and can also be purchased through mail-order catalogs or sex shops.

Topical medications such as minoxidil are effective for some men. Other topical products that show promise contain glyceryltrinitrate, nitroglycerine, alprostadil, or papavarine. Little is known about potential adverse effects of vaginal absorption of these products during intercourse.[39]

Oral medications such as Viagra, Levitra, and Cialis are effective for many men. These medications have demonstrated effectiveness in men whose erectile dysfunction is associated with prostatectomy, radiation therapy, diabetes, certain neurologic disorders, and drug therapies such as SSRIs.[38] Be sure to rule out contraindications such as use of organic nitrate therapy, and the manufacturer warns that Viagra should not be generally used in men for whom sexual activity is inadvisable because of underlying cardiovascular status.[37]

Yohimbine, another oral product made from the bark of the yohimbe tree, is available in health food stores or by prescription as Yocon. Other oral products hold promise for the future, and oral agents have emerged as a first line option for many patients.[39]

Intraurethral suppositories containing the vasoactive drug alprostadil (Prostaglandin E_1), such as Muse and Alibra, have been successful for some men. Intracavernosal injection is one of the most effective ways to obtain and maintain erection, and alprostadil products Caverject and Edex are among the most commonly used. Penile injections are considered safe, but the idea of giving oneself a shot in this area may be hard for some men.[39]

SENSATE FOCUS FOR MALE AND FEMALE AROUSAL DISORDERS

Simple pleasuring exercises can increase or enhance the arousal process. Masters and Johnson called these exercises sensate focus. First, the couple sensually touch each other over their entire bodies, except for the genital and breast areas. This is often difficult, because when the couple is experiencing sexual difficulties, one or both often take on spectator roles and try to think about what is going on in their partner's head. They lose the focus on their own pleasure as participants.

Once partners have been able to focus on their own pleasurable experiences, they can explore the breasts and genitals and determine which touches are pleasurable, threatening, or irritating. What many couples do not realize is that different areas on the breasts and genitals can be more erotic and sensitive than other spots. Next the couple caresses the breasts and genitals to produce arousal. If either of the partners experiences arousal, they may go on to non-coital orgasm, unless the dysfunction is directly related to orgasm.

Before trying intercourse when he is able to gain an erection consistently, the man should deliberately lose his erection by having his partner stop stimulating him. Once his erection has gone down, his partner should then restimulate him until he has another erection. The important lesson here is that if there has been no orgasm, he can lose his erection several times and regain it with further erotic stimulation. Too often a man incorrectly believes that if he loses his erection once, the experience is over for him. After the man has accomplished losing and regaining an erection, his partner can stimulate him while he is lying on his back and then mount him and just hold his penis near her labia and clitoris. When she does this and he holds the erection, she can then insert the penis into her vagina without doing any thrusting, so he can experience being contained in her vagina without stimulation. He will then lose his erection and she can restimulate him. When he gets an erection again, she can put his penis into her vagina and begin slowly thrusting. They can continue this exercise until they are having satisfying intercourse.

ORGASMIC DISORDERS

The psychological issues involved in orgasmic disorders usually involve issues of power and control. Other issues include an inability to relax, let go, and let the tension of the sexual response take over. Being vulnerable, fearing failure, or fearing success can affect orgasmic potential.

Female orgasmic disorder. A woman who has never been orgasmic should begin with self-exploration and stimulation to experience her sexual response cycle without having to perform in front of her partner. The books *For Yourself*,[1] *Sex for One: The Joys of Self-loving*,[40] or *Becoming Orgasmic: A Sexual and Personal Growth Program for Women*[41] are helpful resources for clients to learn about masturbation and orgasm. A vibrator also can be a useful aid in helping the woman experience her orgasmic potential. Once she has become orgasmic, it is easier for her to share with her partner the type of touch that helps her reach an orgasm. As she develops her orgasm response, she can then introduce the experience into intercourse by touching herself or by using a vibrator while her partner's penis is inside her. Women should not get discouraged if orgasm does not occur during the first few lovemaking encounters. It takes time, practice, patience, and comfort. Many women are not orgasmic through intercourse alone.

Male orgasmic disorder. A man who cannot have an orgasm with intercourse is rare and usually has difficulty giving of himself in a relationship. It is most helpful to have him masturbate with his partner so she can experience him having an orgasm. During intercourse, when either partner is ready for orgasm, he should withdraw and masturbate until he feels himself on the brink of orgasm and then again insert his penis in the vagina. The goal is to have him experience having an orgasm. Once this occurs it may be easier for him to get to the point of orgasm through intercourse. A lot of patience and practice are needed for this dysfunction. If he works on his ability to give of himself generally to the relationship, it will help him have an orgasm inside his partner.

Another possibility is that the male orgasm is inhibited because of a fear of an unwanted pregnancy or STI. These men need information about contraception and safer sex methods. Feeling safe can enhance his orgasmic release.

Premature ejaculation. Premature ejaculation has been successfully treated with both the "stop-start" method and the "squeeze" technique. The "stop-start" method is often the easier and preferred procedure. After the man is aroused, his partner should stimulate (masturbate) him until he is almost ready to ejaculate. He should signal his partner, who then stops any further stimulation until the feeling of ejaculatory inevitability subsides. His partner then resumes stimulation until he again feels he is going to ejaculate, and then the partner stops. After stopping three or four times, he should go ahead and have an ejaculation. This process should be repeated several times a week until the client is able to hold back ejaculation for as long as he likes. Next, he can try intercourse, using the female superior position, going through the same process. When his penis is in her vagina, she should begin moving up and down on the penis, until he feels he is going to ejaculate. She should stop until he loses that feeling, and when he does, start moving up and down again. After repeating this exercise several times, the couple can proceed to have an orgasm. With patience and practice, this method will work.

It is also possible to treat premature ejaculation with antidepressants. Combining the use of one of these medicines with the above exercises can bring about more rapid results.[42]

SEXUAL PAIN DISORDERS

When a client suffers from dyspareunia (painful intercourse), vaginismus (inability to insert the penis into the vagina because of spasms), or vulvodynia (sensitive or painful areas in the vagina), it may be best to refer the client to a certified sex therapist or to a specialist, such as a gynecologist who is trained to help with these dysfunctions. (See Chapter 6 on Menstrual Problems and Common Gynecologic Concerns).

REFERENCES

1. Barbach L. For yourself: the fulfillment of female sexuality. Garden City NY: Doubleday, 1976.
2. United Nations. Programme of Action. Reproductive rights and reproductive health. Proceedings of the International Conference on Population and Development, September 5-13, 1994; Cairo, Egypt, 1994; section 7.2:43.

3. Laumann EO, Gagnon JH, Michael RT, Michaels S. The social organization of sexuality—sexual practices in the United States. Chicago IL: University of Chicago Press, 1994.
4. Coles R, Stokes F. Sex and the American teenager. New York: Harper and Row, 1995.
5. Roper Starch Worldwide. Teens talk about sex: adolescent sexuality in the 90's. New York: SIECUS, 1994.
6. Haffner DW, National Commission on Adolescent Sexual Health. Facing facts: sexual health for America's adolescents. New York: SIECUS, 1995.
7. Newcomer S, Udry J. Oral sex in an adolescent population. Arch Sex Behav 1985;14:41-46.
8. Brooks-Gunn J, Furstenberg FF. Coming of age in the era of AIDS. Puberty, sexuality, and contraception. Millbank Quart 1990;68(Suppl 1).
9. Alan Guttmacher Institute. Sex and America's teenagers. New York: The Alan Guttmacher Institute, 1994.
10. U.S. Centers for Disease Control and Prevention. National and state-specific pregnancy rates among adolescents — United States, 1995-1997. MMWR, 2000;49(27): 605.
11. Zelnik M. Shah FK. First intercourse among young Americans. Fam Plann Perspect 1983;15:64-68.
12. National Center for Health Statistics. Contraceptive use in the United States: 1982-1990. Advance Data 1995.
13. U.S. Centers for Disease Control and Prevention. Youth risk behavior surveillance. MMWR 2000;49(ss-5).
14. Cates W. Teenagers and sexual risk taking: the best of times and the worst of times. JAMA 1991;12:84-94.
15. Kinsey AC, Pomeroy WB, Martin CE. Sexual behavior in the human male. Philadelphia: WB Saunders, 1948.
16. Kinsey AC, Pomeroy WB, Martin CE. Sexual behavior in the human female. Philadelphia: WB Saunders, 1953.
17. Schwartz P, Gillmore M, Civic D. The social context of sexuality. In: Cates W, Hansfield and Holmesk (ed). Sexually transmitted diseases. New York: McGraw Hill, 1996.
18. National Victims Center. Rape in America: a report to the nation. Arlington VA: National Victims Center, 1992.
19. Polit DF, White CM, Morton TD. Child sexual abuse and premarital intercourse among high risk adolescents. JAHC 1990;11:231-234.
20. Child Welfare League of America. A survey of 17 Florence Crittenton agencies serving minor mothers. Washington DC: Child Welfare League of America, 1994.
21. Boyer D, Fine D. Sexual abuse as a factor in adolescent pregnancy and child maltreatment. Fam Plann Perspect 1992;24:4-11.
22. Ladas AK, Whipple B, Perry JD. The G spot: and other recent discoveries about human sexuality. New York: Holt, Rinehart and Winston, 1982.
23. Singer J, Singer I. Types of female orgasm. In: LoPiccolo J, LoPiccolo L (ed). Handbook of sex therapy. New York: Plenum Press, 1987.
24. Masters W, Johnson V. Human sexual response. Boston: Little, Brown & Co., 1966.
25. Kaplan HS. Active treatment of sexual dysfunctions. New York: Brunner/Mazel, 1981.
26. Kaplan HS. Sex aversion, sex phobias and panic disorders. New York: Brunner/Mazel, 1987.
27. Kaplan HS. The evaluation of sexual disorders: psychological and medical aspects. New York: Brunner/Mazel, 1983.
28. Kaplan HS. Disorders of sexual desire: and other new concepts and techniques in sex therapy. New York: Brunner/Mazel, 1979.
29. Stayton WR. A theology of sexual pleasure. American Baptist Quarterly 1989;8:94-108.
30. Forrest JD, Frost JJ. The family planning attitudes and experiences of low-income women. Fam Plann Perspect 1996;28:246-255, 277.

31. National Guidelines Task Force. Guidelines for comprehensive sexuality education: kindergarten–12th grade. Second edition. New York: SIECUS, 1996.
32. Annon JS. The behavioral treatment of sexual problems. Vol. 1, Brief therapy. Honolulu HI: Mercantile Printing, 1974:100-105.
33. Laumann EO, Paik A, Rosen RC. Sexual dysfunction in the United States: prevalence and predictors. In: Laumann EO, Michael RT (eds). Sex, Love, and Health in America. Chicago IL: University of Chicago Press, 2001, 352-376.
34. Masters WH, Johnson VE. Human sexual inadequacy. Boston: Little, Brown & Co., 1970.
35. Satterfield S, Stayton W. Understanding sexual function and dysfunction. In: Stayton W (ed). Topics in clinical nursing 1980;1:21-32.
36. Rae S. Rx: desire: there's new hope for women with a loss of libido—and it's NOT Viagra. Modern Maturity. March-April 2001.
37. Physicians' desk reference. 56th edition. Montvale NJ:Medical Economics Company, Inc. 2002:2732-2735.
38. Boyce EG, Umland EM. Sildenafil citrate: a therapeutic update [review]. Clinical Therapeutics 2001;23:2-23.
39. Rowland DL, Burnett AL. Pharmacotherapy in the treatment of male sexual dysfunction. J Sex Research 2000;37:226-243.
40. Dodson B. Sex for one: the joys of self-loving. New York: Harmony Books, 1987.
41. Heiman J, LoPiccolo J. Becoming orgasmic: a sexual and personal growth program for women. Englewood Cliffs NJ: Prentice-Hall, 1988.
42. Crenshaw TL, Goldberg JP. Sexual pharmacology. New York: WW Norton, 1996.

Female Genital Tract Cancer Screening

Michael S. Policar, MD, MPH

- Early detection of pre-invasive lesions by Papanicolaou (Pap) smear prevents at least 70% of potential cervical cancers.

- The goal of Pap smear screening is to detect and treat high-grade squamous intraepithelial lesions (HSIL). Low grade SIL is a benign lesion with a high regression rate, especially in adolescents.

- Pap smear screening should begin 3 years after the onset of sexual activity (or by age 21) and should be discontinued after total hysterectomy for benign disease or in women older than 65 to 70 years old who have a history of normal Pap smears in the prior 10 years.

- Women 30 and older should receive Pap smears every 2 to 3 years, while women under 30 should have conventional Pap smears annually or liquid-based Pap smears every 2 years.

- Oral contraceptive use for 10 years or longer reduces the risk of ovarian cancer by as much as 80%.

- Most guidelines recommend breast cancer screening by mammography at least every 2 years for women age 50 and older. Newer guidelines recommend that women between 40 to 49 years old who choose to have mammograms do so yearly.

A reproductive health care visit represents an ideal opportunity to offer periodic health screening services, including screening for genital tract cancers. As early as the 1920s, the prevalent philosophy of the American medical community was that individuals of all ages should receive an annual physical examination and a battery of routine screening tests to detect early, asymptomatic disease.[1] Over the past decade, however, the wisdom of this practice has been challenged, and research studies and health policy discussions have focused upon the optimal content of periodic health screening: which tests should or should not be performed, how often each screening test should be done, and whether each test should be performed universally or limited to persons of certain age or risk factors. While many approaches to periodic health screening have been proposed, the recommendations of the United States Preventive Services Task Force (USPSTF) are considered the blueprint for the screening guidelines developed by most state Departments of Health, professional specialty societies, and health plans.[2] Using an evidence-based methodology, the USPSTF guidelines gauged both the strength of each recommendation and the quality of the research studies used to develop each guideline. The guidelines emphasize that the most cost-effective approach to maximizing health status is by avoiding the development of disease through primary prevention based on focused risk assessment and counseling interventions, rather than on periodic physical examination or laboratory testing. (See Chapter 1 on Expanding Perspectives on Reproductive Health.)

Over the years, annual periodic health screening has been linked with the provision of prescription hormonal contraceptives. In many cases, a woman could get a prescription for oral contraceptives (OCs) only when she underwent an annual examination, which necessarily included a breast exam and a Papanicolaou (Pap) smear. In this way, women have been compelled to receive desirable public health screening tests as a by-product of their need for contraception. However, many reproductive health programs no longer require genital tract cancer screening for the provision of prescription-based contraceptives, based on the position that beneficial screening tests must be supported on their own merits, and any unnecessary barriers to contraceptive services should be removed.[3-5] Regardless of one's attitude on this issue, genital tract cancer screening is a desirable, and in some cases, lifesaving measure, irrespective of a woman's contraceptive method. Furthermore, hormonal methods should never be restricted or withheld from a woman solely because she has an abnormal Pap smear. There is no reason to believe that the use of any contraceptive method will hasten the progression of an existing cervical lesion. All too often, the unfortunate result of withholding contraceptive methods from a woman with cervical dysplasia is unintended pregnancy, which makes diagnosis more difficult and often delays treatment.

SCREENING FOR CERVICAL CANCER

The Pap smear, more than any other screening test, has proven its cost effectiveness over the years.[6] Although negative press reports in the mid-1980s shed doubts upon Pap smear quality, in the United States early detection and treatment of pre-invasive lesions by Pap smears prevents at least 70% of potential cervical cancers. Of the 13,000 American women who develop new cases of cervical cancer each year:[7,8]

- One-half had not had a Pap smear in the past 3 to 5 years.

- One-half had received a Pap smear within 3 to 5 years that was falsely negative.
  - One-half of these falsely negative smears occurred in women whose initial smears were re-read as normal. Precursor lesions were missed either because the pre-malignant or malignant lesion had too little exfoliation to be detected, the lesion grew rapidly and so did not exist at the time of the initial Pap smear, or there was a sampling error.
  - The other half occurred in women whose initial smears were re-read as abnormal, suggesting a screening or interpretive error in the cytopathology lab.

In 1996 the U.S. Food and Drug Administration (FDA) approved a number of new technologies aimed at improving the detection rate of SIL lesions, thereby reducing the rate of false negatives. One approach, liquid based cytology (LBC) with thin layer preparation technique (Thin Prep Pap Test, AutoCyte Prep), improves accuracy by increasing the number of cells sampled and by removing blood, mucus, and debris from the background of the smear. Another approach is to evaluate the Pap smear by routine microscopy and then re-screen the negative smears with computer-based evaluation techniques (AutoPap QC System) to detect abnormal smears that should be re-evaluated microscopically.

Each of these newer approaches improves Pap smear accuracy over current practices;[9,10] however, controversy persists whether the additional cost associated with these tests justifies their use or, in contrast, if the increased cost of screening actually may lead to fewer Pap smears being performed.[11,12] Because of the greater accuracy of LBC smears, a longer screening interval is recommended when this method of Pap screening is used.

PATHOPHYSIOLOGY

The cervix consists of two types of epithelium:

- Squamous epithelium, which covers the vagina and the portio vaginalis of the cervix
- Columnar epithelium, which covers the endocervical canal, and in younger women, the area around the external cervical os

At menarche, the vaginal pH drops into an acidic range and causes the fragile columnar epithelial cells around the cervical os to be replaced by squamous epithelium, a process referred to as squamous metaplasia. As this process proceeds over decades, the advancing edge of the squamous epithelium (referred to as the squamocolumnar junction) migrates centrally toward the cervical os and ultimately into the endocervical canal.

Because squamous cell cancers and their precursors virtually always develop within the field of metaplasia (also called the transformation zone), both cytological and colposcopic evaluation focus upon this area.

There is now widespread agreement that the cause of cervical dysplasia is an accumulation of DNA mutations in immature metaplastic cells as a consequence of human papilloma virus (HPV) infection in concert with other carcinogenic co-factors. Although more than 100 DNA-types of HPV have been identified, only a limited number are associated with premalignant and malignant epithelial lesions of the lower genital tract: HPV types 16, 18, 45, and 56 are known to have the highest potential for malignant transformation.[13] The high-risk HPV types exert their cancer-causing effects through a series of events leading to the degradation of the p53 tumor suppressor protein in infected cells, reducing the host's ability to reject cells with random DNA mutations. However, HPV infection alone is insufficient to initiate this process. A facilitating agent, or co-factor, appears to be necessary to act in concert with HPV to initiate these premalignant changes. For example, cigarette smoking has been identified as a powerful co-factor, doubling a smoker's risk of cervical cancer.[14,15] Infections due to HPV types 6 and 11, the cause of genital warts and most low-grade cervical lesions, are felt to exhibit very low or no malignant potential.

HPV infections are widespread among sexually active adults, costly to characterize virologically, and cannot be eradicated with anti-viral drugs. The duration of HPV infection remains controversial; while older studies inferred that HPV infection is lifelong, newer studies suggest that HPV infections are transient in a majority of infected individuals.[16,17] In addition, the role of evaluating and treating the male sexual partner in preventing recurrences of cervical dysplasia in treated women and in preventing spread of the virus to uninfected women is uncertain.[18] From a public health viewpoint, it makes more sense to detect and treat pre-invasive lesions, before life-threatening invasive cervical cancers have a chance to develop, rather than to rely on a strategy that focuses on the transmissibility of HPV.

RISK FACTORS FOR CERVICAL CANCER

Epidemiological observations are consistent with the biological mechanism of cervical cancer. The following are primary epidemiological risk factors for the development of cervical cancer:

- Early onset of intercourse (defined as a sexual debut before 20 years old). Metaplasia is most active during adolescence, making a young woman more vulnerable to cell changes.

- Three or more sexual partners in one's lifetime. The greater the number of sexual partners, the greater the risk of acquiring a high-risk type of HPV.

- Male sexual partner who has had other partners, especially if a previous partner had cervical cancer.

- Clinical history of condyloma acuminata. Infection with a low-risk type of HPV is a risk marker for co-infection with a high-risk type.[18]

- Infection with the human immunodeficiency virus (HIV) and other medical conditions associated with immunodeficiency. These illnesses decrease the ability of the immune system to recognize and reject abnormal cells.

Protective factors include virginity, long-term celibacy, life-long mutual monogamy, and long-term use of condoms. Factors that appear to have no effect on cervical cancer risk include history of herpes simplex virus infection, circumcision status of the male partner, religious background, or number of pregnancies. The effect of race and socioeconomic status are controversial. Studies show higher rates of cervical cancer among black women and women of lower socio-economic status;[19] however, it is unclear whether the higher rates are related to poor access to medical care and, consequently, Pap smear services, or other undetermined factors.

HIV Infection and Cervical Cancer Risk

Studies have demonstrated that the natural history of genital tract HPV infection, as well as that of pre-invasive and invasive cervical lesions, is different in HIV-seropositive women when compared to HIV seronegative women.[20] While the prevalence of dysplasia in reproductive-age women is below 3%, its prevalence is 36% among HIV-positive women and 64% among women with acquired immune deficiency syndrome (AIDS). Although an early uncontrolled study suggested that HIV-positive women had substantially higher rates of falsely negative Pap smears, more recent studies show that the accuracy of Pap smears is the same in HIV-positive as in HIV-negative women.[21,22] When cervical dysplasia occurs in an HIV-infected woman, the lesion may progress more rapidly, especially if she is immunocompromised. It also has been observed that HIV-positive women treated for cervical dysplasia have loop electrosurgical excision (LEEP) failure rates of 40% to 60% (even higher if the woman is immuno-compromised) compared with failure rates of 10% for HIV-negative women.[23] In 1992, the Centers for Disease Control and Prevention changed its surveillance definition of AIDS to include cervical cancer in an HIV-positive woman as an indicator of AIDS.[24] Women with HIV also are more likely to develop multifocal vulvar intraepithelial neoplasia (VIN), as well as pre-invasive and invasive squamous cell cancers of the anus.[21] Three clinical recommendations can be made:

1. Because of more rapid progression rates of CIN in HIV-seroposi-tive women, immunocompetent women should receive Pap smears twice in the first year after diagnosis, then annually, while

those who are immunocompromised or who have been treated for dysplasia since the time of HIV diagnosis should receive Pap smears more frequently. No major organization recommends that baseline colposcopy should be performed routinely for all HIV-seropositive women.

2. There is no role for expectant management when an HIV-positive woman has an abnormal Pap smear result. Perform a colposcopy after a single reading of atypical squamous cell of undetermined significance (ASC-US) or squamous intraepithelial lesion (SIL). During this examination, check the vagina, vulva, and anus for neoplastic changes.

3. Do not assume that treatment is futile for the woman who has both HIV and premalignant or malignant cervical disease. Aggressive treatment of cervical disease will prolong life in most cases.

TECHNICAL ASPECTS OF CYTOLOGICAL SCREENING

High accuracy in cytological screening depends on a good quality cervical sample, appropriately performed slide preparation, and competent cytopathologic interpretation.

- **Timing.** A Pap smear may be performed whenever heavy menstrual bleeding is not present. However, the optimal timing is at midcycle in a woman who has not had intercourse for 24 hours and has not placed any substances in her vagina for at least 48 hours.

- **Sampling.** Moisten the speculum with warm water. Avoid the use of other lubricants because they may cause cell clumping on the slide and interfere with cytological interpretation. Using a large cotton-tipped applicator in a gentle wiping motion, remove excess cervical mucus. The order in which cervical specimens are obtained is critical, in that samples most easily contaminated by blood should be taken early in the sampling sequence. DNA probe and amplification tests (LCR, PCR) for chlamydia and gonorrhea should be performed before the Pap smear. If non-DNA tests are used, take the Pap sample first, collect the sample for gonorrhea culture next, and sample for chlamydia testing last.

- **Slide preparation.** First sample the exocervix by rotating a wooden or plastic spatula 360 degrees around the exocervix. Immediately place the sample on a glass slide, creating a monolayer covering most of the slide's surface. Second, sample the endocervical canal, preferably using a brush sampling device, or if one is not available, a saline-moistened cotton-tipped applicator. Plate this sample directly over the first sample by gently rolling the brush or swab over the surface of the slide, again attempting to achieve a monolayer of material. Fix the sample immediately in order to avoid air drying. Unless specifically requested by the cytopathology laboratory, separate slides are not needed for each sample, nor is segmenting the slide into a section for the exocervical sample and another for the endocervical sample. Sampling of the vaginal pool is not helpful and actually may decrease the quality of the sample by adding degenerating cells and other debris.

CYTOLOGICAL SCREENING INTERVALS

The issue of Pap smear screening intervals has been a contentious one, often resulting in inconsistent practices among providers in various specialty groups. Until recently, most providers followed the 1987 Pap Smear Consensus Statement:

> All women who are or who have been sexually active or who have reached 18 years old (should) have an annual Pap test and pelvic exam. After a woman has had three or more consecutive, satisfactory, normal annual exams, the Pap test may be performed less frequently at the discretion of the physician and the patient.

Consequently, most national women's health care organizations, including ACOG and the U.S. Title X Family Planning Program,[25] recommended Pap smear intervals based upon a woman's risk factors for cervical cancer; that is, high-risk women were screened annually while low-risk women were screened less frequently. However, compelling evidence from mathematical modeling shows that time interval of disease progression and screening error rates are the most important factors in computing screening intervals, and that risk factors for cervical cancer should not be considered, as long as the woman is not immunocompromised.[26] This is biologically plausible, as the presence or absence of behavioral or clinical risk factors does not affect the *rate* at which cervical disease progresses in immunocompetent women.

A growing number of high quality studies support 2 to 3 year Pap screening intervals in all immunocompetent women, regardless of the number or degree of risk factors[27,28] and many industrialized countries, including the United Kingdom, Canada, and Japan, have recommended 3-year Pap screening intervals for decades. However, this represents an important departure from the longstanding U.S. public health recommendation that women receive annual Pap smear screening, and both clinician-initiated discussions and public educational campaigns will be necessary to re-educate consumers regarding the reason for this change.[29] In December 2002, The American Cancer Society (ACS) published its updated cervical cancer screening guidelines[30] (Table 3-1), integrating this important change in philosophy.

Table 3-1 Pap smear screening intervals

	2002 American Cancer Society screening recommendation	Rationale
When to start	• Three years after the onset of vaginal intercourse	• HSIL and cervical cancer are extremely rare within 3 years of sexual debut
	• Start no later than 21 years old, unless reliable history of virginity	• Upper age limit (21) needed for providers who do not take a sexual history or for adolescents unwilling to disclose sexual history
	• Virginal women should be counseled regarding the benefits and risks of screening	• HSIL and cervical cancer are extremely rare in the absence of vaginal intercourse
When to stop	• Women 70 and older with intact cervix and 3 normal Paps within 10 years prior to 70 years old	• Cervical cancer in older women is almost entirely confined to the unscreened and underscreened
		• If sexually active, very low risk of new lesion since little active metaplasia
	• Women with total hysterectomy for benign condition	• Squamous cell cancer of the vagina is extremely rare
		• Abnormal vaginal smears are uncommon and rarely important
Interval	Until age 30:	
	• Conventional smears: annually	• Progression to HSIL may be more rapid in younger women
	• LBC smears: every 2 years	• Greater accuracy of LBC smears permits longer screening interval
	30 years old and older:	
	• If three consecutively normal smears, screen every 2-3 years	• Progression to HSIL may be slower in women over 30 years old
	Screen more often if:	
	• HIV seropositive	• Immunocompromise can hasten
	• Immunocompromised by transplant, chemotherapy, chronic steroid use	progression rate from SIL to cancer
	• DES exposure in utero	• Reduced sensitivity for glandular cancers (DES)

Source: Saslow D, et al. (2002)[30]

The ACS guidelines specify that these recommendations apply to asymptomatic women who are being screened for cervical cancer, while those who are "under surveillance" for prior abnormal Paps or who are in the first year after treatment of a pre-invasive cervical lesion should be followed under other protocols.[31]

PAP SMEAR REPORTING SYSTEMS

In the original Pap smear reporting system, premalignant squamous epithelial changes were referred to as dysplasia, with increasing degrees of involvement of the cervical epithelium graded in severity as mild, moderate, and severe dysplasia; full-thickness epithelial lesions were termed carcinoma-in-situ (CIS). In the 1970s, this terminology was replaced with three categories of cervical intraepithelial neoplasia nomenclature (CIN I, II, and III). Since then, the Bethesda Classification System[32] (TBS) for cervical cytological screening (Table 3-2) has become the international standard for cervical cytopathological reporting. One of the most controversial aspects of TBS was the inclusion of 'HPV atypia' and CIN I in the same category of low-grade squamous intraepithelial lesions (LSIL). Some observers who considered these to be two separate entities feared that placing them in the same category would lead to over-aggressive management of atypia or under-evaluation of potentially high-grade CIN lesions.[33] Convincing evidence, however, shows that HPV atypia and CIN I represent the same entity:[34]

- Virologically, both HPV atypia and CIN I are found to have HPV types 6 and 11, although the lesion also may contain high-risk HPV types.

- Morphologically, the two lesions appear colposcopically as acetowhite epithelium with few or no vascular changes.

- Histologically, the nuclear and cytoplasmic characteristics of the lesions are very similar and commonly are indistinguishable under the microscope.

Finally, and most important, the natural history of the two lesions appears to be the same in that 15% to 20% of untreated lesions progress, while the remainder either regress or remain unchanged for long periods of time.[35,36] CIN II and CIN III were combined into the category of high-grade SIL for similar reasons: the lesions are difficult to differentiate histopathologically, and if they are comparable in size, treatment is the same for the two lesions.

Table 3-2 Comparison of Papanicolaou reporting, CIN classification, and The Bethesda System Classification

Bethesda System	CIN System	Papanicolaou System
Low Grade SIL (LSIL)	Condyloma	Condyloma
	CIN I	Mild dysplasia
High Grade SIL (HSIL)	CIN II	Moderate dysplasia
	CIN II	Severe dysplasia
		CIS

MANAGEMENT OF ABNORMAL PAP SMEAR RESULTS

The classification system recommended by the third Bethesda workshop (the 2001 Bethesda System)[32] contained a number of modifications to include new screening technologies, as well as to remedy points of confusion between pathologists and clinicians. Cervical cytology reports conforming to the 2001 Bethesda System format include comments in each of the following categories, as applicable:

— Specimen type (conventional smear vs. liquid-based vs. other)

— Specimen adequacy (satisfactory or unsatisfactory for evaluation)

— General categorization (Negative, Epithelial cell abnormality, Other)

— Interpretation/ Result (see Table 3-3)

— Automated review and ancillary testing (including HPV reflex results, if done)

— Educational notes and suggestions (optional)

Negative, with Comments Regarding Specimen Adequacy

While the 2001 Bethesda System has eliminated the category of "satisfactory, but limited by. . ." (SBLB), comments regarding suboptimal specimen quality still may be made. The finding that most often limits interpretation is a paucity of endocervical cells. Their presence confirms that in the process of sampling the transformation zone, the active squamocolumnar junction was included. Even with the best of sampling efforts, however, endocervical cells are absent in up to 10% of Pap smears obtained from premenopausal women and as many as 50% from postmenopausal women.[37] In addition, fewer endocervical cells may be present in smears from women who use oral contraceptives or are pregnant. If a negative result is reported, take the next Pap smear at a routine interval. A result that describes inadequate or absent endocervical cells but provides no other general categorization or result must be managed as an unsatisfactory smear (see the next subsection).

The proportion of Pap smears with this reading provides an important opportunity to monitor Pap smear technique. If the percentage of Pap smears with no endocervical cells present exceeds 10% to 15%, remedial action is necessary. If clinician education regarding Pap smear technique and a switch to brush sampling devices does not result in improvement, the laboratory's cytopathologist should be consulted in order to determine whether the problem lies with the laboratory or the provider and to define further steps necessary to rectify the problem.

Table 3-3 2001 Bethesda System interpretation/result categories

Negative for intraepithelial lesion or malignancy	
Organisms	• Trichomonas vaginalis
	• Fungal organisms morphologically consistent with Candida sp.
	• Shift in flora suggestive of BV
	• Bacteria morphologically consistent with Actinomyces sp.
	• Cellular changes consistent with herpes simplex virus
Other non-neoplastic findings	• Reactive cellular changes associated with inflammation, radiation, or intrauterine contraceptive device
	• Glandular cells status post hysterectomy
	• Atrophy

Other	
Endometrial cells	• Endometrial cells, cytologically benign, in a woman ≥40 years of age

Epithelial cell abnormalities	
Squamous cell	• Atypical squamous cells (ASC)
	— of undetermined significance (ASC-US)
	— cannot exclude HSIL (ASC-H)
	• Low-grade SIL (LSIL)
	• High-grade SIL (HSIL)
	• Squamous cell carcinoma
Glandular cell	• Atypical glandular cells (AGC)
	— specify endocervical, endometrial, or glandular cells NOS (not otherwise specified)
	• Atypical glandular cells, favor neoplastic
	— specify endocervical or NOS
	• Endocervical adenocarcinoma in situ (AIS)
	• Adenocarcinoma
	— specify: endocervical, endometrial, extrauterine, or NOS

Unsatisfactory for evaluation. Inadequate sampling, air drying, excessive red or white blood cells, or other factors make interpretation impossible. Because unsatisfactory smears have a greater likelihood of being abnormal,[38] repeat the smear, preferably when the woman is at midcycle and has not had intercourse or used vaginal products for at least 24 hours. Do not repeat the Pap smear earlier than 6 weeks from the previous smear; repetitive sampling over short periods of time may increase the risk of falsely negative smears due to decreased exfoliation of abnormal cells and a greater likelihood of reparative changes. Postmenopausal women with one or more unsatisfactory Pap smears due to vaginal atrophy should apply topical vaginal estrogen cream for 4 to 6 weeks, then receive a repeat Pap smear no earlier than 1 week after completing the medication. Unless a woman has a history of endometrial hyperplasia, progestin withdrawal is not necessary after this short course of estrogen exposure. If the proportion of unsatisfactory smears within a practice is greater than 5%, remedial action in consultation with the cytopathologist is recommended.

Negative for Intraepithelial Lesion or Malignancy: Organisms

Trichomonas vaginalis. While the Pap smear is a relatively insensitive test for the detection of Trichomonas (it detects trichomonads in only about one-half of infected women), its specificity is as high as 98%.[39] When the Pap report indicates presence of Trichomonas, review the woman's medical record to determine whether the infection was recently treated. If it has been, no further action is required. If it has not been treated, offer treatment to avoid horizontal transmission to a new sexual partner and to prevent conversion of asymptomatic Trichomonas colonization into an uncomfortable case of symptomatic vaginal trichomoniasis. The practice of requiring microscopic saline suspension confirmation of trichomonads is illogical because such a relatively insensitive test (about 60%) should not be used to confirm a test with a high positive predictive value. Repeat the Pap smear after the next routine screening interval, unless the narrative report mentions obscuring inflammation and indicates the need to repeat the Pap smear after treatment.

Fungus morphologically consistent with Candida *spp.* In most cases, Candida detected on Pap smear is due to normal vaginal colonization with low levels of Candida, rather than frank vaginal candidiasis. Candida colonization is not dangerous to the affected woman or her sexual partner. Repeat the Pap only if the inflammation due to the candidiasis is of sufficient severity that the cytopathologist recommends that the Pap smear be repeated after treatment is complete.

Shift in flora suggestive of bacterial vaginosis. This reading refers to changes detected in the bacterial flora of the vagina in which the normal Lactobacillus are not abundant but coccobacilli are seen in numbers greater than normal. While this description was devised to suggest the possibility of bacterial vaginosis (BV), it is both an insensitive and nonspecific indicator of BV. The clinical diagnosis of BV is made solely on clinical findings (see Chapter 8 on Reproductive Tract Infections), and neither vaginal culture nor Pap smear findings have any role in the diagnosis of this condition. Management is controversial. Many clinicians feel that no further evaluation is necessary and that the next Pap smear should be performed at the routine interval, while others feel that the woman should be informed that BV is inferred from findings on the smear and be offered clinical evaluation for BV.

Bacteria morphologically consistent with Actinomyces *spp.* *Actinomyces israelii* is an anaerobic bacteria capable of causing a severe pelvic infection, especially in long-term IUD users over 35 years of age. A large majority of IUD wearers with Actinomyces on their Pap smears have asymptomatic cervical colonization (not infection) that does not require antibiotic therapy. Examine IUD users with Actinomyces on their Pap smear to determine whether they have evidence of pelvic infection. If symptoms or physical findings suggest pelvic actinomycosis, remove the IUD and initiate intensive antibiotic therapy. Advise the woman to use another method of contraception. While no definitive evidence supports a particular course of action for patients with asymptomatic Actinomyces colonization, some experts recommend removal of the IUD, followed by insertion of a replacement IUD only after a repeat Pap smear performed 3 months later shows the absence of Actinomyces. (See Chapter 21 on Intrauterine Devices.)

Cellular changes consistent with herpes simplex virus (HSV). Although an insensitive indicator of cervical herpes simplex shedding, the Pap smear is a specific indicator. A confirmatory HSV culture will be wasteful of resources, since viral shedding is intermittent and unpredictable. Advise the infected woman to tell her obstetrical care provider so that precautions may be taken to minimize the risk of vertical transmission to a newborn. Unless inflammation interferes with the interpretation of the Pap smear, the next Pap smear should be performed at the routine interval.

Negative for Intraepithelial Lesion or Malignancy: Other Non-Neoplastic Findings

Reactive cellular changes associated with inflammation. Nonspecific reactive inflammatory changes may be associated with benign metaplasia, mechanical or chemical irritation, post-traumatic repair, chlamydial or gonococcal endocervicitis, trichomoniasis, viral infection, invasive cervical cancer, or other unknown factors. Of these possibilities, the only infectious conditions amenable to antibiotic therapy are gonococcal and chlamydial endocervicitis and vaginal trichomoniasis. Women who recently have been evaluated for these organisms and found to be uninfected do not require further evaluation or antibiotic therapy. Evaluate women who have not been screened recently. Either provide empirical antibiotic treatment for women diagnosed with mucopurulent cervicitis or perform gonorrhea and chlamydia tests and treat women who test positive. Empirically treating women with inflammatory Pap smears with topical antibiotic sulfa creams is of no value in either the treatment of cervical infection or the resolution of abnormal Pap smears and is to be condemned.[40]

Rarely, the only Pap smear finding in a woman with an invasive cervical carcinoma is the persistent finding of inflammation. Although not evidenced-based, some experts recommend that women who have had consecutive Pap smears with unexplained inflammation should be evaluated by colposcopy; others contend that this practice is unnecessary because of the extremely low likelihood of detecting a cervical cancer in this circumstance.

Cytological changes associated with the use of an IUD detected on Pap smear are of a benign nature and do not require further investigation.

Atrophy. Atrophy is most common in postmenopausal women or those with estrogen-deficiency states. Treatment of the vaginal atrophy is indicated only if the woman has symptomatic atrophic vaginitis; it is not necessary for the asymptomatic woman. Pap smear screening intervals do not need to be modified, and the woman does not need to be notified.

Other

Endometrial cells, cytologically benign, in a woman ≥40 years of age. Endometrial cells found on Pap smear are an insignificant finding in premenopausal women with normal ovulatory cycling. However, because the endometrium normally is atrophic in postmenopausal women, the finding of endometrial cells may be the result of exfoliation from a focus of endometrial hyperplasia or adenocarcinoma. For this reason, consider the finding of endometrial cells in a postmenopausal woman as a danger sign and sample the endometrium. Because a premenopausal woman with chronic anovulation also is at risk for endometrial hyperplasia, manage the finding of endometrial cells in the same way.

Epithelial Cell Abnormalities: Squamous Cell

Atypical squamous cells of undetermined significance (ASC-US). The ASC category refers to the finding of cells with nuclear atypia that are not normal, yet not diagnostic of SIL. The large majority of ASC-US smears are due to benign HPV infections, although 2.5% of women over 40 years old and 11% under 40 years old with this reading have HSIL, and very rarely, invasive cancer.[41] Because of confusion regarding the meaning of the ASC reading, the 2001 Bethesda System encourages the cytopathologist to further qualify the reading as either ASC-undetermined significance (ASC-US) and ASC-cannot exclude HSIL (ASC-H). ASC-US refers to findings that suggest LSIL, but not meeting criteria, and ASC-H is suggestive of HSIL, but which lack criteria for definitive interpretation.

The ASCCP 2001 Consensus Guidelines[42,43] describe three acceptable options for the management of women with ASC-US results: perform colposcopy, follow with a shorter Pap screening interval, or use HPV typing to differentiate women who are at high risk for having, or progressing to, HSIL (also called intermediary triage).

1. *Immediate colposcopy.* There are a number of advantages to colposcopic evaluation in the management of ASC-US: it represents the "gold standard" for high sensitivity; it often provides an immediate answer regarding the condition of the cervix, permitting reassurance if normal; and it minimizes the risk of loss to follow up. However, the drawbacks to this approach include the fact that most women either will have normal colposcopy or a low-grade lesion destined to resolve quickly; there may be an increased physical and psychological burden owing to colposcopy; and it is associated with high cost in fee-for-service environments.

This option is most reasonable if there is high availability of colposcopic services without additional costs to the patient or health care system, as in some managed care delivery systems.

If colposcopy shows no CIN or cancer, women with unknown or negative HPV results should have a repeat smear in 1 year. If a HPV test is positive for high-risk virus, either cytology can be repeated at 6 and 12 months or an HPV test can be repeated in 1 year. If at follow-up a Pap smear result of ASC or worse occurs, or if the repeat HPV test is positive, colposcopy should be repeated. Those with negative smears or negative HPV testing can return to routine screening intervals.

2. *Repeat cytology with shorter screening intervals.* In this option, cytosmears are repeated twice at 4- to 6-month intervals. If both smears are negative, colposcopy is unnecessary and the woman can return to routine screening intervals. Alternatively, if either smear shows ASC or worse, the woman should undergo colposcopy and managed as described above.

   The advantages of this approach are that it may reduce unnecessary colposcopic procedures and it permits follow-up visits at a clinical site where colposcopy is not available. Arguments against this approach include the potential for loss to follow up which increases with more visits required, as well as the fact that multiple follow-up Pap visits may burden some clinics.

3. *Intermediary triage with HPV testing.* The third option for triage of ASC-US results is to perform reflex HPV testing (for high-risk viral types only) on the stored material contained in liquid-based cytology media. In a large study performed by Kaiser Permanente in Northern California,[44] this regimen resulted in both a high pick-up rate of HSIL and the avoidance of colposcopy in over 50% of the women with ASC-US. With this approach, women with ASC-US who test positive for high-risk HPV should undergo colposcopy, while women who are HPV negative are advised to repeat cytology in 1 year. This approach is not cost-effective for women with ASC-US findings on conventionally performed Pap smears, owing to the necessity of an extra visit for HPV testing.

   Post-menopausal women with an ASC-US result can be managed either with immediate colposcopy, reflex HPV testing, or because of the possibility of epithelial atrophy, given intravaginal estrogen therapy for 4 to 6 weeks, followed by repeat cytology 1 week after completion of treatment. If the repeat smear shows ASC or worse, she should undergo colposcopy, but if negative, cytology should be repeated once more in 4 to 6 months.

ASC-H. Because 24% to 94% of women with ASC-H will have SIL, colposcopic management is recommended. If no lesion is identified, follow-up includes either cytology at 6 and 12 months or HPV testing in

1 year. If at follow-up a Pap smear result of ASC or worse occurs, or if the repeat HPV test is positive, colposcopy should be repeated. Those with negative smears or negative HPV testing can return to routine screening intervals. ASC-H readings should account for 5% to 10% of all ASC results.

Low-grade SIL. Most women with LSIL should undergo colposcopic evaluation, owing to the 10% to 17% risk of an underlying HSIL. If no lesion is seen at colposcopy, surveillance consists of either performing Pap smears at 6 and 12 months or high-risk HPV DNA testing at 12 months. If at follow-up a Pap smear result of ASC or worse occurs, or if the repeat HPV test is positive, colposcopy should be repeated. Those with negative smears or negative HPV testing can return to routine screening intervals. Adolescents with LSIL are more likely to have acute HPV infections that resolve without treatment. Options for adolescents with LSIL on Pap smear include immediate colposcopy, repeat cytology 6 and 12 months after the index Pap, or HPV DNA testing in 1 year.

Post-menopausal women with LSIL can be managed with repeat cytology 6 and 12 months after the index Pap smear, HPV DNA testing in one year, or intravaginal estrogen therapy if there is cytological evidence of atrophy and no contraindication to estrogen. The Pap smear should be repeated one week after completion of therapy, and if negative, again in 4 to 6 months. If at follow-up a Pap smear result of ASC or worse occurs, or if the HPV test is positive, colposcopy should be done. Those with negative smears or negative HPV testing can return to routine screening intervals.

High-grade SIL. Refer women with HSIL for colposcopic evaluation, even if the Pap smear was obtained during pregnancy, a benign Pap smear has been obtained since the SIL reading, or no visible cervical lesion is present. A comprehensive list of indications for colposcopy is included in Table 3-4.

Refer women with Pap smear results reporting squamous cell or adenocarcinoma of the cervix for immediate expert consultation with a physician experienced in the management of gynecologic cancers.

Table 3-4 Indications for colposcopy

- Papanicolaou (Pap) smear showing HSIL or ASC-H
- Pap smear showing atypical glandular cells (AGC)
- Pap smear showing ASC-US or LSIL:
  - Women who are unlikely or unwilling to return for frequent follow-up
  - Women not entering HPV testing or repeat cytology management pathways
  - Finding of ASC or worse on Pap smear performed during observation period
  - High-risk HPV DNA present at initial or subsequent testing
- Cervical leukoplakia (white lesion visible to the naked eye without the application of acetic acid) or other unexplained cervical lesion, regardless of Pap smear result
- Unexplained or persistent cervical bleeding, regardless of Pap smear result

Epithelial Cell Abnormalities: Glandular Cell

Atypical glandular cells (AGC). AGC may result from HPV infection of glandular cells, adenocarcinoma-in-situ (AIS), adenocarcinoma, or in some cases, a SIL lesion. Because adenocarcinomas of the cervix are associated with a rate of false-negative Pap smears as high as 40%,[45] women with AGC require aggressive evaluation in order to exclude a cancer diagnosis. There is no role for observation (repeat Pap smear) in this situation. Management of AGC consists of colposcopic evaluation of the exocervix and thorough endocervical curettage. If atypical endometrial cells are reported, or if the patient is older than 35 years old or has abnormal vaginal bleeding, the endometrium should be sampled as well. If the initial Pap smear result was AGC-NOS (not otherwise specified) and no neoplasia is found at colposcopy, four Pap smears should be repeated at 4 to 6 month intervals. If any of the follow-up Pap smears return as HSIL or AGC, a diagnostic excisional procedure (such as LEEP cone or 'cold knife' cone) is necessary. If any of the Pap smears return as LSIL or ASC, a repeat colposcopy is indicated. If the initial Pap smear result was AGC favor neoplastic, or AIS, and no lesion is found at colposcopy, a diagnostic excisional procedure is recommended to exclude an occult cancer.

TREATMENT OF SQUAMOUS INTRAEPITHELIAL LESIONS

Since the early 1990s, management protocols have become much more conservative, due to the recognition that most LSIL lesions will regress without treatment, rather than progress to higher-grade lesions or cancer. Once a diagnosis of CIN I (LSIL) is made in a patient with a fully visible cervical lesion, she should be followed until there is evidence of HSIL or persistence of LSIL over the period of 1 year. The preferred approach to follow-up is either cytology alone at 6 and 12 months or HPV DNA test* at 12 months, although an acceptable alternative is colposcopy cytology at 12 months. If any of these alternatives is chosen, h provider and the patient must be diligent with follow-up. Alte the patient is uncomfortable with being observed and reque or if she is a poor follow-up risk, immediate treatment choice.

Typical papillary condyloma accuminata of the cally proven by cervical biopsy, should be trea* This aggressive approach decreases the amo which will reduce receptivity to HIV infec of viral transmission to a partner. Cry most inexpensive treatment modalit ations may require the use of LEEP topical 5-fluorouracil (FU), or i condyloma and SIL is considere mended.

54

There is universal agreement that high-grade SIL must be treated, because the risk of progression to cervical cancer is both more likely and more immediate. Consensus guidelines for the management of CIN lesions have been published by the American Society for Colposcopy and Cervical Pathology.[46]

OVARIAN CANCER SCREENING

In the United States in 2003, about 24,500 women were diagnosed with ovarian cancer, making this cancer the fifth most common among American women. However, because of the low 5-year survival rates with this disease, especially in the later stages when it is more commonly diagnosed, it is the leading cause (53%) of gynecologic cancer deaths, accounting for 14,300 deaths in the United States. The average age at diagnosis is 60 years. A woman's lifetime risk of ovarian cancer is about 1 in 70.

Although some risk factors for ovarian cancer are well known, a majority of women diagnosed with this condition have none.[47] Geographic differences are marked; rates in Sweden and the United States are 13 to 15 cases per 100,000 women per year, while the rate in Japan is 3 cases per 100,000 women per year. This difference in part may be related to dietary fat intake, which is higher in the United States and Scandinavia and lower in Japan. A long interval of ovulatory cycles also is associated with ovarian cancer, and low parity, delayed childbearing, and infertility are weak risk factors. Familial predisposition accounts for 5% to 10% of cases, and the risk of ovarian cancer is 5% if one first-degree relative had ovarian cancer and 7% if two or more first-degree relatives had the condition. A site-specific familial ovarian cancer syndrome also has been described, which is mediated through a highly penetrant autosomal dominant gene; in these cases, the risk to a first-degree relative is up to 50%. In addition, women with BRCA-1 and BRCA-2 mutations are at greater risk of both ovarian and breast cancer. Because there is no accurate method to detect early ovarian cancer in these high-risk women, some experts recommend prophylactic oophorectomy for women who have two or more first degree relatives with ovarian cancer and who have completed childbearing.[48]

Inversely, oral contraceptive use reduces the risk of ovarian cancer by much as 80% in women age 40 to 59 years. Not only does longer of use provide more protection, but the effect lasts for as long as after oral contraceptives are discontinued.[49] There is a decreased ovarian cancer in women who are chronic anovulators (also called cystic ovary syndrome); protection also is seen with increasing greater duration of lactation. Contraceptive sterilization is with a 40% to 50% reduction in the risk of ovarian cancer, and (without oophorectomy) with a 35% reduction.

OVARIAN CANCER SCREENING TECHNIQUES

Ovarian cancer typically is diagnosed during an evaluation of a symptomatic woman, but may be detected as a mass found incidentally during pelvic examination or ultrasound. While early ovarian cancer has been long considered a "silent cancer," a recent study showed that 70% of women recalled having symptoms for 3 months or longer before their diagnosis. Ovarian cancer can be associated with pelvic pain, abdominal discomfort and distention, bloating after meals, indigestion, constipation, nausea, urinary frequency, and irregular vaginal bleeding. In advanced stages, ovarian cancer is often accompanied by fatigue, non-specific gastrointestinal symptoms, poor appetite and weight loss, increased abdominal girth, or shortness of breath due to pleural effusion. Currently, it appears that the best way to promptly diagnose ovarian cancer is for both the patient and her clinician to have a high index of suspicion when characteristic symptoms occur.[50]

A number of techniques have been suggested to screen for the early stages of asymptomatic ovarian cancer: periodic bimanual pelvic examination, serum CA-125 measurement, and transvaginal ultrasound examination. Conducting a bimanual pelvic examination as part of periodic health examination is inexpensive and safe and may provide valuable information, but it is insensitive and has not been found to be cost-effective when the visit and examination are done for the sole purpose of ovarian cancer screening. Screening with the serum tumor marker CA-125 will detect up to 80% of women with advanced non-mucinous ovarian cancers, but the test is only 50% to 70% sensitive for early-stage cancers and has poor specificity (many false positives), which may lead to unnecessary invasive and costly workups. Screening with this test is not cost-effective because of the low prevalence of ovarian cancer and the test's moderate sensitivity, poor specificity, and high cost. Vaginal-probe pelvic ultrasound also has been suggested as a screening test because of its high sensitivity (98%), but it has poor specificity and the highest cost of any of the screening modalities. While there is general agreement that asymptomatic low-risk women should not be screened routinely with any of these interventions, either alone or in combination, many experts believe that they should be offered annually to women who have familial risk factors for ovarian cancer, starting at 25 to 30 years old. The current USPSTF guidelines make the following recommendations regarding ovarian cancer screening:[2]

- Screening asymptomatic women for ovarian cancer with ultrasound, tumor markers, or physical exam is not recommended. [D recommendation]

- There is insufficient evidence to recommend for or against testing in asymptomatic women at increased risk of ovarian cancer. [I recommendation]

BREAST CANCER SCREENING

In 2003, breast cancer was the second leading cause of cancer deaths in women in the United States, accounting for one-third of all cancer cases and 15% of cancer deaths in women (40,000 deaths per year). Incidence rates of breast cancer have increased 1% per year since 1973, although mortality rates have remained stable. A woman's lifetime risk of breast cancer, assuming she lives to old age, is about 1 in 9. Risk factors are helpful indicators of risk, but do not predict the development of breast cancer in the majority of cases. Of women with breast cancer, 21% of women age 30 to 54 years have risk factor(s), as do 29% of women between 55 and 84 years old (Table 3-5).[51]

BREAST CANCER SCREENING TECHNIQUES

Breast self-examination (BSE). The longstanding recommendation that all adult women practice monthly BSE is now being questioned.[53] Although BSE may provide women with a sense of empowerment and occasionally may result in earlier detection of a breast mass than might occur by coincidence, two very large randomized clinical trials have shown that breast cancer survival is no greater in women who practice BSE than in those who do not. The larger study, involving 266,000 women in Shanghai, China, concluded that BSE actually may cause more hazard than benefit, owing to the many false positives that result from BSE.[54] From a public health standpoint, these studies suggest that financial and educational resources should not be used to implement population-based BSE programs. For individual women, the message in these studies is that a formal, timed regimen of BSE is no more effective in preventing death from breast cancer than the incidental discovery of unusual breast changes. Nonetheless, women still should be counseled to take note of changes in their breasts, and when they occur, to bring the finding to the attention of their clinician.

For women who continue to practice BSE, the optimal time for performing BSE is 1 to 7 days after the end of the menses. Performing the exam after a shower, while the skin still is wet, may improve accuracy. After inspecting her breasts while she is sitting or standing in front of a mirror, the woman should palpate each breast in turn, with her hand on the side of the breast being examined placed behind her head. The objective of BSE is to detect a significant change in the breasts from one month to the next, not necessarily the finding of a dominant nodule.

Clinical Breast Examination (CBE). While most consensus guidelines include CBE as a component of the periodic health examination in adult women, there is disagreement regarding age of initiation and frequency of screening. The USPSTF states that evidence is insufficient to recommend CBE alone (without mammography), while the American Cancer Society recommends that CBE should be performed at least every 3 years from 20 to 39 years old and annually thereafter. CBE is not a highly

Table 3-5 Risk characteristics of breast cancer

Factor	High-Risk Group	Low-Risk Group
Relative risk >4.0		
Age	Old	Young
Country of birth	North America, Northern Europe	Asia, Africa
Two first-degree relatives with breast cancer diagnosed at an early age	Yes	No
History of cancer in one breast	Yes	No
Relative risk = 2.1-4.0		
Nodular densities on mammogram (postmenopausal)	Densities occupy >75% of breast volume	Parenchyma composed entirely of fat
One first-degree relative with breast cancer	Yes	No
Biopsy-confirmed atypical hyperplasia	Yes	No
High-dose radiation to chest	Yes	No
Oophorectomy before age 35	No	Yes
Relative risk = 1.1-2.0		
Socioeconomic status	High	Low
Place of residence	Urban	Rural
Race/ethnicity		
—Breast cancer at ≥40 years	Caucasian	Asian
—Breast cancer at < 40 years	Black	Asian
Religion	Jewish	Adventist, Mormon
Age at first full-term pregnancy	≥ 30 years	< 20 years
Age at menarche	< 12 years	> 14 years
Age at menopause	> 55 years	< 45 years
Obesity (postmenopausal)	Obese	Slender
Breastfeeding	None	Several years
Hormonal contraceptives —Breast cancer < 45 years	Yes	No
Hormone replacement therapy > 10 years	Yes	No
Height	Tall	Short
History of primary cancer in endometrium, ovary, or colon	Yes	No
Alcohol consumption	Yes	No

Source: Hulka BS, et al. (1995).[52]

accurate screening test, having a sensitivity of only 54% and a false positive rate of 6%. However, one benefit of CBE is that about 5% to 15% of breast cancers missed on mammography are found on CBE, the combination thereby improving detection rates. Consequently, it is reasonable to offer CBE to all women starting as early as 20, but no later than 40 years old, as it is safe, non-invasive, and adds little extra time to the periodic health examination.

When performing CBE,[55] examine the breasts while the woman is sitting with her hands on her hips or behind her head. Repeat the exam while the woman is lying down. Examine each breast in vertical strips. Palpate with flat portion of your fingers rather than your fingertips. If a woman has very pendulous breasts, place your hand between her breast and chest wall, then palpate tissue between your hands. Be sure to include the axillary tail of the breast in the examination. Lymph node examination of the supraclavicular and axillary nodes is an integral component of the examination. Draw a diagram in the medical record indicating the position and size of abnormalities, noting that dominant nodules have measurable dimensions, while fibrocystic change does not.

Mammography

When used as a screening test, the purpose of mammography is to detect pre-clinical breast cancer before a mass can be palpated clinically. Large-scale studies show that in women who receive at least biennial mammograms over a 10-year period, breast cancer mortality is reduced by an average of 24%, with an even greater reduction in women over 50 to 69 years old. The accuracy of mammography as a screening test has improved over the last two decades, resulting in a false-negative rate of 5% to 15% and a false-positive rate of 3% to 6%.

The USPSTF recommends screening mammography every 1 to 2 years for women aged 40 and older,[56] while the American Cancer Society recommends annual mammography beginning at age 40.[57] Both guidelines are in agreement that women 40 to 49 years of age who choose to have screening mammograms should do so annually, given that breast cancer grows more rapidly among younger women and mammograms are more likely to be falsely negative in this age group. However, the benefit of mammography in younger women must be balanced against a lower prevalence of breast cancer among women in their 40s, as well as a higher rate of false positive mammograms because of a greater breast density and a higher likelihood of benign breast conditions.[58–60]

For women 50 and older, USPSTF guidelines state there is no advantage of annual over biennial (every other year) screening, because in older women breast cancers grow more slowly than in younger women.[56] Additionally, mammography has a lower false negative rate in post-menopausal women, since tumors more are surrounded by fatty tissue and therefore are more detectable. ACS guidelines recommend that women under 40 years of age who have increased risk for breast cancer might benefit from additional screening strategies, including initiation of mammographic screening at 30 years old, shorter screening intervals, and the addition of ultrasound or MRI screening.

When used as a diagnostic test in a woman with a breast abnormality, mammography can suggest malignancy at the location of the finding and exclude malignancy elsewhere in the same or opposite breast. In the presence of a dominant breast nodule, a negative diagnostic mammogram does not exclude the diagnosis of breast cancer. In this case, tissue sampling, either by fine-needle aspiration cytology or open biopsy, is the only definitive procedure to exclude cancer.

REFERENCES

1. American Medical Association. Periodic health examination: a manual for physicians. Chicago: American Medical Association, 1940.
2. U.S. Preventive Services Task Force. Guide to clinical preventive services: report of the United States Preventive Services Task Force (2nd edition) Baltimore MD: Williams & Wilkins, 1996.
3. Stewart FH, Harper CC, Ellertson CE, Grimes DA, Sawaya GF, Trussell J. Clinical breast and pelvic examination requirements for hormonal contraception: Current practice vs evidence. JAMA 2001;285(17):2232-9.
4. Grimes DA. Over-the-counter oral contraceptives—an immodest proposal? [editorial]. Am J Public Health 1993;83:1092-1094.
5. Trussell J, Stewart F, Potts M, Guest F, Ellertson C. Should oral contraceptives be available without prescription? Am J Public Health 1993;83:1094-1099.
6. Koss LG. The Papanicolaou test for cervical cancer detection. A triumph and a tragedy. JAMA 1989;261:737-743.
7. Harlan LC, Bernstein AB, Kessler LG. Cervical cancer screening: who is not screened and why? Am J Public Health 1991;81:885-891.
8. Kristensen GB, Skyggebjerg KD, Holund B, et. al. Analysis of cervical smears obtained within 3 years of the diagnosis of invasive cervical cancer. Acta Cytol 1991;35: 47-50.
9. Hessling JJ, et. al. Effectiveness of thin-layer preparations vs. conventional Pap smears in a blinded split-sample study. Extended cytologic evaluation. J Repro Med 2001;46:880-886.
10. Wertlake P. Results of AutoPap system-assisted and manual cytologic screen comparison. J Reprod Med 1999;44:11-17.
11. Hutchinson ML. Assessing the costs and benefits of alternative rescreening strategies [editorial]. Acta Cytol 1996;40-48.
12. Sawaya GF, Grimes DA. New technologies in cervical cytology screening: A word of caution. Obstet Gynecol 1999; 94:304-307.
13. Gross G, Ikenberg H, Gissman L, Hagedorn M. Papillomavirus infection of the anogenital region: correlation between histology, clinical picture and virus type. A proposal of a new nomenclature. J Invest Dermatol 1985;85:147-152.
14. Brinton LA, Schairer C, Haenszel W, Stolley P, Lehman HF, Levine R, Savitz DA. Cigarette smoking and invasive cervical cancer. JAMA 1986;225(23):3265-3269.
15. Winkelstein W, Jr. Smoking and cervical cancer—current status: a review. Am J Epidemiol 1990;131:945-957.
16. Ho, GY et. al. Natural history of cervicovaginal HPV in young women. NEJM 1998;338:423.
17. Moscicki, et. al. The Natural History of HPV Infection as Measured by Repeated DNA Testing in Adolescent and Young Women. J Pediatrics 1998;132:277.
18. Centers for Disease Control and Prevention. Sexually transmitted diseases treatment guidelines 2002. Centers for Disease Control and Prevention. MMWR Recomm Rep. 2002 May 10;51(RR-6):1-78.

19. Centers for Disease Control. Black-white differences in cervical cancer mortality— United States, 1980-1987. MMWR 1990;39:245-248.
20. Korn AP, Landers DV. Gynecologic disease in women infected with human immunodeficiency virus type 1. J Acq Immune Defic Syndr Hum Retrovirol 1995;9:361-370.
21. Korn AP, Autry M, DeRemer PA, Tan W. Sensitivity of the Papanicolaou smear in HIV-infected women. Obstet Gynecol 1994;83:401-404.
22. Adachi A, Fleming I, Burk RD, Ho GY, Klein RS. Women with human immunodeficiency virus infection and abnormal Papanicolaou smears, a prospective study of colposcopy and clinical outcome. Obstet Gynecol 1993;81:372-377.
23. Wright TC, Koulos J, Schnoll F, Swanbeck J, Ellerbrock T, Chaisson M, Richart RM. Cervical intraepithelial neoplasia in women infected with the human immunodeficiency virus: outcome after loop electrosurgical excision. Gynecol Oncol 1994;55:253-258.
24. Centers for Disease Control. 1993 revised classification system for HIV infection and expanded surveillance case definition for AIDS among adolescents and adults. MMWR 1992;41(RR-17):1-19.
25. U.S. Department of Health and Human Services. Improving the quality of clinician Pap smear technique and management, client Pap smear education, and the evaluation of Pap smear laboratory testing: a resource guide for Title X family planning projects. Washington DC: U.S. Department of Health and Human Services, Public Health Service, Office of Population Affairs, Office of Family Planning, 1989:3-4, 59.
26. Frame PS, Frame JS. Determinants of cancer screening frequency: the example of screening for cervical cancer. J Am Board Fam Pract 1998 Mar-Apr;11(2):87-95.
27. Eddy DM. Screening for cervical cancer. Ann Intern Med 1990 Aug 1;113(3):214-226.
28. Sawaya GF, Kerlikowske K, Lee NC, Gildengorin G, Washington AE. Frequency of cervical smear abnormalities within 3 years of normal cytology. Obstet Gynecol 2000;96(2):219-223.
29. Rolnick SJ, LaFerla JJ, Jackson J, Akkerman D, Compo R. Impact of a new cervical Pap smear screening guideline on member perceptions and comfort levels. Prev Med 1999 May;28(5):530-534.
30. Saslow D, Roncowicz CD, et al. American Cancer Society Guideline for the Detection of Cervical Neoplasia and Cancer. CA Cancer J Clin 2002;52:342-362.
31. American Society for Colposcopy and Cervical Pathology. Algorithms from the consensus guidelines for the management of women with cervical cytological abnormalities, 2002. Accessed at: http://www.asccp.org/consensus/cytological.shtml.
32. Solomon D, Davey D, et al. The 2001 Bethesda System: terminology for reporting results of cervical cytology. JAMA 2002:287:2114-2119.
33. Herbst AL. The Bethesda System for cervical/vaginal cytologic diagnosis: a note of caution [editorial]. Obstet Gynecol 1990;76:4049-4050.
34. Kurman RJ, Malkasian GD, Sedlis A, Solomon D. From Papanicolaou to Bethesda: the rationale for a new cervical cytologic classification. Obstet Gynecol 1991;77:779-782.
35. Montz FJ, Monk BJ, Fowler JM, Nguyen L. Natural history of the minimally abnormal Papanicolaou smear. Obstet Gynecol 1992;80:385-388.
36. Nasiell K, Roger V, Nasiell M. Behavior of mild cervical dysplasia during long term follow-up. Obstet Gynecol 1986;67:665-669.
37. Kivlahan C, Ingram E. Papanicolaou smears without endovervical cells. Are they inadequate? Acta Cytol 1986;30:258-260.
38. Ransdell JS, Davey DD, Zalesky S. Clinicopathologic correlation of the unsatisfactory Papanicolaou smear. Cancer 1997;81:139-143.
39. Krieger JN, Tam MR, Stevens CE, et al. Diagnosis of trichomoniasis: comparison of conventional wet mount examination with cytologic studies, cultures, and monoclonal antibody staining of direct specimens. JAMA 1988;259:1223-1227.
40. Reiter RC. Management of initial atypical cervical cytology: a randomized, prospective study. Obstet Gynecol 1986;68:237-240.

41. Kinney WK, Manos MM, Hurley LB, et. al. Where's the high grade cervical neoplasia? The importance of minimally abnormal Papanicolaou diagnoses. Obstet Gynecol 1998;91:973-976.
42. American Society for Colposcopy and Cervical Pathology. Algorithms from the consensus guidelines for the management of women with histological abnormalities, 2003. Accessed at: http://www.asccp.org/consensus/histological.shtml.
43. Wright TC, Cox JT, et al. 2001 Consensus guidelines for the management of women with cervical cytological abnormalities. JAMA 2002;287:2120-2129.
44. Manos, MM, Identifying women with cervical neoplasia using HPV testing for equivocal results. JAMA 1999;281:1605.
45. Hurt WG, Silverberg SG, Frable WJ, Belgrad R, Crooks LD. Adenocarcinoma of the cervix: histopathologic and clinical features. Am J Obstet Gynecol 1977;129:304-315.
46. Wright TC, Cox JT, et al. 2001 consensus guidelines for the management of women with cervical intraepithelial neoplasia. Am J Obstet Gynecol 2003:189:295-304.
47. Whittemore AS, Harris R, Itnyre J. Characteristics relating to ovarian cancer risk. Collaborative analysis of 12 US case-control studies. II. Invasive epithelial ovarian cancers in white women. Am J Epidemiol 1992;136:1184-1203.
48. National Institute of Health Consensus Development Panel on Ovarian Cancer, NIH consensus conference. Ovarian cancer. Screening, treatment, and follow up. JAMA 1995;273:491-497.
49. Rosenberg L, Palmer JR, Zauber AG. A case control study of oral contraceptive use and invasive epithelial ovarian cancer. Am J Epidemiol 1994;139:654-661.
50. American College of Obstetricians and Gynecologists Committee on Gynecologic Practice. The Role of the Generalist Obstetrician-Gynecologist in the Early Detection of Ovarian Cancer. ACOG Committee Opinion number 280. Obstst Gynecol 2002;100:1413-1415.
51. Hoskins KF, Stopfer JE, Calzone KA, et. al. Assessment and counseling for women with a family history of breast cancer: a guide for clinicians. JAMA 1995;273:577-585.
52. Hulka, BS, Stark AT. Breast cancer: cause and prevention. Lancet 1995;346:883-887.
53. Ellman R, Moss SM, Coleman D, et al. Breast self-examination programmes in the trial of early detection of breast cancer: ten year findings. Br J Cancer 1993;65:208.
54. Thomas DB, Gao DL, Self SG, et al. Randomized trial of breast self-examination in Shanghai. Final Results. J Natl Cancer Inst 2002;94:1445-1457.
55. Barton MB, Harris R, Fletcher S. Does this patient have breast cancer? The screening clinical breast exam: should it be done? How? JAMA 1999;282:1270.
56. U.S. Preventive Services Taskforce. Screening for Breast Cancer; 2002 Release. Accessed at http://www.ahcpr.gov/clinic/uspstf/uspsbrca.htm.
57. Smith RA, Saslow D, et al. American Cancer Society guidelines for breast cancer screening: Update 2003. CA Cancer J Clin 2003;54:141-169.
58. Esserman L, Kerlikowski K. Should we recommend screening mammography to women aged 40-49? Oncology 1996; 10:357-364.
59. Kerlikowski K, Grady D, Barclay J, Sickles E, Ernster V. Effect of age, breast density, and family history on the sensitivity of first screening mammography. JAMA 1996;276:33-38.
60. Sox H. Screening mammography in women younger than 50 years of age. Ann Intern Med 1995; 122:550-552.

The Menstrual Cycle

Robert A. Hatcher, MD, MPH
Anne Brawner Namnoum, MD

- Normal ovulatory cycles require the integration of hormones and peptides from the hypothalamus, pituitary gland, and ovaries. When a woman's cycles are irregular, it is usually due to differences in the length of the follicular phase of the cycle.

- The perfect 28-day cycle is the most common pattern, but it occurred in only 12.4% of more than 30,000 cycles recorded by 650 women.[1]

- Hormonal contraceptives have many desirable effects on the cyclic symptoms women experience during their menstrual cycles.

A thorough understanding of the menstrual cycle is fundamental to the discussion of contraception. The ovaries are the source of oocytes (eggs) as well as the hormones that regulate female reproduction. In contrast to the male reproductive system where large numbers of gametes are produced continuously, in women only one gamete is released each month from the time of menarche to the time of menopause. During each monthly interval, or menstrual cycle, a series of events occur that culminates in ovulation and the preparation of the endometrium for implantation of an embryo. The corpus luteum begins to atrophy 9 to 11 days after ovulation if pregnancy does not occur. Shortly thereafter the process of oocyte maturation and endometrial preparation begins anew. Under complex regulation by the hypothalamus, the pituitary gland, and the ovaries, cyclic changes in gonadotropins and steroid hormones induce the development of a dominant follicle, resulting in ovulation and corpus luteum formation.[2] Responding to the cyclic changes in ovarian steroids, the endometrium prepares for implantation should fertilization occur. If pregnancy does not occur, the endometrium sloughs, resulting in menstrual bleeding.

Most women have cycles lasting from 24 to 35 days. Only 0.5% of cycles are shorter than 21 days and 0.9% of cycles are longer than 35 days. At least 20% of women experience irregular cycles.[3] The normal ovulatory menstrual cycle can be divided into four functional phases: follicular (pre-ovulatory), ovulatory, luteal, and menstrual.

MENSTRUAL CYCLE REGULATION
HYPOTHALAMUS AND ANTERIOR PITUITARY

Gonadotropin-releasing hormone (GnRH), a neurohormone synthesized in the hypothalamus, travels via the portal circulation to the anterior pituitary gland. GnRH is secreted in a pulsatile fashion every 60 to 90 minutes, stimulating cells in the anterior pituitary (gonadotropes) to produce follicle-stimulating hormone (FSH) and luteinizing hormone (LH).[4,5] FSH and LH are secreted in a pulsatile manner in response to GnRH pulses. The pulse frequency varies, depending on the phase of the menstrual cycle. FSH plays a dominant role in the promotion of ovarian follicular growth by causing the granulosa cells that line each follicle to proliferate and produce estrogen. LH stimulates androgen production in theca cells adjacent to the granulosa cells. These androgens are the substrates for estrogen production. LH also promotes ovulation and final oocyte maturation and converts estrogen-secreting granulosa cells to progesterone-secreting cells after ovulation.

STEROID PRODUCTION IN THE OVARIES

Together, theca cells and granulosa cells synthesize steroid hormones. According to the two-cell, two-gonadatrophin theory, at the beginning of an ovulatory cycle the outer theca cells can only be stimulated by luteinizing hormone (LH) and the inner granulosa cells can only be stimulated by follicle stimulating hormone (FSH). Theca cells respond to LH by producing the androgens testosterone and androstenedione. These androgens diffuse from the theca cells across the basement membrane of the follicle into granulosa cells, where they are converted to estrogens by the enzyme aromatase. Theca cells have little intrinsic aromatase activity, and granulosa cells are relatively deficient in the enzymes necessary to synthesize androgens; thus the two cell types depend on each other to produce estrogen in the developing follicle. Androgens are critical to follicular development because they are the precursors of estrogens, but if androgens exist in excess amounts, they induce follicular atresia. At low levels, androgens in granulosa cells have two effects: they are the substrate for conversion into estrogen, and they stimulate aromatase activity. Androgen production therefore must be delicately balanced to allow for normal ovarian function.

Moderate levels of estrogen produced by the follicles act on both the hypothalamus and the anterior pituitary to inhibit FSH and LH secretion in a classic negative feedback effect.[6] Progesterone and androgens have a negative feedback effect as well, but theirs is not as prominent as that of estrogen. Paradoxically, higher levels of estrogen have a positive feedback effect on gonadotropin secretion during the middle of a cycle, which initiates the preovulatory surge of LH and FSH.[3] When levels of estradiol in the range of 200 to 300 picograms/milliliter (ml) are present for 2 to 3 days, a gonadotropin surge is elicited. Low levels of progesterone produced before ovulation amplify this positive estrogen feedback effect. The pituitary is the major site of such estradiol action, but there may be a hypothalamic site of action as well. This positive feedback effect of estrogen is critical for ovulation and regular menstrual cycles.

PEPTIDE HORMONES IN THE OVARIES

A variety of peptide hormones produced in the ovary help modulate follicular development and steroid production. One of the more important of these substances is inhibin, a protein composed of alpha and beta subunits. Synthesized in granulosa and theca cells, inhibin suppresses FSH secretion.[7] Activin, composed of two of the beta subunits of inhibin, has the opposite effect and enhances FSH secretion. Ovarian follicular fluid contains more inhibin than activin, thus inhibin from the dominant follicle has a negative feedback effect on FSH secretion. Inhibin and activin also act directly within the ovary to regulate androgen and estrogen production. A third peptide, follistatin, also suppresses FSH, probably by binding activin.

Insulin and insulin-like growth factors also seem to play a significant role as regulators within the ovary. Insulin-like growth factor 1 (IGF-1) stimulates cell division and growth in many tissues. The ovary is now known to be a site of IGF-1 production and action. IGF-1 has been shown to amplify LH-stimulated androgen production in theca cells and to amplify FSH action in granulosa cells. It may also serve to communicate messages between granulosa cells and theca cells.

Oocyte maturation inhibitor (OMI), a peptide hormone present in follicular fluid, prevents final maturation of the oocyte until the time of ovulation. OMI suppression ends within hours following the midcycle LH surge just prior to ovulation.

ENDOMETRIUM

The endometrium responds to the cyclic changes in ovarian steroids. Estrogen increases the thickness of the endometrium by increasing the number and size of endometrial cells. Estrogen also stimulates the formation of progesterone receptors on endometrial cells and increases the blood flow (via spiral arterioles) to the endometrium. Progesterone causes the proliferated endometrium to differentiate and secrete proteins that are important in the survival and implantation of an early embryo if pregnancy occurs. Progesterone and exogenous progestins also decrease the proliferative effects of estrogens on the endometrium by causing down-regulation of estrogen receptors. Withdrawal of estrogen and progesterone results in the orderly and controlled sloughing of the functional zone of the endometrium. This monthly shedding of the lining of the uterus occurs from 400 to 500 times during a woman's reproductive years.[8]

CERVIX

The cervix and cervical mucus also change in response to estrogen and progesterone. The cervical mucus facilitates selective sperm penetration from the vagina to the fallopian tube during the periovulatory period; at other times, the mucus prevents microorganisms and sperm from entering the uterine cavity. When estradiol levels increase during the mid to late follicular phase, the cervical mucus becomes clear, thin, more profuse, and extrudes from the cervical os into the vagina. The cervix itself swells and softens, and the cervical os dilates. After ovulation, progesterone causes the cervix to become more firm, the cervical os to close, and the cervical mucus to become scant, thick, and turbid. Progesterone and exogenous progestins produce a contraceptive effect by causing a thick cervical mucus that sperm cannot penetrate.

THE INTEGRATED CYCLE

FOLLICULAR PHASE

Pulsatile GnRH release by the hypothalamus results in pulses of FSH and LH. FSH stimulates the proliferation of granulosa cells, which produce estradiol from androgen precursors synthesized in theca cells.[3] In the first half of the follicular phase (days 1 to 5), many follicles are "recruited" and begin to grow. The increasing local estradiol levels induce more FSH receptors on the largest follicle, thus producing greater amounts of estradiol. Estradiol and inhibin begin to provide negative feedback on FSH secretion by the anterior pituitary. (See Figures 4-1 and 4-2.)

During days 5 to 7 of the cycle, one of the recruited follicles becomes "dominant," producing the most estradiol, the largest number of granulosa cells and developing the most FSH receptors.[2] As FSH levels decline, the dominant follicle survives while the non-dominant follicles undergo atresia. After day 7, the dominant follicle is selected. The dominant follicle continues to mature and produce high levels of estradiol in the latter half of the follicular phase.[9] The length of the follicular phase is variable from individual to individual, but usually ranges from 10 to 17 days.

Very late in the follicular phase LH activity stimulates stromal tissue causing a rise in androgen levels: a 15% increase in androstenedione and a 20% increase in testosterone. Libido can be stimulated by androgens, and a peak in sexual behavior initiated by women occurs in the ovulatory phase of the cycle. The mid-cycle rise in androgens may therefore increase sexual activity at the time most likely to lead to a pregnancy.[3]

OVULATORY PHASE

Once the estradiol level has exceeded a critical level for 2 to 3 days, a positive feedback occurs in the pituitary, resulting in a surge of LH and FSH.[10] The estradiol level reaches its peak about 24 hours before ovulation. The LH surge leads to resumption of meiosis I in the dominant oocyte, luteinization of granulosa cells, and resultant progesterone production. Prostaglandins, proteolytic enzymes, and the contraction of smooth muscle cells within the follicle result in a break down of the follicular wall. The oocyte and follicular fluid exude about 32 to 44 hours after the onset of the LH surge and 10 to 12 hours after the LH peak. The onset of the LH surge appears to be the most reliable indicator of impending ovulation, and ovulation predictor kits detect this increasing surge of LH.

LUTEAL PHASE

Following the rupture of the follicle, the granulosa and theca cells take up steroids and lutein pigment to give the corpus luteum ("yellow body") a yellow appearance. The hallmark of the luteal phase is the shift from the estrogen-dominated follicular phase to one of progesterone dominance. Progesterone suppresses new follicular growth and causes secretory changes in the endometrium.[11] Peak progesterone production occurs 7 to 8 days after the LH surge, at the approximate time of implantation if fertilization has occurred. The length of the luteal phase tends to be more constant than the follicular phase, approximately 14 days unless pregnancy occurs.

Because progesterone causes an elevation in basal body temperature, daily measurement of basal body temperature can be used to determine whether or not ovulation has occurred. (See Chapter 15 on Fertility Awareness.) Basal body temperatures cannot be used to predict ovulation, as the temperature rise does not occur until after ovulation, but can confirm that ovulation has occurred.

MENSTRUAL PHASE

If a woman does not become pregnant, the corpus luteum rapidly declines 9 to 11 days after ovulation, resulting in a decline of progesterone and estrogen levels.[3] The withdrawal of these hormones initially shrinks endometrial height, decreases blood flow, and begins vasodilation followed by rhythmic vasoconstriction of the spiral arterioles. Ischemia and stasis are followed by interstitial hemorrhage and tissue disorganization, resulting in menstrual flow.[12]

The normal amount of blood lost during a normal menstrual period is 20 to 80 ml. Seventy percent of the blood will slough by the second day, and 90% by the third day.[8] The average duration of the menstrual phase is 4 to 6 days.

Thrombin-platelet plugs limit blood loss, and rising estrogen levels of the new cycle induce clot formation and regrowth of the endometrium. Delayed, asynchronous, or incomplete shedding of the endometrium, as might occur in anovulatory cycles, can be associated with heavier and longer bleeding.

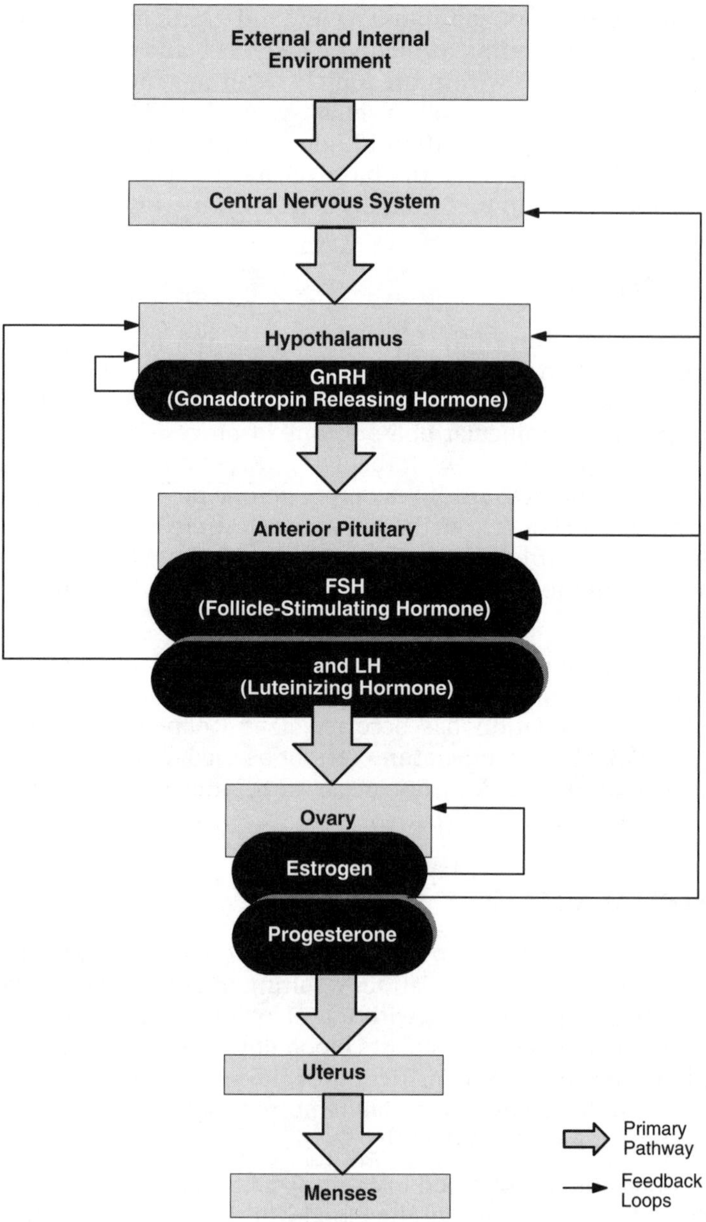

Primary hormone pathways (⇨) in the reproductive system are modulated by both negative and positive feedback loops (→). Prostaglandins, secreted by the ovary and by uterine endometrial cells, also play a role in ovulation, and may modulate hypothalamic function as well.

Figure 4-1 Regulation of the menstrual cycle

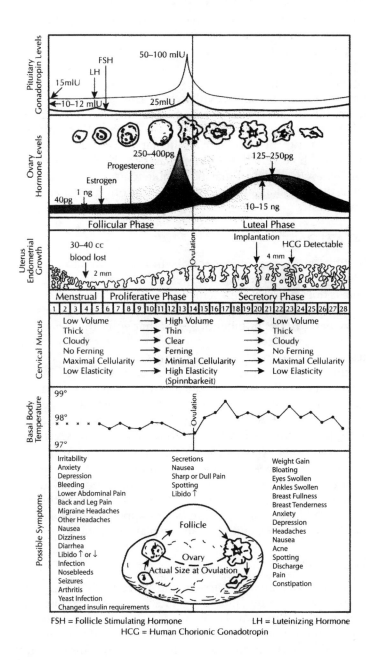

Figure 4-2 Menstrual cycle events: hormone levels, ovarian, and endometrial patterns and cyclic temperature and cervical mucus changes

FERTILIZATION AND IMPLANTATION

A woman is most likely to conceive if fresh sperm are present in the upper reproductive tract when ovulation occurs. The oocyte retains potential for fertilization for 12 to 24 hours, and sperm usually remain viable in the reproductive tract for 72 hours. The extreme intervals at which women have achieved pregnancy after a single act of coitus are 6 days prior to and 3 days after ovulation.[13] The several days prior to ovulation are thus the most fertile cycle days, or the days that conception is most likely to occur. (See Chapter 27 on Impaired Fertility.) After ovulation and during the very early follicular phase, the likelihood of pregnancy is much lower. If a woman has very regular cycles and is monitoring her cycle closely, it may be feasible to use periodic abstinence during the fertile period as a means of contraception. (See Chapter 17 on Fertility Awareness.)

IMPLANTATION

During intercourse, the man deposits into the woman's vagina as many as 300 million spermatozoa suspended in seminal fluid. Because cervical mucus does not mix with semen, the sperm have to pass into the mucus, but this occurs within minutes. Under optimal conditions (in the pre-ovulatory period), the number of sperm that enter the mucus within the first few minutes is often sufficient to accomplish fertilization. Within 30 minutes, several hundred thousand sperm can be found in the cervical canal, and this number remains stable for approximately 24 hours. Because cervical mucus allows easier passage of normal sperm, the sperm population improves over that present in the ejaculate. Sperm pass through the fallopian tubes fairly rapidly, but spermatozoa in the cervical crypts can supply sperm to the upper reproductive tract for several days.

Following extrusion of the oocyte and cumulus complex at the time of ovulation, the oocyte is swept into the lumen of the tube by the fimbria within minutes to hours. Fertilization occurs in the ampullary region of the fallopian tube, and the early embryo is then transported to the uterine cavity within 2 to 3 days. Implantation begins approximately 6 to 7 days after fertilization, when the embryo is at the blastocyst stage.

ANOVULATION

Because normal ovulatory cycles require the integration of hormones and signals from the hypothalamus, pituitary gland, and ovaries, problems at any of these sites may result in anovulation. Inadequate GnRH secretion by the hypothalamus inhibits normal FSH and LH production and results in anovulation. Problems such as weight loss, extensive exercise, stress, depression and anorexia nervosa can interfere with GnRH secretion. Hyperprolactinemia may also result in ovulatory dysfunction or anovulation.

Alterations in the critically balanced factors in the ovary may also lead to anovulation. Excessive concentration of androgens in ovarian follicles may inhibit the emergence of a dominant follicle and result in follicular atresia. As in individuals with polycystic ovarian syndrome, hyperinsulinemia may contribute to the excessive androgen production in the ovaries.

THE MENSTRUAL CYCLE AND AGING

Menstrual cycle length varies as a woman ages. Cycles tend to be longer when a woman is under age 20 and over age 40. It may be several years after menarche before regular, ovulatory cycles are achieved. Several years prior to menopause, menstrual cycles tend to lengthen and anovulatory cycles become more frequent again.[14]

HORMONAL CONTRACEPTIVE EFFECTS

Hormonal contraceptives prevent fertilization in part by disrupting the menstrual cycle. Combined oral contraceptives contain both estrogen and progestin. Progestin-only contraceptives include Depo-Provera injections, Norplant implants, minipills, and intrauterine devices (IUDs) such as the Progestasert System and the Levonorgestrel Intrauterine System. Estrogens and progestins act upon many different organ systems and produce a broad range of effects.[3] Among the most important noncontraceptive benefits of pills are their beneficial effects on the cyclic symptoms women may experience as a result of their menstrual cycles.

Estrogenic Effects

- Ovulation is inhibited because estrogen suppresses FSH and LH, thus preventing the pituitary gland from releasing ovary-stimulating hormones.
- The endometrial secretions and cellular structure are altered.
- Altered local levels of prostaglandins contribute to the degeneration of the corpus luteum.

Progestational Effects

- Ovulation is inhibited by suppression of the midcycle peak of LH and FSH.
- Thickened cervical mucus decreases sperm penetration.
- The activity of the cilia in the fallopian tubes is reduced.
- The endometrium becomes atrophic and impairs implantation.

REFERENCES

1. Vollman RF, The menstrual cycle, In: Friedman E, ed. Major problems in obstetrics and gynecology, W.B. Saunders Co., Philadelphia, 1977.
2. Henderson KM. Gonadotrophic regulation of ovarian activity. Br Med Bull 1979;35:161.
3. Speroff L, Glass RH, Kase G. Clinical gynecologic endocrinology and infertility. 6th edition. Baltimore MD: Lippincott Williams & Wilkins, 1999.

4. Filicori M, Santoro N, Merriam GR, Crowley WF Jr. Characterization of the physiological pattern of episodic gonadotropin secretion throughout the human menstrual cycle. J Clin Endocrinol Metab 1986;62:1136.

5. Reame N, Sauder SE, Kelch RP, Marshall JC. Pulsatile gonadotropin secretion during the human menstrual cycle: evidence for altered frequency of gonadotropin-releasing hormone secretion. J Clin Endocrinol Metab 1984;59:384.

6. Kase NG, Speroff L. The ovary. In: Bondy P, Rosenberg L (eds). Metabolic control and disease. 8th edition. Philadelphia PA: WB Saunders, 1980.

7. Bicsak TA, Tucker EM, Cappel S, Vaughan J, Rivier J, Vale W, Hseuh AJW. Hormonal regulation of granulosa cell inhibin biosynthesis. Endocrinology 1986;119:2711.

8. Swartz DP, Butler W. Normal and abnormal uterine bleeding. In: Thompson JD, Rock JA (eds). TeLindeÕs operative gynecology. 7th edition. Philadelphia PA: J.B. Lippincott, 1992.

9. Clark JR, Dierschke DJ, Wolf RC. Hormonal regulation of ovarian folliculogenesis in rhesus monkey. III. Atresia on the preovulatory follicle induced by exogenous steroids and subsequent follicular development. Biol Reprod 1981;25:332.

10. Hoff, JD, Quigley ME, Yen SSC. Hormonal dynamics at midcycle: a reevaluation. J Clin Endocrinol Metab 1983;57:792.

11. Kase NG, Weingold AB, Gershenson DM. Principles and practice of clinical gynecology. 2nd edition. New York: Churchill Livingstone, 1990.

12. Sixma JJ, Cristiens GCML, Haspels AS. The sequence of hemostasis events in the endometrium during normal menstruation. In: Diczfalusy E, Fraser IS, Webb WTG (eds). WHO symposium on steroid contraception and endometrial bleeding. London: Pittman Press Ltd, 1980.

13. France JT, Graham FM, Gosling L, Hair P, Knox BS. Characteristics of natural conception cycles occurring in a prospective study of sex preselection: fertility awareness symptoms, hormone levels, sperm survival, and pregnancy outcome. Int J Fertil 37:244, 1992.

14. Gosden RG. Follicular status at menopause. Human Reprod 1987;2:617.

Menopause

Anita L. Nelson, MD
Felicia H. Stewart, MD

- Many perimenopausal women need effective contraception. Although women over age 40 have significantly lower baseline fertility than do women in their 20s, an unintended pregnancy at this time in life can be devastating.

- The single greatest health threat for postmenopausal women is cardiovascular disease (CVD). The most important therapeutic recommendation for menopausal women is to adopt healthy lifestyles.

- Routine "replacement" of physiologic doses of hormones for postmenopausal women is not warranted. Hormone treatment can, however, be offered as a targeted therapy to treat specific conditions, such as hot flashes or urogenital atrophy, and as osteoporosis prevention. Provide treatment at the lowest doses needed for the shortest duration needed.

PERIMENOPAUSAL ISSUES

Each woman travels her own unique course through perimenopause. Women who experienced regular cycling in their 20s and 30s often notice subtle changes in their menstrual cycles starting in their late 30s and early 40s. At first, they may note a reduction in the interval between their menstrual periods and, later, an irregular spacing between withdrawal bleeds, as more cycles are anovulatory. Because of anovulation, menses can become heavy and prolonged enough to require evaluation, intervention, and occasionally, surgical therapy.

The earliest manifestations of functional ovarian changes begin by age 35 to 40; fertility per cycle starts to decline in this age group, usually even before menstrual disorders or hot flashes develop. In Hutterite populations with unregulated fertility, 11% of women had their last pregnancy before age 34, and 33% completed childbearing before age 40; only about 13% had any pregnancies after age 45.[1] In donor insemination programs, women under age 31 had annual pregnancy rates of 74%; women over age 35 had rates of 54%.[2] In a U.S. study, women over age 35 required 9 to 10 cycles to conceive, rather than the average 6 cycles for younger women. In addition, the risk of clinically recognized spontaneous abortions increases dramatically as women age: the rate is 10% for women under 30 years versus the 34% for women over 50. Autosomal trisomy contributes significantly more to pregnancy losses in older women.

Early in a woman's life, her ovarian follicles are very responsive to stimulation by follicle-stimulating hormone (FSH). By age 35 to 40, remaining follicles require higher gonadotropin levels to stimulate maturation. FSH levels are able to increase to stimulate remaining follicles because decreased inhibin B production by the fewer stimulated follicles reduces negative feedback from the ovary to the hypothalamus and pituitary. This explains why, in women over age 35 to 40, FSH levels on Cycle Day 3 are used to predict fertility potential, independent of other possible causes of infertility. High FSH levels show that the ovaries must be hyper–stimulated to get follicular activity and that the woman's chance of conception is low even with in vitro fertilization (see Chapter 27 on Impaired Fertility).

No one symptom or laboratory test is accurate enough to rule in or out perimenopause,[3] and there is rarely any clinical utility in making that diagnosis. The transition from fertile cycling to non-cycling, non-fertile status after menopause has recently been formalized into phases using the STRAW (Stages of Reproductive Aging Workshop) system.[4] (See Figure 5-1.) In contrast to the *postmenopausal* period (Stages +1 and +2), which is characterized by low estrogen levels, the 2 to 8 *perimenopausal* years (Stages –2 and –1) are notable for fluctuating, "irregularly irregular" hormone levels.[5]

Recommendations of Stages of Reproductive Aging Workshop (STRAW), Park City, Utah, USA. July 2001.

Stages:	–5	–4	–3	–2	–1	0	+1	+2
Terminology:		Reproductive		Menopausal Transition		FMP	Postmenopause	
	Early	Peak	Late	Early	Late*		Early*	Late
				Perimenopause				
Duration of Stage:		Variable			Variable	Final Menstrual Period	1 yr	4 yrs	Until demise
Menstrual Cycles:	Variable to regular	Regular		Variable cycle length (≥ 7 days; different from normal)	≥ 2 skipped cycles and an interval of amenorrhea (≥ 60 days)		Amenorrhea x 12 months	None
Endocrine:	Normal FSH		↑ FSH	↑ FSH			↑ FSH	

* Stages most likely to be characterized by vasomotor symptoms   ↑ = elevated

Source: Soules MR, et al. (2001).[4]

Figure 5-1 Stages/nomenclature of normal reproductive aging in women

Perimenopause Symptoms and Treatment

At least 15% to 40% of menstruating women in their 40s experience hot flashes, which are often as disturbing as those that occur after menopause.[6] Hot flashes in this age group do not necessarily result from low serum estrogen levels, but occur in the context of dramatically fluctuating estrogen levels.[7] Although we do not completely understand the etiology of hot flashes, women (and men) tend to become symptomatic when their estrogen levels decline rapidly. Absolute estrogen levels in themselves do not explain hot flashes: there is no difference in average estrogen levels between symptomatic and asymptomatic women.[8] The trough estradiol levels can be associated with poor sleep, hot flashes, higher anxiety and depression, even in cycling reproductive-age women.[9]

Perimenopausal women with persistent or severe vasomotor symptoms can be treated with combined hormonal contraception[10] or with postmenopausal doses of estrogen/progestin treatments, although the latter can worsen menstrual abnormalities. If a woman becomes symptomatic during the hormone-free week of hormonal contraceptive use, she can try reducing or eliminating the placebo period. Other approaches include combining postmenopausal estrogen therapy with either depot medroxyprogesterone acetate (DMPA) or the levonorgestrel-releasing intrauterine system. Non-hormonal treatment options, such as those discussed below for postmenopausal women, are also helpful for symptomatic perimenopausal women.

Most women in their perimenopausal years consider themselves to be in reasonably good health, however, they may need to make significant changes prior to menopause to optimize their health after menopause. Encourage them to adopt or maintain long-term healthy lifestyles. Obesity is increasingly a major health problem: 56% of women age 20 to 34 and 75% age 35 to 44 are overweight or obese. Obesity in older women is most often due to inadequate exercise and/or overeating. A decrease in ovulatory cycling may make it more challenging for women in their 40s and 50s to lose weight. During the luteal phase, basal metabolic rates (BMR) increase. Without that change in BMR in the second half of the cycle, caloric intake is stored as fat rather than burned as energy. Promote exercise, not only to contribute to weight control and improve cardiovascular health, but also to enhance bone remodeling and muscle strength for balance. As many as 70% to 80% of older U.S. women have physical activity levels that are lower than recommended.[11]

Contraceptive Options for Perimenopausal Women

Many perimenopausal women need effective contraception. Although women over age 40 have significantly lower baseline fertility than do women in their 20s, an unintended pregnancy at this time in life can be devastating. In the United States, nearly one-third of pregnancies among women aged 40 or older are electively terminated; this proportion approximates that for young (< 14 years) adolescents.[12]

The most common method of contraception used by U.S. couples over age 30 is sterilization. For women still at risk for pregnancy, the full range of contraceptive choices is available. Long-term efficacy and convenience are critical features to consider, as are the women's health problems. Remind women who still have menses that hormone regimens used for hot flash treatment do not prevent ovulation.[13] Provide all at-risk women with emergency contraception (EC). (See Chapter 12 on Emergency Contraception.)

Intrauterine devices (IUD). The copper IUD provides convenient and excellent pregnancy protection without hormones. The levonorgestrel intrauterine system (LNG IUS) is also a particularly attractive alternative for women in the perimenopause, because the endometrial suppression offered by the LNG IUS controls erratic, anovulatory bleeding and reduces the risk for endometrial hyperplasia.

Combined hormonal contraceptives. When non-contraceptive benefits are factored into the equation, combined hormonal contraceptives (pills, patches, and vaginal rings) may be appropriate and appealing options for healthy, nonsmoking, perimenopausal women. Used cyclically, combined hormonal methods cause predictable withdrawal bleeding and prevent the endometrial consequences of unopposed estrogen, such as hyperplasia and endometrial cancer. Combined hormonal contraceptives also stabilize (at least 3 out of every 4 weeks) the woman's hormone levels and reduce hot flashes. There is also evidence that use of low-dose OCs may slow some of the bone loss characteristic of these years.[14] Continuous use of combined oral contraceptives achieves all of these objectives and eliminates menses, dysmenorrhea, and hormonal fluctuations that occur during the placebo pill week.

In the wake of the WHI studies, women are often confused by the apparently conflicting information they hear about hormones. On the one hand, perimenopausal women are being reassured that even long-term use of pharmacologic doses of hormones in contraceptives does not increase their risk of breast cancer or significantly increase their risk of cardiovascular disease if they are healthy and normotensive. On the other hand, women are told that use of estrogen-progestin therapy (EPT) after the menopause increases the risk of myocardial infarction (MI) in the short run (first year of use) and of breast cancer in the long run (after 5 years of use). The answer is not the formulation (OCs versus EPT), but the woman. A woman who has delayed menopause (age 55) has the same increase in risk of breast cancer as a 55-year-old woman who went through menopause at age 49 and who has used EPT for over 5 years. If the women in the WHI trials had been given OCs instead of EPT, they would probably have experienced more adverse health risks than were demonstrated by EPT use. Healthy perimenopausal women obtain contraceptive benefits to offset the small health risks associated with OC use.

Progestin-only contraceptives. For perimenopausal women who have relative contraindications (e.g., smoking) to the pharmacologic doses of estrogen found in combined hormonal contraceptives, a progestin-only contraceptive, such as the LNG-IUS, progestin-only pills, or DMPA, can be used for contraception. Menopausal treatment doses of estrogen may be added to DMPA to reduce losses in bone mineralization and to help control hot flashes as well as to reduce breakthrough bleeding due to endometrial atrophy. This combination may also be continued through the early menopausal years until it is reasonably likely that the woman is no longer at risk for pregnancy. Progestin-only pills should not be combined with estrogen for contraception.

Barrier methods. Barrier methods may be an appropriate choice for women who are willing to accept a lower efficacy rate, especially if they are needed for prevention of sexually transmitted infections (STI).

Sterilization. Sterilization is feasible but costly, and it subjects women to operative risks for only a few years of contraceptive protection.

M ENOPAUSE

Menopause means permanent cessation of menses following or in association with loss of ovarian follicular activity. Menopause can be diagnosed in women in the following circumstances:

- Women who have had surgical removal of their ovaries
- Women with intact ovaries who have been amenorrheic for 1 year with no other cause (no need for laboratory confirmation if these changes occur during an appropriate age range [> 47 years])
- Women who had a hysterectomy with ovarian preservation when ovarian estradiol production has decreased to a menopausal level

After menopause, women are no longer at risk for pregnancy since they have no more recruitable follicles, but this lack of follicles also results in decreased ovarian production of estrogen.

The median age of menopause is 51.3 years. Approximately 1% of women undergo menopause before age 40; at the other extreme, 2% of women are still not menopausal at age 55. Menopause before age 30 can be associated with chromosomal abnormalities (e.g., gonadal dysgenesis), so a genetic evaluation is appropriate in this situation.[15] Premature menopause (< 40 years old) and early menopause (< 45 years old) are strongly influenced by family history,[16] but otherwise, the age of menopause does not follow a clear familial pattern and is generally not predictable. Women who smoke, have type-1 diabetes, live at high altitudes, or are undernourished or vegetarian undergo menopause at younger ages than do women without these risk factors. Premature menopause is a risk factor for significant medical problems, including osteoporosis and cardiovascular disease, and can be a personal tragedy for a woman who has not yet completed her desired childbearing.

DIAGNOSIS OF MENOPAUSE

There are no blood tests to diagnose menopause early and reliably enough to guarantee a woman that she is no longer at risk for pregnancy.[17] During the perimenopausal years (Stages -3 to 0), day-to-day fluctuations of both gonadotropins and hormones can be quite extreme:[7] FSH levels can temporarily crest to very high levels, and estradiol (E2) levels can plunge into the menopausal range. There is no need to order FSH or luteinizing hormone (LH) levels to test for menopause in a woman with hot flashes who is still menstruating; her cycling verifies that she still has ovarian steroidogenesis and her symptoms classify her as perimenopausal. At best, tests of gonadotropins could confirm her premenopausal state; at worst, they could confuse the picture and put her at risk for unintended pregnancy with a false diagnosis of menopause. In some situations, it may be helpful to determine her level of thyroid-stimulating hormone (TSH), and rule out other diagnoses.[19]

For the same reason, hormone tests also are not reliable indicators of when to discontinue hormonal contraceptive methods that may mask the symptoms of menopause. Fortunately, the diagnosis of menopause need not be made precisely. Some experts recommend that healthy women continue their hormonal contraceptives until age 53 to 55, when the likelihood of pregnancy is very slight.[10]

On the other hand, it is not necessary to wait for 1 year of amenorrhea to initiate treatment for symptomatic women. The women who chose not to use hormonal contraception should not be required to suffer hot flashes and related symptoms or to undergo accelerated loss of bone mineralization for 12 months before therapy is initiated. It is quite feasible to provide symptomatic women who have had less than a year of amenorrhea with postmenopausal hormonal treatments or other therapies listed below, along with the advice that they continue to use nonhormonal contraception until the diagnosis of menopause is secure.

HEALTH RISKS IN THE MENOPAUSE

Most women over age 50 are not well informed about their long-term health risks. In a recent telephone survey of U.S. women, 34% reported that breast cancer is the greatest health problem confronting women, while less than 8% reported that cardiovascular disease or stroke is a major concern.[20] Cardiovascular disease caused 34% of all deaths in women over age 65 in 1999, whereas breast cancer accounted for only 4%.[21] At every age after 55, more women die of heart disease than of any other cause. The distortion of the real health hazards is dangerous. Health care provider recommendations for smoking cessation, exercise promotion, and dietary modification may be ignored because those lifestyle issues have no impact on breast cancer susceptibility and because they may require profound, and often challenging, lifestyle modifications. On the other hand, women may be reluctant to use EPT even in the short term, because they harbor an inflated estimate of their baseline risk of developing breast cancer. Inform women of their true health risks, design appropriate interventions, and make referrals as needed. Risk assessment for cardiovascular disease, bone fracture, diabetes, and breast cancer may identify targeted interventions that will be particularly important for at-risk women.

Because cardiovascular disease (CVD) is such an enormous health problem,[22] it is important to identify risk factors for CVD, including diabetes, hypertension, dyslipidemia, smoking, obesity, and a family history of CVD. Diabetic women and women with Syndrome X (See Chapter 6 on Menstrual Problems and Common Gynecologic Concerns) enter menopause with the same probabilities for heart attack and stroke as similarly aged men and should be treated a *priori* as if they have coronary artery disease (CAD).[22] Many women have other risk factors for CVD. In the United States, 25% of women are sedentary, 20% smoke, 52% over age 45 have hypertension, and 40% over age 55 have high cholesterol.[23] New guidelines have been published for estimating the 10-year risk of CAD in women and for controlling those risks.[24,25] For example, blood pressure control is critical in forestalling premature MI and stroke; the upper limit for normal blood pressures is now 120 mm Hg systolic and 80 mm Hg diastolic. Statins have been shown to improve life expectancy. For every 2-point drop in low-density lipoprotein (LDL) cholesterol, the risk of heart attack in men decreases by 1%. The data for women appear to be similarly impressive.

Women at high risk for breast cancer ($\geq$1.7% risk of developing breast carcinoma in the next 5 years) may wish to use chemoprophylaxis with appropriate selective estrogen receptor modulators (SERMs). Osteoporotic women and osteopenic women with risks factors can combine exercise, calcium, and Vitamin D with prescription therapies to reduce their risk of future fracture.

The most important therapeutic recommendation for menopausal women to help them improve both the quantity and the quality of their remaining years is to adopt healthy lifestyles. Smokers should be provided realistic estimates of the effects that their smoking will have on their health. All women should avoid second-hand smoke exposure. Overweight women need to learn the impact that their excess pounds may have on their risk for CVD and diabetes. Controlled weight and avoidance of visceral obesity contribute greatly to reducing a woman's risk for fatal and non-fatal MI. Similarly, women should be told that exercise could improve their quality of life. Women who exercise have an extended CVD-free life and a reduced risk of respiratory disease.[26] By the same token, providers must recognize that almost 1 out of every 5 women age 40 to 55 reports some limitation in physical functioning (e.g., hypertension, arthritis, cancer, obesity, stress or poverty)[27] and should tailor individual health promotion programs to meet the individual constraints of their patients.

POSTMENOPAUSAL HORMONE THERAPY: A NEW PARADIGM

The results of the randomized clinical trials (RCTs) of postmenopausal hormone therapies have changed the paradigm used in treating post-menopausal women. These studies have demonstrated that routine "re-placement" of physiologic doses of hormones for postmenopausal women is not warranted. Instead, offer hormone treatment to women as a targeted therapy intended to treat identified conditions, such as hot flashes and urogenital atrophy, and to prevent osteoporosis. Provide treatment at the lowest doses needed for the shortest duration of time needed. On an individual basis, help the woman weigh the benefits of hormone therapy against her potential risks. Because her benefits may diminish over time and her risks may increase, help her periodically reassess her candidacy. Accompany each assessment of the benefits and risks of such therapy with a discussion of the benefits and risks of the ever-growing list of nonhormonal therapies.

HOT FLASHES AND RELATED SYMPTOMS OF ESTROGEN DEFICIENCY

The hallmark of the "menopausal syndrome" is the hot flash, but the full range of symptoms is much broader. Women may be troubled by fatigue, moodiness, depression, difficulty sleeping, decreased libido and orgasmic response, anxiety, changes in memory and cognition, weight gain, joint pain, scalp hair loss, hair growth or acne on face, skin changes, palpations, nausea, headaches, and urinary tract infections. Hot flashes, which affect 68% to 90% of recently menopausal women in the United States,[28] can be quite uncomfortable and embarrassing. During a flash, women radiate heat from all parts of their bodies; even toe temperatures have been observed to increase by up to 7 degrees Fahrenheit.[29] At night, the flashes can disrupt a woman's normal sleep cycle. Even if a woman is not completely awakened, the quality of her sleep may be diminished by hot flashes. Chronic sleep deprivation can cause mood disturbances, irritability, anxiety, and tearfulness.[30,31] Sleep disruptions also can signifi-cantly reduce a woman's ability to concentrate and remember. In one study, reproductive-aged women who were tested prior to bilateral oophorectomy and again 2 months postoperatively demonstrated significantly decreased scores on immediate and delayed recall of paired associates compared to hormone users who retained their abilities in those areas.[32] The biological plausibility of this functional impairment is supported by a wide variety of imaging studies. Perfusion studies clearly demonstrate significantly reduced blood flow to the brain during the 20 to 30 minutes that each hot flash lasts.[33]

Recent analyses have shown that only women who are symptomatic from vasomotor symptoms can expect postmenopausal EPT to offer a net long-term improvement (benefits minus side effects) in overall quality of life.[34]

Hormonal Therapy for Hot Flashes

The most effective therapy currently available for hot flashes is estrogen treatment (ET) for hysterectomized women or estrogen-progestin therapy (EPT) for women with an intact uterus. Well-designed, randomized, prospective, placebo-controlled, cross-over trials comparing estrogen treatment to placebo indicate the following:[35–38]

- Placebo treatments can have a very strong effect (a 30% to 60% reduction in hot flash frequency and severity). For this reason, it is not appropriate to endorse any therapy that has not proven itself superior to placebo in clinical trials.

- Estrogen shows a significantly greater clinical effect than placebo for treatment of hot flashes. Depending upon the dose used, ET and EPT reduced hot flash frequency by 80% to 96% compared to a 50% reduction observed with placebo use.

- ET may have a relatively slow onset of action. Decreases in hot flash intensity and frequency can be observed within 1 week of ET initiation, but the maximal effect is generally not achieved for at least 1 month of use. Do not rush to increase ET dose, unless the woman experiences no improvement.

- A rapid discontinuation in estrogen treatment dose can result in a return of symptoms. Often, within 1 to 3 months, a rebound occurs in which the woman experiences more frequent hot flashes than she had prior to therapy.

New studies have found that EPT and ET with 50% to 75% of the doses previously considered "conventional" can reduce hot flash frequency and severity almost as well as the conventional doses.[38] Given these results, it would be prudent to start with the lowest dose feasible and raise the dose only if needed. For women using conventional doses, consider lowering the dose over time in women who continue to use hormone therapy. There is no arbitrary limit to the number of years a woman may use hormone therapy to control bothersome symptoms as long as the benefits of ET/EPT outweigh her health risks.

Non-hormonal Therapy for Hot Flashes

Other interventions may be helpful as first-line therapies for women unable or unwilling to use hormonal therapy or as adjunctive measures for women who do not have adequate relief with initial doses of hormonal therapy.

Lifestyle Measures for Hot Flashes:

- Smoking cessation reduces hot flashes and is imperative for good overall health.

- Avoiding triggers may help reduce hot flashes. A woman may notice that certain things (such as spicy foods, computer screens, or chocolate) spark her symptoms.
- Wearing layered clothing may help. Removing a jacket during a hot flash may reduce heat discomfort, and the jacket can be put back on if a post-flash chill occurs.
- Controlling room temperature and humidity may help.
- Using relaxation techniques and self-hypnosis may reduce hot flashes by up to 50%.[39,40]
- Exercising may not alter the frequency or intensity of hot flashes, but it improves sleep quality (and cardiac and bone health).

Other Prescription Medications Superior To Placebo

- **Clonidine.** Applying one patch (0.05 to 0.1 mg) each week reduced hot flashes by 46% in clinical trials, but 40% of women discontinued clonidine because of side effects such as dizziness and dry mouth.[41] As with other alpha adrenogenic agonists (lofexidine and methyldopa) that alter neurotransmitters in the hypothalamus to regulate the neuroregulatory center, clonidine reduced hot flashes about 20% to 65%.[42–44] Clonidine raises the sweating threshold in symptomatic, but not asymptomatic, postmenopausal women.[45]

- **Selective serotonin reuptake inhibitors (SSRIs).** Short courses of treatment, such as venlafaxine 37.5 to 75 mg daily, paroxetine 10 to 20 mg daily, or fluoxetine 20 mg daily, have demonstrated significantly larger reductions in hot flashes than placebo in small scale studies.[46–48] However, 2% to 23% of SSRI users experience sexual dysfunction.

- **Bellergal-S.** This is a combination of belladonna alkaloids, ergotamine tartrate, and phenobarbital. As an "autonomic system stabilizer," Bellergal-S inhibits the sympathetic-parasympathetic pathway. Early studies showed a 66% reduction in menopausal symptoms with Bellergal-S compared to a 24% reduction with placebos.[49] A more recent study showed that all benefits were seen at 2 and 4 weeks of treatment, but by 8 weeks, there was no difference between women treated with Bellergal or placebo.[50] Bellergal often sedates, which may be helpful if it is used only at night. There is some potential for addiction.

- **Progestin compounds.** DMPA 150 mg IM or MPA 10 mg daily led to an 85% to 87% reduction in hot flashes in postmenopausal women. Side effects can include mastalgia, mood changes, bloating, and weight gain. Micronized progestin, off-label, has also been recognized to reduce hot flashes.

- **Megestrol acetate.** Studies showed that 74% of women had ≥ 50% reduction in hot flashes compared to 20% of women using placebo.[51]

- **Soy.** Capsules (60 g of soy protein) taken daily reduced hot flashes 45% vs. a 30% placebo effect.[52] These capsules are not available in the United States.

- **Androgen supplements** (with estrogen). Preparations with low-dose estrogen plus androgen may provide more relief than low-dose estrogen alone but achieve the same effect as higher dose estrogen.[53] Some small studies with estrogen and androgen showed that the combination reduced lack of concentration, depressive moods, and fatigue more than estrogen alone.[54] Androgens reduce sex hormone binding globulin (SHBG) and may alter lipids or increase acne. (Hair loss may occur when women take 5 mg or more of methyltestosterone.)

- **Tibolone** (not available in the United States). This compound, with estrogenic, progestogenic and androgenic properties, is used in Europe for treating vasomotor symptoms in menopausal women.[55]

- **Gabapentin.** In one small study, gabapentin, 900 mg, reduced hot flashes by 45% compared to a 29% placebo effect.[56] The drug is related to GABA neurotransmitter, but the mechanism of action is not well defined. Gabapentin use is associated with anorgasmia.

Over-the-Counter Agents for Hot Flashes

Nearly 1 out of every 3 Americans uses complementary therapies. In the United States, annual expenditures for such treatments total 5 to 6 billion dollars each year. Although few clinical studies exist, more data are becoming available about the effectiveness of alternative treatment approaches.[57,58] The following over-the-counter therapies have been evaluated in clinical trials that included placebo. Little information, however, is available about possible adverse effects or long-term risks.

- **Soy isoflavones.** Phytoestrogens are derived from soy, garbanzo beans, and legumes. The active ingredients in many isoflavones are genistein and daidzein. Early studies found short-term reduction in hot flash frequency of 45%,[59,60] although a long-term study showed return of symptoms later.[61] One randomized trial with 100 mg of soy isoflavones daily for 4 months showed a statistically significant improvement above the placebo arm,[62] but other studies with 72 mg and 114 mg did not show improvement.[143,144] Epidemiologic studies have shown that women who have high soy intake have fewer hot flashes.[63] If plant proteins are substituted for animal proteins, there can be a beneficial effect on lipid profiles, but soy protein supplements do not show beneficial effects.[64] If soy supplements are added as medication to a woman's routine diet, she must be advised to significantly decrease her routine dietary intake to accommodate the soy calories. Modest intake throughout the day is better than a larger single dose.[145]

- **Red clover isoflavones.** Two placebo-controlled studies of 40 mg/d showed a 54% to 75% reduction of hot flashes vs. a 30% reduction with placebo, but two other placebo-controlled studies showed no effect above that provided by placebo.[65,66,74]

- **Black cohosh** (20 to 40 mg/day). Six major efficacy studies have been published on black cohosh, the most commonly used herbal therapy. One large study reported a reduction in "menopausal symptoms" in 80% of women by 4 weeks of treatment. The other studies reported improvements in symptoms but did not include placebo controls. Black cohosh may be 25% to 30% more effective than placebo for symptoms.[67,68] The German Commission E recommends limiting use of black cohosh to 6 months.

Treatments with No Evidence of Efficacy in Hot Flashes

- **Evening primrose oil.** One randomized, double-blinded 6-month clinical trial showed no significant benefit.[69] In addition, the agent causes gas and bloating and may increase activity of anticoagulants.

- **Chasteberry.** No clinical studies have been conducted in menopausal women.

- **Dong Quai.** One double-blinded placebo-controlled study using 4.5 g dong quai root as monotherapy showed no difference from placebo.[70]

- **Ginseng.** One randomized, double-blinded, placebo-controlled study of Ginsana (200 mg) for 16 weeks found no significant improvement in 3 out of 3 quality-of-life scales.[71] Drug-drug interactions include anti-platelet and anticoagulation medications.

- **Vitamin E.** A 4-week trial found no difference in hot flashes in women using 800 IU compared to placebo.[72,73]

SYMPTOMS RELATED TO MENOPAUSAL SYNDROME

Many women (especially those with hot flashes) complain of difficulties with sleep around the time of menopause.[75] In an RCT, women on ET reported significant improvement in sleep and fewer awakenings; they also reported feeling less tired the next day.[76] Interestingly, both women with and without hot flashes reported significant improvement in sleep quality. In the WHI, symptomatic women were found to have a small but significant improvement in sleep quality for the 3 years of study on EPT.[34]

Women who suffer hot flashes in the perimenopausal period may develop depressive symptoms that cause significant morbidity, even though they may not be due to clinical depression. In one RCT, ET lowered depression symptom scores more than placebo and also lowered menopausal-related symptoms.[77] In another study, EPT given to reduce vasomotor symptoms improved mood, as measured by the Kupperman Index, beyond that provided by placebo.[36] Another approach to treating women with perimenopausal depressive symptoms due to estrogen deficiency is to use SSRIs, which will directly address their depression and, incidentally, reduce vasomotor symptoms.

GENITOURINARY ATROPHY

With time, most postmenopausal women who do not use ET develop genitourinary atrophy. The vagina, the trigone of the bladder, and the urethra have the highest concentrations of estrogen receptors in the body.

Vagina. The most common problems that result from urogenital atrophy are dyspareunia and vaginal infections. Women with low estrogen levels (especially those who do not engage in vaginal intercourse) experience a thinning of the vaginal epithelium. As its ruggations flatten, the vagina becomes considerably less elastic. The underlying vessels and lymphatic system regress, resulting in loss of lubrication. Vaginal dryness is reported as a frequent sexual problem by 44% of postmenopausal women compared to 14% of premenopausal women.[78] This is an important issue today as more older men are being treated for erectile dysfunction; their partners may not be physically prepared for coitus. Water-soluble and silicone-based lubricants can provide coital lubrication. However, hormone therapy reverses all the underlying physiologic problems;[79] tissue elasticity and thickening generally is evident within 6 weeks of therapy. More prolonged treatment (up to 12 months) may be required to restore underlying vessels and lymphatic structures, which provide lubrication. Creams placed on the outer third of the vagina optimizes outcome.[146] Atrophy of the vagina also decreases natural vaginal defenses against infection. Vaginal fluid loses its protective acidity; the rise in vaginal pH (pH = 6.5-7.5) results from the loss of glycogen in the vaginal epithelium transudate that is needed to support lactobacillus in the vaginal ecosystem.

Urinary tract. After menopause, bladder infections also increase. Constriction of the estrogen-sensitive vaginal tissues causes the urethral meatus to rotate downward, closer to the vagina. Estrogen may effectively treat irritative urinary symptoms such as frequency and urgency and to reduce the risk of recurrent urinary tract infections.[80] Dysuria in postmenopausal women can be due to the increased incidence of cystitis, to the thinned tissue surrounding the urethral tissue, or to the development of urethral caruncles. Caruncles form when tissues surrounding the urethral meatus contract and evert the distal portion of the urethral externally. This creates a red, tender, fleshy halo surrounding the meatus. The caruncle tissue may not sufficiently epithelialize to tolerate external exposure and can be easily irritated, although many women with caruncles are asymptomatic.

Pelvic relaxation. Earlier investigators hypothesized that problems such as cystoceles, rectoceles, and uterine prolapse might be caused or worsened by lack of estrogen. Similarly, since genuine stress incontinence tends to worsen after menopause, low estrogen levels were blamed for this problem. Today, however, we recognize that estrogen deficiency does not cause these problems. Postmenopausal hormone therapy does not cure incontinence,[81] and may even increase the risk.[147] Topical estrogen (creams, rings, suppositories) is often used to treat atrophy because it results in low serum levels of estrogen. For example, a cystocele that protrudes from the vagina can become easily eroded as it rubs against the labia when a woman walks. Locally applied estrogen can help thicken the epithelium and reduce erosion. Estrogen used with vaginal pessaries can reduce the incidence of friction erosions in the vault. Finally, pre-treatment of the vagina with local estrogen is used to improve the outcome of postmenopausal surgical repair.

OSTEOPENIA, OSTEOPOROSIS, AND FRACTURE

In the 5 to 6 years following a woman's last menses, her bone mineral density (BMD) decreases at the fastest rate in her life. Each year, a recently menopausal woman can lose 4% to 8% of her trabecular BMD and 1% to 2% of cortical BMD. The rate of bone loss decreases after that time. Unless she takes measures, virtually every woman is at risk for becoming osteopenic or even osteoporotic if she lives long enough. Lifetime bone loss is about 35% of cortical bone and 50% of trabecular bone.[82]

Over half of U.S. women over age 50 studied in the NHANES III study had osteoporosis or osteopenia.[83] African-American women had the lowest rates of osteopenia and osteoporosis (28% and 8%), while non-Hispanic white women had the highest rates (42% and 17%), and Mexican-American women were intermediate (37% and 13%). Low BMD puts a woman at a higher risk for bone fracture. The most common fracture among women under 65 is wrist or forearm fracture, which usually results when women extend their arms to try to break falls when they slip. Later in life, women can experience spontaneous vertebral crush fractures, which not only create painful spinal deformities, but also result in the loss of mobility, loss of height, and increases in respiratory problems as well as abdominal protrusion. The average American woman loses more than 1 inch of height after menopause; each inch represents 2.5 vertebral fractures.

The most serious fracture site is the hip. Women with osteopenia have a doubled risk for hip fracture compared to women with normal BMD, and women with osteoporosis have a nearly 9-fold increased risk.[84] A 70-year-old woman who suffers a hip fracture faces an added 8% to 18% increase in mortality above her baseline risk during the 6 months following fracture. One year after the hip fracture, only 50% of the survivors that age are healed; 25% are dependent on family members for care and the remaining 25% are living in nursing homes. Older women have even worse outcomes. Hip fracture is the second most common reason older women are placed in nursing homes, exceeded only by Alzheimer's disease.

Prevention Measures

Bone health measures should begin early in life. Weight-bearing exercise in moderation is critical to initiate the skeletal remodeling process. Smoking cessation is important, as is moderation in alcohol use. Adequate calcium intake at all ages is needed to provide the building blocks to build new bone. Menopausal women not using estrogen treatment require 1200 mg of calcium a day; those taking hormones need only 1000 mg. The typical American diet is deficient in calcium; therefore, most women require daily supplements. Calcium should be taken with food to maximize absorption. People who live above latitude 52°, where the ultraviolet B radiation is filtered by the earth's atmosphere, require vitamin D supplementation with 400 to 800 IU/day during October to March. Elderly women everywhere and women who are housebound or unable to synthesize vitamin D may routinely need vitamin D supplementation. Smoking worsens the state of vitamin D in postmenopausal women.[148] One placebo-controlled, British trial in which people age 15 to 85 were mailed 100,000 IU Vitamin D or placebo every 4 months for 5 years showed a 22% overall reduction in all fracture risk and a 33% lower rate for fracture of the hip, wrist or forearm, or vertebra.[85]

Offer prophylactic measures to all menopausal women, even women who enter menopause with robust bone. Therapies to prevent osteoporosis are most effective when initiated early in menopause, because the goal is to preserve the maximum BMD to prevent fractures.[86,87] In addition to recommending adequate intake of calcium and vitamin D and smoking cessation, advise exercise to increase muscle strength, balance and bone architecture. To help prevent older women from falling, recommend home safety improvements such as removing loose rugs, rerouting wiring out of the pathways, installing lights over all stairways, and ensuring that all porches and stairways have guardrails. Avoid prescribing treatments that create problems such as hypotension or dizziness. The role of hip protectors is questionable.

Screening

There is still no clear consensus about screening recommendations for osteoporosis. The National Osteoporosis Foundation (NOF) recommends that all caucasian women over age 65, women who have experienced at least one fracture, and post-menopausal women with other risk factors (see Table 5-1) should be screened.[88] Few data are available for other groups of women. Other sets of risk factors have been tested and found to be slightly superior to the NOF list in predicting bone mineral loss.[89] However, regardless of the list of risk factors used, only half of women with osteoporosis will be identified on the basis of risk factors.[84]

Dual-energy X-ray absorptiometry (DEXA) is the most specific and sensitive screening approach for measuring BMD. Ultrasound scans of the calcaneus also play a role in screening.[149] Women found to have osteopenia/osteoporosis on ultrasound should be referred for DEXA scans for confirmation. X-rays are not sensitive enough to detect early signs of bone loss.

Table 5-1   Risk factors for osteoporosis and related fractures in Caucasian postmenopausal women

MAJOR RISK FACTORS
- Personal history of fracture as an adult
- History of fragility fracture in a first-degree relative
- Low body weight (< 127 lbs)
- Current smoking
- Use of oral corticosteroid therapy for more than 3 months

ADDITIONAL RISK FACTORS
- Impaired vision
- Estrogen deficiency at an early age (< 45 yrs)
- Dementia
- Poor health/frailty
- Recent falls
- Low calcium intake (lifelong)
- Low physical activity
- Alcohol in amounts > 2 drinks per day

MEDICAL CONDITIONS THAT MAY BE ASSOCIATED WITH AN INCREASED RISK OF OSTEOPOROSIS

AIDS/HIV	Insulin-dependent diabetes mellitus
Amyloidosis	Lymphoma and leukemia
Ankylosing spondylitis	Malabsorption syndromes
Chronic obstructive pulmonary disease	Mastocytosis
Congenital porphyria	Multiple myeloma
Cushing's syndrome	Multiple sclerosis
Eating disorders (e.g., anorexia nervosa)	Pernicious anemia
Female athlete triad	Rheumatoid arthritis
Gastrectomy	Severe liver disease, especially primary
Gaucher's Disease	biliary cirrhosis
Hemochromatosis	Spinal cord transsection
Hemophilia	Sprue
Hyperparathyroidism	Stroke (CVA)
Hypogonadism, primary and secondary	Thalassemia
(e.g., amenorrhea)	Thyrotoxicosis
Hypophosphatasia	Tumor secretion of parathyroid
Idiopathic scoliosis	hormone-related peptide
Inadequate diet	Weight loss
Inflammatory Bowel Disease	

DRUGS THAT MAY BE ASSOCIATED WITH REDUCED BONE MASS IN ADULTS

Aluminum	Immunosuppressants
Anticonvulsants (phenobarbital,	Lithium
phenytoin)	Long-term heparin use
Cytotoxic drugs	Progesterone, parenteral, long-acting
Glucocorticosteroids and	Supraphysiologic thyroxine doses
adrenocorticotropins	Tamoxifen (premenopausal use)
Gonadotropin-releasing hormone agonists	Total parenteral nutrition

Source: Physician's Guide to Prevention and Treatment of Osteoporosis (2003).

The DEXA T score compares a woman's BMD to the average BMD of women in the peak years of BMD. If a woman's T score is between 1 and 2.5 standard deviations below normal, she has osteopenia. Osteoporosis is defined as a BMD at least 2.5 standard deviations below normal.

The DEXA Z score compares a given woman's BMD to the BMD of aged-matched controls. A low Z score requires a work-up for acute bone loss (e.g. hyperparathyroidism, Paget's disease, etc.). A postmenopausal woman should not be reassured by a normal Z score; it means that she has lost as much bone as other women her age, not that she has healthy bone.

Treatment of Osteoporosis

The medications listed in Table 5-2 have proven effective in preserving bone mineral density. Treatment is generally recommended for post-menopausal women with no risk factors whose T scores are below -2.0 and women with one or more risk factors with T scores below -1.5,[88] as well as for post-menopausal women with vertebral or hip fracture, regardless of T scores.

Estrogens, bisphosphonates, and SERMs reduce fracture risk. Five years of estrogen therapy, with or without progestins, reduced the risk of vertebral fractures by 50% to 80% and reduced the incidence of non-vertebral fracture by 25%; by 10 years, EPT reduced hip fracture rates in one study by nearly 75%.[90] Although one analysis found that the EPT impact on fracture was greatest in women under age 60, the WHI demonstrated a 39% reduction in hip fractures with EPT[91] and ET[150] among women with a median age of 63.2 at enrollment.

Alendronate (a bisphosphonate) prevents vertebral and non-vertebral (including hip) fractures in women with established osteoporosis, and also in women with osteopenia. Once-a-week dosing has made this a first-line therapy. Risedronate is a newer bisphosphonate that has proven to be effective in reducing both vertebral and non-vertebral fractures in osteoporotic postmenopausal women.[92]

Both biphosphonates reduce vertebral fractures by over 40% and hip fractures by 40% to 50% in three-year chemical trials. Safety and efficacy with alendronate have been shown for up to 10 years of use.[151] Biphosphonates provide residual protection; 1 year after discontinuation, there was not loss of BMD. Both agents also demonstrate synergy with HT use.[93]

The SERM, raloxifene, increases BMD, decreases bone turnover, and reduces vertebral fracture rates by 49% in 4 years of use by osteopenic women without inducing any increase in the risk of endometrial cancer.[94] A secondary analysis of breast cancer in osteoporotic women treated with raloxifene showed a decrease in the risk of breast cancer; comparative RCTs are currently studying this possible application.[97] Because of short study times, there is currently no evidence that raloxifene reduces the risk of hip fracture although BMD may improve in the hip.[95-96]

Calcitonin and parathyroid hormone are used only for the treatment, not prevention, of osteoporosis.[98] Despite early interest in statins to protect bone, subsequent studies failed to find any protection against bone loss.[99,152] Androgens added to estrogen not only decrease osteoclast activity to decrease bone resorption, but also stimulate osteoblast activity to promote more bone mineralization. Testosterone therapy increased bone strength and resistance to mechanical stress as well as increasing BMD. DHEA, 50 mg, increased total and lumbar spine BMD.[100]

Table 5-2 Bone mineralization medications

Drug	Dose
Prophylaxis	
Estrogens with or without progestin	CEE equivalent 0.3 – 1.25 mg/day
Alendronate[a,b]	5 mg daily or 35 mg weekly
Risedronate[b]	5 mg daily
Raloxifene	60 mg daily
Therapy (established osteoporosis)	
Alendronate[a]	10 mg daily or 70 mg weekly
Risedronate	5 mg daily
Raloxifene	60 mg daily
Calcitonin	200 IU daily intranasally; 100 IU/daily subcutaneous or IM
Teriparatide (parathyroid hormone)	20 mcg daily subcutaneous

a. Studies show that addition of estrogen increases BMD above levels seen with bisphosphonate therapy.
b. Risedronate is approved for prophylaxis (prevention) of osteoporosis only for corticosteroid-induced osteoporosis. It is approved for the treatment of osteoporosis of any etiology.

COLORECTAL CANCER: IMPACTS OF HT

Colon cancer is the third leading cause of cancer deaths in U.S. women. Screening with 3 fecal occult blood samples annually and colonoscopy every 5 to 10 years is important in disease detection. High-risk women may need more frequent tests. HT has been shown to reduce the risk of colorectal cancer. In the WHI, EPT users had a hazard ratio of 0.63 (0.43 – 0.92) in 5 years of study, but ET users had no protection.[91] These results are consistent with earlier observations from the Nurses Study that demonstrated that current users of hormone therapy had a statistically significant reduction in the risk of colorectal cancer and large adenoma development.[101] The magnitude of these benefits is similar to the reductions that would be realized if women underwent routine colonoscopy as recommended. However, EPT did not reduce colon cancer mortality.[153]

COGNITION: IMPACTS OF HT

Cognition requires multiple mental processes, including attention, perception, working memory, executive function, learning, and memory. Over time, the function of each of these processes is affected by natural aging, disease, drugs, sleep deprivation, and hormonal changes. Dementia is a significant decline in memory accompanied by a decline in at least one other cognitive domain (aphasia, apraxia, agnosia, or disruption in the ability to abstract). The decline must be significant enough to interfere with occupational or social functioning in order to meet diagnostic criteria of dementia.[102]

Women given estrogen in prospective nonrandomized trials had better regional perfusion to the hippocampus and performed better on memory tests.[103,104] Reproductive-aged women who had estrogen production halted by treatment with leuprolide acetate depot for 3 months had significant declines in the verbal memory functioning, which was restored when estrogen was added to the GnRH agonist.[105]

The effect of ET on older women is more complex. When estrogen was given to women with Alzheimer's Disease (AD), it did not slow the progression of the disease.[106,107] In older women (mean age 72) tested at baseline and 6 years later, women who were past users of hormone therapy had less decline in scores over time, but current users experienced the same declines as never users.[108] A prospective study done in Cache County, Utah, similarly showed that women who had previously used hormone therapy for 10 years had the lowest risk of developing AD, but current hormone therapy users, even women who had used hormone therapy for more than a decade, showed no protection against AD.[109]

In the largest RCT to date, the Women's Health Initiative Memory Studies (WHIMS) of women over age 65, the risk of developing probable dementia was doubled in the EPT group versus controls; however, all the statistically significant increased risk was found in women over age 75.[110] This finding verified that starting EPT in elderly women increases the risk of all-cause dementia, especially vascular dementia. There was no evidence that EPT increased the risk of developing mild cognitive impairment. In a parallel study, WHIMS showed that EPT given to women over age 65 did not improve global cognitive function as measured by the modified mini mental state exam (MMMSE). In fact, twice as many EPT users as placebo users suffered a significant decline (> 2 standard deviations) in their scores.[111]

At this time, we can make the following conclusions:

1. Providing EPT to older (> 75 years) women increases their risk of developing dementia.

2. There is no evidence of any improvement in global cognitive function in older (> 65 years) women started on EPT and some suggestion of adverse effects.

3. Younger women should not take EPT to reduce their risk of developing dementia, but there is no evidence that EPT increases their risk of AD later in life.

During the clinical RCT of fracture rates in women treated for 3 years with the SERM raloxifene or placebo, the cognitive test scores of participants were studied in a secondary analysis. The raloxifene group tended to have a lower risk of decline on tests of attention and verbal delayed recall although overall scores of cognition were not different.[112]

RISKS AND SIDE EFFECTS OF POSTMENOPAUSAL HORMONAL THERAPY

Table 5-3 shows hazards ratios from the WHI study of a population of women whose average age was 63 years.

Table 5-3 Women's Health Initiative (WHI) results

	EPT		ET	
	Hazard Ratio	95% CI	Hazard Ratio	95% CI
CHD	1.29	1.02–1.63	0.91	0.75–1.12
Stroke	1.31[1]	1.02–1.68[1]	1.39	1.10–1.77
Thrombosis	2.11	1.58–2.82	1.33	0.99–1.79
DVT	2.07	1.44–2.87	1.47	1.08–2.08
PE	2.13	1.39–3.25	1.34	0.87–2.06
Invasive breast cancer	1.26[2]	1.00–1.59[2]	0.77	0.59–1.01
Colorectal cancer	0.63	0.43–0.92	1.08	0.75–1.53
Hip fractures	0.66	0.45–0.96	0.61	0.41–0.91
Vertebra fractures	0.66	0.44–0.96	0.62	0.42–0.93
Total mortality				

1 Estimate updated Wassertheil-Smoller S, et al (2003).[114]
2 No increase in risk was seen in women who had never used HT prior to study enrollment

Modified from: Rossouw JE (2002),[91] WHI Study Group (2004).[151]

Cardiovascular Risks

After years of observational study data suggesting ET and EPT use reduced reduction in the risk and morbidity of MI in EPT users, the results of the randomized clinical trials showing an increase in risk of MI during the first 12 to 18 months of use were initially quite surprising.[91] ET had no protective effect on coronary heart disease.[151] As a result, the National Institutes of Health, the FDA, the American Heart Association, and other leading organizations have all advised that clinicians not suggest to patients that EPT and ET reduces a woman's risk of CVD. All women seem to be at risk for this early increased risk of MI associated with EPT initiation, but women with elevated LDL may be at even higher risk.[113]

VTE and Stroke Risk

The risk of stroke with HT use increased progressively with duration of study. Over the complete study periods, EPT users had 31% more risk of stroke than non-users, and ET users had a hazard ratio of 1.39 (RR 1.10–1.77).[114] EPT-associated thromboembolic events (deep vein thrombosis and pulmonary embolus) were in the range anticipated from previous studies (RR 2.11); ET use was associated with a lower risk (RR 1.47).

Uterine Cancer

For women with intact uteri, using estrogen without progestin significantly increases the risk for endometrial hyperplasia and cancer. In the 3-year PEPI study, women randomized to receive only estrogen were more likely to develop simple, complex, or atypical hyperplasia, compared to women receiving HT.[115] Metaanalysis of long-term epidemiologic studies has found a relative risk of 2.3 (95% CI 2.1 -2.5), about 1 additional woman in 1,000, for endometrial cancer in women with uteri who use ET.[116] Women who have undergone endometrial ablation are also at risk, because there remain isolated islands of residual endometrial tissue.

The increased risk for endometrial cancer can be reduced if the estrogen is supplemented with cyclic[117] or continuous progestin.[118] The WHI found no increase in risk for uterine cancer with EPT use for up to 5 years of use compared to placebo.[119] Progestin can be given cyclically (at least 12 to 14 days per month), continuously (with daily estrogen), in a pulsed pattern (combined with estrogen for 3 days, then removed for 3 days),[120] or by an independent route (progestin-releasing IUS). Less frequent dosing of progestin (such as every 3 to 4 months) may not provide the same protective effect on the endometrium as do the more conventional therapies. For example, one study found that women who had withdrawal periods only quarterly had a 1.5% rate of hyperplasia compared to a baseline rate of 0.9%.[121]

Breast Cancer

Breast cancer is the second most common cancer that occurs in postmenopausal women (after skin cancer) and the second most frequent cause of cancer deaths (after lung cancer). A Caucasian women's risk for developing breast cancer increases every year she lives until she is age 80; her lifetime risk will approach 12.5%. Risks are somewhat lower among African American women.

Risk Assessment and Prophylactic Treatment

Calculate each individual woman's risk. In most cases, use the Gail model (available at http://bcra.nci.nih.gov/brc/start.htm) to estimate the patient's 5-year and lifetime risks for developing breast cancer. The Gail model is not appropriate for estimating risk in high-risk women or unscreened women. Discuss chemoprophylaxis with high-risk women. Tamoxifen 20 mg per day for 5 years reduced the risk of developing breast cancer by 49% in women with a 5-year risk greater than 1.66%.[122] Prophylaxis with this agent is most appropriate in premenopausal women who are less likely to be at risk for endometrial cancer or venous thromboembolism. The International Breast Cancer Intervention Study (IBIS) raised concerns about prophylaxis in postmenopausal women because older women experienced higher total mortality rates on tamoxifen.[123] Other agents that may reduce the risk of breast cancer, such as raloxifene and aromatase inhibitors, are in clinical trials now.

Hormone Exposure and Risk of Breast Cancer

Many factors link development of breast cancer to sex steroids. Factors that reduce a woman's lifetime exposure to hormones reduce her risk for breast cancer: early menopause, bilateral oophorectomy, and the use of antiestrogens (tamoxifen). Women who undergo early menarche or late menopause are at higher than average risk for developing breast cancer, as are women with the higher than average endogenous levels of estrogen production. Hormone exposure may act indirectly by increasing cell proliferation or by increasing the chances that a mutant cell line might emerge. It is therefore not surprising that continuing a woman's exposure to estrogen and progestin for longer periods of time into the post-menopausal years might increase her risk of breast cancer.

In the WHI study, long-term use (> 5 years) of estrogen with progestins increased a woman's risk of developing invasive breast cancer but not ductal carcinoma in situ (DCIS).[124] In the WHI, EPT users with diagnosed breast cancer were more likely to have more advanced (i.e., regional or metastatic) and larger (1.7 cm vs 1.5 cm) cancers than women using placebo (25.4% vs 16.0%). The observational Million Women Study (England) reported that even a few months of EPT use increased the risk of developing breast cancer as well as breast cancer mortality.[125] However, in the WHI study, EPT use for less than 5 years did not increase the risk of invasive cancer. Several studies suggest that EPT use, particularly continuous EPT use, blocks the natural decrease in breast density in the early years of menopause or may even increase density in older women, both of which would diminish mammographic sensitivity. The WHI also found that EPT users were more likely to have abnormal mammograms than women taking placebo, thus requiring more follow-up.[124]

Advise patients of the following:

- Short-term use of EPT has not been shown to increase the risk of breast cancer;[126] use for more than 5 years has been associated with an increased risk. Estrogen alone does not increase risk.
- The absolute risk a woman faces when using EPT depends upon her baseline risk. The 8 excess invasive cancers per 10,000 women per year reported in the WHI reflect the older age of women in that study (63.2 years old on average). Over the same period of use, fewer 50-year-old women would get breast cancer as a result of EPT use.
- In long-term clinical trials, the increase in breast cancer risk induced by EPT had disappeared within 2 to 4 years after the hormone was stopped.
- Mammographic density returns to baseline within 2 to 4 weeks of stopping EPT.[127] Periodic vacations from EPT prior to mammography may be helpful in maintaining the sensitivity of the screening.

Early short-term studies of women given EPT after breast cancer did not show any increased risk in the development of a second breast cancer.[128–130]

However, a large prospective study was cancelled because the recurrence rates were higher in cancer survivors using hormone.[154] Caution is advised when considering ET/EPT for these women.[131]

Other Health Risks

The current use of hormones increases the risk of gallbladder disease by 2 to 3 times (for all women, not just those at high risk). One observational study indicated an increased risk of ovarian cancer in EPT users compared to non-users,[132] but the WHI has reported no statistically significant increase (RR 1.58; CI 0.77-3.24).[119]

SIDE EFFECTS OF HT

Irregular Spotting and Bleeding

Most menopausal women who begin cyclic HT experience regular withdrawal bleeding, which they often find undesirable.[133] Combined continuous formulations of hormone treatments were designed to reduce this bothersome event. However, over one-third of women using continuous HT at conventional doses experienced breakthrough bleeding during the first 3 months. Lower dose HT achieves cumulative amenorrhea faster than conventional doses.[134]

Other Side Effects

Breast tenderness is a common side effect of ET and EPT. Slowing the introduction of hormones (e.g., one-half dose every 3 days, then increasing frequency of use, and then increasing doses) can reduce this problem. Generally, mastalgia resolves, but some women may benefit from significantly lower dose therapy or may need weekend "holidays" to control their breast symptoms. Some women experience nausea; taking estrogen transdermally may help. Headaches, bloating, and fatigue are other issues that can arise in hormone users. Try changing doses, formulations, or route of administration.

CONTRAINDICATIONS TO POSTMENOPAUSAL HORMONE THERAPY

Product labeling lists the following conditions as contraindications to menopausal estrogen treatment:

- Pregnancy
- Unexplained vaginal bleeding
- Active liver disease; chronic, impaired liver function
- Active thrombophlebitis or thromboembolic disorder
- Carcinoma of the breast
- Known or suspected estrogen-dependent neoplasia

Cautions (relative contraindications) to hormone treatment include seizure disorder, hypertension, familial hyperlipidemia, migraine headache with aura, and gallbladder disease. The risk estrogen may pose for a woman with a history of thrombosis is unknown. Although a history of estrogen-dependent cancer is listed as a contraindication to estrogen treatment, it is unknown whether HT use increases a woman's risk for recurrence of endometrial cancer. The risk of squamous cell cervical carcinoma recurrence is believed to be unaffected by post menopausal hormone therapy. Little is known about the impact on women with a prior history of ovarian cancer.[136] ET could aggravate endometriosis or cause growth of uterine leiomyomata, but in practice, these effects are not commonly clinically significant.

POSTMENOPAUSAL ESTROGEN/PROGESTIN THERAPY CHOICES

Table 5-4 lists the products available for postmenopausal hormone therapy. Today, oral therapies are most frequently used. Conjugated equine estrogen (CEE) has been available for over 40 years and was the formulation studied by the WHI. Estradiol-containing products have been available in the United States for decades and have been used even more extensively in Europe. Ethinyl estradiol (EE), the estrogen used in birth control pills, is being used in some combination hormone treatment products.

Transdermal estrogen (estradiol), which avoids first-pass hepatic effects, has been used for more than a decade and may have less impact on thrombosis.[135] Products containing estrone (E$_1$) and estriol (E$_3$) have been developed, building on the fact that the estrogens are rapidly interconverted, both in the circulation and intracellularly. Compounding pharmacies offer to design specific combinations of the various estrogens for individual women in combinations of 2 or 3 of these basic estrogens. There is no evidence of clinical superiority of these products or even of their clinical equivalence to FDA-approved products, and there is concern that they are being actively promoted for women with contraindications to ET.

Because most postmenopausal women do not want to have monthly cycles, combination estrogen/progestin pills were developed to induce amenorrhea. Combination estrogen and progestin transdermal products are also available.

Topical ET/EPT. Estrogen vaginal cream can be used for treatment of urogenital atrophy—either alone or in combination with systemic hormone therapies. An estradiol-releasing vaginal ring is approved for hot flash reduction as well as urogenital atrophy therapy in hysterectomized women. In the future, estrogen/progestin releasing vaginal rings may be feasible for EPT for women with intact uteri. A percutaneous estrogen cream has been developed for topical application once a day; the slow absorption permits control of vasomotor symptoms. Clinical trials are underway testing the efficacy of percutaneous progestin creams for hot flash control.

Progesterone. Progesterone is needed to provide endometrial protection for women with intact uteri, but it also contributes to symptom relief in combination with estrogen or as a sole agent. Oral progestins, such as medroxyprogesterone acetate, have traditionally been used due to their long half-lives. Micronized progesterone can be used daily, orally or vaginally, with a more favorable impact on high-density lipoprotein (HDL) and glucose tolerance.[137] Some of the progestins from oral contraceptives, such as levonorgestrel, norethindrone, and norgestimate, are being used in products for menopause treatment. The LNG-IUS has been used as the progestin source of progestin-estrogen therapy in postmenopausal women, although this is not an FDA-approved indication and is based on a limited number of small studies.[138] A levonorgestrel-releasing IUS sized for postmenopausal uteri is being tested in Europe. Compounded progesterone creams have been popularized as sole hormone therapies, with very little scientific testing; the NIH is currently investigating the safety and efficacy of these products in clinical trials.

Table 5-4   FDA-Approved Hormone Therapy Prescription Drugs
(Not necessarily approved for these indications)

Generic Name (Description; Source)

Brand Name	Strengths
Oral Estrogen Therapy Products	
Natural conjugated estrogen tablets (estrogen sulfates-estrone, equilin, 17 l-dihydroequilenin and small amounts of other estrogen sulfate esters; blended to match material obtained from pregnant mares' urine)	
Premarin®	0.3, 0.45, 0.625, 0.9, 1.25, 2.5 mg
Synthetic conjugated estrogen tablets	
Cenestin®	0.3, 0.625, 0.9, 1.25 mg
Esterified estrogens tablets (sodium salts of sulfate esters of estrogenic substances of the type excreted by pregnant mares: 75–85% sodium estrone sulfate, 6–15% sodium equilin sulfate)	
Menest®	0.3, 0.625, 1.25, 2.5 mg
Estradiol tablets	
Estrace®	0.5, 1, 2 mg
Gynodiol®	0.5, 1, 1.5, 2 mg
Innofem®	0.5, 1, 2 mg
Estradiol tablets	0.5, 1, 2 mg
Estropipate tablets (prepared from crystalline estrone-estrone sulfate)	
Ogen®	0.625, 1.25, 2.5, 5 mg
Ortho-est®	0.625, 1.25 mg
Estropipate tablets	0.75, 1.5, 3 mg*
Estropipate tablets	0.75, 1.5, 3, 6 mg**
	* Calculated as 0.625, 1.25, 2.5 mg sodium estrone sulfate
	** Calculated as 0.625, 1.25, 2.5, 5 mg sodium estrone sulfate
Ethinyl estradiol tablets	
Estinyl®	0.02, 0.05, 0.5 mg

(continued)

Table 5-4 FDA-Approved Hormone Therapy Prescription Drugs—*(cont'd)*

Generic Name (Description; Source)

Brand Name	Strengths

Oral Combination Hormonal Therapy Products

17ß-estradiol and micronized norgestimate tablets

Prefest®   1 mg estradiol x 3 days and
                    1 mg estradiol + 0.09 mg norgestimate x 3 days

Conjugated estrogens and medroxyprogesterone acetate (MPA) tablets

Premphase®   0.625 Premarin x 14 days and
                    0.625 Premarin + 5 mg MPA x 14 days

Prempro®   0.3, 0.45 Premarin + 1.5 mg MPA or
                    0.625 Premarin + 2.5, 5 mg MPA

Esterified estrogens and androgen tablets (FDA reevaluating approval)

Estratest®   1.25 Estratab + 2.5 mg methyltestosterone

Estratest® H.S. (Half-Strength) 0.625 Estratab + 1.25 mg methyltestosterone

Ethinyl estradiol (EE) and norethindrone acetate (NA) tablets

femhrt®   0.005 mg EE + 1 mg NA

Estradiol and norethindrone acetate (NA) tablets

Activella®   1 mg estradiol + 0.5 mg NA

Oral Progestin Therapy Products

Medroxyprogesterone acetate tablets

Provera®   2.5, 5, 10 mg

Medroxyprogesterone acetate   2.5, 5, 10 mg

Medroxyprogesterone acetate   10 mg

Megestrol acetate oral suspension

Megace®   40 mg

Megestrol acetate   40 mg

Megestrol acetate tablets

Megace®   20, 40 mg

Megestrol acetate   20, 40 mg

Megestrol acetate   40 mg

Norethindrone acetate tablets

Aygestin®   5 mg

Norethindrone acetate   5 mg

Micronized progesterone capsules

Prometrium®   100, 200 mg

Transdermal Estrogen Therapy Products

Matrix estradiol transdermal systems

Alora®   0.025, 0.05, 0.075, 0.1 mg/day, 2/week

Climara®   0.025, 0.0375, 0.05, 0.06, 0.075, 0.1 mg/day, 1/week

Ecslim®   0.025, 0.0375, 0.05, 0.075, 0.1 mg/day, 2/week

Vivelle®   0.025, 0.0375, 0.05, 0.075, 0.1 mg/day, 2/week

Vivelle Dot®   0.0375, 0.05, 0.075, 0.1 mg/day, 2/week

Estradiol   0.05, 0.1 mg/day

(continued)

Table 5-4 FDA-Approved Hormone Therapy Prescription Drugs—*(cont'd)*

Generic Name (Description; Source)

Brand Name	Strengths
Reservoir estradiol transdermal systems	
Estraderm®	0.05, 0.1 mg/day, 2/week
Estradiol topical emulsion	
Estrasorb™	0.75 mg/day
EstroGel™	0.75 mg/day

Transdermal Combination Hormonal Therapy Products

Matrix estradiol (E2)/ norethindrone acetate (NETA) transdermal systems

CombiPatch®	0.05 mg/day E2 + 0.14 mg/day NETA, 2/week or
	0.05 mg/day E2 + 0.25 mg/day NETA, 2/week

Matrix estradiol (E2)/ levonorgestrel (LNG) transdermal system

ClimaraPro	0.045 mg E2/day + 0.015 mg LNG/day, once a week

Vaginal Estrogen Therapy Products

Vaginal creams	
Premarin®	0.625 mg/g natural conjugated estrogen
Ogen®	1.5 mg/g estropipate
Estrace®	0.01% estradiol
Vaginal rings (3 months)	
Estring®	2 mg (0.0075 mg/day) 17 beta-estradiol
Femring®, Menoring®	0.05, 0.1 mg/day estradiol acetate
Vaginal tablets	
Vagifem®	0.025 mg estradiol (estradiol hemihydrate)

Vaginal Progestin Therapy Products

Progesterone vaginal gels	
Crinone®	45 mg (4%), 90 mg (8%)

Injectable Estrogen Therapy Products

Estradiol cypionate injections	
Depo-Estradiol	5 mg/ml, 1-5 mg/3-4 weeks
Estradiol cypionate	5 mg/ml, 1-5 mg/3-4 weeks
Estradiol valerate injections	
Delestrogen®	10, 20, 40 mg/ml
Estradiol valerate	20, 40 mg/ml

Injectable Progestin Therapy Products

Progesterone injections	
Progesterone	50 mg/ml

POSTMENOPAUSAL ANDROGEN THERAPY

Ovarian androgen production slows over the years. A 40-year-old woman has only half the androgen levels than a 20-year old woman has. During the years immediately following menopause, testosterone production varies—a few women have higher levels, most stay relatively stable, and some fall. However, 4 to 5 years into menopause, androgens levels uniformly fall. Much of the early research work on androgens focused on libido. Studies have found that testosterone replacement often increases sexual fantasies and other measures of libido but has no measurable effect on the frequency of intercourse or orgasm. More recently, however, placebo-controlled studies have shown that androgen treatment may also enhance a woman's sense of well-being and energy as measured by standardized indices.[139] Testosterone is also important for bone preservation. Within the bone, some testosterone is converted to estrogen, which reduces osteoclastic activity; testosterone also directly stimulates osteoblastic cells to rebuild bone. Endogenous testosterone levels are especially likely to be low in oophorectomized women and older menopausal women.[140] Today, only one product is available for testosterone treatment, but a matrix transdermal patch for testosterone therapy for postmenopausal women has completed clinical trials.[141] In prescribing androgens, consider the potential adverse impact on lipids.

Studies of the safety and efficacy of dehydroepiandrosterone (DHEA) and related compounds are also underway. One study found that DHEA replacement in elderly women with very low serum DHEAS levels could reverse age-related changes in fat mass, fat-free mass, and BMD.[142] Unfortunately, DHEA is not subject to FDA regulations, so the potency and purity of any given product is not monitored. However, small clinical studies indicate that the maximum dose of DHEA should be limited to 25 mg/day to minimize adverse effects on lipids.

SUMMARY

Emphasize lifestyle issues in promoting long-term health for all perimenopausal and postmenopausal women. Women with menopause symptoms may also want to consider using estrogen or estrogen-progestin treatment. Help the patient make an informed therapeutic choice by weighing the benefits against possible adverse effects and risks.

Provide therapy at the lowest dose for the shortest duration of time needed. Other therapy benefits include a reduced risk of osteoporosis and bone fracture. For women with osteoporosis or osteopenia, both SERMs (raloxifene) and bisphosphonate (alendronate, risedronate) provide BMD protection and have variable but growing data about fracture protection. Bisphosphonates, now with more convenient weekly dosing, provide longer residual protection of the bone, with no decrease in BMD for at least 1 year after discontinuation of therapy. This suggests that a pulsed therapy with "vacations" from medication may be feasible. Exercise and calcium are also essential for bone health.

For women with risk factors for CVD (such as hypertension, diabetes, obesity, hyperlipidemia, elevated C-reactive protein, elevated homocysteine), directed therapies are most appropriate. Consistent use of antihypertensive agents is challenging, but blood pressure normalization extends years of life. Use of ACE inhibitors in appropriate candidates not only reduces stroke and MI risk, but also protects against renal failure. Statins combined with diet and exercise help reduce cardiovascular events. For diabetic women, good glucose control with diet and oral hypoglycemic agents and/or insulin is the healthiest approach and improves longevity as well as quality of years (delayed onset of blindness, renal failure, etc.).

Mental exercise and social connectedness are key recommendations for the mental activity and psychological health of the patient. Advise all women to keep healthy, get involved, stay alert, and keep in contact with others—sage advice to maintaining long-term vivaciousness and quality of life.

REFERENCES

1. Tietze C. Reproductive span and rate of reproduction among Hutterite women. Fertil Steril 1957;8(1):89-97.
2. van Noord-Zaadstra BM, Looman CW, Alsbach H, Habbema JD, te Velde ER, Karbaat J. Delaying childbearing: effect of age on fecundity and outcome of pregnancy. BMJ 1991;302(6789):1361-1365.
3. Bastian LA, Smith CM, Nanda K. Is this woman perimenopausal? JAMA 2003;289:895-902.
4. Soules MR, Sherman S, Parrott E, Rebar, Santoro N, Utian W, Woods N. Executive summary: stages of reproductive aging workshop (STRAW). Fertil Steril 2001; 76:874-878.
5. World Health Organization. Report of a WHO scientific group: Research on the menopause. Geneva: WHO Technical Report Series 670, 1981.
6. Oldenhave A, Jaszmann LJ, Haspels AA, Everaerd WT. Impact of climacteric on well-being. A survey based on 5213 women 39 to 60 years old. Am J Obstet Gynecol 1993;168:772-780.
7. Santoro N, Brown JR, Adel T, Skurnick JH. Characterization of reproductive hormonal dynamics in the perimenopause. J Clin Endocrinol Metab 1996;81(4):1495-1501.
8. Freedman RR. Menopausal hot flashes. In Lobo RA, Kelsey J, Marcus R. Menopause: Biology and Pathobiology. San Diego: Academic Press, 2000:219.
9. Hollander LE, Freeman EW, Sammel MD, Berlin JA, Grisso JA, Battistini M. Sleep quality, estradiol levels, and behavioral factors in late reproductive age women. Obstet Gynecol 2001;98:391-397.
10. Kaunitz AM. Oral contraceptive use in menopause. Am J Obstet Gynecol 2001; 185 (2 Suppl): 532-537.
11. Buchner DM. Physical activity and quality of life in older adults. JAMA 1997;277:64-66.
12. Henshaw SK. Unintended pregnancy in the United States. Fam Plann Perspect 1998;30:24-29, 46.
13. Gebbie AE, Glasier A, Sweeting V. Incidence of ovulation in perimenopausal women before and during hormone replacement therapy. Contraception 1995;52:221-222.
14. Kuohung W, Borgatta L, Stubblefield P. Low-dose oral contraceptives and bone mineral density: an evidence-based analysis. Contraception 2000;61(2):77-82.
15. Rebar RW. Premature ovarian failure. In Lobo RA, Kelsey J, Marcus R. Menopause: Biology and Pathobiology. San Diego: Academic Press, 2000:142.
16. de Bruin JP, Bovenhuis H, van Noord PA, Pearson PL, van Arendonk JA, te Velde ER, Kuurman WW, Dorland M. The role of genetic factors in age at natural menopause. Hum Reprod 2001;16:2014-2018.

17. Burger HG, Dudley EC, Hopper JL, Groome N, Guthrie JR, Green A, Dennerstein L. Prospectively measured levels of serum follicle-stimulating hormone, estradiol, and the dimeric inhibins during the menopausal transition in a population-based cohort of women. J Clin Endocrinol Metab 1999;84:4025-4030.

19. Mohyi D, Tabassi K, Simon J. Differential diagnosis of hot flashes. Maturitas 1997;27(3):203-214.

20. Mosca L, Jones WK, King KB, Ouyang P, Redberg RF, Hill MN. Awareness, perception, and knowledge of heart disease risk and prevention among women in the United States. American Heart Association Women's Heart Disease and Stroke Campaign Task Force. Arch Fam Med 2000;9(6):506-515.

21. Anderson RN. Deaths: Leading Causes for 1999. National vital statistics reports; vol 59 no 11. Hyattsville, Maryland: National Center for Health Statistics, 2001. http://www.cdc.gov/nchs/data/nvsr/nvsr49/nvsr49_11.pdf

22. CDC. Major cardiovascular disease (CVD) during 1997-1999 and major CVD hospital discharge rates in 1997 among women with diabetes—United States. MMWR Morb Mortal Wkly Rep 2001;50:948-954.

23. Mosca L, Grundy SM, Judelson D, King K, Limacher M, Oparil S, Pasternak R, Pearson TA, Redberg RF, Smith SC Jr, Winston M, Zinberg S. Guide to Preventive Cardiology for Women. AHA/ACC Scientific Statement Consensus panel statement. Circulation 1999;99:2480-2484.

24. Mosca L, Appel LJ, Benjamin EJ, Berra K, Chandra-Strobos N, Fabunmi RP, et al. Evidence-based guidelines for cardiovascular disease prevention in women. Circulation 2004;109:672-693.

25. Executive Summary of The Third Report of The National Cholesterol Education Program (NCEP) Expert Panel on Detection, Evaluation, And Treatment of High Blood Cholesterol In Adults (Adult Treatment Panel III). JAMA 2001;285:2486-2497.

26. Kushi LH, Fee RM, Folsom AR, Mink PJ, Anderson KE, Sellers TA. Physical activity and mortality in postmenopausal women. JAMA 1997;277:1287-1292.

27. Pope SK, Sowers MF, Welch GW, Albrecht G. Functional limitations in women at midlife: the role of health conditions, behavioral and environmental factors. Womens Health Issues 2001;11:494-502.

28. Kronenberg F. Hot flashes: epidemiology and physiology. Ann N Y Acad Sci 1990; 592:52-86; discussion 123-133.

29. Molnar GW. Body temperatures during menopausal hot flashes. J Appl Physiol 1975;38:499-503.

30. Baker A, Simpson S, Dawson D. Sleep disruption and mood changes associated with menopause. J Psychosom Res 1997;43(4):359-369.

31. Kronenberg F, Cote LJ, Linkie DM, Dyrenfurth I, Downey JA. Menopausal hot flashes: thermoregulatory, cardiovascular, and circulating catecholamine and LH changes. Maturitas 1984;6(1):31-43.

32. Phillips SM, Sherwin BB. Effects on memory function in surgically menopausal women. Psychoneuroendocrinology 1992;17:485-495.

33. Greene RA. Estrogen and cerebral blood flow: a mechanism to explain the impact of estrogen on the incidence and treatment of Alzheimer's disease. Int J Fertil Womens Med 2000;45:253-257.

34. Hays J, Ockene JK, Brunner RL, Kotchen JM, Manson JE, Patterson RE, Aragaki AK, Shumaker SA, Brzyski RG, LaCroix AZ, Granek IA, Valanis BG. Effects of estrogen plus progestin on health-related quality of life. N Engl J Med 2003;348:1839-1854.

35. Coope J, Thomson JM, Poller L. Effects of "natural oestrogen" replacement therapy on menopausal symptoms and blood clotting. Br Med J 1975;4:139-143.

36. Derman RJ, Dawood MY, Stone S. Quality of life during sequential hormone replacement therapy—a placebo-controlled study. Int J Fertil Menopausal Stud 1995;40(2):73-78.

37. Greendale GA, Reboussin BA, Hogan P, Barnabei VM, Shumaker S, Johnson S, Barrett-Connor E. Symptom relief and side effects of postmenopausal hormones: results from the Postmenopausal Estrogen/Progestin Interventions Trial. Obstet Gynecol 1998;92:982-988.

38. Utian WH, Shoupe D, Bachmann G, Pinkerton JV, Pickar JH. Relief of vasomotor symptoms and vaginal atrophy with lower doses of conjugated equine estrogens and medroxyprogesterone acetate. Fertil Steril 2001;75:1065-1079.

39. Freedman RR, Woodward S. Behavioral treatment of menopausal hot flushes: evaluation by ambulatory monitoring. Am J Obstet Gynecol 1992;167(2):436-439.
40. Wijma K, Melin A, Nedstrand E, Hammar M. Treatment of menopausal symptoms with applied relaxation: a pilot study. J Behav Ther Exp Psychiatry 1997;28(4):251-261.
41. Laufer LR, Erlik Y, Meldrum DR, Judd HL. Effect of clonidine on hot flashes in postmenopausal women. Obstet Gynecol 1982;60:583-586.
42. Clayden JR, Bell JW, Pollard P. Menopausal flushing: double-blind trial of a non-hormonal medication. Br Med J 1974;1(905):409-412.
43. Hammond MG, Hatley L, Talbert LM. A double blind study to evaluate the effect of methyldopa on menopausal vasomotor flushes. J Clin Endocrinol Metab 1984;58:1158-1160.
44. Jones KP, Ravnikar V, Schiff I. A preliminary evaluation of the effect of lofexidine on vasomotor flushes in post-menopausal women. Maturitas 1985;7(2):135-139.
45. Freedman RR, Dinsay R. Clonidine raises the sweating threshold in symptomatic but not in asymptomatic postmenopausal women. Fertil Steril 2000;74(1):20-23.
46. Loprinzi CL, Kugler JW, Sloan JA, Mailliard JA, LaVasseur BI, Barton DL, Novotny PJ, Dakhil SR, Rodger K, Rummans TA, Christensen BJ. Venlafaxine in management of hot flashes in survivors of breast cancer: a randomised controlled trial. Lancet 2000;356:2059-2063.
47. Stearns V, Isaacs C, Rowland J, Crawford J, Ellis MJ, Kramer R, Lawrence W, Hanfelt JJ, Hayes DF. A pilot trial assessing the efficacy of paroxetine hydrochloride (Paxil) in controlling hot flashes in breast cancer survivors. Ann Oncol 2000;11:17-22.
48. Loprinzi CL, Sloan JA, Perez EA, Quella SK, Stella PJ, Mailliard JA, Halyard MY, Pruthi S, Novotny PJ, Rummans TA. Phase III Evaluation of Fluoxetine for Treatment of Hot Flashes. J Clin Oncol 2002;20:1578-1583.
49. Lebherz TB, French L. Nonhormonal treatment of the menopausal syndrome. A double-blind evaluation of an autonomic system stabilizer. Obstet Gynecol 1969;33:795-799.
50. Bergmans MG, Merkus JM, Corbey RS, Schellekens LA, Ubachs JM. Effect of Bellergal Retard on climacteric complaints: a double-blind, placebo-controlled study. Maturitas 1987;9(3):227-234.
51. Loprinzi CL, Michalak JC, Quella SK, O'Fallon JR, Hatfield AK, Nelimark RA, Dose AM, Fischer T, Johnson C, Klatt NE, et al. Megestrol acetate for the prevention of hot flashes. N Engl J Med 1994;331:347-352.
52. Albertazzi P, Pansini F, Bonaccorsi G, Zanotti L, Forini E, De Aloysio D. The effect of dietary soy supplementation on hot flushes. Obstet Gynecol 1998;91:6-11.
53. Simon J, Klaiber E, Wiita B, Bowen A, Yang HM. Differential effects of estrogen-androgen and estrogen-only therapy on vasomotor symptoms, gonadotropin secretion, and endogenous androgen bioavailability in postmenopausal women. Menopause 1999;6:138-146.
54. Sarrel PM. Psychosexual effects of menopause: role of androgens. Am J Obstet Gynecol 1999;180:S319-324.
55. Albertazzi P, Di Micco R, Zanardi E. Tibolone: a review. Maturitas. 1998;30:295-305.
56. Guttuso T Jr, Kurlan R, McDermott MP, Kieburtz K. Gabapentin's effects on hot flashes in postmenopausal women: a randomized controlled trial. Obstet Gynecol 2003;101:337-345.
57. Taylor M. Alternatives to conventional hormone replacement therapy. Contemp Ob/GYN 1999 May:23-50.
58. Hudson T. Managing perimenopausal symptoms: an integrative medicine approach. The Female Patient 2001;26:33-40.
59. Upmalis DH, Lobo R, Bradley L, Warren M, Cone FL, Lamia CA. Vasomotor symptom relief by soy isoflavone extract tablets in postmenopausal women: a multicenter, double-blind, randomized, placebo-controlled study. Menopause 2000;7(4):236-242.
60. Brzezinski A, Adlercreutz H, Shaoul R, Rösler A, Shmueli A, Tanos V, and Schenker JG. Short-term effects of phytoestrogen-rich diet on postmenopausal women. Menopause 1997;4:89-94
61. St Germain A, Peterson CT, Robinson JG, Alekel DL. Isoflavone-rich or isoflavone-poor soy protein does not reduce menopausal symptoms during 24 weeks of treatment. Menopause 2001;8:17-26.

62. Han KK, Soares JM Jr, Haidar MA, de Lima GR, Baracat EC. Benefits of soy isoflavone therapeutic regimen on menopausal symptoms. Obstet Gynecol 2002;99:389-394.
63. Nagata C, Takatsuka N, Kawakami N, Shimizu H. Soy product intake and hot flashes in Japanese women: results from a community-based prospective study. Am J Epidemiol 2001;153:790-793.
64. Teede HJ, Dalais FS, Kotsopoulos D, Liang YL, Davis S, McGrath BP. Dietary soy has both beneficial and potentially adverse cardiovascular effects: a placebo-controlled study in men and postmenopausal women. J Clin Endocrinol Metab 2001;86:3053-3060.
65. Baber R, Templeman C, Morton T, et al. Randomized, placebo-controlled trial of an isoflavone supplement and menopausal symptoms in women. Climacteric 1999;2:85-92.
66. Knight D, Howes J, Eden J. The effect of Promensil, an isoflavone extract, on menopausal symptoms. Climacteric 1999;2:79-84.
67. Taylor M. Botanicals: medicines and menopause. Clin Obstet Gynecol 2001;44: 853-863.
68. McKenna DJ, Jones K, Humphrey S, Hughes K. Black cohosh: efficacy, safety, and use in clinical and preclinical applications. Altern Ther Health Med 2001;7(3):93-100.
69. Chenoy R, Hussain S, Tayob Y, O'Brien PM, Moss MY, Morse PF. Effect of oral gamolenic acid from evening primrose oil on menopausal flushing. BMJ 1994;308(6927):501-503.
70. Hirata JD, Swiersz LM, Zell B, Small R, Ettinger B. Does dong quai have estrogenic effects in postmenopausal women? A double-blind, placebo-controlled trial. Fertil Steril 1997;68:981-986.
71. Wiklund IK, Mattsson LA, Lindgren R, Limoni C. Effects of a standardized ginseng extract on quality of life and physiological parameters in symptomatic postmenopausal women: a double-blind, placebo-controlled trial. Swedish Alternative Medicine Group. Int J Clin Pharmacol Res 1999;19(3):89-99.
72. Emmert DH, Kirchner JT. The role of vitamin E in the prevention of heart disease. Arch Fam Med 1999;8(6):537-542.
73. Barton DL, Loprinzi CL, Quella SK, Sloan JA, Veeder MH, Egner JR, Fidler P, Stella PJ, Swan DK, Vaught NL, Novotny P. Prospective evaluation of vitamin E for hot flashes in breast cancer survivors. J Clin Oncol 1998;16:495-500.
74. Fugh-Berman A, Kronenberg F. Red clover (Trifolium pratense) for menopausal women: current state of knowledge. Menopause 2001;8(5):333-337.
75. Oldenhave A, Jaszmann LJ, Haspels AA, Everaerd WT. Impact of climacteric on well-being. A survey based on 5213 women 39 to 60 years old. Am J Obstet Gynecol 1993;168(3 Pt 1):772-780.
76. Polo-Kantola P, Erkkola R, Helenius H, Irjala K, Polo O. When does estrogen replacement therapy improve sleep quality? Am J Obstet Gynecol 1998;178(5): 1002-1009.
77. Soares CN, Almeida OP, Joffe H, Cohen LS. Efficacy of estradiol for the treatment of depressive disorders in perimenopausal women: a double-blind, randomized, placebo-controlled trial. Arch Gen Psychiatry 2001;58(6):529-534.
78. Rosen RC, Taylor JF, Leiblum SR, Bachmann GA. Prevalence of sexual dysfunction in women: results of a survey study of 329 women in an outpatient gynecological clinic. J Sex Marital Ther 1993;19(3):171-188.
79. Sarrel PM. Sexuality and menopause. Obstet Gynecol 1990;75(4 Suppl):26S-30S; discussion 31S-35S.
80. Hextall A, Cardozo L. The role of estrogen supplementation in lower urinary tract dysfunction. Int Urogynecol J Pelvic Floor Dysfunct 2001;12:258-261.
81. Zullo MA, Oliva C, Falconi G, Paparella P, Mancuso S. Efficacy of estrogen therapy in urinary incontinence. A meta-analytic study. Minerva Ginecol 1998;50:199-205.
82. Riggs BL, Melton LJ 3rd. Involutional osteoporosis. N Engl J Med 1986;314:1676-1686.
83. Looker AC, Orwoll ES, Johnston CC Jr, Lindsay RL, Wahner HW, Dunn WL, Calvo MS, Harris TB, Heyse SP. Prevalence of low femoral bone density in older U.S. adults from NHANES III. J Bone Miner Res 1997;12:1761-1768.

84. Siris ES, Miller PD, Barrett-Connor E, Faulkner KG, Wehren LE, Abbott TA, Berger ML, Santora AC, Sherwood LM. Identification and fracture outcomes of undiagnosed low bone mineral density in postmenopausal women: results from the National Osteoporosis Risk Assessment. JAMA 2001;286:2815-2822.

85. Trivedi DP, Doll R, Khaw KT. Effect of four monthly oral vitamin D3 (cholecalciferol) supplementation on fractures and mortality in men and women living in the community: randomised double blind controlled trial. BMJ 2003;326:469.

86. Lindsay R, Cosman F. Estrogen in prevention and treatment of osteoporosis. Ann N Y Acad Sci 1990;592:326-333; discussion 334-345.

87. Torgerson DJ, Bell-Syer SE. Hormone replacement therapy and prevention of nonvertebral fractures: a meta-analysis of randomized trials. JAMA 2001;285:2891-2897.

88. Physician's Guide to Prevention and Treatment of Osteoporosis. Washington DC: National Osteoporosis Foundation, 2003. http://www.nof.org/professionals/clinical/ clinical.htm

89. Cadarette SM, Jaglal SB, Murray TM, McIsaac WJ, Joseph L, Brown JP. Evaluation of decision rules for referring women for bone densitometry by dual-energy x-ray absorptiometry. JAMA 2001;286:57-63.

90. Cauley JA, Seeley DG, Ensrud K, Ettinger B, Black D, Cummings SR. Estrogen replacement therapy and fractures in older women. Study of Osteoporotic Fractures Research Group. Ann Intern Med 1995;122:9-16.

91. Rossouw JE, Anderson GL, Prentice RL, LaCroix AZ, Kooperberg C, Stefanick ML, Jackson RD, Beresford SA, Howard BV, Johnson KC, Kotchen JM, Ockene J. Risks and benefits of estrogen plus progestin in healthy postmenopausal women: principal results from the Women's Health Initiative randomized controlled trial. JAMA 2002;288:321-333.

92. Harris ST, Watts NB, Genant HK, McKeever CD, Hangartner T, Keller M, Chesnut CH 3rd, Brown J, Eriksen EF, Hoseyni MS, Axelrod DW, Miller PD. Effects of risedronate treatment on vertebral and nonvertebral fractures in women with postmenopausal osteoporosis: a randomized controlled trial. Vertebral Efficacy With Risedronate Therapy (VERT) Study Group. JAMA 1999;282:1344-1352.

93. Ettinger MP. Aging bone and osteoporosis: strategies for preventing fractures in the elderly. Arch Intern Med 2003;163:2237-2246.

94. Ettinger B, Black DM, Mitlak BH, Knickerbocker RK, Nickelsen T, Genant HK, Christiansen C, Delmas PD, Zanchetta JR, Stakkestad J, Gluer CC, Krueger K, Cohen FJ, Eckert S, Ensrud KE, Avioli LV, Lips P, Cummings SR. Reduction of vertebral fracture risk in postmenopausal women with osteoporosis treated with raloxifene: results from a 3-year randomized clinical trial. Multiple Outcomes of Raloxifene Evaluation (MORE) Investigators. JAMA 1999;282(7):637-645.

95. Prestwood KM, Gunness M, Muchmore DB, Lu Y, Wong M, Raisz LG. A comparison of the effects of raloxifene and estrogen on bone in postmenopausal women. J Clin Endocrinol Metab 2000;85:2197-2202.

96. Umland EM, Rinaldi C, Parks SM, Boyce EG. The impact of estrogen replacement therapy and raloxifene on osteoporosis, cardiovascular disease, and gynecologic cancers. Ann Pharmacother 1999;33:1315-1328.

97. Cummings SR, Eckert S, Krueger KA, Grady D, Powles TJ, Cauley JA, Norton L, Nickelsen T, Bjarnason NH, Morrow M, Lippman ME, Black D, Glusman JE, Costa A, Jordan VC. The effect of raloxifene on risk of breast cancer in postmenopausal women: results from the MORE randomized trial. Multiple Outcomes of Raloxifene Evaluation. JAMA 1999;281:2189-2197.

98. Downs RW Jr, Bell NH, Ettinger MP, Walsh BW, Favus MJ, Mako B, Wang L, Smith ME, Gormley GJ, Melton ME. Comparison of alendronate and intranasal calcitonin for treatment of osteoporosis in postmenopausal women. J Clin Endocrinol Metab 2000;85:1783-1788.

99. van Staa TP, Wegman S, de Vries F, Leufkens B, Cooper C. Use of statins and risk of fractures. JAMA 2001;285:1850-1855.

100. Villareal DT, Holloszy JO, Kohrt WM. Effects of DHEA replacement on bone mineral density and body composition in elderly women and men. Clin Endocrinol (Oxf) 2000;53:561-568.

101. Grodstein F, Martinez ME, Platz EA, Giovannucci E, Colditz GA, Kautzky M, Fuchs C, Stampfer MJ. Postmenopausal hormone use and risk for colorectal cancer and adenoma. Ann Intern Med 1998;128:705-712.
102. American Psychiatric Association. Diagnostic and Statistical Manual of Mental Disorders 4th Ed Washington DC APA 1994.
103. Maki PM, Resnick SM. Longitudinal effects of estrogen replacement therapy on PET cerebral blood flow and cognition. Neurobiol Aging 2000;21(2):373-383.
104. Resnick SM, Maki PM, Golski S, Kraut MA, Zonderman AB. Effects of estrogen replacement therapy on PET cerebral blood flow and neuropsychological performance. Horm Behav 1998;34(2):171-182.
105. Sherwin BB, Tulandi T. "Add-back" estrogen reverses cognitive deficits induced by a gonadotropin-releasing hormone agonist in women with leiomyomata uteri. J Clin Endocrinol Metab 1996;81(7):2545-2549.
106. Henderson VW, Paganini-Hill A, Miller BL, Elble RJ, Reyes PF, Shoupe D, McCleary CA, Klein RA, Hake AM, Farlow MR. Estrogen for Alzheimer's disease in women: randomized, double-blind, placebo-controlled trial. Neurology 2000;54(2):295-301.
107. Mulnard RA, Cotman CW, Kawas C, van Dyck CH, Sano M, Doody R, Koss E, Pfeiffer E, Jin S, Gamst A, Grundman M, Thomas R, Thal LJ. Estrogen replacement therapy for treatment of mild to moderate Alzheimer disease: a randomized controlled trial. Alzheimer's Disease Cooperative Study. JAMA 2000;283(8):1007-1015.
108. Matthews K, Cauley J, Yaffe K, Zmuda JM. Estrogen replacement therapy and cognitive decline in older community women. J Am Geriatr Soc 1999;47(5):518-523.
109. Zandi PP, Carlson MC, Plassman BL, Welsh-Bohmer KA, Mayer LS, Steffens DC, Breitner JC; Cache County Memory Study Investigators. Hormone replacement therapy and incidence of Alzheimer disease in older women: the Cache County Study. JAMA 2002;288(17):2123-2129.
110. Shumaker SA, Legault C, Rapp SR, Thal L, Wallace RB, Ockene JK, Hendrix SL, Jones BN 3rd, Assaf AR, Jackson RD, Kotchen JM, Wassertheil-Smoller S, Wactawski-Wende J; WHIMS Investigators. Estrogen plus progestin and the incidence of dementia and mild cognitive impairment in postmenopausal women: the Women's Health Initiative Memory Study: a randomized controlled trial. JAMA 2003;289(20):2651-2662.
111. Rapp SR, Espeland MA, Shumaker SA, Henderson VW, Brunner RL, Manson JE, Gass ML, Stefanick ML, Lane DS, Hays J, Johnson KC, Coker LH, Dailey M, Bowen D; WHIMS Investigators. Effect of estrogen plus progestin on global cognitive function in postmenopausal women: the Women's Health Initiative Memory Study: a randomized controlled trial. JAMA 2003;289(20):2663-2672.
112. Yaffe K, Krueger K, Sarkar S, Grady D, Barrett-Connor E, Cox DA, Nickelsen T; Multiple Outcomes of Raloxifene Evaluation Investigators. Cognitive function in postmenopausal women treated with raloxifene. N Engl J Med 2001;344(16):1207-1213.
113. Manson JE, Hsia J, Johnson KC, Rossouw JE, Assaf AR, Lasser NL, Trevisan M, Black HR, Heckbert SR, Detrano R, Strickland OL, Wong ND, Crouse JR, Stein E, Cushman M; Women's Health Initiative Investigators. Estrogen plus progestin and the risk of coronary heart disease. N Engl J Med 2003;349(6):523-534.
114. Wassertheil-Smoller S, Hendrix SL, Limacher M, Heiss G, Kooperberg C, Baird A, Kotchen T, Curb JD, Black H, Rossouw JE, Aragaki A, Safford M, Stein E, Laowattana S, Mysiw WJ; WHI Investigators. Effect of estrogen plus progestin on stroke in postmenopausal women: the Women's Health Initiative: a randomized trial. JAMA 2003;289(20):2673-2684.
115. PEPI Trial Writing Group. Effects of hormone replacement therapy on endometrial histology in postmenopausal women. The Postmenopausal Estrogen/Progestin Interventions (PEPI) Trial. JAMA 1996;275:370-375.
116. Grady D, Gebretsadik T, Kerlikowske K, Ernster V, Petitti D. Hormone replacement therapy and endometrial cancer risk: a meta-analysis. Obstet Gynecol 1995;85: 304-313.
117. Persson I, Yuen J, Bergkvist L, Schairer C. Cancer incidence and mortality in women receiving estrogen and estrogen-progestin replacement therapy—long-term follow-up of a Swedish cohort. Int J Cancer 1996;67:327-332.
118. Weiderpass E, Adami H-O, Baron JA, Magnusson C, Bergstrom R, Lindgren A, Correia N, Persson I. Risk of endometrial cancer following estrogen replacement with and without progestins. J Natl Cancer Inst 1999;91:1131-1137.

119. Anderson GL, Judd HL, Kaunitz AM, Barad DH, Beresford SA, Pettinger M, Liu J, McNeeley SG, Lopez AM; Women's Health Initiative Investigators. Effects of estrogen plus progestin on gynecologic cancers and associated diagnostic procedures: the Women's Health Initiative randomized trial. JAMA 2003;290(13):1739-1748.

120. Casper RF. Regulation of estrogen/progestogen receptors in the endometrium. Int J Fertil Menopausal Stud 1996;41:16-21.

121. Ettinger B, Selby J, Citron JT, Vangessel A, Ettinger VM, Hendrickson MR. Cyclic hormone replacement therapy using quarterly progestin. Obstet Gynecol 1994; 83(5 Pt 1):693-700.

122. Fisher B, Costantino JP, Wickerham DL, Redmond CK, Kavanah M, Cronin WM, Vogel V, Robidoux A, Dimitrov N, Atkins J, Daly M, Wieand S, Tan-Chiu E, Ford L, Wolmark N. Tamoxifen for prevention of breast cancer: report of the National Surgical Adjuvant Breast and Bowel Project P-1 Study. J Natl Cancer Inst 1998; 90:1371-1388.

123. IBIS investigators. First results from the International Breast Cancer Intervention Study (IBIS-I): a randomised prevention trial. Lancet 2002;360:817-824.

124. Chlebowski RT, Hendrix SL, Langer RD, Stefanick ML, Gass M, Lane D, Rodabough RJ, Gilligan MA, Cyr MG, Thomson CA, Khandekar J, Petrovitch H, McTiernan A; WHI Investigators. Influence of estrogen plus progestin on breast cancer and mammography in healthy postmenopausal women: the Women's Health Initiative Randomized Trial. JAMA 2003;289(24):3243-3253.

125. Beral V; Million Women Study Collaborators. Breast cancer and hormone-replacement therapy in the Million Women Study. Lancet 2003;362(9382):419-427.

126. Li CI, Malone KE, Porter PL, Weiss NS, Tang MT, Cushing-Haugen KL, Daling JR. Relationship between long durations and different regimens of hormone therapy and risk of breast cancer. JAMA 2003;289(24):3254-3263.

127. Colacurci N, Fornaro F, De Franciscis P, Mele D, Palermo M, del Vecchio W. Effects of a short-term suspension of hormone replacement therapy on mammographic density. Fertil Steril 2001;76(3):451-455.

128. DiSaia PJ, Grosen EA, Kurosaki T, Gildea M, Cowan B, Anton-Culver H. Hormone replacement therapy in breast cancer survivors: a cohort study. Am J Obstet Gynecol 1996;174:1494-1498.

129. O'Meara ES, Rossing MA, Daling JR, Elmore JG, Barlow WE, Weiss NS. Hormone replacement therapy after a diagnosis of breast cancer in relation to recurrence and mortality. J Natl Cancer Inst 2001;93:754-762.

130. Brewster WR, DiSaia PJ, Grosen EA, McGonigle KF, Kuykendall JL, Creasman WT. An experience with estrogen replacement therapy in breast cancer survivors. Int J Fertil Womens Med 1999;44(4):186-192.

131. Chlebowski RT, McTiernan A. Elements of informed consent for hormone replacement therapy in patients with diagnosed breast cancer. J Clin Oncol 1999; 17(1):130-142.

132. Rodriguez C, Patel AV, Calle EE, Jacob EJ, Thun MJ. Estrogen replacement therapy and ovarian cancer mortality in a large prospective study of US women. JAMA 2001;285:1460-1465.

133. den Tonkelaar I, Oddens BJ. Preferred frequency and characteristics of menstrual bleeding in relation to reproductive status, oral contraceptive use, and hormone replacement therapy use. Contraception 1999;59:357-362.

134. Archer DF, Dorin M, Lewis V, Schneider DL, Pickar JH. Effects of lower doses of conjugated equine estrogens and medroxyprogesterone acetate on endometrial bleeding. Fertil Steril 2001;75(6):1080-1087.

135. Scarabin PY, Oger E, Plu-Bureau G. Differential association of oral and transdermal oestrogen-replacement with venous thromboembolism risk. Lancet 2003;362:428-432.

136. Guidozzi F, Daponte A. Estrogen replacement therapy for ovarian carcinoma survivors: A randomized controlled trial. Cancer 1999;86:1013-1018.

137. The Writing Group for the PEPI Trial. Effects of estrogen or estrogen/progestin regimens on heart disease risk factors in postmenopausal women. The Postmenopausal Estrogen/Progestin Interventions (PEPI) Trial. JAMA 1995;273(3):199-208.

138. Andersson K, Mattsson LA, Rybo G, Stadberg E. Intrauterine release of levonorgestrel—a new way of adding progestogen in hormone replacement therapy. Obstet Gynecol 1992;79:963-967.

139. Shifren JL, Braunstein GD, Simon JA, Casson PR, Buster JE, Redmond GP, Burki RE, Ginsburg ES, Rosen RC, Leiblum SR, Caramelli KE, Mazer NA. Transdermal testosterone treatment in women with impaired sexual function after oophorectomy. N Engl J Med 2000;343:682-688.

140. Simon JA. Safety of estrogen/androgen regimens. J Reprod Med 2001;46:281-290.

141. Mazer NA. Testosterone deficiency in women: etiologies, diagnosis, and emerging treatments. Int J Fertil Womens Med 2002;47(2):77-86.

142. Villareal DT, Holloszy JO, Kohrt WM. Effects of DHEA replacement on bone mineral density and body composition in elderly women and men. Clin Endocrinol (Oxf) 2000;53:561-568.

143. Penotti M, Fabio E, Modena AB, Rinaldi M, Omodei U, Vigano P. Effect of soy-derived isoflavones on hot flushes, endometrial thickness, and the pulsatility index of the uterine and cerebral arteries. Fertil Steril. 2003;79(5):1112-1117

144. Nikander E, Kilkkinen A, Metsa-Heikkila M, Adlercreutz H, Pietinen P, Tiitinen A, Ylikorkala O. A randomized placebo-controlled crossover trial with phytoestrogens in treatment of menopause in breast cancer patients. Obstet Gynecol. 2003;101(6): 1213-1220

145. Setchell KD, Brown NM, Desai PB, Zimmer-Nechimias L, Wolfe B, Jakate AS, Creutzinger V, Heubi JE. Bioavailability, disposition, and dose-response effects of soy isoflavones when consumed by healthy women at physiologically typical dietary intakes. J Nutr. 2003;133(4):1027-1035

146. Cicinelli E, Di Naro E, De Ziegler D, Matteo M, Morgese S, Galantino P, Brioschi PA, Schonauer A. Placement of the vaginal 17beta-estradiol tablets in the inner or outer one third of the vagina affects the preferential delivery of 17beta-estradiol toward the uterus or periurethral areas, thereby modifying efficacy and endometrial safety. Am J Obstet Gynecol. 2003;189(1):55-58

147. Grodstein F, Lifford K, Resnick NM, Curhan GC. Postmenopausal hormone therapy and risk of developing urinary incontinence. Obstet Gynecol. 2004;103(2): 254-260

148. Valimaki MJ, Laitinen KA, Tahtela RK, Hirvonen EJ, Risteli JP. The effects of transdermal estrogen therapy on bone mass and turnover in early postmenopausal smokers: a prospective, controlled study. Am J Obstet Gynecol. 2003;189(5):1213-1220

149. Khaw KT, Reeve J, Luben R, Bingham S, Welch A, Wareham N, Oakes S, Day N. Prediction of total and hip fracture risk in men and women by quantitative ultrasound of the calcaneus: EPIC-Norfolk prospective population study. Lancet. 2004;363(9404):197-202

150. Women's Health Initiative Steering Committee. Effects of conjugated equine estrogen in postmenopausal women with hysterectomy: the Women's Health Initiative randomized controlled trial. JAMA. 2004;291(14):1701-1712

151. Bone HG, Hosking D, Devogelaer JP, Tucci JR, Emkey RD, Tonino RP, Rodriguez-Portales JA, Downs RW, Gupta J, Santora AC, Liberman UA; Alendronate Phase III Osteoporosis Treatment Study Group. Ten years' experience with alendronate for osteoporosis in postmenopausal women. N Engl J Med. 2004;350(12):1189-1199

152. LaCroix AZ, Cauley JA, Pettinger M, Hsia J, Bauer DC, McGowan J, Chen Z, Lewis CE, McNeeley SG, Passaro MD, Jackson RD. Statin use, clinical fracture, and bone density in postmenopausal women: results from the Women's Health Initiative Observational Study. Ann Intern Med. 2003;139(2):97-104

153. Chlebowski RT, Wactawski-Wende J, Ritenbaugh C, Hubbell FA, Ascensao J, Rodabough RJ, Rosenberg CA, Taylor VM, Harris R, Chen C, Adams-Campbell LL, White E; Women's Health Initiative Investigators. Estrogen plus progestin and colorectal cancer in postmenopausal women. N Engl J Med. 2004;350(10):991-1004

154. Holmberg L, Anderson H; HABITS steering and data monitoring committees. Related Articles, Links HABITS (hormonal replacement therapy after breast cancer—is it safe?), a randomised comparison: trial stopped. Lancet. 2004;363(9407): 453-455

Menstrual Problems and Common Gynecologic Concerns

Anita L. Nelson, MD

- Take a systems approach when evaluating menstrual problems:
  - For primary amenorrhea, determine the status of uterine and breast development;
  - For secondary amenorrhea, start with progestin-challenge test after pregnancy has been excluded;
  - For dysfunctional uterine bleeding, rule out all other causes first.
- About 3% to 10% of reproductive-age women in the United States have endometriosis. Nearly 25% to 35% of infertile women have endometriosis.
- Pelvic masses are fairly common; the relative frequencies of different types of masses changes with a woman's age. Rule out ectopic pregnancy immediately.
- As many as 50% of married couples experience some sexual dissatisfaction, but few women present sexually related complaints to their health care providers.

Reproductive health care providers help women with a wide range of gynecologic problems in conjunction with providing family planning services. Many of these problems, including sexually transmitted infections (STIs) and vulvovaginitis, are addressed in other chapters. This chapter focuses on menstrual cycle disorders and some of the more common gynecologic problems such as breast and vulvar lesions, pelvic masses, endometriosis, and sexual dysfunction. Contraceptive methods often serve dual purposes of providing contraception and relieving troublesome symptoms.

MENSTRUAL PROBLEMS

During their reproductive years, women frequently experience disorders in menstrual cycling such as excessive bleeding, infrequent bleeding, or painful menses. In addition, even normal menstrual cycling can be associated with other problems such as premenstrual syndrome (PMS) and menstrual migraine.

DYSMENORRHEA

Dysmenorrhea, Greek for painful menstruation, is classified as primary (intrinsic and usually of early onset) or secondary (due to some other physical cause and usually of later onset). In a study of young women attending a family planning clinic, 72% of those surveyed reported having experienced dysmenorrhea; for 15%, the symptoms were severe enough to interfere with their normal activities.[1]

In addition to painful uterine cramping with menses, many women with dysmenorrhea also experience nausea, vomiting, diarrhea, headaches, or lightheadedness. Symptoms may vary in severity from cycle to cycle but generally continue throughout the reproductive years. Dysmenorrhea can be an incapacitating problem, causing significant disruption each month. Young women lose days at school, and older women are hampered at home and in the workplace.

Primary Dysmenorrhea: Etiology

Primary dysmenorrhea has physiologic, not psychological, causes. Despite the fact that early investigators held that dysmenorrhea occurred in "maladjusted women who were intensely rejecting their feminine role and suffered from deep hostility,"[2] it is understood today that the problem is not in the woman's head but in her uterus. Measurements with intrauterine catheters demonstrate that women with primary dysmenorrhea generate intrauterine pressures similar to those seen during the second stage of labor.[3–5]

Women with primary dysmenorrhea are generally ovulatory and thus produce progesterone in the luteal phase. Progesterone stimulates the production of prostaglandins in the base of the endometrium. When the endometrium sloughs, women with primary dysmenorrhea have been found to produce excessive amounts of prostaglandins,[6] which increase the force of uterine contractions. These contractions reduce uterine blood flow, causing ischemia and intensifying pain. In addition, intermediates in the production of prostaglandins (e.g., cyclic endoperoxides) in the presence of high prostaglandin levels can directly cause pain. When injected into the general circulation by uterine contractions, prostaglandins can also precipitate systemic symptoms such as headache, nausea, vomiting, and diarrhea. Other etiologies of primary dysmenorrhea, such as structural abnormalities of the uterus (blind horns), cervix (stenotic os), or vagina (transverse septa), usually present with amenorrhea or can usually be ruled out by a careful pelvic examination.

Primary Dysmenorrhea: Therapies

Symptomatic therapies include rest, applying a heating pad, or taking teas or over the counter medications to treat the discomfort. Usually, however, women seeking medical care have already tried these measures without success and are in need of therapies targeted to treat the pathophysiology underlying their complaints. Two complementary objectives are to reduce the thickness of the endometrial lining and to reduce prostaglandin production.

Endometrial thinning. Hormonal therapies reduce the thickness of the endometrium, the amount of blood loss, and the production of prostaglandins.[7] Combination oral contraceptives (OCs) generally decrease menstrual blood flow at least 40% within 3 months when used in cyclic fashion. Within 3 to 4 months of beginning oral contraceptive therapy, 90% of women experience marked decreases in the severity of pain.[7,9,10] Oral contraceptive formulations with a higher ratio of progestin to estrogen are more effective in thinning the endometrium than are formulations with a more estrogenic balance.[9] Women can achieve additional relief with OCs by reducing their number of withdrawal bleeds, thereby reducing the number of days of discomfort each year. Continuous use of active pills for 6 weeks (eliminating the placebo pills in the first of two packages) or for 9 weeks (eliminating the placebo pills in the first two sequential packages) can be very helpful.[11] These approaches, referred to as "bicycling" and "tricycling," use only monophasic pill formulations. (See Chapter 19 on Combined Hormonal Contraceptive Methods.) Ultimately, continuous OC use can be to prevent menses for prolonged intervals with no known adverse impacts. Depot-medroxyprogesterone acetate (DMPA) is also helpful in treating dysmenorrhea. After their third injection, nearly half of DMPA users become amenorrheic and avoid dysmenorrhea altogether. The levonorgestrel-releasing intrauterine system (LNG-IUS, manufactured by Berlex) is also an excellent choice for women with dysmenorrhea because, after initial months of frequent spotting and bleeding, users 12 months have a 70% to 90% reduction in menstrual blood loss and enjoy a marked reduction of dysmenorrhea. Extended use of other combined hormonal methods, such as the hormonal contraceptive patch or vaginal ring, are under investigation and are expected to be both safe and effective.

Other medications are also available to achieve amenorrhea, but their use is limited due to side effects and cost. Danazol, an androgen used to treat endometriosis, effectively induces amenorrhea but can be used for only 4 to 6 months due to androgenic side effects including acne, hirsutism, oily skin, clitoral enlargement, and voice deepening. Gonadotropin releasing hormone (GnRH) agonists, also used for treatment of endometriosis, induce amenorrhea and, therefore, eliminate dysmenorrhea. However, use is also limited to 4 to 6 months because these agents cause hypoestrogenic side effects such as vasomotor symptoms (hot flashes), vaginal dryness, and osteoporosis. GnRH agonists have been combined with estrogen/progestin "add-back" therapy for treating endometriosis, but not for treating primary dysmenorrhea alone.

Prostaglandin inhibition. Prostaglandin synthetase inhibitors such as NSAIDs and COX-2 inhibitors are more effective than placebo in treating dysmenorrhea.[12] Taken at the onset of menses or just prior to menses, NSAIDs reduce prostaglandin release into the menstrual fluid and significantly reduce dysmenorrhea as well as menstrual blood loss.[12] Aspirin is no more effective than placebo and can increase menstrual blood loss.[13]

Rule out other causes of pain in women who fail to respond to these therapies. Some women who have primary dysmenorrhea early in life may subsequently develop other problems, adding to their dysmenorrhea later in life (see secondary dysmenorrhea). Women with persistent complaints may benefit from a psychological evaluation and treatments for chronic pain. Some investigators report that a transcutaneous electrical nerve stimulation (TENS) unit reduces dysmenorrhea. Some investigators have suggested that dietary manipulations such as supplementing omega-3 polyunsaturated fatty acids may decrease dysmenorrhea in adolescents.[14] Surgical interventions including a presacral nerve ablation, endometrial ablation, and hysterectomy are treatments of last resort, reserved for patients who do not respond to medical and other approaches.

Secondary Dysmenorrhea

Women with secondary dysmenorrhea also complain of painful uterine cramping with menses but may have other accompanying complaints, such as dyspareunia or non-menstrual pelvic pain. The pain that women with secondary dysmenorrhea experience is, by definition, due to uterine or pelvic pathology. The most common causes are adenomyosis, endometriosis, and pelvic adhesions. Adenomyosis is the presence of endometrial glands and stroma embedded in the myometrium (the deep muscle layer of the uterus). Adenomyosis, most commonly found in parous women, is thought to develop most frequently during labor. Heavy menses and dyspareunia can also accompany the dysmenorrhea of adenomyosis. Monthly ovarian hormonal swings stimulate this ectopically located endometrium and irritate the surrounding uterus. On examination, women with adenomyosis have enlarged, perhaps somewhat boggy, uteri that tend to be tender during menses. Implantation of endometrial tissue outside the uterus is called endometriosis (see the section on Endometriosis). Women with endometriosis experience painful menses due to the cyclic sloughing of material from the implants and adhesions. Pelvic adhesions from previous pelvic inflammatory disease (salpingitis or tubo-ovarian abscesses), appendicitis, and pelvic or abdominal surgery can also cause dysmenorrhea. Other pelvic pathology, including uterine fibroids, cervical stenosis, and some types of pelvic masses may also cause painful menses. Copper intrauterine devices (IUDs) sometimes are associated with heavier or more uncomfortable menses but are an unusual cause of clinically significant secondary dysmenorrhea.

Full evaluation into the causes of the patient's pain may require diagnostic laparoscopy.

The treatment of secondary dysmenorrhea should be targeted to the underlying problems considering other factors, including the patient's desire for fertility. In the absence of problems requiring surgical intervention, the treatments outlined for primary dysmenorrhea (especially those that eliminate menses) are often at least partially successful for treatment of symptoms of secondary dysmenorrhea. If these interventions are not sufficiently effective, or if there are other issues, such as infertility, more definitive surgical treatments may be needed. For example, secondary dysmenorrhea caused by pelvic scarring may benefit from surgical lysis of adhesions. For women with fibroids, a myomectomy might more effectively reduce menstrual flow and discomfort. Consider more significant therapies such as endometrial ablation and hysterectomy only to treat incapacitating, intractable dysmenorrhea unresponsive to more conservative measures and only for women who do not desire future childbearing.

AMENORRHEA

Amenorrhea, the absence of menses, is also classified as primary or secondary. The workup for primary amenorrhea can begin when there is a lack of any secondary sexual characteristics by age 14, the lack of menses by age 16, or no menses within 2 years after the breasts develop (thelarche) or the appearance of pubic or axillary hair (pubarche or adrenarche). Secondary amenorrhea occurs only in women who have previously menstruated. Technically, secondary amenorrhea is the absence of menses for at least 3 months in a woman who previously has had regular monthly menses and for at least 6 to 12 months in a woman who normally experiences irregular menses. The absence of menses for a shorter period is referred to as "delayed menses."

Begin the evaluation of amenorrhea in a sexually active reproductive-age woman with a pregnancy test. History may be helpful in identifying women at risk for pregnancy, but it is not always reliable. Once you have ruled out pregnancy as a cause of the patient's amenorrhea, the evaluation of amenorrhea further depends upon its classification. Both primary and secondary amenorrhea have a multitude of causes, so take a systematic approach to find answers in a cost-effective manner.

Primary Amenorrhea

Usually the evaluation of primary amenorrhea involves consultation with specialists, but a fundamental understanding of the possible etiologies can be helpful to advise the young patient and her often anxious family. An efficient evaluation of primary amenorrhea relies on two physical findings: the presence of a uterus and breast development (Figure 6-1)[15] in the absence of any male genitalia suggestive of a hermaphrodite.

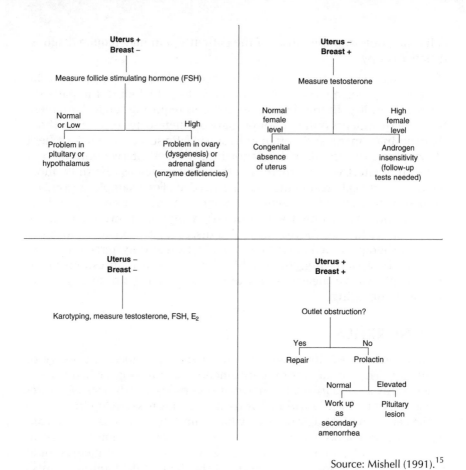

Source: Mishell (1991).[15]

Figure 6-1 Diagnostic evaluation for primary amenorrhea

Uterus present, no breast development. If the patient has a uterus but no breast development, it can be assumed that she is genetically female but that she is not producing estrogen. The problem may reside in her hypothalamus, pituitary, or ovary. A helpful test to distinguish among the causes is her serum level of follicle stimulating hormone (FSH).

- **Low FSH level.** If her FSH is low, her ovaries are not being stimulated and the problem lies in the functioning of her pituitary or hypothalamus. Isolated pituitary failure is extremely rare. Hypothalamic failure can be demonstrated by administering a GnRH stimulation test. If the patient responds to GnRH stimulation by making FSH and luteinizing hormone (LH), she proves that her pituitary can function and that her problem is at the hypothalamic level. The problem may be primary failure or result from an eating disorder or excessive exercise.

- **Elevated FSH level.** If her FSH is consistently elevated with low estradiol, she has gonadal failure. Genetic causes often underlie gonadal failure: Turner's syndrome, mosaicism, pure gonadal dysgenesis, autoimmune disease or life-threatening 17alpha-hydroxylase deficiency. Occasionally, chemotherapy or radiation treatments for carcinoma early in life can destroy ovarian function. Whatever the cause, once you have confirmed the diagnosis of ovarian failure and counseled the patient about infertility, give her estrogen and progestin therapy to establish female secondary sexual characteristics and to mitigate the effects of hypoestrogenism on her bone. Additional therapy may be needed to control other aspects of her disorder.

Uterus absent, breast development. If a woman has breasts but no uterus, check her serum testosterone levels. If her testosterone levels are within the range for a normal woman, her diagnosis is usually a congenital absence of the uterus. If her levels are in the male range, she may have androgen-resistance syndrome (testicular feminization). Further tests will be needed to confirm that she is genetically 46 XY. However, since she is phenotypically a woman and has been raised as a woman, her sexual identity should not be altered. She needs counseling about her infertility, since she has no uterus and her ovaries are abnormal. Her gonads have a high potential for malignancy; after puberty, she should undergo a gonadectomy and receive hormone therapy.[16]

Uterus absent, no breast development. Women without breasts or uterus need to undergo genetic testing since many of these women have male karyotypes.

Uterus present, breast development. Thirty percent of women with primary amenorrhea have both breasts and uterus. Rule out outlet obstruction such as imperforate hymen, transverse vaginal septa. Also consider pituitary adenoma, even in women without galactorrhea, and other causes commonly found in women with secondary amenorrhea. Evaluate these last women as per secondary amenorrhea.

Secondary Amenorrhea

The absence of menses is an important symptom because it can indicate a serious systemic medical problem or it can represent a problem confined to the reproductive system. Even if a woman does not desire fertility, she must be evaluated because the underlying problem and/or its consequences justify prompt therapy.

Conduct a thorough history and physical examination. Take a careful menstrual history, checking for ovulatory symptoms (mittelschmerz), moliminal complaints (bloating, cramping, or breast changes that typically herald the onset of menses), and any vasomotor symptoms she may be experiencing. Question her about recent changes in weight, dietary habits, acne, hair growth, cold or heat intolerance, galactorrhea, recent pregnancy, genital tract procedures, known medical problems, stress, and exercise patterns. On examination, pay close attention to signs of androgen excess (hirsutism, acne), hypoestrogenism (dry, flattened vaginal mucosa), pro-lactin excess (galactorrhea), or thyroid dysfunction (skin, pulse, and reflex changes). Obtain a complete drug history because many classes of medi-cations (prescription, OTC, or street drugs) can induce amenorrhea or oligomenorrhea. Perform a pregnancy test to rule out pregnancy.

If an obvious reason for the woman's amenorrhea emerges from this initial screening, order specifically targeted diagnostic tests to confirm the diagnosis. For example, if the patient has spontaneous galactorrhea, measure her prolactin and thyroxin stimulating hormone (TSH) levels. A 48-year-old woman who complains of hot flashes and has had no menses for a year needs no specific tests to confirm menopause. A woman using DMPA needs no further workup when she develops amenorrhea in the absence of other symptoms. On the other hand, a 20-year-old woman with a recent onset of hirsutism and amenorrhea will need to have her androgen status evaluated to rule out a tumor.

Frequently, however, no single cause is discovered on the basis of the history and physical examination. Several systematic approaches have been developed by experts in the field, but one particularly cost-effective protocol[17] evaluates the components of the reproductive system in order: uterus and lower genital tract, ovaries, pituitary and hypothalamus (see Figure 6-2).

Uterus and lower genital tract. Evaluation begins with the uterus and lower genital tract. A physical examination will have already ruled out functional blockage of menstrual flow from the vagina such as an imper-forate hymen or transverse septum. (These commonly cause primary amenorrhea, but not secondary amenorrhea.) First test the functional capacity of the uterus and the patency of the lower genital tract with a progestin challenge test. Give the patient medroxyprogesterone acetate 5 milligrams (mg) per day for 10 days.

- If the patient experiences a withdrawal bleed, then it is estab-lished that her cervix is patent, she is producing estrogen, and her endometrium is functioning. She next needs an evaluation of the upper compartments to determine why she is not ovulating and producing progestin (see the next section).

- If she does not experience a withdrawal bleed, she needs a de-tailed evaluation of her uterus and cervix. Check for cervical stenosis by passing a uterine sound or a cervical os finder. Assess the responsiveness of the endometrium by priming her uterus with estrogen (such as conjugated equine estrogen 0.625 mg) for 25 days, adding progestin the last 10 to 12 days.

- If the patient experiences a withdrawal bleed after estrogen/pro-gestin cycling, her endometrium is functioning, and her cervix is patent. Therefore, her higher compartments will need to be tested to determine why she is not making estrogen.

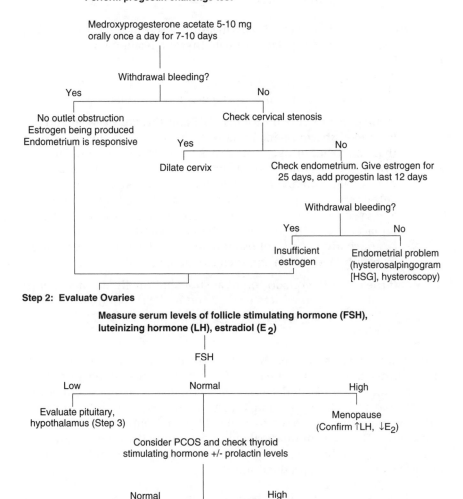

Step 1: Evaluate Uterus and Lower Genital Tract
Perform progestin challenge test

Medroxyprogesterone acetate 5-10 mg
orally once a day for 7-10 days

Withdrawal bleeding?

Yes — No outlet obstruction
Estrogen being produced
Endometrium is responsive

No — Check cervical stenosis

Yes — Dilate cervix

No — Check endometrium. Give estrogen for
25 days, add progestin last 12 days

Withdrawal bleeding?

Yes — Insufficient estrogen

No — Endometrial problem
(hysterosalpingogram
[HSG], hysteroscopy)

Step 2: Evaluate Ovaries

Measure serum levels of follicle stimulating hormone (FSH),
luteinizing hormone (LH), estradiol (E$_2$)

FSH

Low — Evaluate pituitary,
hypothalamus (Step 3)

Normal — Consider PCOS and check thyroid
stimulating hormone +/- prolactin levels

High — Menopause
(Confirm ↑LH, ↓E$_2$)

Normal — Cycle to prevent
hyperplasia

High — Target treatment

Step 3: Evaluate Function of Pituitary Gland and Hypothalamus
Consider imaging. Consider GnRH challenge test.

Source: Modified from Speroff et. al. (1999).[17]

Figure 6-2 Systematic diagnostic evaluation for secondary amenorrhea

- If she does not have withdrawal bleed, she may have a disorder in her uterine lining, such as Asherman's syndrome. She will benefit from direct endometrial evaluation by hysteroscopy or hysterosalpingogram (HSG).

Ovaries. Evaluate the ovaries by measuring serum levels of FSH, LH, and, perhaps, estradiol (E_2), and evaluate thyroid dysfunction by measuring a TSH.

- If her TSH is abnormal, treat her thyroid dysfunction. Re-evaluate her menstrual status after TSH levels have normalized.

- If the patient's gonadotropins (FSH and LH) are elevated and her E_2 is low, she most likely has ovarian failure. If she is younger than 25 years of age, obtain a karyotype to rule out Turner's Syndrome or gonadal dysgenesis. If she is between 25 and 40 years of age, conduct a more detailed evaluation of other possible autoimmune endocrinopathies such as thyroid dysfunction. In any event, treat her as if she were menopausal. Offer sex steroid replacement with hormone therapy, combination hormonal contraceptives, or bisphosphonates to reduce the long-term effects of hypoestrogenism, such as osteoporosis.

- If the patient's gonadotropins are not abnormally elevated, her E_2 is within the reproductive range and her TSH is normal, consider polycystic ovary syndrome (see the section on Polycystic Ovary Syndrome)

Pituitary and hypothalamus. If the gonadotropins are low or normal and no other abnormalities are identified, the patient's pituitary or hypothalamus may be implicated. Draw a prolactin level. If her prolactin levels are elevated into the tumor range (usually above 70 to 100), consider ordering magnetic resonance imaging (MRI) or computerized axial tomography (CT) of the pituitary gland to determine the presence and size of a prolactinoma. Bromocriptine therapy is usually successful in controlling excessive prolactin production.

If there is no evidence of hyperprolactinemia, consider an eating disorder. Eating disorders can disrupt menstrual cycling, even in a woman of normal weight. One study found that 55% of amenorrheic women had an eating disorder.[18] If you suspect an intracranial neoplasia, obtain appropriate imaging studies. A woman who has stress due to extreme exercise, eating disorders, or situational factors should have her underlying problems addressed; she also needs hormonal modulation to maintain adequate estrogen levels to prevent osteoporosis and to protect her endometrium.[19] Young women with hypothalamic amenorrhea have improved bone mineralization when they are given oral contraceptives but not when given medroxyprogesterone or placebo.[8,20] Naltrexone can also be used to treat women with weight-loss-related amenorrhea.[21]

OLIGOMENORRHEA

Oligomenorrhea is appropriately viewed as a being on a continuum between normal, ovulatory cycling and secondary amenorrhea. Many of the causes of amenorrhea can, in milder forms, present as oligomenorrhea. When the interval between a woman's menses exceeds 35 days but is not long enough to qualify as being amenorrhea, she has oligomenorrhea. It is important to identify the etiology of the oligomenorrhea to reduce other consequences of an underlying endocrinopathy or other medical problems and to help improve fertility potential when she is ready to conceive. Most women with oligomenorrhea have anovulatory cycles. Often this menstrual pattern is life-long; many women with polycystic ovary syndrome (PCOS) have consistently irregular and infrequent menses (see the next section). Sometimes oligomenorrhea develops because of excessive weight gain or after significant weight loss.

Medical problems such as hypothyroidism, hyperprolactinemia, and liver dysfunction can cause oligomenorrhea, as can certain medications. Women with stress and those who engage in extreme exercise or excessive dieting often develop oligomenorrhea, which can progress to amenorrhea. Cheerleaders and women involved in seasonal sports may have irregular menses during the months they participate in those activities. In these women, oligomenorrhea results from suppressed estrogen production. Adequate sex steroid levels can be maintained with estrogen-containing contraceptives. On the other hand, women with other causes of oligomenorrhea, such as extreme increases in weight and PCOS usually have excessive amounts of unopposed estrogen. Unopposed estrogen leads to uninterrupted endometrial stimulation and increases the risk for endometrial hyperplasia and carcinoma. These women need a source of progesterone to offset the estrogen stimulation. Cyclic administration of progestin or combined hormonal contraceptives (pills, rings, patches), or endometrial suppression with progestin-only pills, DMPA or the LNG-IUS, are reasonable alternatives. Continuous administration of combination oral contraceptives protects the endometrium without inducing cyclic bleeding.

Polycystic ovary syndrome (PCOS). Previously called Stein-Leventhal syndrome, PCOS is the most frequent cause of oligomenorrhea. It is also the most common endocrinopathy of reproductive aged women. In textbook descriptions, women with PCOS are obese, hirsute, oligomenorrheic, and subfertile. In reality, many women with PCOS are not overweight and many do not have hirsutism.[22] Even its name is not defining; many women with polycystic-appearing ovaries (PAOs) do not have PCOS.[23] The common characteristics of PCOS are hyperandrogenism and chronic anovulation.

The diagnosis of PCOS is usually made clinically. According to the 1990 National Institutes of Health (NIH) consensus conference, a woman with PCOS has anovulatory cycles (either >35 day intervals or fewer than 8 periods a year) with either hyperandrogenism (hirsutism, acne, male pattern balding, clitoromegaly, voice deepening) or hyperandrogenemia (elevated free or total testosterone or elevated DHEAS) in the absence of any other etiology. Therefore, most of the laboratory tests needed to confirm the diagnosis are ones used to rule out other etiologies, such as thyroid dysfunction, adrenal insufficiency, or androgen-producing tumors. Women with hirsutism in particular should have morning levels of 17-hydroxy progesterone measured to rule out adult-onset congenital adrenal hyperplasia (CAH). The newer 2004 Rotterdam PCOs criteria focus on hirsuit women who may have oligomenorrhea and infertility problems. Ultrasound findings of 12 antral follicles are used to support their diagnosis. Older approaches, such as measuring LH/FSH ratios, are not helpful in establishing the diagnosis.

PCOS can result from disruptions in the hypothalamic-pituitary axis, the adrenal glands, and/or the ovary.[24] These dysfunctions cause overproduction of androgens (testosterone and DHEAS), which are responsible for the classic PCOS-related problems such as hirsutism and acne. The excessive androgen levels, paradoxically, also cause relatively high levels of estrogen found in PCOS due to peripheral conversion of androgens to estrone (E_1) in adipose, skin and muscle. Estrone stimulates endometrial proliferation and, simultaneously, suppresses pituitary production of FSH. In the absence of FSH stimulation, ovulation and subsequent luteal progesterone production cease. Endometrial proliferation continues unchecked, resulting in irregular, uncoordinated endometrial sloughing and an increased risk of endometrial cancer. With anovulatory cycles, fertility is also compromised. However, women with PCOS can have ovulatory cycles on an unpredictable, intermittent basis and should not be considered to be protected against unintended pregnancy by their condition.

There are other associated health risks for which women with PCOS should be monitored. Many women with PCOS have insulin resistance, which increases their risk of developing overt diabetes;[26] both obese (BMI >27) and lean PCOS women are at risk, but overweight women are at higher risk. Insulin-like growth factors are produced by the ovary in PCOS, which can contribute to coronary artery disease.[27] Many women with PCOS have unhealthy lipid profiles with high LDL and triglyceride levels; androgenized women with polycystic ovaries have lipid profiles similar to male profiles.[28,29] Both the lipid and insulin abnormalities are independent risk factors for cardiovascular disease.[27,30] Therapy is designed to reduce long-term adverse health consequences of PCOS and to address the patient's immediate complaints. Encourage weight reduction, exercise, and sensible diets to reduce cardiovascular disease risks. Both hyperinsulinemia and hyperandrogenemia in obese women with PCOS can be reduced with a loss of at least 5% of their current weight.[31] Weight distribution is also important. Women with PCOS tend to have more visceral obesity, which is defined by a waist-to-hip ratio greater than 1.2 ("apple shape"), as opposed to gynecoid obesity, with a waist-to-hip ratio less than 0.75 ("pear shape").[32] Hormonal contraceptives with low androgenicity can be used to treat certain aspects of the condition. OCs, patches and vaginal rings with low androgenicity can deal with hirsutism and acne (see below), prevent unopposed endometrial proliferation, and provide contraceptive protection.[33] DMPA or the LNG-IUS can prevent endometrial proliferation and reduce pregnancy risks. Cyclic progestin with 5 mg medroxyprogesterone acetate 12 days each month can reduce the risk of endometrial hyperplasia.

Women with acne or hirsutism may be offered estrogenic oral contraceptives to suppress ovarian production of androgens and increase sex human binding globulin (SHBG). Increases in SHBG reduce serum levels of the biologically active, unbound androgens. With lower circulating levels of androgen, further hair growth is reduced, and sebum production is blocked, which helps reduce future acne outbreaks. Topical agents and antibiotics can be used first line to treat acne or can be combined with OCs to provide better treatment for mild to moderate acne. Continuous OC administration is superior to cyclic oral contraceptive use in controlling LH and testosterone levels.[34] Other indicated therapies to slow the progression of new hair growth include spironolactone or corticosteroids (if adrenal androgen overproduction is implicated by levels of dehydroepiandrosterone sulfate [DHEAS] greater than 75 mg/ml). Studies show that drospirenone-containing OCs are also helpful for acne treatment. Cyproterone acetate-estrogen regimens have been reported to be as effective as spironolactone, although that agent is not available in the United States.[35] Anti-androgens such as flutamide and finasteride, which directly inhibit hair growth without serious side effects, represent a new approach to the treatment of hirsutism in women with PCOS.[36,37] Gonadotropin-releasing agonists with estrogen add-back therapies have also been used to block new hair growth, but this approach is still considered experimental. Some women benefit from bleaching of their facial hair to reduce its visibility. Removal of existing hair by electrolysis or newer laser treatments is also often advocated after new hair growth stimulation has been slowed. The clinical response to any hormonal therapy is usually slow. Maximal oral contraceptive impact on acne was seen at 6 months;[33] however, treatment for hirsutism may not achieve its full potential for 1 to 2 years. There is an important PCOS support group at http://www.pcosupport. org/.

EXCESSIVE OR IRREGULAR UTERINE BLEEDING

Menorrhagia and hypermenorrhea refer to periods that occur at regular intervals but are marked with prolonged bleeding (>7 days) or excessive blood loss (>80 cc). Metrorrhagia is irregular but frequent uterine bleeding of variable amounts. Menometrorrhagia is used to describe prolonged uterine bleeding occurring irregularly. Polymenorrhea is uterine bleeding occurring at short intervals (<21 days). Intermenstrual bleeding is bleeding of variable amounts occurring between regular menses. Postcoital bleeding occurs after sexual intercourse.

The "normal" values for the frequency and duration of menses as well as the amount of blood loss each cycle vary widely (see Table 6-1). A woman's history of her menses may not be clinically accurate. Common pitfalls are that women may report bleeding-free days rather than cycle length measured from first day of bleeding in one cycle to the next. Some women report that their menses occur on exactly the same date each month and become concerned if they have 2 periods in one month even if one starts on the first of the month and the second on the last day. Quantifying actual blood loss may also be quite challenging.[38-40] Estimates derived from numbers of pads or tampons used are complicated by variations in fastidiousness among women. By the time excessive menstrual bleeding causes anemia, a woman has suffered very significant blood loss. At least as important as the absolute numbers of days or amounts of blood loss is any *change* the patient may perceive from what has been established as normal for her. A woman who has historically bled 3 days per cycle and now notices that she bleeds for 6 to 7 days may still be within an arbitrary range for normal, but she merits an evaluation since she is experiencing a significant change from her baseline pattern.

Table 6-1 Range of normal values for menses

	Range	Average
Frequency	21 – 35 days	28 days
Duration	2 – 6 days	4 days
Blood Loss	20 – 80 ml	30 – 35 ml

Causes of excessive uterine bleeding may be classified into several categories to facilitate evaluation (see Table 6-2). Organic gynecologic disease is the first concern when women present with abnormal bleeding. Pregnancy and pregnancy-related complications (e.g., threatened abortion or ectopic pregnancy) and infection of the cervix, endometrium, or fallopian tubes are primary differential diagnoses for sexually active women. Endometrial and cervical polyps and uterine leiomyoma and adenomyosis can cause menorrhagia. Endometrial hyperplasia and carcinoma are often associated with heavy and prolonged menses as well as intermenstrual bleeding. Cervical infection or carcinoma more classically present with postcoital bleeding.

Table 6-2 Etiologies of excessive uterine bleeding

Consider causes
- Obstetrical: pregnancy or pregnancy complications (a sensitive pregnancy test can rule out)
- Medication: phenytoin, anticoagulants, digitalis, unopposed estrogen, copper IUDs
- Systemic diseases: coagulation disorders, endocrinopathies (e.g., thyroid or adrenal disorders); hepatic or renal failure, trauma
- Cervical abnormalities: infection, polyp, cancer, trauma
- Abnormalities: fibroids, infection, hyperplasia, polyp, cancer, adenomyosis
- Dysfunctional uterine bleeding (DUB) = diagnosis of exclusion

Systemic diseases such as thyroid dysfunction, liver cirrhosis, active hepatitis, adrenal hyperplasia, incipient renal failure, and hypersplenism can cause prolonged or heavy menses by altering estrogen metabolism or coagulation factor production. Similarly, women with intrinsic blood dyscrasias such as Von Willebrand's disease, idiopathic thrombocytopenia purpura (ITP), aplastic anemia, or platelet dysfunction often have chronic menorrhagia. Acute problems such as leukemia, severe sepsis, or disseminated intravascular coagulation (DIC) may also induce menorrhagia. Medications such as digitalis, phenytoin, anticoagulants, and plastic and copper IUDs are associated with increased menstrual flow. Heavy menstrual bleeding can result from trauma such as sexual abuse or the presence of a foreign body in the vagina.

Dysfunctional uterine bleeding (DUB) is a diagnosis of exclusion. DUB generally results from anovulatory cycling and usually develops during the extremes of reproductive life—adolescence and perimenopause.[41] Within the first year of menarche, approximately 55% of cycles are anovulatory.[42] Anovulation results in unopposed estrogen stimulation of the endometrium, which produces a thick lining. Without progesterone, there is an uncoordinated endometrial sloughing, an imbalance in prostaglandins, with a relative excess of PGE (the vasodilating prostaglandin) and a relative paucity of PGF_2 (the vasoconstricting prostaglandin). Under these influences, women develop heavy and prolonged bleeding.

Evaluation of Excessive Uterine Bleeding

Take a complete menstrual history, emphasizing the last several months. The age of the patient and the pattern of her bleeding guide the evaluation. Perform pregnancy tests for all reproductive-age women who have abnormal bleeding. If anemia is a concern, determine the patient's hemoglobin or hematocrit. Rule out vaginal and cervical abnormalities (infection, carcinoma, or polyps) by examination, testing as indicated for gonorrhea and chlamydia, and test for cervical cytology, if not done recently. Perform a bimanual examination to rule out cervical motion tenderness, to determine the size and shape of the uterus, and to detect ovarian or adnexal masses. Perform thyroid function tests for women with suggestive signs or symptoms. If a menarcheal woman has bleeding severe enough to require transfusion, evaluate her for blood dyscrasias.[43] Women with a life-long history of heavy and prolonged menses should also be evaluated for Von Willebrand's disease, especially if her female relatives have had prolonged menses. Women with risk factors such as advanced reproductive age (over 35), obesity, or unopposed estrogen exposure from either exogenous sources (medications) or intrinsic sources (PCOS) who present with heavy or new onset irregular menses should have an endometrial biopsy to rule out endometrial hyperplasia or carcinoma. Some practitioners use hysteroscopically-directed biopsy in the initial evaluation of vaginal bleeding, but the technique is more frequently used to evaluate women whose abnormal bleeding persists after endometrial sampling fails to provide a diagnosis.

Treatment of Excessive or Abnormally Timed Uterine Bleeding

Treat any identified problem causing vaginal bleeding, such as infection, polyps, miscarriage, etc. For women with bleeding due to fibroids, initial therapy can be the same as for DUB unless surgery is indicated for other reasons. The treatment for dysfunctional uterine bleeding depends on the severity and acuteness of the problem.

Acute, severe dysfunctional uterine bleeding. Women with significant acute bleeding that causes anemia may need hospitalization. Perform a dilation and curettage (D&C) for any woman who is hypovolemic or hemodynamically unstable. Sample the endometrium if the patient has risk factors for hyperplasia. For other women, a trial of medical therapy is appropriate. The goal in the acute setting is to promptly heal the denuded areas of the endometrium. The drug of choice is estrogen, because it will initiate endometrial proliferation and seal over the active bleeding sites within the uterus. Administer estrogen orally using either high-dose estrogen therapy preparations such as 2.5 mg conjugated equine estrogen or high-dose oral contraceptive preparations with 50 μg ethinyl estradiol 2 to 4 times a day for 1 to 2 days. Success rates for these preparations are comparable, in the 80% to 85% range.[44,45] NSAIDS are useful as adjunctive therapeutic agents in the acute phase.

Bleeding generally stops or dramatically slows after 12 to 24 hours of estrogen therapy. If the patient does not respond promptly to initial estrogen therapy, she should have a diagnostic dilation and curettage. Once the acute bleeding slows, support endometrial growth by adding progestin (typically, medroxyprogesterone acetate 5 mg per day). No additional progestin is needed if OCs were used initially. Taper the hormonal doses rapidly in the following days. Then maintain endometrial suppression by continuing maintenance doses of sex steroids (one OC a day or routine hormone therapy doses) for at least 2 to 3 weeks to allow recovery of normal hemoglobin levels. When the hormonal support is withdrawn, the patient should undergo a coordinated (and, hopefully, limited) endometrial sloughing.

Acute, prolonged but less significant bleeding. For hemodynamically stable women with significantly less bleeding, outpatient therapy with OCs or NSAIDs can be sufficient.[46] The need for endometrial sampling will be determined by the presence of risk factors for endometrial carcinoma and the chronicity of her abnormal bleeding. Methergine has no demonstrated efficacy in controlling uterine bleeding in nonpregnant women.[47]

Long-term medical therapies. After an acute bleeding event, or after a report of prior menorrhagia, the goal is to prevent future bleeding episodes. Therapy depends on the etiology of the woman's dysfunctional uterine bleeding (see Table 6-3) and her desire for future childbearing.

Table 6-3 Characteristics and types of dysfunctional uterine bleeding

Type of DUB	Characteristics	Treatment
Anovulatory (90% of DUB)	• Occurs at extremes of reproductive ages • No moliminal symptoms • Irregular, unpredictable bleeding, sometimes excessive • Underlying problems: — Unopposed estrogen stimulation — Lack of progesterone priming of prostaglandins — Excessive vasodilating prostaglandins	• Cycle endometrium — Oral contraceptives monthly — Cyclic progestin (last 12 days of cycle) • Suppress endometrium — DMPA — Oral contraceptives (bicycling/tricycling) — Danazol — GnRH agonists — Progestin IUS • Provide vasoconstrictive prostaglandins — NSAIDS starting first day of menses x 3 days
Ovulatory (10% of DUB)	• Occurs in peak reproductive years • Bleeding predictable but excessive and prolonged • Bleeding due to imbalance in prostaglandins — Inadequate vasoconstrictive prostaglandins	• Suppress endometrium — Oral contraceptives monthly, bicycling/tricycling — DMPA — Danazol — GnRH agonists — Progestin IUS • Correct prostaglandin imbalances — NSAIDS starting first day of menses x 3 days

- *Medical therapies.* For women with an ongoing problem with anovulatory uterine bleeding as a cause of menorrhagia, prevent a recurrence by pharmacologically inducing cyclic withdrawal bleeding with cyclic combined hormonal contraceptives (pills, patches, or rings) or progestins (medroxyprogesterone 5 mg daily for 10 to12 days each month) or by suppressing her endometrium altogether with progestin only OCs, DMPA, combined continuous OCs, and the LNG-IUS.[48] Women with heavy monthly menses can be started on NSAIDS for the first 3 days of flow each month. Ibuprofen 200 to 400 mg every 4 to 6 hours, mefenamic acid 500 mg initially, and 250 mg every 6 hours, or naproxen 275 mg every 8 hours have all demonstrated efficacy; hormonal contraceptives, including OCs (combined or progestin-only) taken cyclically or continuously, DMPA, and the LNG-IUS, can each be very helpful, significantly reducing menstrual blood loss either as sole agents or combined with hormonal therapies. Women with

Von Willebrand's disease require therapy targeted to their coagulation defect, unless their menses are hormonally eliminated.

- *Surgical therapies.* Many women with significant bleeding undergo a D&C for the immediate control of bleeding as well as for diagnosis. However, the effects of a D&C are only temporary. Initiate medical care to avoid the recurrence of the problem. Other surgical interventions such as endometrial ablation with laser, resectoscope, thermal balloon or roller ball,[49] and hysterectomy are reserved for women who have other pelvic pathology and for those who fail to improve with medical therapy.

MENSTRUALLY INDUCED EXACERBATIONS OF OTHER MEDICAL PROBLEMS

Migraine headaches are quite common, especially in reproductive-age women; approximately 1 in 6 women suffers migraine headaches. Sex steroid hormones have been implicated as a cause of migraines because over two-thirds of adults with migraines are women, and cyclic oral contraceptives may worsen the symptoms or frequency of migraine headaches in 15% to 50% of women. In general, women who have migraines without aura should use combined oral contraceptive pills with caution, and those who have migraines with aura should avoid estrogen-containing contraceptive methods.

However, there is one type of migraine that may be treated with appropriately timed hormonal contraception. Menstrual migraines are a special subset of migraines; they start 2 to 3 days before menses and continue into the menses but occur at no other time. Pure menstrual migraines comprise 7% to 9% of all migraines. In addition, another 35% of women suffer a worsening of migraine symptoms during menses. An intriguing set of experiments demonstrated the causal links between decreases in estrogen levels and the onset of menstrual migraine headaches. Administering estrogens premenstrually delayed the headaches but did not alter menses; in contrast, administering progesterone delayed menses but did not affect headaches.[50] Some investigators have suggested that suppressing ovulation with oral contraceptives may be helpful in blocking estrogen-withdrawal headaches.[51,52] Continuous use of active oral contraceptives may eliminate withdrawal headaches for long stretches of time.[11,53] If the patient desires to have monthly menses, make every cycle a first-day start with combination OCs, patches or rings to minimize the menstrual estrogen withdrawal. Alternatively, severe menstrual migraines have been shown to respond well to treatment with GnRH agonist and estrogen/progestin add-back therapy.[54] DMPA can also be used to reduce estrogen fluctuations.

Nonhormonal treatments for menstrual migraine include NSAIDS or judicious use of narcotics and injectable agents such as dihydroergotamine or sumatriptan. If those fail to treat the pain adequately and the pain keeps a woman from her usual productivity at least 2 days a month, most physicians would recommend preventive therapy. Prophylactic agents include beta blockers (Inderal), calcium channel blockers, and selective anti-depressants. Other important self-help measures include regular physical exercise and avoidance of headache triggers (food and other sensory stimuli). Some women have reported that incipient menstrual migraines can be curtailed by sexual activity and orgasm. The National Headache Foundation maintains a headache hotline at 1-800-843-2256 and a website at www.headaches.org.

Other diseases that worsen with menstrual cycling, such as some seizure disorders, asthma, and Behcet's disease (oral and genital ulcers as well as ophthalmia), may respond to hormonal manipulations.[55] Some women with seizure disorders suffer seizures exacerbated by or occurring only during menses. In the past, authors have suggested that treatment with progestogenic oral contraceptives might be helpful,[56] but little clinical data support these ideas. Oral contraceptives alleviate the symptoms of Behcet's disease in some resistant cases.

Hormonal contraceptive methods to suppress menstrual blood loss can also aid women with anemia caused by sickle cell disease, renal failure, and coagulopathies (such as hemophilia or Von Willebrand's disease). Other women taking medications that increase menstrual blood loss, such as anticoagulants, long-term NSAIDS, and some anticonvulsants, may distinctly benefit from oral contraceptives, DMPA or LNG-IUS to reduce or eliminate monthly drains of their hemoglobin reserves. Adjust the doses of estrogen and progestin for women using anticonvulsants. Women who are anticoagulated by medication or blood dyscrasias also need protection from ovulation, which poses the threat of internal hemorrhage with monthly ovulation.[56,57]

PREMENSTRUAL SYNDROME (PMS)

Premenstrual syndrome (PMS) is a heterogeneous collection of signs and symptoms that share one common characteristic: a temporal relationship to the menstrual cycle. By definition, PMS is the cyclic appearance of at least one symptom prior to menses followed by an entirely symptom-free time starting near the first day of menses. To be considered clinically significant, the problem must be of a magnitude sufficient to affect a woman's work, lifestyle, or interpersonal relationships.[58] The most common symptoms of PMS include abdominal bloating, anxiety, breast tenderness, crying spells, depression, fatigue, irritability, thirst, appetite changes, and edema. Women with PMS rarely have only physical complaints; they also often have behavioral and psychological complaints. A related syndrome called premenstrual dysphoric disorder (PMDD) has been defined by the American Psychiatry Association (see Table 6-4) to focus more on affective disorders of PMS.[59]

About 20% to 30% of women have moderate to severe PMS, and another 1% to 10% have debilitating symptoms.[60] Premenstrual dysphoria affects

3% to 8% of North American women during their reproductive years.[61-63] PMS can increase relationship strain, sexual dysfunction, social isolation, work absenteeism, suicide, and psychotic behavior. Some law courts around the world have accepted PMS as a mitigating factor for criminal behavior and, in some cases, as grounds for a plea of temporary insanity. Many PMS symptoms can persist even after hysterectomy. Women with functioning residual ovaries can experience symptoms, as can women using cyclic post-menopausal hormone therapy.

After a thorough history and a complete examination have ruled out other causes, the key to diagnosing PMS is a prospective charting of symptoms for at least 2 to 3 cycles. A woman who is overwhelmed by a series of complaints should chart only the 3 to 5 complaints that most profoundly bother her. This chart should also include her weight and, if possible, a record of her basal body temperatures. (See Chapter 15 on Fertility Awareness Methods.) No laboratory tests are needed to diagnose PMS although, in some cases, hypothyroidism or other endocrinopathies may need to be ruled out. Panels to measure sex steroid hormonal levels are completely unnecessary,[64] and their use reflects a basic misunderstanding of the underlying pathophysiology of PMS.

Table 6-4 DSM-IV criteria for premenstrual dysphoric disorder (PMDD)

Need at least five symptoms including:

- At least one of the following:
  — Affective lability
  — Persistent and marked anger or irritability
  — Marked anxiety and tension
  — Markedly depressed mood, feeling of hopelessness

- With 1 to 4 of the rest from the following:
  — Decreased interest in usual activities
  — Easy fatigability or marked lack of energy
  — Subjective sense or difficulty in concentration
  — Marked change in appetite
  — Sleep disorders
  — Physical symptoms—breast tenderness, headache, edema, joint or muscle pain, weight gain

Source: American Psychiatric Association (2000).[59]

Carefully study the patterns of the patient's symptoms. Symptoms do not need to reappear with equal intensity in each cycle; different symptoms may occur during different cycles. It is the timing that is critical. PMS symptoms peak in the luteal phase and completely disappear with the onset of menses. For many women, clinical depression and other serious problems worsen premenstrually, but this is not PMS, because those women never have a symptom-free interval.[65] As many as half the women with self-diagnosed PMS have other problems, which require careful evaluation and therapies different from those for PMS.[66] Even women with

PMS-like symptoms verified by daily charting frequently may have underlying or concomitant psychiatric problems. In one study, 59% of women with PMS also had clinical depression or an anxiety disorder.[67]

The cause of PMS is unknown. Early investigators suggested that PMS was due to a lack of progesterone, and many therapies were developed to provide progesterone supplements to women with PMS.[68,69] Subsequent investigations failed to find a difference in any significant hormone levels between PMS sufferers and controls; FSH, LH, estradiol, progestin, prolactin, SHBG, and testosterone were equivalent.[70] Similarly, in placebo controlled studies, women using progesterone supplements did no better than controls.[71] However, women whose symptoms vary from cycle to cycle appear to have variation in the ratio of their ovarian hormones. Researchers have suggested that some women with PMS have a central opioid abnormality resulting in lower beta endorphin levels,[72] although other studies have challenged this hypothesis.[73] PMS sufferers have no deficiencies in magnesium, zinc, vitamin A, vitamin E, thiamine, or vitamin B6; nutritional deficiencies are not a cause of PMS.[74] One investigator found low adrenocorticotropin levels in women with PMS.[75] Other hypotheses include the suggestion that women with PMS have abnormal prostaglandin production, endogenous hormone allergies, or psychosomatic influences.

Increasing evidence suggests that serotonin dysregulation may be important in the pathogenesis of many of the psychological elements in PMS such as tension, irritability, and dysphoria.[76–82] In clinical trials, half of women with premenstrual dysphoria improved with treatment to selectively inhibit the reuptake of serotonin.[83] However, many women did not improve, so serotonin disorders are not an etiology for all PMS sufferers. It is likely that several mechanisms are involved in PMS. Therapy needs to be individualized for each woman's specific problems.

Treatment for PMS

PMS treatment is strongly influenced by a placebo effect. In a wide range of studies, researchers report that 40% to 94% of patients will improve in the short term regardless of the treatment used. This reinforces the need to rely on placebo controlled studies rather than case reports and personal testimonials to determine the true efficacy of a particular drug or treatment for PMS.

Overall, a comprehensive approach to treatment is needed. Reassure the woman with physiologic menstrual changes. Give her emotional support, education, reassurance, and perhaps, dietary manipulation. Both the patient and her family benefit from discussion of hormonal changes and PMS. Charting the symptoms can help the patient gain more insight into her problem and more control over the situation, even if she decides not to take medication. Cognitive behavioral therapy may be helpful for some women. Self-help groups formed within a clinic or private practice can help women learn coping skills from experts and from one another. Although exogenous stress does not cause PMS, women with PMS have less tolerance for stress and may benefit from stress-reduction strategies. Relaxation, biofeedback, and acupuncture have all been reported to be helpful.[84-86] Regular exercise can reduce stress and physical complaints, but it does not alter the emotional components of PMS.[87] There has been some suggestion that aerobic exercise may be more helpful than body-building exercise.[88] When recommending exercise, set a realistic achievable program to avoid additionally burdening a woman with a sense of failure.

Diet. Dietary manipulations have been recommended for years in the treatment of PMS. Traditionally, women have been advised to resist carbohydrate cravings premenstrually. Newer evidence suggests that carbohydrate-rich, low-protein foods consumed during the luteal phase may improve mood swings.[89] Caffeine may worsen PMS symptoms, increasing nervous tension, heart rate, and a general body awareness. Avoiding caffeine and related compounds from all sources (coffee, tea, chocolates, over-the-counter medications, and so on) may be helpful. Be sure to advise the patient to abstain from caffeine throughout her cycle to avoid monthly symptoms of acute caffeine withdrawal.

Vitamins. Vitamin therapy has been recommended to reduce PMS symptoms. Pyridoxin (vitamin B_6) is important in the biosynthesis of neurotransmitters. One prospective placebo-controlled study found significant improvement of PMS symptoms among women taking vitamin B_6.[90] However, several subsequent studies failed to detect any differences.[91] Some companies market multivitamin PMS supplements with daily doses of high levels of vitamins B_6, A, and E in addition to magnesium and calcium. Peripheral neuropathy can occur when vitamin B_6 is taken at daily doses as low as 200 mg, so patients should use moderation if taking these supplements. Both vitamin E and primrose oil are prostaglandin precursors used routinely to treat PMS in other countries, based primarily on the results of uncontrolled studies. Primrose oil can be relatively expensive ($2.00 per day) but otherwise poses no known dangers. If a patient is interested in vitamin therapy, recommend she take a daily multivitamin supplemented with calcium and 50 mg or less of vitamin B_6.[25,92] The addition of primrose oil should not be harmful.

Medical therapy. Medical therapy is useful for women whose symptoms are severe or who do not respond to education, counseling, or stress-reduction and related techniques. The mainstay of medical treatment today is selective serotonin reuptake inhibitors (SSRIs). About 60% of women with PMS, especially those with emotional or behavioral changes, improve on SSRIs. Even some women with physical complaints improve. SSRIs differ, so carefully select the agent. For example, fluoxetine may be more appropriate for women with complaints of depression and fatigue, because it has activating properties, whereas sertraline may be a better choice for women who suffer from insomnia, irritability, or anxiety.[93] If one agent is not successful, try another before abandoning SSRIs as a class.

SSRIs at doses used to treat depression on a chronic basis may be relatively expensive and may be associated with higher incidence of side effects, such as decreased libido, anorgasmia, and weight gain. Many women with PMS improve on lower doses,[83] and some do not require daily dosing despite the known delay in onset of action. Several options for administration are outlined in Figure 6-3.

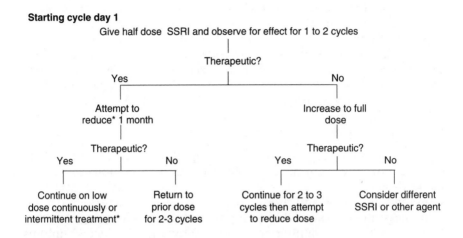

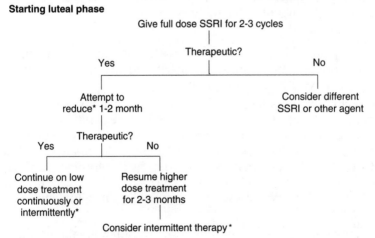

* Intermittent therapy options:
• Administer SSRI only during luteal phase or
• Administer low-dose SSRI during follicular phase, increase to therapeutic dose during luteal phase

Source: Freeman EW (1996).[92]

Figure 6-3 Flexibility in SSRI use for premenstrual syndrome (PMS)

For women whose symptoms do not respond to SSRIs, consider prescribing anxiolytics. For PMS sufferers, the preferred agent is alprazolam.[71] Begin therapy at low doses (e.g., 0.25 mg three times a day), and progressively increase the dose (e.g., 1 mg to 2.5 mg a day) until the patient improves. Alternatively, try increasing the morning and evening doses while holding the mid-day dose low or dividing the dose into a four-times-a-day regimen. The most effective pattern of use for alprazolam in the treatment of PMS has not been defined. Some studies have found therapeutic response with intermittent use (e.g., 4 to 5 days preceding menses) while other studies have found such protocols no better than placebo. It is likely that individualizing therapies will be the key. To avoid withdrawal symptoms, taper the alprazolam doses each time it is discontinued. Be careful when prescribing these agents, because they have potential for abuse; women with histories or current problems with alcoholism or other substance abuse are not appropriate candidates. Buspirone HCl, 10 mg three times a day, may be an effective alternative.

Ovulation suppressants may also be helpful in the treatment of PMS. Oral contraceptives are beneficial for women with complaints of dysmenorrhea, irritability, and anger. For some oral contraceptive users, PMS symptoms are milder and shorter, but others have an increase in depression, breast tenderness, and bloating. Several studies have suggested that the drospirenone-containing oral contraceptives may reduce symptoms of PMS.[94] Carefully select patients who may benefit, and monitor the results. Similarly, Danazol and GnRH agonists may provide relief,[95] but side effects limit their use to 4 to 6 months. Symptoms return once these agents are discontinued.

The 150 or more symptoms associated with PMS have been grouped into five categories to help target therapy. Some therapies have been shown to be effective in subsets of symptoms:

- **Anxiety.** Nervous tension, mood swings, irritability, restlessness, and impatience. If the patient's symptoms are debilitating, complement counseling and supportive measures with other efforts to reduce stress, including tips on organization. Unfortunately, studies have failed to demonstrate the efficacy of physical exercise. Serotonergic antidepressants and benzodiazepines have proven effective. Premenstrual use of prostaglandin inhibitors may also be helpful.

- **Depression.** Crying, confusion, social withdrawal, and insomnia must be carefully evaluated to rule out an underlying depressive or thyroid disorder. Antidepressants administered on a daily basis with prostaglandin inhibitors are most successful as short-term therapy.

- **Pain.** Severe uterine cramping, backache, and breast pain. Problems with menstrual cramping and backache respond well to the therapies outlined under the discussion of dysmenorrhea, especially those therapies that eliminate menses. Breast tenderness can be eased with a fitted support bra (sized for the luteal phase, when breast volume may increase 20%). Avoidance of methylxanthines found in coffee, tea, chocolate, and many prepared foods may be helpful. Bromocriptine has not been found to be a useful agent in any of the reported studies. Danazol is effective with mastalgia but can be taken for only a few months.

- **Water retention.** Weight gain, swelling, breast tenderness, and abdominal bloating. Many women experience no absolute increase in weight, but have fluid shifts. Spironolactone 25 mg taken orally two to four times a day for 14 days has efficacy in some studies. The role of drospirenone-containing OCs for this indication is well documented. Other diuretics, most notably hydrochlorothiazide, are inappropriate for this problem.
- **Hypoglycemia.** Headaches, cravings for sweets, increased appetite, fatigue, and reduced coordination can be treated by eliminating sex steroid cycling or by dietary manipulations such as avoiding simple sugars and fats, eating several small meals of complex carbohydrates, and consuming fresh foods.

GYNECOLOGIC PROBLEMS
VULVAR LESIONS

Vulvar lesions present both diagnostic and therapeutic challenges. Since the vulva is composed of squamous epithelium with a full range of underlying structures, virtually any pathology found anywhere on the skin can also be found on the vulva.[96] Psoriasis, eczema, vitiligo, moles, freckles, basal cell carcinoma, melanoma, and squamous cell carcinoma can occur on the vulva. Often because of moisture and other local influences, common lesions have a different appearance on the vulva than they do elsewhere on the body. For example, psoriasis on the vulva often has a more velvety appearance with less scaling. Sexually transmitted lesions such as condyloma lata, condyloma acuminata and molluscum contagiosum present in the vulva and other genital areas. Paget's disease of the vulva, hidradenitis suppurativa, and Bartholin's cysts involve the vulva due to the relatively unique glandular structures adjacent to or underlying the vulva. The epidermis of the vulva is at risk for developing changes such as dystrophy, hyperplasia and lichen sclerosis. Allergic reactions are increasingly common. The vulva can also be a site for metastasis and spread of diseases from other areas. For example, the vulva can be a site of fistula for Crohn's disease and for metastasis of choriocarcinoma.

The patient can play a pivotal role in diagnosing and detecting vulvar disease. If she does serial vulvar self-examinations, she may be able to draw a clinician's attention to a new lesion or to reassure the clinician that an existing lesion has had no growth for years. Every woman should be encouraged to do self-examination as a part of a comprehensive program of preventive health care. The clinician can help her learn more about this traditionally taboo area of her body by providing her a mirror during routine pelvic exam.

The key to successful treatment of vulvar lesions is early detection. Carefully examine all the surfaces of the vulva under adequate illumination. Use a hand-held magnifying lens if needed to study the borders and coloration of the lesion. Colposcopy is not as useful for grading the severity of the vulvar changes (as it can on the cervix) because the vulva epithelium can be too thick to permit an analysis of underlying vascular changes.

Vulvar lesions are often categorized by their color: white, red, or pigmented.

White Lesions

White lesions often represent structural changes in the epidermis and dermis. Lichen sclerosis is a generalized thinning of the epidermis with loss of the dermal papilla. It can occur at any age and is independent of hormone status. Patients may complain of pruritus, which can at times be intense. Over time as more of the vulva becomes involved, the skin loses elasticity and can split painfully (fissure) and bleed during intercourse or a pelvic examination. In contrast, hyperplasia, which involves a profound thickening of the epidermis with no nuclear changes, also appears as a white lesion but often with a brighter color and a coarser texture without the linear crinkling characteristic of lichen sclerosis. The differences between the two lesions may not be obvious on inspection; it is also possible to have a mixture of both hyperplasia and lichen sclerosis. Dystrophy can induce a chronic burning sensation of the vulva. Lesions may not be immediately obvious on inspection, but after a 5-minute exposure to 5% acetic acid-soaked gauze, characteristic sharp-bordered, bright, white lesions appear. Biopsy is necessary for diagnosis of any of these lesions. On the other hand, the whitened areas of vitiligo are quite evident and often parallel changes occurring elsewhere on the body.

In women who have been sexually active, condyloma are relatively common. Condyloma acuminata, caused by HPV, first appear as sessile, fleshy lesions. At this stage, they are easily treated with topical chemotherapeutic agents such as podophyllin, bichloracetic acid (BCA), or trichloracetic acid (TCA) or imiquimod. (See Chapter 8 on Reproductive Tract Infections.) Mature condyloma with thicker epithelia may require local destruction with cryotherapy, laser, LEEP, or surgical excision. Biopsy is required only if the diagnosis is unclear or if the lesion is large, growing, unusual appearing, or fails to respond to conventional treatments. Recurrences are common, especially as the so-called "ring-around-the-lesion." Newer topical immuno-boosting agents (e.g., imiquimod) can reduce wart reoccurrence. Women with vulvar condyloma acuminata may have warts on other exposed surfaces, including the vagina, cervix, anus, urethra and buccal mucosa. They are also at higher risk for cervical dysplasia and require cervical cytology testing. Condylomata lata are vulvar warts that develop in secondary syphilis, when the blood tests for syphilis will be positive. The lesions teem with spirochetes and are very contagious. Systemic antibiotic therapy is needed. Molluscum contagiosum appears as dome-shaped papules with central umbilication. Over time, the papules may resolve on their own and form skin tag-like lesions; however, most experts recommend removing the central core and touching the base of each lesion with silver nitrate to control oozing or treating off label with topical imiquimod.[97] (See Chapter 8 on Reproductive Tract Infections.)

Red Lesions

Red lesions are usually characteristic of infection but also may be associated with general skin changes or with neoplasms. The initial lesion of primary syphilis is a painless clean, shining, indurated chancre. Painful inguinal adenopathy can develop days to weeks after the chancre. Serology tests will be negative, but darkfield microscopy can demonstrate corkscrew-shaped spirochetes. In the absence of darkfield microscopy, treatment can be initiated on the basis of the lesion's classic appearance. Lymphogranuloma venereum (LGV) also first presents as a painless, raised lesion that the patient may not notice. It has a more injected, necrotic appearance compared with the glistening surface of the chancre. If LGV is untreated, painful inguinal adenopathy can develop in 1 to 3 weeks. The adenopathy is usually unilateral and can have a characteristic "double groove" sign in women. Granuloma inguinale starts as a relatively painless nodule that ruptures and creates an open, fleshy, oozing lesion that slowly fibroses, eventually constricting the surrounding tissue. (See Chapter 8 on Reproductive Tract Infections.)

In contrast to these relatively painless ulcers, herpes simplex and chancroid generally produce extremely painful lesions. Herpetic lesions start as vesicles that rupture and leave clearly defined, isolated ulcers. Chancroid may start as isolated ring-shaped lesions, but rapidly spreads by autoinoculation to form serpiginous (snake-like) bilateral lesions on each labia. If a chancroid is untreated, a tender inguinal bubo can form and rupture, leaving an open, weeping ulcer in the groin. While some of these lesions are relatively uncommon in the United States, their incidence is increasing and is contributing to the spread of HIV. For more information, see Chapter 8 on Reproductive Tract Infections.

Candida vulvovaginitis presents with erythema, edema, and often, excoriation. Characteristic satellite lesions dot the periphery of the lesion. Similarly tinea ("jock itch") can infect the labia. Today many women use a wide range of feminine hygiene products that incite painful or pruritic allergic reactions that can mimic fungal infections. If the offending agent is on a pad, the vulvar erythema may have a classic hourglass shape reflecting the areas of contact. The lack of satellite lesions helps distinguish delayed allergic reactions from candidal infections. Other infections such as trichomoniasis, nits, Bartholin's abscesses, hidradenitis suppurativa, and folliculitis tend to present with more localized erythema and purulence. Non-infectious problems such as eczema and psoriasis generally appear as red lesions on the vulva. Trauma to the vulva also presents with red lesions. Paget's disease of the vulva usually has a red, velvety appearance. Deep biopsies of this last lesion are needed because an underlying adenocarcinoma occurs in about 10% of cases. An evaluation is also needed to rule out associated (colon, breast, uterine) carcinoma. Isolated small (1 to 3 mm) fiery-red dots in the peri-introital area in the vestibule called vestibulitis can cause extreme pain on touch or with attempted intercourse.[98]

Pigmented Lesions

Pigmented lesions range from benign lentigo (freckles) to invasive squamous cell carcinoma of the vulva. These lesions present the greatest diagnostic challenges. Lesions may have distinctly different and more subtle presentations in women with darker pigmentation. Even in women with lighter-colored skin, it is often difficult to be confident that a compound nevus is not an early melanoma. Carefully examine the lesion with a hand-held magnifying lens to ensure the nevus has clear borders, smooth surface contours, and no variegation in color. If any suspicious features are present, biopsy is mandatory. Basal cell lesions have a characteristic round, cored out "rat-bite" lesion with raised pearly edges. Vulvar intraepithelial neoplasia (VIN) is usually multicentric in premenopausal women and may appear as darkened areas with a rougher surface. It is usually not possible to distinguish VIN from early squamous cell carcinoma by inspection alone. Determining the full extent of the disease is crucial, so multiple biopsies are often necessary.

Other Vulvar Problems

Although not associated with a visible lesion, many women suffer from vulvodynia (burning vulvar syndrome),[99] which is a constant neurologic type of pain in the vulva and which can involve the perianal area.[100] Vulvodynia may result from nerve irritation due to previous laser therapy or from topical treatments such as corticosteroids or antibiotics. Pudendal neuralgia can result from previous damage to the pudendal nerve such as diabetes, infection with the herpes simplex virus, degenerative disc disease or tumor, and obstetrical, surgical, or other trauma. Treatment with low-dose tricyclic antidepressants is helpful in dealing with this peripheral neuropathy.[101]

ENDOMETRIOSIS

Endometriosis is the presence of endometrial implants (glands and stroma) outside the uterus.[102] Endometriosis most frequently involves the peritoneal surfaces of pelvic organs—the cul de sac, ovaries, fallopian tube, uterus, broad ligament, ureters, rectovaginal septum, and uterosacral ligaments. The bowel, including the appendix, is often involved both superficially and in the deeper layers. Other more unusual sites include surgical scars, the bladder, the vulva, and the lungs. Endometriosis has many different appearances. The classical implant is nodular and brown, black, or reddish in color with a puckering of the surrounding tissue in a "powder burn" pattern. However, papular implants that are white, yellow, or nonpigmented are common, as are implants buried deep within pelvic adhesions. Endometriomas are cystic masses of endometriosis contained within the ovary; these cysts are filled with thick brownish fluid, which give the lesions their popular name, "chocolate cysts."

Endometriotic implants are transported out of the uterus primarily by retrograde menstruation. As the uterus contracts to expel the sloughed endometrial lining, some of the material is compressed out the fimbria and into the pelvic cavity. Other mechanisms such as hematogenous and lymphatic spread create more distal implants. The initial red endometriotic implants have been thought to respond to monthly sex steroid stimuli the same way the endometrial lining does—by proliferating, hypertrophying, and ultimately sloughing at the end of the cycle. The "local" menstrual blood, as well as the implants themselves, incites an inflammatory response creating adhesions to adjacent structures. Ultimately, the inflammatory reaction leads to fibrosis characterized by black and white lesions.[102] If the cyst on the ovary does not perforate early, large endometriomas can form. On the uterosacral ligament or within the sigmoid colon, the same process leads to creation of the deep nodules.

Endometriosis is a common problem: about 3% to 10% of reproductive-age women in the United States have endometriosis. Women undergoing laparotomy for gynecologic diseases have higher rates: ranging from 14% to 21%. Nearly 25% to 35% of infertile women have endometriosis.[103,104] Rates may be twice as high in Asian women, in women who delay childbearing, and in women with a family history of endometriosis.

Clinical Presentation of Endometriosis

The symptoms associated with endometriosis are variable. Over 50% of affected women complain of secondary dysmenorrhea; the pain often precedes the onset of vaginal bleeding each month. Dyspareunia is quite common; dyschezia (painful defecation) and dysuria may also occur. At least 15% of pelvic pain is caused by endometriosis. Lower abdomen pain, back pain, or even loin pain can be due to endometriosis.[105] Some women complain of pain with exercise. In addition to pain, the patient may present with complaints of fatigue, malaise and sleep difficulties. Advanced endometriosis can cause infertility (see Chapter 27 on Fertility Impairment). There is no consistent relationship between the extent of endometriosis and a woman's symptoms; even small implants can cause significant pain. On physical examination, a fixed retroverted uterus and tender nodular uterosacral ligaments, with or without an adnexal mass, are findings consistent with advanced endometriosis. However, a definitive diagnosis requires direct visualization, usually via laparoscopy. Biopsies help confirm the visual impression at the time of surgery. A formal classification system has been developed by the American Society for Reproductive Medicine to help stage the extent of disease and guide therapy and counseling.[106]

Treatment of Endometriosis

Treatment is determined by the nature and severity of the patient's symptoms and disease as well as her desire for fertility. Women with ovarian endometriomas greater than 2 cm in diameter require surgical removal because large endometriomas are not amenable to medical therapy and because they can rupture and cause an acute abdomen. Surgery is also appropriate for women whose endometriosis is resistant to medical management. Cystectomy is appropriate for isolated endometria. More extensive surgery involving excision of adhesions and ablation of implants may be added for infertile women and those desiring future fertility whose advanced disease does not respond to medical therapy. However, the relationship between mild endometriosis and infertility is unclear. A 90% 5-year cumulative pregnancy rate has been reported for women with untreated minimal to mild endometriosis.[107] Treatment of women with mild endometriosis has not been shown to increase fertility rates (see Chapter 27 on Fertility Impairment).[108,109] Hysterectomy and bilateral oophorectomy may be needed to treat more advanced disease unresponsive to medical therapies.

Women with endometriosis presenting with dysmenorrhea and pelvic pain can be treated with medical therapy. About 80% to 85% of women improve with any of the medical therapies; selection of treatment often depends upon side effects.[110] NSAIDS may reduce dysmenorrhea, especially if combined with oral contraceptives. Combined continuous use of oral contraceptives is particularly helpful in creating a pseudopregnancy state, shrinking the implants and inducing amenorrhea. (See Chapter 19 on Combined Hormonal Contraceptive Methods.) Progestins have long been a mainstay of therapy. Significant symptomatic relief from endometriosis-related pain can be obtained with DMPA use.[112] Danazol and GNRH agonists (such as buserelin, goserelin, leuprorelin acetate, nafarelin, and triptorelin) are FDA approved medications that are particularly helpful in shrinking and softening the implants to make them more amenable to surgical excision or ablation. They are also useful after surgery to treat residual disease and to prevent re-seeding. As stand-alone therapy, however, they can be used only for limited times. Danazol is an androgen that blocks gonadotrophins and directly suppresses ovarian hormone production. It can be used for only 6 to 9 months because it causes side effects: acne, hirsutism, and virilization. GNRH agonists block gonadotrophin production and reduce circulating estrogen levels to shrink implants.[111] Its use as a single agent is limited by its hypoestrogenic side effects. In this case, however, prolonged therapy is possible, if after initial therapy with GnRH agonists alone for 3 to 6 months, low doses of estrogen and progestin are added to the therapy.

PELVIC MASS

Pelvic masses are fairly common, but their evaluation may be somewhat challenging. The differential diagnosis of a pelvic mass varies with the woman's age and includes not only gynecologic causes (ovarian, tubal, and uterine masses) but also non-gynecological sources (a pelvic kidney and masses arising from the bowel, bladder, peritoneum, omentum, kidney and the blood vessels and nerves of the pelvis).[113] Although pelvic masses may cause symptoms, they are often found incidentally during examination of asymptomatic women.

- **Prepubertal girls.** A pelvic mass usually presents with pain and is frequently related to gastrointestinal problems (appendicitis or volvulus) or urinary pathology (bladder distension, Wilms' tumor, or neuroblastoma). The most common gynecological cause for a pelvic mass in young girls is a germ cell tumor of the ovary, followed closely by a simple ovarian cyst.

- **Reproductive-age women.** Consider pregnancy (intrauterine and ectopic) and infection (pyosalpinges or hydrosalpinges) as well as hormonally related cysts and the full range of benign and malignant neoplasms of the ovary, fallopian tube, and uterus. Uterine malformations such as bicornuate uterus, as well as paratubal and paraovarian cysts, can present as masses. Non-gynecological causes other than appendiceal abscesses and surgical adhesions are relatively rare.

- **Post-menopausal women.** Gynecological causes of pelvic masses are more likely to be malignant in this age group; 40% of ovaries that can be palpated in women more than 2 years after menopause are malignant.[114] The most common non-gynecological causes are diverticular abscesses and colon cancer. Colon cancer occurs more frequently than ovarian or endometrial cancer in this age group.

Common Masses in Reproductive-Age Women

Promptly rule out pregnancy when a reproductive-age woman appears with an adnexal mass. Ectopic pregnancy may be suggested by a history of missed menses or irregular vaginal spotting or bleeding, pelvic pain, and symptoms of pregnancy. The cervix may be cyanotic, and the uterus will be slightly enlarged and globular. Cervical motion tenderness may localize the lesion to one side, where an adnexal mass may be palpable. However, the pelvic mass that is palpated often is not the ectopic pregnancy itself but the corpus luteum cyst. Perform a pregnancy test. The remainder of the evaluation depends on her clinical status. Acutely ill women require surgical evaluation and treatment. A stable, minimally symptomatic patient may be evaluated with serial ß-hCG titers and transvaginal ultrasound of the uterus once the levels of hCG reach the discriminatory zone (usually 1400 to 2000 mIU/ml). A dilation and curettage (D&C) in a pregnant woman that fails to yield products of conception can also point to an ectopic pregnancy. Treatment for small, non-acute ectopic pregnancies is usually medical and can be offered on an outpatient basis. (See Chapter 26 on Pregnancy Testing and Management of Early Pregnancy.)

Other masses related to pregnancy include the corpus luteum cyst or a luteoma of pregnancy. The latter may cause significant androgenic changes. Fibroids may grow rapidly in pregnancy to form palpable masses and may cause extreme pelvic pain as they outgrow their blood supply and undergo necrosis.

Infection Related Masses

If a woman is sexually active or has recently had a pelvic procedure performed, consider the possibility of an infection (See Chapter 8 on Reproductive Tract Infections). The classic presentation of gonorrhea-associated pelvic inflammatory disease (PID) is high fever, gastrointestinal complaints, and severe lower abdominal pain developing near the end of menses. The affected woman walks bent over with a slow gait (the "PID shuffle") and has both abdominal tenderness and bilateral rebound in the lower quadrants. Her cervix is edematous and has a purulent discharge. On bimanual exam, she has marked cervical motion tenderness and, if she is able to tolerate abdominal pressure, may be found to have bilateral masses.

Today, however, the most common cause of salpingitis is chlamydia, which has a more subtle presentation. Its onset can be anytime in the menstrual cycle and it can cause significant tubal damage but produce only mild clinical symptoms. Therefore, the minimum criteria needed to diagnose PID have been reduced to two: cervical motion tenderness, and uterine/adnexal tenderness with no other etiology. The CDC suggests that if the patient does not have white cells on her wet mount, however, other etiologies should be sought. Other infectious causes of salpingitis are less common but include actinomycosis and tuberculosis. Post-operative infections (such as after C-section, hysterectomy, or D&C) account for nearly 40% of the pelvic abscesses.

Benign Adnexal Masses

Asymptomatic ovarian masses in reproductive-age women are most likely to be physiological (follicular or luteal) cysts. A woman who uses hormonal methods of contraception may still be vulnerable to follicular cysts but because ovulation is blocked, will rarely develop a corpus luteum cyst (CLC). However, the progestin-only pill and the LNG-IUS do not protect against CLCs. Moderately sized, asymptomatic, physiological cysts may be permitted to resolve spontaneously. Follicular cysts in an asymptomatic patient using low-dose progestin methods, such as levonorgestrel-releasing implants or IUD or progestin-only pills, may not undergo atresia for 6 to 8 weeks.

The most common ovarian neoplasm in young women is a cystic teratoma (dermoid). Teratomas usually present as a mobile mass that floats near the anterior abdominal wall and are characterized on ultrasound by internal echoes representing fat, hair or teeth. Also on the list of differential diagnoses are other common neoplasms including endometrioma, mucinous cystadenoma, and serous cystadenoma. Carcinoma, including borderline lesions, are a rare but ever-present possibility in the reproductive age woman.

Surgical therapy is usually necessary for diagnosis as well as for therapy for any mass that persists for longer than 4 to 8 weeks or is larger than 8 to 10 cm. Laparoscopic removal of adnexal masses has decreased the costs, physical discomfort, and recovery time of abdominal surgery. Ovarian preservation is the goal for women in their reproductive years. Therefore, cystectomy is the standard procedure unless malignancy is discovered, surgical difficulties present, or bleeding is not otherwise controllable.

A woman who has a pelvic mass accompanied by intermittent severe pain, fever, or gastrointestinal complaints may have torsion of a pre-existing pelvic mass (e.g., dermoid, physiologic ovarian cyst, paratubal cyst or distal portion of previously transected tube). The ovary can twist on its pedicle intermittently, causing intermittent severe pain separated by hours or days of dull aching. Although ultrasound Doppler flow studies can suggest torsion, the diagnosis of torsion requires surgical evaluation and treatment. Prompt diagnosis is important, because once the torsion has completely cut off blood supply to the involved structures, they will necrose and have to be removed. If the torsion can be diagnosed early, it may be possible to untwist the pedicle and save the involved ovary and tube. Other causes of acutely symptomatic pelvic masses include rupture of an endometrioma or a ruptured hemorrhagic corpus luteal cyst.

Benign Uterine Masses

Uterine tumors such as fibroids (leiomyoma) and adenomyosis also present as pelvic masses, especially during the reproductive years. About 20% of women in their late 30s to 40s have fibroids. All fibroids start within the walls of the muscle layer of the uterus as intramural fibroids. Subserosal fibroids are fibroids that grow to the outer surface of the uterus and present in physical exam as a markedly irregular shaped uterus. Submucosal fibroids grow toward the endometrial surface and protrude into that cavity.

Both intramural and submucosal fibroids may cause significantly heavier menses but only a minimally enlarged uterus. Aborting fibroids, pediculated fibroids and parasitic fibroids are all possible but relatively uncommon.

It is sometimes difficult to distinguish uterine masses from ovarian masses. If the ovary can be felt as distinct from the pelvic mass, then the mass is more likely to be uterine. If, during a bimanual exam, the mass can be moved without moving the uterus, an adnexal mass is more likely. Ultrasound is helpful but not mandatory to characterize and to determine the size and locations of fibroids; sonography can also document the normalcy of the ovaries and permit conservative management in almost all asymptomatic women. If women with fibroids have abnormal bleeding, it may still be necessary to perform endometrial biopsies to rule out hyperplasia or carcinoma. Surgery such as myomectomy or hysterectomy is generally reserved for women who are symptomatic and refractory to medical therapy and those who have rapidly growing masses.

Another cause of uterine enlargement is adenomyosis. The endometrial glands and stroma embed in the muscular layer of the uterus and cause a generalized enlargement and tenderness of the uterus, especially during menses. Women with adenomyosis usually experience heavy and often painful menses.

Pelvic Malignancies

Cervical cancer rates dropped dramatically in the United States after the introduction of routine Pap smear testing in the 1950s. In the United States, most women developing cervical cancer these days have not had appropriate screening. However, in developing countries, cervical cancer is still the most common gynecologic cancer. Early disease may be asymptomatic and diagnosed only on cytological testing. More advanced cervical cancer usually presents as persistent or postcoital vaginal bleeding or discharge and, on examination, as a pelvic mass.

Uterine cancers span the spectrum of lethality. Endometrial carcinoma (cancer of the lining of the uterus) is the most common gynecologic cancer. Early diagnosis and treatment of endometrial cancer is more likely than with other gynecologic cancers because endometrial cancer usually causes abnormal uterine bleeding, which prompts women to seek help. On the other hand, uterine sarcoma (cancer of the myometrial elements) has a dismal prognosis, not only because of its inherent lethality, but also because it produces very few symptoms until it is quite advanced.

Ovarian cancer strikes over 30,000 women each year in the United States, and nearly half of that number die each year. Survival rates, stage for stage, are equivalent to other gynecologic cancers, but ovarian carcinoma is the leading cause of death due to gynecologic cancer because the most cases are diagnosed only in advanced stages. The bimanual exam is the standard screening test for ovarian cancer in asymptomatic, low-risk women. Only women with family histories suggesting a high risk or genetic predispositions to breast/ovarian carcinoma (BRCA mutation carriers) should be screened every 6 to 12 months by transvaginal ultrasonography and serum tumor markers, such as CA 125.[115] (See Chapter 3 on Breast and Genital Tract Cancer Screening.)

Special attention is required for postmenopausal women. Two or 3 years after menopause, a woman's ovaries should be significantly atrophied and difficult to detect on pelvic exam. A palpable postmenopausal ovary merits evaluation.[116] Perform transvaginal ultrasound to characterize and measure the volume of the ovary[117] and measure serum tumor markers such as CA 125 if you suspect an ovarian mass. Color-flow Doppler may be of assistance. If the ultrasound image shows that the mass is a small simple cyst and the patient's CA 125 level is low, conservatively manage the condition by repeated testing or explore the pelvis by laparoscopy.[118] If the ultrasound image demonstrates any complexity within the mass or if the patient's CA 125 levels are elevated, surgery is usually required to rule out carcinoma.[119] These new non-invasive testing modalities have reduced the need for surgery to diagnose ovarian cancer.[120] However, inappropriate use of them (especially of ultrasound and CA 125) to screen low-risk women results in a large increase in costly testing and unnecessary surgery.

SEXUAL DYSFUNCTION

Intercourse is needed for human reproduction, but as a broader concept, sexuality also serves many other purposes in human interaction. Sexuality can form a bond between people. It can relieve tension and promote relaxation. Sexual dysfunction can deprive couples of many of its benefits. Women's health care providers are in a pivotal position to identify women with sexuality problems, to develop diagnoses and to guide the couple to more complete sexual functioning or to refer them to appropriate resources to help them.

Sexual dysfunction is a relatively common problem. As many as 50% of all married couples experience some sexual dissatisfaction or dysfunction.[121] Despite the widespread prevalence of sexual problems, women often hesitate to volunteer their complaints to health care providers. In one study, only 3% of women seen in a typical gynecological practice presented with sexually related complaints, but another 16% acknowledged problems when directly asked during a comprehensive review of systems.[122] The most common complaint was dyspareunia (48%), followed by decreased sexual desire (21%), partner problems or dysfunction (8%), vaginismus (6%), anorgasmia (4%), and other problems (13%).

Once a sexual problem has been identified, it has to be more completely characterized and placed within the context of the woman's complete sexual history. Make no assumptions about the patient's sexual orientation. Be aware of your own comfort with the topic and any non-verbal messages you may be communicating. Ask open-ended questions in a non-judgmental manner to reduce the patient's embarrassment or discomfort in discussing these topics (See Chapter 2 on Sexuality and Reproductive Health).[123]

DYSPAREUNIA

Dyspareunia accounts for nearly half of all women's sexual complaints. The causes are widespread but can be generally grouped into four categories: pain on intromission, mid-vaginal pain, pain with deep thrusting, and postcoital pain.

Pain on intromission. Some vulvar problems can be easily identified on careful inspection: the small exquisitely tender "red dot" characteristic of vestibulitis; the shallow ulcer of Bechet's disease; herpetic lesions; vulvovaginal candidiasis with its red, swollen, excoriated appearance; the smooth, reddened areas of allergic reactions; the white cigarette paper changes of lichen sclerosus; and the inadequate orifice of an imperforate hymen. Vulvodynia, more likely present as chronic pain, is less obvious but may also cause pain on initiation of intercourse. Severe, prolonged hypoestrogenism and lichen sclerosis can result in inelastic tissue that does not expand to accommodate penile penetration or other sexual manipulations. Therapy in each of these cases initially targets the underlying pathology and then attempts to break the pain-aversion cycle that is often caused by the first problem.

A special cause of pain on intromission is vaginismus, which is the involuntary contraction of the introital structures. Although vaginismus is a relatively infrequent problem in the general population, it accounts for a disproportionately large proportion of women with sexual problems. Women with extreme vaginismus may not be able to tolerate touch of their genitalia during either sexual encounters or physical examination. A desensitizing program of progressive vaginal dilatation may be helpful but it often needs to be complemented with counseling to deal with the woman's underlying fears and misperception of her reproductive organs.[124,125] (See Chapter 2 on Sexuality and Reproductive Health.)

Pain in mid-vagina. Pain that starts immediately after intromission can be due to problems in the vagina or in any of the adjacent structures. An episiotomy scar may be sensitive due to tender granulation tissue or may have entrapped nerve endings that trigger pain when touched. An overly corrected colporrhaphy may create too constricted an orifice to permit comfortable vaginal contact. Intrinsic anatomical defects such as a congenital septum may be painful during thrusting against its leading edge. Infections may cause dyspareunia, so test for urethral or bladder tenderness to help rule out urethritis, urethral diverticula, cystitis or interstitial cystitis as causes of mid-vaginal dyspareunia. Lack of adequate lubrication can cause pain during early thrusting. Lack of lubrication can be due to sexual practices (such as inadequate foreplay or lack of arousal) or to hypoestrogenism (with menopause, breast feeding, or use of DMPA).

Pain with deep thrusting. Dyspareunia that occurs during deep thrusting usually involves upper tract pelvic organs or other intraperitoneal structures. Intercourse during active salpingitis can be quite uncomfortable, but usually the longer-term consequences of infection are responsible for chronic deep-thrust dyspareunia. Adhesions formed by PID, endometriosis, and previous pelvic or abdominal surgery fix the pelvic organs and do not allow for movement to accommodate the pressure exerted against them during intercourse. The stretch placed on the adhesions can cause a tearing or ripping sensation, which can be quite painful. Interestingly, there is no observable relationship between the amount of adhesions and the severity of a woman's symptoms. Gossamer-thin adhesions cause profound pain while dense adhesions may not cause any noticeable discomfort. Women who have undergone hysterectomy occasionally have an ovary adherent to the vaginal cuff; this condition is quite sensitive to forceful contact during intercourse. Piriformis sensitivity has been reported to cause pain that can be reproduced during bimanual exam by pressing against the lateral vaginal fornix. For acute infections, a history and physical exam supported by limited laboratory testing is generally sufficient to make a diagnosis. In more chronic conditions, a thorough digital exam of the entire vault can help define the problem: a fixed uterus suggests adhesions while nodules along the uterosacral ligament point to endometriosis. Posterior tenderness may be the result of a fractured coccyx or bowel pathology. Adjunctive testing with ultrasound and, often, diagnostic laparoscopy may be needed to make a definite diagnosis. During the workup suggest using different coital positions to direct the penis away from sensitive areas to provide some degree of relief.

Postcoital pain. Some women suffer pain with orgasm due to painful uterine or abdominal muscle contractions. Others develop severe headaches after orgasm. Prophylactic administration of nonsteroidal agents 1 hour prior to intercourse can reduce or eliminate these problems. If a woman has been unable to achieve orgasm to release the venous pressure built up during the arousal phase, she may experience a dull aching or throbbing sensation in her pelvis postcoitally. This is referred to as pelvic congestion syndrome. Some women with this problem will benefit from couples' counseling on coital timing; others may benefit from instructions about masturbation.

Sexual Disinterest

Complaints about decreased libido have only recently achieved attention as medical concerns. They were not even addressed in the Masters and Johnson work in the 1970s. However, sexual disinterest is apparently widespread. In one survey, 2 out of every 10 women reported difficulty becoming sexually aroused; one-third said they had difficulty maintaining excitement and another one-third expressed a complete disinterest in sex.[126] However, 83% of these couples rated their marriages as happy or very happy. While perfect sexual function is not a prerequisite for marital happiness, sexual disinterest can create stresses within the relationship. In addition, the obverse is also true; relationship stresses frequently present themselves first in the bedroom.

Medical problems and medications can affect libido.[127] Chronic diseases, such as diabetes, are often associated with decreased sexual activity. People recovering from myocardial infarction may be extremely apprehensive about engaging in strenuous activities. Women who have had mastectomy, colostomy, or vulvectomy may feel unattractive and have diminished libido. Pain from arthritis and other diseases that limit motion may dampen sexual interest. Psychological problems, such as pronounced depression, may first manifest as decreased libido. A history of sexual abuse can leave deep psychological scars and can transform pleasurable sexuality into repeated reminders of former nightmares. Pregnancy can introduce difficulties with sexual relations. Patients can benefit from reassurance as well as explicit advice about safer and more comfortable coital positioning.[128] (See Chapter 2 on Sexuality and Reproductive Health.)

Medications such as sedatives, narcotics, hypnotics, anticonvulsants, centrally acting antihypertensives, tranquilizers, anorectics, and some antidepressants may interfere with sexual desire and/or sexual function.[129] Estrogen has a more complex set of effects; while it increases vaginal lubrication, it also increases sex hormone binding globulin, which may decrease free serum androgen levels and thus may decrease libido over time. In small amounts, alcohol may decrease inhibition, but, primarily, it is a depressant and decreases a woman's arousal.

Lifestyle issues are pivotal to a woman's sexuality.[130] Fatigue and stress over finances or other issues rob her of libido as profoundly as medications. Distraction by daily tasks or lack of privacy can subdue passion. Over time, predictability combined with a limited sexual menu can replace anticipation and excitement with sheer routine and boredom; diminished desire is the end result. Stresses within the relationship are also strong deterrents to libido. At a practical level, a partner's sexual techniques can profoundly affect a woman's libido; rapid, self-centered, or rough sexual practices may leave the woman unaroused. In retrospect, these influences are obvious but in a clinical setting they may not be as clear. Use open-ended questions to carefully and sensitively inquire about the couple's sexual dynamics.

REFERENCES

1. Andersch B, Milsom I. An epidemiologic study of young women with dysmenorrhea. Am J Obstet Gynecol 1982;144:655-660.
2. Berry C, McGuire F. Menstrual distress and acceptance of sexual role. Am J Obstet Gynecol 1972;114:83-87.
3. Smith RP. Cyclic pelvic pain and dysmenorrhea. Obstet Gynecol Clin North America 1993;20:753-764.
4. Tolman EL, Partridge R. Multiple sites of interaction between prostaglandins and nonsteroidal anti-inflammatory agents. Prostaglandins 1975;9:349-359.
5. Wilson L, Kurzrok R. Uterine contractility in functional dysmenorrhea. Endocrinology 1940;27:23-28.
6. Pickles VR, Hall WJ, Best FA, Smith GN. Prostaglandins in endometrium and menstrual fluid from normal and dysmenorrheic subjects. J Obstet Gynaecol Br Comm 1965;72:185-192.
7. Creatsas G, Deligeoroglou E, Zachari A, Loutradis D, Papadimitriou T, Miras K, Aravantino D. Prostaglandins PGF2u, PGE2, 6-Keto-PGF1μ, TXA2 and TXB2 serum levels in dysmenorrheic adolescents before, during and after treatment with oral contraceptives. European J Obstet Gynecol and Repro Biol 1990;36:292-298.
8. Ayers JWT, Gidwana GP, Schmidt IMV, Gross M. Osteopenia in hypoestrogenic young women with anorexia nervosa. Fertil Steril 1984;41:224-228.
9. Milsom I, Sundell G, Andersch B. The influence of different combined oral contraceptives on the prevalence and severity of dysmenorrhea. Contraception 1990;42:497-506.

10. Robinson JC, Plichta S, Weisman CS, Nathanson CA, Ensminger M. Dysmenorrhea and use of oral contraceptives in adolescent women attending a family planning clinic. Am Obstet Gynecol 1992;166:578-583.

11. Sulak PJ, Cressman BE, Waldrop E, Holleman S, Kuehl TJ. Extending the duration of active oral contraceptive pills to manage hormone withdrawal symptoms. Obstet Gynecol 1997;89:179-183.

12. Dawood MY. Nonsteroidal anti-inflammatory drugs and reproduction. Am J Obstet Gynecol 1993;169:1255-1265.

13. Chan WY. Prostaglandin inhibitors and antagonists in dysmenorrhea therapy. In: Dawood MY (ed). Dysmenorrhea. Baltimore: Williams & Wilkins, 1981.

14. Harel Z, Biro FM, Kottenhahn RK, Rosenthal SL. Supplementation with omega-3 polyunsaturated fatty acids in the management of dysmenorrhea in adolescents. Am J Obstet Gynecol 1996;174:1335-1338.

15. Mishell DR. Infertility, contraception and reproductive endocrinology. Boston: Blackwell Scientific Publications, 1991.

16. Doody KM, Carr BR. Menstrual cycle disorders. Obstetrics and gynecology clinics of North America. Philadelphia: W.B. Saunders Co., 1990;17:361-387.

17. Speroff L, Glass RH, Kase NG. Clinical gynecologic endocrinology and infertility. 6th edition. Baltimore: Williams & Wilkins, 1999.

18. Warren MP, Holderness CC, Lesobre V, Tzen R. Hypothalamic amenorrhea and hidden nutritional insults. J Soc Gynecol Invest 1994;1:84-88.

19. Shangold M, Rebar RW, Colston Wentz A, Schiff I. Evaluation and management of menstrual dysfunction in athletes. JAMA 1990;263:1665-1669.

20. Hergenroeder AC, Smith EO, Shypailo R, Jones LA, Klish WJ, Ellis K. Bone mineral changes in young women with hypothalamic amenorrhea treated with oral contraceptives, changes in young women with hypothalamic amenorrhea treated with oral contraceptives, medroxyprogesterone or placebo over 12 months. Am J Obstet Gynecol 1997;176:1017-1025.

21. Genazzani AD, Petraglia F, Gastaldi M, Volpogni C, Gamba O, Genazzani AR. Naltrexone treatment restores menstrual cycles in patients with weight loss-related amenorrhea. Fertil Steril 1995;64:951-956.

22. Franks S. Polycystic ovary syndrome: a changing perspective. Clin Endocrinol 1989;31:87-120.

23. Givens JR. Polycystic ovaries—a sign, not a diagnosis. Semin Reprod Endocrinol 1984;2:271-280.

24. Rebar RW. Gonadotropin secretion in polycystic ovary disease. Seminars Reprod Endocrinol 1984;2:223-230.

25. Thys-Jacobs S, Ceccarelli S, Bierman A, Weisman H, Cohen MA, Alvir J. Calcium supplementation in premenstrual syndrome: a randomized crossover trial. J Gen Intern Med 1989;4:183-189.

26. Dunaif A, Green G, Phelps RG, Lebwohl M, Futterweit W, Lewy L. Acanthosis nigricans, insulin action, and hyperandrogenism: clinical, histological, and biochemical findings. J Clin Endocrinol Metab 1991;73:590-595.

27. Mason HD, Margara R, Winston RL, Seppala M, Koistinen R, Franks S. Insulin-like growth factory-I (IGF-I) inhibits production of IGF-binding protein-1 while stimulating estradiol secretion in granulosa cells from normal and polycystic human ovaries. J Clin Endocrinol Metab 1993;76:1275-1279.

28. Graf MJ, Richards CJ, Brown V, Meissner L, Dunaif A. The independent effects of hyperandrogenemia, hyperinsulinemia, and obesity on lipid and lipoprotein profiles in women. Clin Endocrinol 1990;33:119-131.

29. Wild RA, Painter PC, Coulson PB, Carruth KB, Ranney GB. Lipoprotein lipid concentrations and cardiovascular risk in women with polycystic ovary syndrome. J Clin Endocrinol Metab 1985;61:946-951.

30. Legro RS. Is polycystic ovary syndrome a genetic disease? Contemporary Ob/Gyn 1996;9:43-57.

31. Pasquali R. Antenucci D, Casimirri F, Venturoli S, Paradisi R, Fabbri R, Balestra V, Melchiondra N, Barbara L. Clinical and hormonal characteristics of obese amenor-rheic hyperandrogenic women before and after weight loss. J Clin Endocrinol Metab 1989;68:173-179.
32. Lapidus L, Bengtsson C, Larsson B, Pennert K, Rybo E, Sjostrom L. Distribution of adipose tissue and risk of cardiovascular disease and death: a 12-year follow up of participants in the population study of women in Gothenburn, Sweden. Br Med J 1984;289:1257-1261.
33. Redmond GP, Olson WH, Lippman JS, Kafrissen ME, Jones TM, Jorizzo JL. Norges-timate and ethinyl estradiol in the treatment of acne vulgaris: a randomized, placebo-controlled trial. Obstet Gynecol 1997;89:615-22.
34. Ruchhoft EA, Elkind-Hirsh KE, Malinak R. Pituitary function is altered during the same cycle in women with polycystic ovary syndrome treated with continuous or cyclic oral contraceptives on a gonadotropin-releasing hormone agonist. Fertil Steril 1996;66:54-60.
35. Erenus M, Yucelten D, Gurbuz, O, Durmusoglu F, Pekin S. Comparison of spirono-lactone-oral contraceptive versus cyproterone acetate-estrogen regimens in the treatment of hirsutism. Fertil Steril 1996;66:216-219.
36. Marcondes JAM, Minnani SL, Luthold WW, Wajchenberg BL, Samojilk E, Kirschner MA. Treatment of hirsutism in women with flutamide. Fertil Steril 1992;57:543-547.
37. Tolino A, Petrone A, Sarnacchiaro F, Cirillo D, Ronsini S, Lombardi G, Nappi C. Finasteride in the treatment of hirsutism: new therapeutic perspectives. Fertil Steril 1996;66:61-65.
38. Chimbira TH, Anderson ABM, Turnbull AC. Relation between measured menstrual blood loss and patient's subjective assessment of loss, duration of bleeding, num-ber of sanitary towels used, uterine weight and endometrial surface area. Br J Obstet Gynaecol 1980;87:603-609.
39. Fraser IS, McCarron G, Markham R. Blood and total fluid content of menstrual discharge. Obstet Gynecol 1985;65:194-198.
40. Haynes PJ, Hodgson H, Anderson ABM, Turnbull AC. Measurement of menstrual blood loss in patients complaining of menorrhagia. Br J Obstet Gynaecol 1977;84:763-768.
41. Neinstein LS. Menstrual problems in adolescents. Med Clin North Am 1990;74;1181-1203.
42. Hillard PA. Heavy uterine bleeding in adolescents. Contemporary Ob/Gyn 1995;40:21-32.
43. Claessens EA, Cowell CA. Dysfunctional uterine bleeding in the adolescent. Pediatr Clin North Am 1981;28:369-371.
44. Magos AL. Management of menorrhagia. Br J Med 1990;300;1537-1538.
45. Shaw RW. Assessment of medical treatments of menorrhagia. Br J Obstet Gynaecol 1994;101 (Suppl 11):15-18.
46. Bonnar J, Sheppard BL. Treatment of menorrhagia during menstruation: random-ized controlled trial of ethamsylate, mefenamic acid, and tranexamic acid. BMJ 1996;313:579-582.
47. Nilsson L, Rybo G. Treatment of menorrhagia. Am J Obstet Gynecol 1971;110:713-720.
48. Bayer SR, DeCherney AH. Clinical manifestations and treatment of dysfunctional uterine bleeding. JAMA 1993;269:1823-1828.
49. Paskowitz RA. "Rollerball" ablation of the uterus. J Reprod Med 1995;40:333-336.
50. Somerville BW. The role of estradiol withdrawal in the etiology of menstrual migraine. Neurology 1972;22:355-365.
51. Mattson RH, Rebar RW. Contraceptive methods for women with neurologic disor-ders. Am J Obstet Gynecol 1993;168:2027-2032.
52. Szigethy A, Dienes L. The relationship between atypical migraine and multiphasic oral contraceptives. Therapia Hungarica 1991;40:185-188.
53. Guillebaud J. The pill and other hormones for contraception. 4th edition. Oxford, England: Oxford University Press, 1991.

54. Murray SC, Muse KN. Effective treatment of severe menstrual migraine headaches with gonadotropin-releasing hormone agonist and add-back therapy. Fertil Steril 1997;67:390-393.

55. Beynon HLS, Harbet NE, Barnes PJ. Severe premenstrual exacerbations of asthma: effect of intramuscular progesterone. Lancet 1988;2:370-372.

56. Boggess KA, Williamson HO, Homm RJ. Influence of the menstrual cycle on systemic diseases. Obstet Gynecol Clin North Amer 1990;17:321-342.

57. Neinstein LS. Issues in reproductive management. New York: Theime Medical Publishers, 1994.

58. Reid RL. Premenstrual syndrome. Curr Probl Gynecol Fertil 1985;8:1-57.

59. American Psychiatric Association. Diagnostic and statistical manual of mental disorders, fourth edition text revision (DSM-IV-TR). Washington DC: American Psychiatric Association, 2000:771-774.

60. Shoupe D. Premenstrual syndrome: diagnosis and management. In: Mishell DR Jr, Brenner PF (eds). Management of common problems in obstetrics and gynecology. Boston: Blackwell Scientific Publications, 1994.

61. Haskett RF, DeLongis A, Kessler RC. Premenstrual dysphoria: a community survey [abstract]. Presented at the 140th annual meeting of the American Psychiatric Association, May 9-15, 1987, Chicago, IL.

62. Johnson SR, McChesney C, Bean JA. Epidemiology of premenstrual symptoms in a nonclinical sample. I. Prevalence, natural history and help-seeking behavior. J Reprod Med 1988;33:340-346.

63. Rivera-Tovar AD, Frank E. Late luteal phase dysphoric disorder in young women. Am J Psychiatry 1990;147:1634-1636.

64. Chihal HJ. Premenstrual syndrome: an update for clinicians. Obstet Gynecol Clinics North Amer 1990;17:457-481.

65. Rubinow DR, Roy-Bryne P, Hoban MC, Gold PW, Post RM. Prospective assessment of menstrually related mood disorders. Am J Psychiatry 1984;141:684-686.

66. Harrison WM, Robkin JH, Endicott J. Psychiatric evaluation of premenstrual changes. Psychosomatics 1985;26:789.

67. Fava M, Pedrazzi F, Guaraldi GP, Romano G, Genazzani AR, Facchinetti F. Comorbid anxiety and depression among patients with late luteal phase dysphoric disorder. J Anx Disorders 1992;6:325-335.

68. Dalton K. The premenstrual syndrome and progesterone therapy. London: William Heimann, 1984.

69. Frank RT. The hormonal causes of premenstrual tension. Arch Mem Psychiatry 1931;26:1053-1057.

70. Rubinow DR, Hoban C, Grover G, Galloway DS, Roy-Byrne P, Andersen R, Merriam GR. Changes in plasma hormones across the menstrual cycle in patients with menstrually related mood disorders and in control subjects. Am J Obstet Gynecol 1988;158:5-11.

71. Freeman EW, Rickels K, Sondheimer SJ, Polansky M. A double-blind trial of oral progesterone, alprazolam, and placebo in treatment of severe premenstrual syndrome. JAMA 1995;274:51-57.

72. Chuong CH, Coulam CB, Kao PC, Bergstrahl EJ, Go VI. Neuropeptide levels in premenstrual syndrome. Fertil Steril 1985;44:760-765.

73. Schmidt PJ, Nieman LK, Grover GN, Muller KL, Meriam GR, Rubinow DR. Lack of effect of induced menses on symptoms in women with premenstrual syndrome. New Engl J Med 1991;324:1174-1179.

74. Mira M, Stewart PM, Abraham SF. Vitamin and trace element status in premenstrual syndrome. Am J Clin Nutr 1988;47:636-641.

75. Redei E, Freeman EW. Preliminary evidence for plasma adrenocorticotropin levels as biological correlates of premenstrual syndrome. Acta Endocrinol 1992;128:536.

76. Eriksson E, Hedberg MA, Andersch B, Sunblad C. The serotonin reuptake inhibitor paroxetin is superior to the noradrenaline reuptake inhibitor maprotiline in the treatment of premenstrual syndrome: a placebo-controlled trial. Neuropsychopharmacology 1995;12:167-176.

77. Lepage P, Steiner M. Gender and serotonergic dysregulation: implications for late luteal phase dysphoric disorder. In: Cassano GB, Akiskal HS (eds). Serotonin-related psychiatric syndromes: clinical and therapeutic links. London: Royal Society of Medical Services, 1991:131-143.
78. Rapkin AJ. The role of serotonin in premenstrual syndrome. Clin Obstet Gynecol 1992;35:629-636.
79. Rojansky N, Halbreich U, Zander K, Barkai A, Goldstein S. Imipramine receptor binding and serotonin uptake in platelets of women with premenstrual changes. Gynecol Obstet Invest 1991;31:146-152.
80. Steiner M. Female-specific mood disorders. Clin Obstet Gynecol 1992;35:599-611.
81. Yatham LN. Is 5HT1A receptor subsensitivity a trait marker for late luteal phase dysphoric disorder? A pilot study. Can J Psychiatry 1993;38:662-664.
82. Yonkers KA, Halbreich U, Freeman EW. Efficacy of sertraline for treatment of premenstrual dysphoric disorder [abstract #NR278]. New research program and abstracts of the American Psychiatric Association 148th annual meeting, May 20-25, 1995, Miami, FL.
83. Steiner M, Steinberg S, Stewart D, Carter D, Berger C, Reid R, Grover D, Streiner D. Fluoxetine in the treatment of premenstrual dysphoria. N Engl J Med 1995;332:1529-1534.
84. Goodale IL, Domar AD, Benson H. Alleviation of premenstrual syndrome with the relaxation response. Obstet Gynecol 1990;75:649-655.
85. Oleson T, Flocco W. Randomized controlled study of premenstrual symptoms treated with ear, hand and foot reflexology. Obstet Gynecol 1993;82:906-911.
86. Van Zak DB. Biofeedback treatments for premenstrual and premenstrual affective syndromes. Int J Psychosom 1994;41:53-60.
87. Prior JC, Vigna Y, Sciarreta D, Alojado N Schulzer M. Conditioning exercise decreases premenstrual symptoms: a prospective controlled 6 month trial. Fertil Steril 1987;47:402-408.
88. Steege JF, Blumenthal JA. The effects of aerobic exercise on premenstrual symptoms in middle-aged women: a preliminary study. J Psychosom Res 1992;37:127-133.
89. Sayegh R, Schiff I, Wurtman J, Spiers P, McDermott J, Wurtman R. The effect of a carbohydrate-rich beverage on mood, appetite, and cognitive function in women with premenstrual syndrome. Obstet Gynecol 1995;86:520-528.
90. Abraham GE, Hargrove JT. Effect of vitamin B6 on premenstrual symptomatology in women with premenstrual tension syndrome: a double-blind crossover study. Infertility 1980;3:155-165.
91. London RS, Bradley L, Chiamore NY. Effect of a nutritional supplement on premenstrual symptomatology in women with premenstrual syndrome: a double-blind longitudinal study. J Am Coll Nutr 1991;10:494.
92. Freeman EW, Kielich AM, Sondheimer SJ. PMS: new treatments that really work. Cont Ob/Gyn 1996;25:44.
93. Rickels K, Freeman EW, Sondheimer SJ, Albert J. Fluoxetine in the treatment of premenstrual syndrome. Curr Ther Res 1990;48:161-166.
94. Freeman EW, Kroll R, Rapkin A, Pearlstein T, Brown C, Parsey K, Zhang P, Patel H, Foegh M. Evaluation of a unique oral contraceptive in the treatment of premenstrual dysphoric disorder. J Womens Health Gend Based Med 2001;10:561-9.
95. Muse KN, Futterman LA, Yen SSC. The premenstrual syndrome: effects of medical ovariectomy. N Engl J Med 1984:1345-1346.
96. Friedrich Jr EG. Major problems in obstetrics and gynecology. Vol. 9. Philadelphia: W.B. Saunders 1983:35-60.
97. Kaufman RH, Faro S, Friedrich Jr EG, Gardner HL. Benign diseases of the vulva and vagina. St. Louis: Mosby 1994.
98. Friedrich EG Jr. Vulvar vestibulitis syndrome. J Reprod Med 1987;32:110-4.
99. Lynch PJ, Edwards L. Genital dermatology. New York: Churchill Livingstone, 1994:237-249.
100. Nunns D. Vulval pain syndromes. BJOG 2000;107:1185-93.
101. McKay M. Dysesthetic ("essential") vulvodynia. Treatment with amitriptyline. J Reprod Med 1993;38:9-13.

102. Brosens IA. Endometriosis—a disease because it is characterized by bleeding. Am J Obstet Gynecol 1997;176:263-267.
103. Cramer DW. Epidemiology of endometriosis. In: Wilson EA (ed). Endometriosis. New York: Alan R. Liss, 1987:5-22.
104. Olive DL, Schwartz LB. Endometriosis. N Engl J Med 1993;328:1759.
105. Mahmood TA, Templeton A. Prevalence and genesis of endometriosis. Hum Reprod 1991;6:544-9.
106. American Society for Reproductive Medicine. Revised American Society for Reproductive Medicine classification of endometriosis:1996. Fertil Steril 1997;67:817-821.
107. Badway SZA, Elbarkry MM, Samuel F, Dizer M. Cumulative pregnancy rates in infertile women with endometriosis. J Reprod Med 1988;33:757-760.
108. Fedele L, Parzzini F, Radici E, Bocciolone L, Bianchi S, Bianchi C, Canadiani GB. Buserelin acetate versus expectant management in the treatment of infertility associated with minimal or mild endometriosis: a randomized clinical trial. Am J Obstet Gynecol 1992;166:1345-1350.
109. Garcia CF, Davis SS. Pelvic endometriosis: infertility and pelvic pain. Am J Obstet Gynecol 1977;129:740-747.
110. Prentice A. Regular review: Endometriosis. BMJ 2001;323:93-5.
111. Prentice A, Deary AJ, Goldbeck-Wood S, Farquhar C, Smith SK. Gonadotrophin-releasing hormone analogues for pain associated with endometriosis. Cochrane Database Syst Rev 2000;(2):CD000346.
112. Vercellini P, DeGiorgi O, Oldani S, Cortesi I, Panazza S, Crosignani PG. Depot medroxyprogesterone acetate versus an oral contraceptive combined with very-low-dose danazol for long-term treatment of pelvic pain associated with endometriosis. Am J Obstet Gynecol 1996;175:396-401.
113. Russell DJ. The female pelvic mass: diagnosis and management. Med Clin N Amer 1995;79:1481-1493.
114. Bennington JL, Fergusen BR, Haber SL. Incidence of relative frequency of benign and malignant ovarian neoplasms. Obstet Gynecol 1968;32:627-632.
115. Seltzer V. Screening for ovarian cancer: an overview of the screening recommendations of the 1994 NIH consensus conference. Prim Care Update.
116. Barber H, Graver E. The PMPO syndrome (postmenopausal palpable ovary syndrome). Obstet Gynecol 1971;38:921-923.
117. Rodriguez MH, Platt LD, Medearis AL, Lacarra M, Lobo RA. The use of transvaginal sonography for evaluation of postmenopausal ovarian size and morphology. Am J Obstet Gynecol 1988;159:810-814.
118. Parker WH. The case for laparoscopic management of the adnexal mass. Clin Obstet Gynecol 1995;38:362-369.
119. Curtin JP. Management of the adnexal mass. Gynecol Oncol 1994;55:S42-S46.
120. Goldstein SR. Postmenopausal adnexal cysts: how clinical management has evolved. Am J Obstet Gynecol 1996;175:1498-1501.
121. Stenchever MA. Counseling the patient. Comprehensive gynecology. St. Louis, MO: Mosby Yearbook, 1992;192.
122. Bachmann GA, Leiblum SR, Grill J. Brief sexual inquiry in gynecological practice. Obstet Gynecol 1989;73:425.
123. Masters WH, Johnson VE. Human sexual response. Boston: Little Brown & Co., 1996:141-168.
124. American College of Obstetricians and Gynecologists. Sexual dysfunction. ACOG Technical Bulletin, No. 211, 1995.
125. Valens L. When a woman's body says no to sex. New York: Penguin Books, 1988.
126. Frank E, Anderson C, Rubinstein P. Frequency of sexual dysfunction in normal couples. N Engl J Med 1978;299:111.
127. Schover LR, Jensen SB. Sexuality and chronic illness. New York: Guilford Press, 1988.
128. Bing E, Colman L. Making love during pregnancy. New York: Bantam Books, 1977.
129. Anonymous. Drugs that cause sexual dysfunction: an update. Med Lett Drugs Ther 1992;34:73.
130. Renshaw DC. When the patient's chief complaint is sexual disinterest. Prim Care Update Ob/Gyns 1994;1:194-198.

HIV/AIDS and Reproductive Health

Felicia Guest, MPH, CHES

- Every patient merits help in building personal skills for preventing infection with the human immunodeficiency virus (HIV). Ask each patient, "What do you do to protect yourself from AIDS?"
- Reproductive health care settings are a critical conduit to HIV testing. Offer counseling and voluntary testing to each patient.
- Reproductive-age women constitute the fastest-growing segment of the U.S. AIDS epidemic. Many are not aware of their infection.
- Ensure access to primary and reproductive health care for HIV-infected women, either by direct treatment or careful referral.
- Preventing unintended pregnancy in HIV-infected women is the most humane and cost-effective approach to preventing perinatal transmission.
- The standard of prenatal care is routine HIV testing for all pregnant women. Be certain HIV-infected pregnant women have access to antiretroviral drug regimens that can improve health status, reduce viral load, and reduce the likelihood of perinatal transmission.

Infection with the human immunodeficiency virus (HIV) is a global pandemic, with 96% of infected people living in resource-poor countries, where only a small percentage of the world's HIV prevention and treatment resources are deployed. Some 40 million people are living with HIV/AIDS (acquired immunodeficiency syndrome), including 19.2 million women. On almost every continent, AIDS is a leading cause of death among young women. Most have been infected via sexual exposure to infected men.[1]

Some 141,000 U.S. women have been reported to have AIDS,[2] and 120,000 to 160,000 infected U.S. women are alive today, 80% of whom are of childbearing age.[3] They are demographically similar to women who seek reproductive health care in family planning, prenatal, abortion, and STI service sites. Several characteristics describe the epidemic in U.S. women:

Young women. Women with HIV are young. About 21% are 20 to 29 years old when their AIDS is reported, suggesting many were infected in their teen years. All states report cases of AIDS, and 34 states and 2 U.S. territories report cases of HIV infection. Through 2000, 80% of women with AIDS and 86% of women with HIV were 13 to 44 years old. Younger groups have higher proportions of infected females than do older groups. Among AIDS cases reported in 2000, 24% of those age 25 and older were women, compared with 40% of 20 to 24-year-olds and 53% of teenagers.[4]

Women of color. Black and Hispanic women are disproportionately represented in reported AIDS cases, particularly in urban areas of the Northeast and the rural South. About 85% of children with perinatally-acquired AIDS are black or Hispanic.[5]

Heterosexual women. Sex with an HIV-infected male accounted for 37% of all AIDS cases in U.S. women reported in 2001. Heterosexual exposure is a major risk factor among younger women, accounting for 55% of cumulative cases among 20- to 24-year-olds and 51% among teenagers.[2] The number of women with heterosexually acquired AIDS may be higher than what is officially reported. Women are twice as likely as men to have their AIDS reported without an established risk factor for transmission, and at least half of these "no identified risk" cases are likely to have been transmitted heterosexually.[2,5]

Women who have sex with women can also be at risk. Although the frequency of woman-to-woman sexual HIV transmission is rare, risk from injecting drug use, heterosexual sex, and other behaviors can be considerable.[6] In San Francisco, for example, 40% of lesbian and bisexual women reported unsafe heterosexual sex practices and 10% of the group reported injecting drug use. The HIV prevalence rate among this study sample was 1.2%.[7]

Injecting drug users. Among U.S. women, injecting drug use played a significant role during the first decade of the AIDS epidemic. About 39% of AIDS cases among U.S. women have involved women who injected drugs with shared and uncleaned injection equipment. Thousands more women were infected by male sex partners who were injecting-drug users.[2,4]

Geographic clustering. States in the Northeast and South have a higher prevalence of HIV in women than do other states, and urban areas are harder hit than small towns and rural areas, except in rural areas of the South where prevalence is high, particularly among childbearing women.[2,4,5]

HIV PREVENTION IN THE REPRODUCTIVE HEALTH CARE SETTING

All reproductive health care patients merit some sort of help with improving their personal skills for HIV prevention. Even the patient in a long-term mutually-faithful relationship is theoretically one risky choice away from HIV, whether that choice is made by her or by her partner. Many patients are not in long-term mutually-faithful relationships. Patients may want and need new HIV prevention skills to help others, including their own children.

HIV prevention for women operates on three levels, beginning with *primary* prevention, the most common. On this level, providers help uninfected women remain uninfected by teaching them about negotiation skills, safer sex techniques, and avoiding IV drug use with shared, uncleaned equipment. In *secondary* prevention, infected women who do not want a pregnancy are helped to choose the best possible contraceptive and to practice safer sex techniques in order to protect uninfected sex partners. And in *tertiary* prevention, infected pregnant women are helped to reduce their likelihood of perinatal transmission with antiretroviral drug regimens and modified labor and delivery procedures.

HIV RISK ASSESSMENT

Providers in the reproductive health care setting are ideally situated to broach HIV risk assessment and behavior change with patients, because, with our contraception and STI services, we already help people reduce health risks in their sexual lives. Our patients expect us to discuss sexual issues, and may even look to us for sexual information. And perhaps most important, reproductive health care clinics may be for many young women the only source of health care.

Ask each and every patient, "What do you do to protect yourself from AIDS?[8] You can always encourage your patient, even during a brief discussion, to take one step further in skill mastery. You may even be able to determine readiness for behavior change by assessing the answer given to your question. The patient who answers, "I thought I would get some condoms while I'm here today" is more ready to try new behavior than is the patient who answers, "Who, me?" (See Chapter 10 on Education and Counseling for more on supporting behavior change.)

With new patients, and with all patients if you provide services in areas of ≥1% HIV prevalence, use a more explicit HIV risk assessment (Table 7-1) whenever time allows.[9] These questions provide a springboard to assess each patient's personal experiences. Although reproductive health physicians are more likely than other primary care physicians to ask about sex and drug behavior,[10] many are reluctant to risk offending patients. It may be helpful to begin with, "I'm going to ask you some personal questions that we ask everyone, because we think it is so important to your health. Is that all right with you?"

Simply ask questions or, if your patient population has good literacy skills and is reasonably comfortable with a frank approach to sexual topics (patients at a college campus health service, for example), give them a questionnaire to complete. Always provide a private setting. Document only what is critical to good patient care, and rigorously protect the written record under lock and key. Some health care providers who use questionnaires choose to return the document to the patient after discussion, with the assurance that only minimal information will be recorded in the chart.

Table 7-1 Assessing HIV risk behaviors

Answer these questions for all the time in your life from 1977 to now.

What are you doing that you think may be putting you at risk for AIDS?

Sex

Have you had an oral, vaginal, or anal sexual experience with another person?

If yes, with about how many different people? 1? 2 or 3? 4 to 10? More than 10?

Have your partners been men, women, or men sometimes and women sometimes? What about your partner's partners?

Have you felt that a sex partner put you at risk for AIDS (injecting drug user, bisexual, lots of partners before you)?

Have you had a sexually transmitted infection, such as herpes, gonorrhea, genital warts, or chlamydia?

Have you felt forced to have a sexual experience when you didn't want to?

What do you do to protect yourself from AIDS?

Do you use male condoms? Female condoms? Other barriers? Please describe how you use them.

Thinking about sex and AIDS, what do you think is the riskiest thing you do?

Drugs

Have you used injecting drugs with shared uncleaned equipment, including street drugs, steroids?

Have you had sex with a person who uses injecting drugs and shares uncleaned equipment?

How many drinks of beer, wine, spritzers, and hard liquor have you had in the last 7 days?

Have you had sex while stoned, high, or drunk, so that you can't remember details?

Have you had sex in exchange for drugs, money, food, or shelter?

Do you think alcohol or drugs ever got you into trouble?

Thinking about drugs and AIDS, what do you think is the riskiest thing you do?

Blood

Have you shared uncleaned equipment for tattooing, body piercing?

Have you had a blood transfusion?

Have you had sex with a person who has had a blood transfusion?

Do you have hemophilia?

Have you had sex with a person with hemophilia?

Have you received donor semen, egg, transplanted organ, or tissue?

Thinking about blood and AIDS, what do you think is the riskiest thing you do?

Other

Have you ever had a test for HIV? What prompted you to have the test?

Avoid making an "ophthalmic" assessment, that is, drawing conclusions about a patient's sexual and other behaviors based on appearances. Avoid assumptions such as:

- Sexually-experienced people know how to use safer sex techniques.
- People with good jobs don't use drugs.
- Single people have lots of partners and risky sex practices.
- Older people have few partners and infrequent sex.
- Married people are heterosexual.

Remember that terminology can sometimes get in the way of clarity with this type of risk assessment. For example, teens may not know the word "monogamous." Lay people may think "sexually active" means vigorous sex, or lots of partners. Many people who engage in same-gender sexual intimacy do not think of themselves as "homosexual."

SUBSTANCE ABUSE ASSESSMENT

Substance use can be intricately connected with sexual risk-taking. A survey of high-school-age students found that in 2001 almost one-third of boys and one-fifth of girls used alcohol or drugs the last time they had intercourse.[11] Abuse of alcohol and drugs increases HIV risk because of potentially self-destructive risk-taking, such as unsafe sex with someone just met or exchanging unsafe sex for drugs, money, food, or shelter. The riskiest substance-using behavior of all is using shared uncleaned injection equipment. Having sex with an injecting-drug user is also extremely risky, and because injecting-drug use in the present or past is often a carefully hidden practice, some patients will not be aware that a sex partner uses injecting drugs.

EXPLICIT SAFER SEX SKILLS

Teach explicit safer sex skills, including correct use of male and female condoms and other latex and plastic barriers, to all at-risk patients (Table 7-2). Be sure to include prevention skills for oral sex, because HIV transmission through unprotected oral sex is possible, especially with activities that expose the mouth to semen.[12–14] Sexual transmission may be especially likely during the weeks of primary HIV infection, when viral load, and thus infectivity, are high.[15,16]

Advise all patients that a crucial time for diligent safer sex practices is the first few months of a new relationship. Delaying intercourse allows for a deeper relationship, a fuller assessment of partner trustworthiness, and an opportunity to get an HIV test together. Using male or female latex or plastic condoms consistently during the more infectious early HIV infection interval protects against what might be a legacy from a recent past relationship.[17]

Table 7-2 Options for sexual intimacy and HIV prevention

Safe

All unprotected sexual activities, when both partners are monogamous, trustworthy, and known by testing to be free of HIV; also

Sexual fantasies

Massage

Hugging

Body rubbing

Dry kissing

Solo masturbation without contact with partner's semen, vaginal secretions, blood, or broken skin

Erotic conversation, books, movies, videos, electronic images

Erotic bathing, showering

Eroticizing feet, hands, hips, abdomen, ears, other body parts

Low But Potential Risk

All sexual activities, when both partners are monogamous, trustworthy, but have not been tested; also

Wet kissing with no broken skin, cracked lips, or damaged mouth tissue

Hand-to-genital touching or mutual masturbation on healthy, intact skin or with a latex or plastic barrier

Vaginal or anal intercourse using latex or plastic condom correctly with adequate lubrication

Oral sex on a man using a latex or plastic condom

Oral sex on a woman using a latex or plastic barrier such as a female condom, dental dam, plastic wrap, or modified male condom (especially if she does not have her period or a vaginal infection with discharge)

Unsafe in the absence of mutual monogamy, trust, and HIV testing of both partners

Blood contact of any kind, including menstrual blood

Any vaginal or anal intercourse without a latex or plastic condom

Oral sex on a woman without a latex or plastic barrier such as a female condom, dental dam, plastic wrap, or modified male condom (especially if she is having her period or has a vaginal infection with discharge)

Oral sex on a man without a latex or plastic condom, especially if associated with semen in the mouth

Oral-anal contact

Shared sex toys or douching equipment

Any sex that causes tissue damage or bleeding, such as rough vaginal or anal intercourse, rape, or fisting

Customize teaching methods for the patient who is with you. Use audiovisual, print, and electronic teaching aids appropriate to the patient's comfort, pleasure, age, language, culture, and learning style. Be sure to make safer sex guidance patient-specific and related to her particular issues, rather than giving her vague, global advice:[9] "Starting today, put condoms on the night stand beside the bed," rather than "always use condoms." "Stop dating Randy, who is also dating other women," rather than "Have fewer, safer partners." "Next time you're out with friends and might have sex, avoid getting high on drugs or alcohol," rather than "Have safer sex."[9]

PARTNER SELECTION AND ASSESSMENT SKILLS

Younger patients may benefit from skill-building on choosing a boyfriend or girlfriend. Consider teaching how to analyze potential partners in categories such as "Don't Even Think About It," "I Deserve Better," and "This Could Work," described in Chapter 10, Education and Counseling, Table 1.

Teach patients to ask about and look for genital tract infections in sexual partners. Genital tract shedding of HIV increases in the presence of other untreated infections,[18] so advise patients to avoid sex or at least use condoms until a health care provider can answer any questions about HIV and other infections.

SKILL-BUILDING

Teach skills, not just facts. Most Americans know what HIV/AIDS is, know it is lethal, and know it is transmitted through sexual fluids and blood. However, sexual decisions and substance-using decisions are not generally based on reason. Human beings tend to act not out of what we know, but out of what we *feel* and *see* and *want*. Patients need our help, therefore, with skills for forging relationships with trustworthy low-risk people, for negotiating sex in relationships, and for operating from an internal value system rather than from external pressures.

POSTEXPOSURE PROPHYLAXIS, SEX, AND DRUGS

In cases of isolated high-risk exposures to HIV—unprotected vaginal or anal intercourse, rape, receptive oral sex with ejaculation, or sharing injection equipment when the partner is known or suspected to be infected—consider postexposure chemoprophylaxis. Because data on efficacy are limited, the U.S. Public Health Service position as of 2003 is that no recommendation can be made either for or against treatment.[19] Nonetheless, an increasing number of health care providers offer treatment to survivors of sexual assault and to other types of patients as well, when treatment can begin as soon as possible, and no later than 72 hours after possible isolated exposure. Treatment usually consists of a 1-month course of drugs combined from 2 or 3 antiretroviral drug groups, much like the combination therapy regimens used by persons with HIV.

Discuss treatment protocol options with your local rape crisis center, or call the Post-Exposure Prophylaxis Hotline operated by the National HIV/AIDS Clinicians' Consultation Center for guidance on individual cases. The hotline is based at the University of California at San Francisco, and can be reached toll-free 24 hours a day, 7 days a week at 1-888-448-4911. Whether to accept any offered treatment is the patient's decision. Treatment may cost $1,000-$1,600, and may not be covered by health insurance plans.[20]

FACTORS AFFECTING SEXUAL TRANSMISSION

The likelihood of sexual HIV transmission is variable. HIV viral load in the infected partner is a major determining factor. In a study of 416 serodiscordant heterosexual couples, each logarithmic increase in viral load was associated with a 2.5-fold increase in the probability of transmission.[21] Risk is influenced by characteristics in both the infected partner and the uninfected partner.[17]

Risk of sexual transmission may be increased:

- During the first months of HIV infection, when infectiousness is high and likely to go unrecognized
- During late HIV infection, when infectiousness often increases as the immune system becomes less effective in controlling the virus, especially in the absence of antiretroviral treatment
- When the infected partner has a concurrent reproductive tract infection

Risk of sexual transmission may be decreased:

- If the infected partner follows an effective antiretroviral drug regimen
- If the uninfected partner has a specific mutation in an HIV receptor gene
- If either the infected or the uninfected partner is circumcised

Contraceptive Choice

Contraceptive method also influences the likelihood of sexual transmission. One powerful reason women of all ages like oral contraceptives, other hormonal methods, intrauterine devices (IUDs), and surgical sterilization is that nothing mechanical or intrusive gets in the way of lovemaking. Therefore, special effort may be needed to encourage at-risk patients to add male or female condoms or other barriers for HIV protection. (The same issues apply when counseling HIV-infected patients. See discussion later in this chapter.) An inverse relationship exists between the use of more effective noncoital contraceptives and concurrent condom use.[22-24] In a Baltimore survey, for example, more than three-fourths of sterilized women never used a condom, compared with 46% of nonsterilized women.[23] Among 12,000 U.S. high school students, 19% of pill users also used condoms at last intercourse, compared with 54% of other sexually active students; pill use was the single strongest predictor of failure to use condoms, even stronger than alcohol or drug use or multiple partners.[25] Pills-plus-condoms is by no means the norm for sexual protection. This behavior is rarely modeled in the media, and pregnancy often feels more like a genuine personal threat than does HIV.[26] Almost everyone knows someone involved in an unplanned pregnancy, while many people have never (to their knowledge) known anyone with HIV.

Male condoms. The take-home message for all patients and their partners is that always using male condoms and always using them correctly works as HIV prevention.[27] Halfway measures do not work.[28,29] The counseling goal is to teach this message without causing patients to conclude, "Nobody's perfect every time, so why bother using them at all?" Help patients clarify their personal barriers to condom use,[30] and support their efforts to come as close to consistent, correct use as they possibly can.

The 2001 National Institutes of Health report on condom effectiveness against STDs concludes that consistent and correct condom use during intercourse prevents HIV infection for women and men.[31,32] In a study of HIV-discordant heterosexual partners, no HIV infections occurred among couples who always used condoms, versus a 10% infection rate in couples who used condoms intermittently.[33] Other studies of HIV-discordant couples have also demonstrated a protective effect from condoms.[28]

Giving patients precise answers about how much protection they can count on remains difficult. One problem is that we do not know how to factor in slippage and breakage effects. (See Chapter 16 on Male Condoms.) Further, other behavioral and biological factors play a role in HIV transmission. Most HIV-infected men shed HIV in semen intermittently, regardless of disease stage or antiretroviral treatment. An infected man can never omit condoms and other safer sex behaviors with complete safety.[34] Help patients understand that male condoms prevent sexual HIV transmission, but more precise quantifying of condom efficacy depends on personal circumstances and behaviors.

Timing when to put on a male condom is a practical issue. Some men leak seminal fluid from the urethral meatus once the penis is fully erect. This clear pre-ejaculatory fluid can contain HIV and other pathogens (although not motile sperm capable of causing pregnancy).[35,36] When a condom is used for safer sex, it must be rolled on the penis well before the penis has any contact with the partner's mouth, vagina, anus, or any broken skin.

Spermicides. For decades, nonoxynol-9-based spermicidal products were the "chicken soup, it can't hurt" of contraceptive care in the United States. Many providers advised users of other methods to add a spermicide for both improved contraceptive efficacy and for STI protection. This advice must be re-evaluated in the context of HIV risk, in part because frequent spermicide use can cause vulvovaginal epithelial disruption, which could theoretically increase susceptibility to HIV. Moreover, discouraging reports of international, multicenter trials of nonoxynol-9 indicate that it does not protect women against HIV infection.[37] Emerging data indicate that nonoxynol-9 may cause more anatomic damage if used during anal intercourse. Finally, use of nonoxynol-9-coated condoms is not recommended.

Epithelial disruption could be affected by spermicide dose, delivery system, or frequency of use,[28] so it is prudent to caution patients who use spermicides routinely and to help them develop the safest possible approach to contraception and HIV prevention. In addition, advise patients concerned about vaginal or penile irritation to avoid spermicidally-lubricated products. (See Chapter 16 on Male Condoms and Chapter 17 on Vaginal Spermicides.)

Oral contraceptives and other hormonal methods. The combined oral contraceptive pill may increase the vascularity of the cervical epithelium, extend the area of cervical ectopy, and alter certain immune parameters.[28,38] In a study of women at high risk of HIV, Depo-Provera was associated with a 2-fold increased risk of HIV.[39] Data on other hormonal methods are limited. It is prudent to advise hormonal method users to use male or female latex or plastic condoms until they are confident both partners are free of HIV and other STIs.

IUDs. Reproductive health clinicians routinely advise against the IUD for the patient at high risk for RTIs, including HIV. However, current data support wider IUD use by women at moderate-to-low risk of RTI. Moreover, data from Kenya indicate IUD use by HIV-infected women carries no higher risks than for uninfected women.[40] A past history of STI, if cured, does not rule out IUD use for women desiring this method. Factors that might increase the risk of HIV transmission by women using IUDs are longer, heavier periods and disrupted endometrial or cervical epithelium.[28] However, HIV-infected women using IUDs shed virus less often than do women using hormonal contraceptives.[41]

Female condoms. In vitro studies show that this condom is an effective barrier against HIV transmission, but no human studies of transmission effects have been published.[28]

Diaphragms and cervical caps. While randomized controlled trials are under way, no data exist on the efficacy of diaphragms or caps for HIV protection. However, the increased proportion of CD4 target cells in the cervix provides a theoretical basis for devices that cover the cervical os protecting against HIV infection.[42] HIV can be heterosexually transmitted to a woman via vaginal exposure alone, so diaphragms and caps that cover the cervix and a small portion of the vagina may offer less protection than consistent use of male condoms.[28,42] (See Chapter 18 on Vaginal Barriers.)

Sterilization. Tubal sterilization has no known effect on HIV transmission risk. HIV persists in semen after vasectomy.[28,43]

Male Circumcision

Lack of circumcision increases the risk of sexual HIV acquisition for both women and men. The foreskin may cause vaginal microabrasions during intercourse,[28] and it may hold HIV, as it does other pathogens, in a moist environment that facilitates acquisition by the male.[21,44,45]

Advice for Contraceptive Patients

Until further data are available, it seems prudent to advise all patients as follows:

- Use male or female latex or plastic condoms each time you suspect even the slightest risk of HIV but choose to have vaginal or anal intercourse anyway.

- Use latex or plastic condoms for men and latex or plastic vulvar barriers for women any time you suspect any risk of HIV but choose to have oral sex anyway.

- Vaginal spermicides using nonoxynol-9 do not protect against HIV.[37]

- Any tissue damage to the vulva or vagina or penis could increase susceptibility to HIV and other RTIs. Avoid intercourse until you are healed. See your care provider for help with healing.

- These directions can be modified for gay male, lesbian, and bisexual patients.

SPECIAL CONSIDERATIONS IN HIV PREVENTION

Romance. It is difficult to hold simultaneously the two thoughts, "I am in love with you," and "You might pose an infection risk to me." Romantic (germ-free) fantasy is a hallmark of midadolescence,[46] and many people never manage to be clear-eyed about romance even when realism pervades other aspects of the adult worldview. Therefore, the reproductive health care provider is frequently in the unenviable position of bubble-burster, attempting to foster self-protective health behavior where there is only desire, emotional need, and single-minded devotion to the idealized romantic relationship.

Effective HIV prevention counseling with patients who are in love does not set up the beloved as a bad person, but stresses that all people can and do harm other people even when they do not intend to, and that people who love each other would certainly try to help each other maintain good health!

Power. Sometimes women make a personal commitment to HIV prevention but have little hope of enlisting the cooperation of the male partner. They say, for example, "You might as well not give me any condoms, because I know he won't use them." In all U.S. cultural groups, women typically lack economic, social, and physical power equal to that of men. Even when couples negotiate and achieve a relationship with equal decision-making power, they are likely to have begun the relationship with a power imbalance.

One direct way to address this issue is to invite women to bring in their partners and to offer prevention skill-building for these men, either together with the female partner or alone. When men cannot or will not come in, offer telephone counseling with a male counselor. When no way exists to speak directly with the patient's partner, give patients audio or print messages to give to men. Remember that community and cultural norms vary substantially in how sexual decisions are made and by whom, so be sure counseling is grounded in the reality of your patient's life. For example, assess her risk of abuse, battering, rape, or abandonment should she try to insist on condom use.

A woman-initiated vaginal microbicide is a high research priority for HIV prevention, but it may be a decade away.[47] Meanwhile, women at risk must be encouraged to use male and female latex or plastic condoms and other safer sex techniques as consistently as they possibly can, even when they are unaccustomed to such expressions of personal power.

Special needs of adolescents. The critical challenge is to implement effective HIV prevention strategies for adolescents who are entering into sexual and perhaps drug-use experimentation. Interventions in the first two decades of the HIV epidemic have increased knowledge (89% of high schoolers have been taught about HIV in school[11]) and sometimes led to modest behavior change. However, in general, adolescents still take many risks. More than 60% of all 12th grade students had had intercourse in 2001, and 49% of them report using a condom the last time they had sex.[11] Among a cohort of urban adolescents moving into young adulthood, risk-taking behaviors remained about the same over a 5-year period, regardless of their knowledge about HIV, number of sources of information, acquaintance with infected people, perception of personal risk, or experience with HIV test counseling.[48] It will not surprise health care providers that most of these young people, like many of our older patients, disliked condoms, did not use them on a regular basis, and did not trust condoms to be protective.

A bold six-step plan for improving HIV-prevention efforts with adolescents is essential:[49]

- Use teenagers as spokespersons, and not as irresponsible stereotypes, in prevention campaigns.

- Replace abstinence-only campaigns with a more balanced approach aimed at delaying first intercourse and other risky sexual experimentation.

- Saturate the adolescent environment with appropriate and explicit risk-reduction messages.

- Link prevention programs with easy access to testing and medical services.

- Help adults learn to deal with sexuality and HIV, including parents, teachers, youth workers, and health care workers.

- Link on-site condom availability with HIV prevention programs in schools and youth agencies.

Deciding to be safe. Deciding to protect oneself (and others) from HIV is not one choice, like flipping a switch, but rather a series of hundreds of choices made day after day in the arenas of sex and drug use. When patients tell their stories, point out to them all their decision points, the places where they made safe and unsafe decisions, and whether they made them actively or passively. An important take-home message for patients is that HIV prevention decisions are made every single day, and we can always learn from our past experiences. (See Chapter 10 on Education and Counseling for more on supporting behavior change.)

H IV TESTING AND COUNSELING

About one-third of U.S. women age 18 to 44 have had an HIV test, excluding those tested as blood donors.[50] No more important conduit to HIV testing services exists for women than the reproductive health care provider, and such providers are urged to offer testing as a standard component of care.

WHEN TO OFFER TESTING

Offer routine counseling and voluntary HIV testing with informed consent to *all* women. With tools to help uninfected women remain uninfected, to help control the advance of HIV-related immunodeficiency and illness, and to markedly reduce the likelihood of perinatal transmission, providers can do no less. Routine, voluntary HIV testing for all pregnant women is the standard of care in the United States.[9]

Certain situations call for the care provider's strong recommendation to seek testing, and extra effort to assure that patients have reasonable access to counseling and testing services. Centers for Disease Control and Prevention (CDC) guidelines[9] advise extra efforts for:

- All pregnant women
- All patients who know they have had exposure to an HIV-infected person
- All patients who know they have shared injection equipment with an HIV-infected person
- All patients with possible recent occupational exposure
- All patients in settings with a ≥1% HIV seroprevalence
- All patients from "populations at increased behavioral or clinical HIV risk," such as those in STI clinics, teen clinics with high rates of STIs, or correctional facilities, regardless of that setting's HIV seroprevalence
- Patients with "clinical signs or symptoms suggesting HIV infection (e.g., fever or illness of unknown origin, opportunistic infection without known reason for immune suppression)"

- Patients with "diagnoses suggesting increased risk for HIV (such as another STI or bloodborne infection)"
- Patients with self-reported HIV risks (Table 7-1)
- Patients who ask for an HIV test

Also urge HIV testing for women who are contemplating pregnancy or who have had sexual exposure to a person whose health history and HIV status are unknown.

TEST COUNSELING

The decision to be tested for HIV belongs to the patient. The structure of testing and counseling services is up to your agency, and must be in accord with local, state, and federal policies that govern provision of HIV services. Current CDC testing guidelines[9] stress flexibility in implementing testing services, and remind care providers to consider characteristics of the patient population, HIV prevalence in the local setting, and available resources as they tailor services. This welcome latitude is markedly different from the rigorous checklist-style test counseling guidance published by the CDC in the early years of HIV testing.

There is neither a uniform, official, "certified" test counseling protocol nor an official certificate-granting counselor training course. This is a notion that persists from the early days of HIV testing when CDC offered the only training information on testing and test counseling that was available for health care providers. Today there are many sources of training, and many useful approaches to test counseling. Current CDC testing guidelines[9] describe a number of creative and carefully studied counseling options that are client-centered and allow flexibility for specific situations. Physicians, midlevel clinicians, nurses, health educators, outreach workers, and other care providers can offer effective and compassionate test counseling.

For pretest services, your role is to explain how the test is done, what the routine screening procedure will and will not reveal, implications of anonymous vs. confidential testing, and instructions on learning test results. Some patients tested with routine (rather than rapid) test technologies do not return for test results, so use the pre-test session to teach personalized and explicit risk-reduction skills. A counselor guide (Table 7-3) for the pre-test session (and for devising an informed consent document) and guides for giving negative and positive test results to patients may be helpful (Tables 7-4 and 7-5). All providers who give positive HIV-antibody test results to patients will need training to master the skills of breaking bad news.[51,52] This special encounter must help support the patient first, and then seek to accomplish no more than one or two critical educational goals. Many patients report that they remember little or nothing the care provider said after hearing the word, "positive."

Counselors who are experienced at HIV test counseling generally allow 10 to 15 minutes for a pre-test session, 10 to 15 minutes for a negative post-test session, and 30 minutes or longer for a positive post-test session. We naturally dread telling a young woman she has a grave illness. Test counseling can be time-consuming. It may require training and mastery of new referral sources. Be careful to provide sensitive staff training and support both before and after your work setting initiates testing and counseling.

COUNSELING AND TESTING ISSUES

Anonymous and confidential testing. CDC guidelines stress the importance of having anonymous testing available for patients.[9] Anonymous testing never links a name to the sample presented for evaluation (although age, county of residence, sex, and other general demographic characteristics are often recorded). The anonymous patient is given a number code for getting test results. In contrast, confidential testing is name-linked, and information is protected to a degree determined by state law and the formal policies and staff commitment to confidentiality at the testing site.

Allow patients to choose the approach they prefer, and be prepared to make a careful referral for anonymous testing if you are unable to provide it on-site. Most laboratories are willing to work out a coding system for anonymous samples, even for private practitioners. Patients not offered anonymous testing and reluctant to have an HIV test on record are likely to go to a test site where they are not known, to use a false name, or both. Another alternative for anonymous testing is home collection of a test sample using an over-the-counter kit, discussed below.

With the possible exception of the very low risk "worried well," discourage patients from donating blood as a way to learn HIV status, and remind them that such donations are not anonymous.

Testing technology. For the past 15 years, HIV testing in the United States typically sampled serum using an enzyme immunoassay (EIA) screening test and Western blot confirmatory test.[9] Results have generally been available in 1 to 2 weeks.

The EIA and Western blot are very sensitive and specific.[9] Yet neither test is perfect, so an HIV test is reported as positive only after at least two EIAs and one Western blot or other confirmatory test (all using the same test sample) are all positive. As with any screening test, population prevalence is the single biggest factor in determining a test's predictive value; the higher the prevalence, the greater the likelihood that a positive test result means that the person is truly infected.[9] Always regard HIV test results in the context of the total patient history and clinical picture, and re-evaluate when the two are not in accord. The injecting-drug-using woman with thrush who tests negative merits further evaluation, as does the healthy woman in a stable, trusting, and monogamous relationship and with no drug use or transfusion history who tests positive.

Table 7-3 Components of pre-test counseling

Reason for considering test

- Elicit patient's reason(s) so counselor can use a client-centered approach to be as helpful as possible

About the HIV antibody test

- What kind of sample is used for testing: blood, oral mucosal transudate, urine
- What antibodies are
- How soon the test is accurate
- Why this is not a test for AIDS

How people get infected with HIV

- Through unprotected oral, vaginal, or anal intercourse with an infected person
- Through bloodstream-to-bloodstream contact with an infected person
    - Sharing uncleaned equipment for injectable drugs, steroids, tattoos, skin piercing
    - Transfusion of blood or blood products before March 1985
- From infected woman to child during pregnancy, labor and delivery, or breastfeeding. Risk depends on amount of virus in woman's body; average 25% risk for untreated U.S. women, but can be markedly reduced with medication

Deciding whether to have the test

- Your right to decide whether to be tested
- Unforced informed consent
- Anonymous versus confidential testing
- Who will see the results if test is done here, including state laws
- Other sites for testing; home collection kit

Benefits of being tested

- Peace of mind; knowing, one way or the other
- If infected:
    - Begin treatment for slowing HIV, managing related problems
    - Prevent transmission to others
    - Make informed childbearing decisions
    - Diagnose illness or symptoms
    - Access assistance programs

Difficulties with being tested

- Anxiety, waiting for results
- If infected:
    - Learning you have a very serious illness
    - Telling sex or injecting-drug-equipment-sharing partners (health care agencies can provide help with this task)
    - Possible relationship difficulties with partner, family, friends
    - Possible threat to job
    - Difficulty getting or keeping insurance
    - Few experienced care providers in some locales

(continued)

Table 7-3 Components of pre-test counseling—*(cont'd)*

What your results will mean

- If antibody positive:
  - — You are infected
  - — You can pass the virus on to other people
- If antibody negative or indeterminate:
  - — You are not infected

    or

  - — You are infected, but your body has not yet made enough antibodies for test to be positive

Reducing risk for HIV

- Develop a personalized risk reduction plan today with counselor (using Tables 7-1, 7-2, and the CDC's Revised Guidelines for HIV Counseling, Testing, and Referral[9] as starting points)

For more information

- National AIDS Hotline 800-342-AIDS
- Local and regional hotlines
- HIV InSite: hivinsite.ucsf.edu
- Go Ask Alice: www.goaskalice.columbia.edu

Assure patient understanding and obtain documentation of voluntary consent if patient chooses testing

---

Table 7-4 Post-test counseling for negative results

Give results promptly. Do not expect people to digest much guidance once they have their results. Allow time for supportive counseling about relief, other personal feelings and concerns, then move to personal risk reduction. Information can be reinforced in print for patients who are comfortable reading the language(s) you have available. Make return appointment for more skill-building if warranted and reasonable.

What the HIV antibody screening test looked for

- Antibodies to HIV, not the virus itself (additional tests can look for the virus itself)
- Evidence of infection acquired longer ago than 1–6 months

What negative results mean

- You may not have been exposed

  or

- You may have been exposed, but did not become infected; you cannot count on this good fortune in the future

  or

- You were infected recently, and it is too soon for the test to be positive; if you have had a possible exposure in the past 6 months, consider getting another test 1-2 months from now, and use safer sex and other prevention measures in the meantime

Reducing risk for HIV

- Develop a personalized risk reduction plan today with counselor (using Tables 7-1,7-2, and the CDC Revised Guidelines for HIV Counseling, Testing, and Referral[9] as starting points)

(continued)

Table 7-4 Post-test counseling for negative results—*(cont'd)*

How this office can help
- Condoms and other safer sex supplies
- Help with a personal risk reduction plan
- Referral for drug, alcohol treatment

For more information
- National AIDS Hotline 800-342-AIDS
- Local and regional hotlines
- HIV InSite: hivinsite.ucsf.edu
- Go Ask Alice: www.goaskalice.columbia.edu

Table 7-5 Post-test counseling for positive results

Give results promptly. Positive results using rapid screening tests are preliminary until confirmatory testing is done. Do not expect people to take in much new information after they hear that they are infected. Allow plenty of time for supportive counseling about feelings, following patient's lead. Consider giving information in print to read later on if the patient is comfortable reading materials in the language(s) you have available, and make a return appointment or referral for ongoing counseling and care. Be sure patients have a reasonable plan of action (where to go when they leave your office, whom they will tell) before leaving your office.

What the positive HIV antibody screening test result means
- You have antibodies for HIV in your blood (or oral transudate, urine, or other tested body fluid)
- You are infected with the virus that causes AIDS
- You can pass the virus on to other people

What the test result does NOT tell you
- How long you have been infected
- Whether you already have AIDS
- The present status of your immune system

Could the test be wrong?
- On rare occasions, a negative person's test result comes back positive
- The chance of this happening is less than 1 in 1,000
- Consider being retested by a different testing laboratory if you believe your test result is wrong

What next?
- Learn about HIV; for many people, knowledge is empowering
- Visit a care provider experienced with HIV for a workup, including
  - T-cell count (CD4 count) to learn the status of your immune system
  - Viral load test to learn how active the HIV is right now
  - TB test
  - Any needed medicines
- Start now to keep your body as healthy as you can
  - Eat well, get plenty of rest, moderate exercise
  - Limit or stop drugs that you drink, inhale, inject, or swallow
  - Avoid new STIs (sexually transmissible infections) and treat any infections you have (these infections can increase the amount of HIV in your body)

(continued)

Table 7-5   Post-test counseling for positive results—*(cont'd)*

How this office can help

- Assist with or refer for immediate needs (housing, financial)
- Help you tell others about your HIV
- Answer your questions, and questions from friends and family
- Assist with finding a care provider experienced with HIV
- Supply contraception for you, partner
- Help you develop a plan of action for this difficult crisis period
- Assist with or refer for emotional support resources
- Help you develop a personalized plan to reduce risk of transmitting your HIV to others
- Supply condoms and other safer sex equipment
- Other services, based on resources available

Whom you should tell

- Medical and dental care providers, so proper care can be offered
- Past and present sex partners and people with whom you shared injecting-drug equipment
- Learn about HIV before you talk to him/her/them
  - Talk in private
  - Avoid casting blame
  - Think ahead of time how to react if the person gets upset
  - Strongly suggest testing for him/her/them as soon as possible
    - For peace of mind, if negative
    - For early access to medicine to control HIV
    - For taking steps to avoid giving HIV to others
    - For informed childbearing decisions

How to avoid giving your HIV to others

This office can help you develop a personalized plan, including:

- Tear up any donor cards
- Do not donate blood, tissue, eggs, semen, organs
- Do not share razors, toothbrushes (in case any blood is on them)
- Clean up spilled blood or bloody body fluids promptly, using bleach and water
- Inform sex partner(s), and negotiate a safer sex plan ahead of time
- Do not share injection drug, tattoo, or body-piercing equipment
- Limit or stop any drug use that impairs your judgment such as alcohol, crack, or cocaine
- Avoid pregnancy, or use medicine during pregnancy, during labor and delivery, and give medicine to your baby in the first weeks of life to reduce risk of HIV for the child
- Avoid breastfeeding

For more information

- National AIDS Hotline 800-342-AIDS
- Local support resources for HIV-infected persons
- Resources to meet personal needs, such as drug treatment
- HIV InSite: hivinsite.ucsf.edu
- Medscape: http://www.health.medscape.com/hivaidscenter

New technologies have added options for testing other body fluids and for providing rapid test results.[53] These newer technologies are FDA-approved and provide sensitivity and specificity comparable to traditional tests.

- Patients reluctant to visit a care provider can purchase a drugstore kit, collect their own finger-prick blood sample, mail off the sample to a lab, and call for anonymous results and telephone counseling a few days later. As of 2003, one FDA-approved brand, Home Access, is available in the United States for about $45 for results in 7 business days and about $60 for results in 3 business days. Concerns about moving HIV testing out of the traditional health care setting will be familiar to reproductive health care providers who remember the advent of home pregnancy testing. What about tester error? How will people find any follow-up care they need? Will telephone counseling be supportive and skilled enough to make appropriate referrals? Early reports are reassuring. One study of home blood collection found that 98% of the time subjects were able to obtain a testable blood specimen and they correctly answered 96% of the questions about HIV risk after receiving pre-test counseling by telephone. Study subjects could elect to use interactive, automated information recordings or live telephone counselors; only one-third of subjects chose a live counselor during the pre-test or post-test call.[54] Product information on Home Access is available at http://www.homeaccess.com.

- As of mid-2004, three rapid HIV screening tests are available in the United States: OraQuick, Reveal, and Uni-Gold. More tests are making their way to market. All three brands provide a definitive negative result and a *preliminary* positive result in a matter of minutes. *Definitive* positive results require a confirmatory test such as a Western Blot. Sensitivity and specificity are comparable to standard EIAs,[56,57] and costs range from $10–14 per test.

  OraQuick is the only rapid test approved to date for use with IgG-rich oral fluid as well as for whole blood and plasma, and may be a good option for patients who fear needles. A Clinical Laboratory Improvements Amendments of 1988 (CLIA) waiver permits OraQuick use (at present, for whole blood samples only) in clinics, labor and delivery areas, and other care settings with appropriate staffing, training, and quality control. A CLIA waiver for oral fluid testing is anticipated. Check the CDC internet site to track developments in the arena of rapid testing at www.cdc.gov/hiv/rapid_testing.

  Rapid test technology makes it easier than ever to offer HIV testing as a routine service in women's health care settings, taking advantage of providers' unique trust relationships and ability to discuss sexual issues and risks with patients.

- Other options for routine screening that avoid needles and blood are urine EIA and Western blot using products from Calypte

Biomedical. Product information is available at 1-877-CALYPTE, or www.calypte.com. This screening test is slightly less sensitive (98.7%) than other EIAs.[53]

Without doubt, more technological refinements will follow, perhaps even home HIV-test kits that supply rapid results without requiring a needle stick, blood, or even a live or automated telephone counselor. Be prepared to encounter patients whose first conversation with a health professional about HIV comes weeks, months, or years after learning positive test results on their own at home, in the dorm, or anywhere at all.

Table 7-6 Possible causes of problematic HIV test results[9]

False-negative EIA
- Recent infection
- Infection with a form of HIV not detectable by standard test, such as HIV-2 or HIV-1 group 0 (alternate tests are available)

Indeterminate or false-negative Western blot
- Recent infection
- End-stage HIV
- Perinatally-exposed uninfected infants who are losing maternal antibody (seroreverting) may have indeterminate results
- Nonspecific reactions in pregnant or parous women
- Patients with "repeated indeterminate Western blot results a month or more apart are unlikely to be HIV-infected and can be provided test results in the same way as patients with negative results, unless recent HIV exposure is suspected"[9]

False-positive Western blot
- Rare

Prenatal testing. The U.S. Public Health Service recommends that all pregnant women in the United States be tested for HIV infection.[9] A joint statement by the American Academy of Pediatrics and the American College of Obstetricians and Gynecologists also supports "universal HIV testing with patient notification as a routine component of prenatal care," and also encourages routine test counseling, "but not as a prerequisite for and barrier to prenatal HIV testing."[58]

Many women learn they have HIV when testing is done as part of routine prenatal care, and acceptance of HIV testing in this setting is fairly high, 74-95% in one multicity study.[59] Women in this study were positively influenced to accept the test because they believed that finding and treating HIV would help both woman and offspring and because their provider strongly endorsed the test. Women who declined testing gave reasons such as not perceiving a risk, having scheduling difficulties, and having a history of previous testing.

Counseling about pregnancy options becomes an important component of post-test counseling if the HIV diagnosis is learned early in pregnancy; the patient may be overwhelmed by the large amount of highly emotional information to absorb at once. Pregnant infected women make the same sorts of reproductive decisions as uninfected women, with similar percentages of terminated pregnancies and live births. For the infected woman who chooses to continue the pregnancy, follow post-test counseling with guidance about her immune status, medicines to help control the advance of her HIV and reduce the likelihood of perinatal transmission, and the potential impact of all these medicines on her developing fetus. (See the following section for more on the care of pregnant women.)

Charting. Charting HIV test results is clearly important for ongoing medical care, although problems with confidentiality may result. This dilemma can be addressed by maintaining HIV-related information in a separate chart, by using a code for HIV test results, or by removing HIV-related information before releasing the chart. This latter practice is required by law in some states. State and local professional associations may offer guidance for appropriate, lawful charting that does not compromise patient, care provider, or health care.

MEDICAL CARE AND PSYCHOSOCIAL SUPPORT FOR INFECTED WOMEN

CHARACTERISTICS OF HIV IN WOMEN

The course of HIV infection in women is similar to the illness in men. Early symptoms, opportunistic infections, treatment response, and duration of illness are consistent with findings in men once access to care and immune status at diagnosis are taken into account. Women may manifest immunologic impairment and CD4 cell depletion at HIV viral load levels 30% to 50% lower than those in men, and recommended treatment threshholds may come to reflect this gender difference.[60]

Acute HIV infection can be identified 40% to 90% of the time.[60] During the primary infection, many people experience a flu-like syndrome lasting 1 to 4 weeks and characterized by fever, generalized lymphadenopathy, skin rash, headache, diarrhea, malaise, and lethargy. Few people recognize this syndrome as HIV, and this lack of awareness can lead to missed opportunities for early treatment, and also to unsafe behaviors in a time of relatively high infectiousness.

After the primary infection period, adults with HIV typically feel well for months or years, then progress (especially in the absence of effective antiretroviral treatment) from minor skin and constitutional symptoms, to discrete opportunistic illness, to a cascade of illnesses, then to end-stage disease. Specific patterns of immune response to HIV in the first few weeks after infection may predict what pattern of progression the illness will follow. CD4 cell count, viral load, and reproductive health concerns differ according to the stage of HIV infection in women (Table 7-7). Whether all people with HIV ultimately progress along this course is not clear.

The current standard of care for HIV is Highly Active Antiretroviral Therapy, or HAART, a combination of oral antiretroviral agents that inhibit different phases of the HIV life cycle. HAART regimens can be composed of drugs from 2, 3, or more classes, including nucleoside analog reverse transcriptase inhibitors (NRTIs), non-nucleoside reverse transcriptase inhibitors (NNRTIs), protease inhibitors (PIs) and fusion inhibitors. About 20 single-drug or combination products constitute the FDA-approved HAART armamentarium. HAART should be initiated and managed by—or in close consultation with—an experienced HIV clinician in order to prevent the development of resistance to single drugs or to entire classes of drugs. Having an experienced care provider has been shown to be a factor in prolonging life for persons with HIV.[61] The HAART daily pill-taking schedule is demanding, side effects are common, and HIV mutation and resistance can occur quickly if the regimen is not followed carefully. The success of this combination drug approach varies from patient to patient and long-term effects continue to emerge. Moreover, HAART regimens are expensive, and some patients cannot tolerate the drugs.

HAART and viral load testing have made it possible to attack HIV with greater success than ever before. Viral load testing uses DNA or RNA detection assays to measure the actual amount of HIV in plasma, permitting an accurate determination of real-time viral activity and a rapid assessment of antiretroviral drug efficacy. For example, a clinician can now assess baseline viral load, start HAART, look at viral load again in a few days or weeks, and quickly alter an ineffective regimen that is not lowering viral load. Much remains to be learned about treating HIV, and many infected people have little or no access to these new technologies. Nonetheless, there is renewed hope that HIV can be a truly manageable disease.

Infected women need high-quality primary care and HIV care from a clinician experienced with and comfortable with HIV medical management. Reproductive health care would ideally be managed in this primary care/HIV care setting also, but in some cases these are two providers in two different sites, so careful attention to shared information, shared decision making, and collaboration is essential.

Advice on medical management of patients with HIV is available from the National HIV/AIDS Clinicians' Consultation Center based at the University of California at San Francisco. This no-cost "warmline" is staffed Monday through Friday from 6:00 a.m. to 5:00 p.m. Pacific Time, and voicemail is available 24 hours a day, 7 days a week. Call 1-800-933-3413.

A natural role for all care providers is to assist HIV-infected patients with health promotion practices that will engender optimism and contribute to well-being. Provide guidance on nutrition, stress management, exercise, rest, and reduction or elimination of tobacco, alcohol, and drugs.[62]

GYNECOLOGIC MANAGEMENT

The keys to successful management of gynecologic infections in women with HIV are high index of suspicion, prompt diagnosis, aggressive treatment (especially for immunocompromised women), and primary or secondary prophylaxis when appropriate.

Table 7-7 Stages of HIV infection and reproductive health concerns

	Primary HIV Infection/ Seroconversion	Symptom-Free	Early Symptoms	Discrete Illness/Cascade of Illness/Endstage
Duration	Average 1–8 weeks	Few months to many years	Few months to several years	Few months to several years
CD4 Cell Count x 10⁶ /L Normal = 500–1600	Normal or slightly low	Typically > 500	Typically < 500	AIDS diagnosis automatic at 200 or less
Viral Load copies/ml	High	Variable	Rising (without HAART*)	High (without HAART)
Characteristics	Some notice a flu-like illness and rash that resolves on its own Would test negative for HIV antibody in "window period" that typically lasts 6–12 weeks post-infection Might test positive for p24 antigen or HIV RNA HAART* may delay progression	Likely to test positive 6–12 weeks after infection Without test, may have no reason to suspect infection With test, difficult to resolve feeling well with grave diagnosis With test, loss of sense of health, and loss of uncomplicated sex Not sure how long feeling well will last May begin HAART, especially if high viral load	Fevers, night sweats, zoster, candida, hairy leukoplakia, skin problems, weight loss, fatigue, loss of appetite Symptoms may cue testing and diagnosis Should begin HAART	Mild or severe multiple opportunistic bacterial, viral, fungal, parasitic infections Neoplastic diseases: Kaposi's sarcoma (uncommon in women), lymphoma, cervical cancer Neurologic: dementia, memory loss, peripheral neuropathy, affect, gait may be affected Many medications daily, side effects likely. Multiple prophylaxes added to HAART. Loss of ability to work or care for self, ability to interact with others Saying goodbye

(continued)

*HAART = Highly Active Antiretroviral Therapy

*Some notice a flu-like illness

Table 7-7 Stages of HIV infection and reproductive health concerns—*(cont'd)*

	Primary HIV Infection/ Seroconversion	Symptom-Free	Early Symptoms	Discrete Illness/Cascade of Illness/Endstage
Reproductive Health Concerns	No screening test available for early diagnosis, and so sex partner(s) and offspring may be placed at risk Assess contraception, safer sex	May not know diagnosis, so may not protect sex partner(s) and offspring Likely to be tested as part of routine prenatal screening Offer anticipatory guidance on future pregnancy planning Frequent Paps, aggressive management of abnormal findings Pregnancy likely to be normal except for transmission risk for offspring Assess contraception, safer sex	Pregnancy likely to be normal except for transmission risk for offspring Frequent Paps, aggressive management of abnormal findings Aggressive management of gynecologic infections Assess contraception, safer sex	Aggressive management of reproductive tract infections (RTIs) Medications may interfere with hormonal contraception; assess drug interactions Assist with short-range and long-range child care plans Pregnancy may result in prematurity, low birth weight, premature rupture of membranes, other complications Frequent Paps, aggressive management of abnormal findings Assess contraception, safer sex
Risk of Transmission to Offspring	Risk may increase above 25% baseline if primary infection occurs during pregnancy.	25% each pregnancy without treatment. Decreased to about 2% with effective HAART.	25% each pregnancy without treatment. Decreased to about 2% with effective HAART.	25% each pregnancy without treatment. Decreased to about 2% with effective HAART.

Source: Modified from Anderson (ed.) (2001)

Vulvovaginal candidiasis. Candidiasis is common in HIV-infected women, and may recur frequently when immune status deteriorates. Non-*albicans* strains are present in 1 in 4 vaginal isolates from women with HIV. First-line treatment is a 7-day course of one of the topical antifungals. If topical treatment proves unsatisfactory, consider oral fluconazole (a single dose, 150mg po). Information about azole resistance with intermittent one-dose fluconazole therapy is limited. Fluconazole should be used with caution in order to protect the availability of the azoles for other indications related to HIV.[63]

Human papillomavirus and cervical disease. Genital warts caused by human papillomavirus (HPV) are common in HIV-infected women and may progress more rapidly in the presence of a declining immune status. These patients have 10 times the rates of Pap smear-detected abnormalities and dysplasia as noninfected women.[64] In a prospective cohort study, 1 in 5 HIV-infected women with no evidence of cervical disease developed biopsy-confirmed squamous intraepithelial lesions (SILs) within 3 years.[65] Consider baseline colposcopy or cervicography, appropriate Pap smear intervals (see below), and prompt colposcopy and excision of any abnormal findings.

One-year Pap smear intervals are appropriate for women with a history of normal results. Screen every 6 months for women who have symptomatic HIV, a CD4 < 200, or both. Shorten the interval to 4 to 6 months for ASCUS/LGSIL findings, and, following treatment of preinvasive lesions, every 3 to 4 months for a year, then 6-month intervals.[63]

Pelvic inflammatory disease (PID). Public Health Service guidelines note that it is not clear whether immunosuppressed women with PID require more aggressive treatment than other women.[66] Others recommend an individualized approach to oral vs. parenteral therapy, hospitalizing patients with inadequate response to outpatient therapy, an unclear diagnosis where emergency surgery cannot be ruled out, pregnancy, inability to use outpatient treatment, immunosuppression, or tuboovarian abscess or other evidence of severe illness.[63] With appropriate treatment, the course of PID in HIV-infected women is similar to PID in other women.

Herpes. Herpes lesions may be more extensive, more painful, atypical in location or appearance, and slower to heal in the presence of immune dysfunction. Treat in accordance with standard guidelines. Women with advanced immunosuppression may need higher doses (acyclovir 400mg po 5 times/day or acyclovir 800mg 3 times/day) and longer treatment. Consider daily suppressive therapy for women with frequent recurrences.[63]

Menstrual problems. Studies of menstrual problems in infected women offer conflicting evidence, and whether HIV itself or related immunosuppression affects menstrual patterns will await further research.[63] Infected women, like other women, cope with menopause and may be appropriate candidates for hormonal replacement therapy with the proper indications.[67] Hormonal intervention also may be offered for heavy bleeding and anemia and to ease discomfort. All menstrual irregularities merit a full evaluation; do not assume HIV is always the culprit.

PSYCHOLOGICAL CARE AND SUPPORT

Women with HIV are likely to be caregivers themselves, accustomed to attending to the needs of children, spouse/partner, parents, and others; they may resist moving into a self-care mode. Women may make sure their children's clinic appointments are kept, for example, but be less diligent about keeping their own appointments. Gently remind the patient that she deserves care as well. Collaborate in establishing family-centered HIV clinics where all family members are cared for at the same time.

Often the infected woman is not the only infected person in her household; her spouse or partner and one or more children may also have HIV, so the disruption of daily life may be profound.

When infected women discuss their biggest worries and concerns, several fundamental needs are often mentioned:

- Having housing
- Earning an income
- Having a caregiver for children when mother is not feeling well
- Worrying about the health of children
- Feeling dread about disclosing illness to loved ones, especially children
- Fearing loss of the ability to care for oneself
- Worrying about the relationship with a spouse/partner
- Coping with addiction

Any guidance, support, and referral you can offer to assist with these fundamental concerns is likely to be welcome and helpful. Remember that for some women—an addicted woman, perhaps, or a woman in poverty—HIV may not be at the top of her list of problems to worry about.

REPRODUCTIVE HEALTH CARE

Women with HIV in their reproductive years may make many active or passive decisions about their reproductive lives, including contraceptive practice, desire for pregnancy, outcome of an unintended pregnancy, and prenatal practices to reduce perinatal transmission of HIV. Infected women are free to make reproductive choices for themselves just as other women do. Support them with information and time to reflect on decisions in an unpressured environment.

Reproductive decision making for infected women is similar to uninfected women, and desire for a child is often profound.[68] Counseling for the infected woman who is pregnant or contemplating pregnancy includes important medical issues:

- Impact of HIV on pregnancy
- Impact of pregnancy on HIV
- Effect of medicines on woman and developing fetus
- Risk of woman-to-offspring transmission
- Options for reducing woman-to-offspring transmission
- Risk of breastfeeding for HIV transmission
- Course of HIV in perinatally-infected infants
- Access to HIV-experienced obstetric and pediatric care
- Access to HIV medications

Counseling for pregnancy optimally includes a full understanding of the patient's personal goals, her support network, an understanding of stressors in her life, and her overall physical and emotional status. Once this groundwork is in place, guide the patient through specific questions to help her predict how she would feel, how others would feel, and what would happen:

- Is she able and willing to love and care for a baby, whether or not the baby is infected?
- Does she have the support of a partner, family members, or friends who can help care for a child?
- Who will care for the child—teach the child about his or her culture, remember his or her mother, and raise the child according to her values—if she becomes sick or dies?
- In what ways (good or bad) will having a baby change her life?
- What are the reasons that she wants (or does not want) to have a child?
- Does she feel pressured by others to have (or not have) a child?
- Does she have enough information to make an informed decision?

Clearly, this is difficult counseling work, best carried out by counselors with experience, compassion, and the ability to help with the feelings of grief and loss that these scenarios will likely generate. The goal is to guide each patient to an uncoerced, thoughtful decision.

HIV-infected women who do not wish to become pregnant, like other women, are more likely to succeed with a contraceptive method they have chosen for themselves and feel comfortable using (Table 7-8). The goal is high contraceptive efficacy, low risk of woman-to-partner HIV transmission (if applicable), and low risk of partner-to-woman STI transmission.[69,70] This goal is met by choices such as oral contraceptives plus male latex or plastic condoms. Despite our best efforts to increase awareness of transmission risks, infected women may choose a contraceptive without regard to disease transmission factors, just as uninfected women sometimes do.

Table 7-8   Contraception for the HIV-infected woman

Method	Possible Benefits	Possible Drawbacks
Oral Contraceptives	Good effectiveness with consistent use	Unclear interaction of steroids and immune function
	Less blood loss to avoid anemia	Possible interaction with certain antibiotics, antiretrovirals, other drugs
		Possible increased shedding of virus from genital tract
		No RTI protection
		No HIV protection for partner
Depo-Provera	Good low-maintenance effectiveness	Unclear interaction of steroids and immune function
		Possible increased shedding of virus from genital tract
		No RTI protection
		No HIV protection for partner
IUD	Good low-maintenance effectiveness	Risk of infection during insertion interval
		No RTI protection
		No HIV protection for partner
		Increased days of bleeding, possible anemia
Diaphragm, Cap, Spermicides	Some RTI protection	Increases vulnerability to UTIs for some users
		Requires good technique
Male, Female Condom	Good RTI protection HIV protection for partner	Male condom requires partner cooperation; partner cooperation helpful with female condom
		Requires good technique
Surgical Sterilization	Good low-maintenance efficacy for women who desire no more children	No RTI protection No HIV protection for partner

Sources: Adapted from Anderson, HIV and reproduction (2001) and Cates W Jr. (2001)

Thousands of U.S. women with HIV give birth each year. Generally, HIV-infected women who are immunocompetent have uneventful pregnancies with normal labor and delivery. Just as with any women with serious systemic illness, immunocompromised women may have complicated pregnancies, including prematurity, low birth weight, and premature rupture of membranes. However, the effects of HIV on pregnancy are hard to differentiate from the effects of poverty, poor health care, or addiction. Pregnancy does not appear to speed HIV progression.[70]

Without HAART, each offspring of an infected woman in the U.S. faces approximately a 25% risk of being infected in utero, during birth, or while breastfeeding. With HAART, the risk falls to 2% or less[9] (see below). Infants will all test positive for HIV antibody at birth because of the presence of maternal antibodies in infant blood. The HIV antibody screening test becomes accurate for the infant's true status at 15 to 18 months. Repeated polymerase chain reaction (PCR) testing is used to reveal the infant's true infection status. PCR testing is performed at birth, 2 weeks, and 6 weeks of age. If all three are negative, the baby is diagnosed as HIV-negative. If any are positive, repeated PCR testing is ordered. If all are positive, the baby is diagnosed as HIV-infected.

Reducing perinatal transmission risk. More than 8,200 U.S. children have developed AIDS because they were born to infected women.[2] A 1994 multicenter controlled trial of 477 HIV-infected pregnant women (called AIDS Clinical Trial Group 076 or ACTG 076) demonstrated that zidovudine (AZT) lowered perinatal transmission from 26% to 8% when given to women during pregnancy and to their newborn children during the first 6 weeks of life.[71] Today, strategies to reduce perinatal HIV transmission continue to evolve rapidly, and some critical data are not yet available. Combination HAART therapy, usually including zidovudine, is recommended for all pregnant women with the goal of suppressing plasma HIV RNA to undetectable levels. This combination regimen reduces perinatal HIV transmission more effectively than zidovudine alone. Antiretroviral treatment is also recommended for the HIV-exposed infants in their first weeks of life.[72] HAART initiation may be delayed until the second trimester.

As with HIV testing, the decision to accept or refuse HAART belongs to the woman. The care provider's role is to teach the facts clearly, neutrally, and thoroughly, and to assure that access to care and quality of care will not be influenced by the patient's decision.

Labor and delivery. In the absence of breastfeeding, an estimated 60% to 75% of perinatal HIV transmissions occur around the time of labor and delivery, and a number of strategies can reduce exposure of the neonate to maternal blood and secretions.[73] Suggested approaches include vaginal disinfection, RTI treatment during pregnancy to lower viral shedding at term, avoidance of intrapartum invasive procedures, and cesarean delivery. Scheduled cesarean delivery before rupture of membranes is recommended for women whose HIV viral load at 36 weeks or later is above 1,000 copies/mL.[74] Avoid delays in delivery once membranes have ruptured. The risk of perinatal HIV transmission can double when fetal membranes rupture more than 4 hours before delivery.[75,76]

Breastfeeding. Advise infected women in the United States to bottle feed infants to reduce the risk of postnatal HIV transmission via breast milk.[9] The precise risk of HIV transmission via breast milk is difficult to quantify, and may be influenced by the woman's HIV status (with high viral loads during primary infection and late stage disease), her use of antiretroviral drugs, breastfeeding patterns, and other factors. Among infected women who breastfeed, perhaps 10% to 15% of all vertical transmissions are associated with breastfeeding.[77] (See Chapter 23 on Postpartum Contraception and Lactation.) Little is known about the impact of breastfeeding on the HIV-infected woman's nutritional status and overall health, or about the immunoprotective qualities of the breast milk produced by immunocompromised women.

WORKPLACE SAFETY

Concern with personal safety is normal when providing care for HIV-infected patients, as with all patients with infectious disease. When agency policies and staff training are managed appropriately, worker safety can be maintained at high levels. Workplace safety procedures regarding HIV and other blood-borne pathogens have these essential components:

- Standard precautions or another infection control system for protecting the worker (and patient) from body fluid exposure
- Hepatitis B vaccination for all workers with any risk of exposure to blood or bloody body fluid
- A post-exposure plan for appropriate management of needle sticks and other accidental exposures (see below)
- Appropriate procedures for prompt evaluation and respiratory isolation for known or suspected tuberculosis

INFECTION CONTROL

In the ambulatory reproductive health care setting, most care providers use standard precautions. This means they treat as potentially infectious (for some type of infection, not necessarily HIV) all body fluids except for sweat. The following precautions are recommended:[78]

- Wash hands before and after every patient contact.
- Dispose of needles and sharps in puncture-resistant containers, and never recap needles.
- Wear latex or vinyl gloves when likely to touch body fluids, mucous membranes, or broken skin.
- Wear protective eye wear and mask when eyes and mucous membranes may be splashed.
- Wear a water-repellent gown when clothing could be soiled with body fluids.
- Cover any broken skin that could come into contact with body fluids.

OCCUPATIONALLY ACQUIRED HIV

Several cases of occupationally acquired HIV are reported annually. Needlesticks and other percutaneous exposures have accounted for 84% of cases.[79] Almost all exposures have been to blood or to concentrated virus in a laboratory setting. No infections have been observed from blood exposure to intact skin, from airborne droplets, or from environmental surfaces. What proportion of occupationally acquired infections are actually reported is unknown.

The rate of occupational HIV infection following a single needlestick or other percutaneous exposure is about 0.3% in 6,498 reported accidental exposures in the U.S. and other countries.[80] Not all exposures are equally likely to transmit HIV, however. Deep injuries, visibly bloody instruments, instruments previously placed in the source patient's artery or vein, and exposure to source patients who died within 60 days (and presumably had a high viral load) appear to increase risk.[81,82]

POST-EXPOSURE MANAGEMENT

In the event of an accidental workplace exposure to blood or another infectious body fluid from a person known or suspected to have HIV, follow these steps promptly:

- Decontaminate the site thoroughly

- Report the exposure to your facility's staff person designated to handle workplace injury (an important step, should you ever seek worker's compensation or other support).

- Seek guidance on appropriate chemoprophylaxis from your facility's designated staff person; or

- Call the National Clinicians' Post-Exposure Prophylaxis Hotline or PEPline at 1-888-448-4911, which is staffed 24 hours a day, 7 days a week. (If possible, have the person designated to treat injuries in your facility make the call.) This service is operated by the National HIV/AIDS Clinicians' Consultation Center and based at the University of California at San Francisco. The no-cost resource also assists with occupational exposures to other blood-borne pathogens such as hepatitis B and C. Before the call, identify the source patient if possible. If the source patient is known, learn what you can from a quick review of medical charts and laboratory results. If the patient is known to have HIV, review antiretroviral medications, recent HIV viral load test results, and any recent HIV drug resistance testing. A post-exposure chemoprophylaxis regimen will be tailored to the specific type of exposure, characteristics of the source patient, and the pregnancy status and wishes of the exposed person. If treatment is recommended, it usually consists of a month-long course of 2 or 3 antiretroviral agents. Treatment should begin as soon as possible, ideally within an hour of exposure. Be sure to have baseline HIV testing done immediately as well.

INFECTED HEALTH CARE PROVIDERS

Many thousands of health care providers have acquired HIV through sex and the other typical transmission routes. Whether HIV-infected health care workers place patients at risk is an important question. Retrospective studies using voluntary HIV testing of patients cared for by 51 infected physicians, surgeons, and dentists found no evidence of transmitted infection in any of the more than 22,000 patients evaluated.[83] Infected dentists, physicians, and other care providers are usually advised to make practice decisions in consultation with the personal physician, supervisor, and other professional groups as appropriate.

PERSONAL PERSPECTIVE ON WORKPLACE SAFETY

The health care workplace is not, and has never been, 100% safe. Ultimately, each care provider is responsible for personal safety and must insist on sound workplace policies and procedures, appropriate safety devices, high-quality barriers, and adequate staff training. In emergency situations, take the extra seconds to protect yourself and your coworkers with barriers and careful disposal of sharps. Most important, find a way to maintain compassionate touching, even when a latex barrier must sometimes come between care provider and patient.

REFERENCES

1. Joint United Nations Programme on HIV/AIDS. AIDS epidemic update: December 2002. Available at http://www.unaids.org. Accessibility verified April 8, 2003.
2. Centers for Disease Control and Prevention. HIV/AIDS surveillance report. 2001;13(2):1-44.
3. Karon JM, Rosenberg PS, McQuillan G, Khare M, Gwinn M, Petersen LR. Prevalence of HIV infection in the United States, 1984-1992. JAMA 1996;276:126-131.
4. Hader SL, Smith DK, Moore JS, Holmberg SD. HIV infection in women in the United States: status at the millennium. JAMA 2001;285:1186-1192.
5. Karon JM, Fleming PL, Steketee RW, DeCock KM. HIV in the United States at the turn of the century: an epidemic in transition. Am J Public Health 2001;91:1060-1069.
6. Stevens PE, Hall JM. Sexuality and safer sex: the issues for lesbians and bisexual women. JOGNN 2001;30:439-447.
7. Lemp GF, Jones M, Kellogg TA, Nieri GN, Anderson L, Withum D, Katz M. HIV seroprevalence and risk behaviors among lesbians and bisexual women in San Francisco and Berkeley, California. Am J Public Health 1995;85:1549-1552.
8. Bush DM. Personal communication to F. Guest, November 10, 1991.
9. Centers for Disease Control and Prevention. Revised guidelines for HIV counseling, testing, and referral and revised recommendations for HIV screening of pregnant women. MMWR 2001;50(No. RR-19):1-86. Available online at http://www.cdc.gov/hiv/dhap/htm. Accessibility verified April 8, 2003.
10. Kerr SH, Valdiserri RO, Loft J, Bresolin L, Holtgrave D, Moore M, MacGowan R, Marder W, Rinaldi R. Primary care physicians and their HIV prevention practices. AIDS Patient Care and STDs 1996;10:227-235.
11. Centers for Disease Control and Prevention. Trends in sexual risk behaviors among high school students–United States, 1991-2001. MMWR 2002;51(38):856-859.
12. Stephenson J. HIV risk from oral sex higher than many realize. JAMA 2000:283:1279.

13. Cohen MS, Shugars DC, Fiscus SA. Limits on oral transmission of HIV-1. The Lancet 2000;356:272.
14. Rothenberg RB, Scarlett M, del Rio C, Reznik D, O'Daniels C. Oral transmission of HIV. AIDS 1998;12:2095-2105.
15. Schacker T, Collier AC, Hughes J, Shea T, Corey L. Clinical and epidemiologic features of primary HIV infection. Ann Intern Med 1996;125:257-264.
16. Daar ES, Little S, Pitt J, Santangelo J, Ho P, Harawa N, Kerndt P, Giorgi JV, Bai J, Gaut P, Richman DD, Mandel S, Nichols S. Diagnosis of primary HIV-1 infection. Ann Intern Med 2001;134:25-29.
17. Royce RA, Seña A, Cates W Jr, Cohen MS. Sexual transmission of HIV. N Engl J Med 1997;336:1072-1078.
18. St. Louis ME, Wasserheit JN, Gayle HD. Editorial: Janus considers the HIV pandemic—harnessing recent advances to enhance AIDS prevention. Am J Pub Health 1997;87:10-12.
19. Centers for Disease Control and Prevention. Management of possible sexual, injecting-drug-use, or other nonoccupational exposure to HIV, including considerations related to antiretroviral therapy. MMWR 1998;47(No. RR-17):1-14.
20. Hirschhorn L, Kunches L, Mayer K. Nonoccupational postexposure prophylaxis: evolving clinical practice. AIDS Clinical Care 2000;12:6-7, 9, 11-12.
21. Quinn TC, Wawer MJ, Sewankambo N, Serwadda D, Li C, Wabwire-Mangen F, Meehan MO, Lutalo T, Gray RH for the Rakai Project Study Group. Viral load and heterosexual transmission of human immunodeficiency virus type 1. N Engl J Med 2000;342:921-929.
22. Cates W Jr. Contraception, unintended pregnancies, and sexually transmitted diseases: why isn't a simple solution possible? Am J Epidemiol 1996;143:311-318.
23. Centers for Disease Control and Prevention. Contraceptive method and condom use among women at risk for HIV infection and other sexually transmitted diseases—selected U.S. sites, 1993-1994. MMWR 1996;45:820-823.
24. Roye CF, Seals B. A qualitative assessment of condom use decisions by female adolescents who use hormonal contraception. J Assn Nurses in AIDS Care 2001;12:78-87.
25. Collins J, Holtzman D, Kann L, Kolbe L. Predictors of condom use among U.S. high school students, 1991. Abstract #WSC134. Presented at the Ninth International Conference on AIDS, June 6-11, 1993, Berlin, Germany.
26. Whaley AL. Preventing the high-risk sexual behavior of adolescents: focus on HIV/AIDS transmission, unintended pregnancy, or both? J Adol Health 1999;24:376-382.
27. American College of Obstetricians and Gynecologists. Statement of the American College of Obstetricians and Gynecologists on a report on condom effectiveness. July 25, 2001. Available at http://www.acog.org/from_home/publications/. Accessibility verified April 8, 2003.
28. Howe JE, Minkoff HL, Duerr AC. Contraceptives and HIV. AIDS 1994;8:861-871.
29. Roper WL, Peterson HB, Curran JW. Commentary: condoms and HIV/STD prevention—clarifying the message. Am J Pub Health 1993;83:501-503.
30. Grady WR, Klepinger DH, Nelson-Wally A. Contraceptive characteristics: the perceptions and priorities of men and women. Fam Plann Perspect 1999;31:168-175.
31. National Institute of Allergy and Infectious Diseases, Workshop summary. Scientific evidence on condom effectiveness for sexually transmitted disease (STD) prevention. July 20, 2001.
32. Cates W Jr. The NIH condom report: the glass is 90% full. Fam Plann Perspect 2001;33:231-233.
33. deVincenzi I. A longitudinal study of human immunodeficiency virus transmission by heterosexual partners. N Engl J Med 1994;331:341-346.
34. Krieger JN, Coombs RW, Collier AC, Ho DD, Ross SO, Zeh JE, Corey L. Intermittent shedding of human immunodeficiency virus in semen: implications for sexual transmission. J Urology 1995;154:1035-1040.
35. Ilaria G, Jacobs JL, Polsky B, Koll B, Baron P, MacLow C, Armstrong D, Schlegel PN. Detection of HIV-1 DNA sequences in pre-ejaculatory fluid. Lancet 1992;340:1469.

36. Pudney J, Oneta M, Mayer K, Seage G, Anderson D. Pre-ejaculatory fluid as a potential vector for sexual transmission of HIV-1. Lancet 1992;340:147.
37. McCormack S, Hayes R, Lacey CJN, Johnson AM. Microbicides in HIV prevention. BMJ 2001;322:410-413.
38. Stephenson JM. Systematic review of hormonal contraception and risk of HIV transmission: when to resist meta-analysis. AIDS 1998;12:545-553.
39. Martin Jr. HL, Nyange PM, Richardson BA, Lavreys L, Mandaliya K, Jackson DJ, Ndinya-Achola JO, Kreiss J. Hormonal contraceptives, sexually transmitted diseases, and risk of heterosexual transmission of human immunodeficiency virus type 1. J Infect Dis 1998;178:1053-1059.
40. Sinei SK, Morrison CS, Sekadde-Kigondu C, Allen M, Kokonya D. Complications of use of intrauterine devices among HIV-1-infected women. Lancet 1998;351:1238-1241.
41. Richardson BA, Morrison CS, Sekadde-Kigondu C, Sinei SK, Overbaugh J, Panteleeff, DD, Weiner DH, Kreiss JK. Effect of intrauterine device use on cervical shedding of HIV-1 DNA. AIDS 1999;13:2091-2097.
42. Moench TR, Chipato T, Padian NS. Preventing disease by protecting the cervix: the unexplored promise of internal vaginal barrier devices. AIDS 2001;15:1595-1602.
43. Peterson G, Akridge RE, Gibson J, Nikolaeva I, Ross S, Lee W, Dragavon J, Nirapathpongporn A, Krieger J, Coombs RW. Detection of HIV-1 in semen and blood by nucleic acid amplification: effect of vasectomy on the recovery of HIV-1 RNA from seminal plasma. Abstract #I017. Presented at the 36th Interscience Conference on Antimicrobial Agents and Chemotherapeutics, 1996.
44. Moses S, Plummer FA, Bradley JE, Ndinya-Achola JO, Nagelkerke NJD, Ronald AR. The association between lack of circumcision and risk for HIV infection: a review of the epidemiological data. Sexually Transmitted Diseases 1994;21:201-210.
45. Halperin DT, Bailey RC. Male circumcision and HIV infection: 10 years and counting. Lancet 1999;354:1813-1815.
46. Hofmann AD. Adolescent growth and development. In: Hofmann AD, Greydanus D (eds). Adolescent Medicine, 3rd ed. Stamford CT: Appleton & Lange, 1997.
47. Wang C, Celum C. Prevention of HIV. In: Anderson JR (ed). A Guide to the Clinical Care of Women with HIV. Rockville MD: HIV/AIDS Bureau, Health Resources and Services Administration, 2001. Available online at http://www.hab.hrsa.gov/. Accessibility verified April 8, 2003.
48. Stiffman AR, Earls F, Dore P, Cunningham R. Changes in acquired immunodeficiency syndrome-related risk behavior after adolescence: relationships to knowledge and experience concerning human immunodeficiency virus infection. Pediatrics 1992;89:950-956.
49. Hein K. "Getting real" about HIV in adolescents. Am J Public Health 1993;83:492-494.
50. Centers for Disease Control and Prevention. HIV testing among women aged 18-44 years—United States, 1991 and 1993. MMWR 1996;45:733-737.
51. Ptacek JT, Eberhardt TL. Breaking bad news: a review of the literature. JAMA 1996;276:496-502.
52. Buckman R, Kason Y. How to break bad news: a guide for health care professionals. Baltimore MD: Johns Hopkins University Press, 1992.
53. Brodie S, Sax P. Novel approaches to HIV antibody testing. AIDS Clinical Care 1997;9:1-5,10.
54. Frank AP, Wandell MG, Headings MD, Conant MA, Woody GE, Michel C. Anonymous HIV testing using home collection and telemedicine counseling. Arch Intern Med 1997;157:309-314.
55. Gallo D, George JR, Fitchen JH, Goldstein AS, Hindahl MS. Evaluation of a system using oral mucosal transudate for HIV-1 antibody screening and confirmatory test. JAMA 1997;277:254-258.
56. Branson BM. Rapid tests for HIV antibody. AIDS Rev 2000;2:76-83.
57. O'Rourke M. Rapid fingerstick testing: a new era in HIV diagnositics. AIDS Clin Care 2003;15:19-23, 30.

58. American Academy of Pediatrics and American College of Obstetricians and Gynecologists. Human immunodeficiency virus screening. Pediatrics 1999;104:128.
59. Fernandez MI, Wilson TE, Ethier KA, Walter EB, Gay CL, Moore J, for the Perinatal Guidelines Evaluation Project. Acceptance of HIV testing during prenatal care. Public Health Rep 2000;15:460-468.
60. Greenblatt RM, Hessol NA. Epidemiology and natural history of HIV infection in women. In: Anderson JR (ed). A Guide to the Clinical Care of Women with HIV. Rockville MD: HIV/AIDS Bureau, Health Resources and Services Administration, 2001. Available online at http://www.hab.hrsa.gov/. Accessibility verified April 8, 2003.
61. Anderson JR. Approach to the patient. In: Anderson JR (ed). A Guide to the Clinical Care of Women with HIV. Rockville MD: HIV/AIDS Bureau, Health Resources and Services Administration, 2001. Available online at http://www.hab.hrsa.gov/. Accessibility verified April 8, 2003.
62. Jewett JE, Hecht FM. Preventive health care for adults with HIV infection. JAMA 1993;269:1144-1153.
63. Abularach S, Anderson JR. Gynecologic problems. In: Anderson JR (ed). A Guide to the Clinical Care of Women with HIV. Rockville MD: HIV/AIDS Bureau, Health Resources and Services Administration, 2001. Available online at http://www.hab.hrsa.gov/. Accessibility verified April 8, 2003.
64. Maiman M. Management of cervical neoplasia in human immunodeficiency virus-infected women. J Natl Cancer Inst Monogr 1998;23:43-49.
65. Ellerbrock TV, Chiasson MA, Bush TJ, Sun X-W, Sawo D, Brudney K, Wright Jr. TC. Incidence of cervical squamous intraepithelial lesions in HIV-infected women. JAMA 2000;283:1031-1037.
66. Centers for Disease Control and Prevention. Sexually transmitted diseases treatment guidelines 2002. MMWR 2002;51(No. RR-6):1-78.
67. Clark RA, Bessinger R. Clinical manifestations and predictors of survival in older women infected with HIV. J Acquir Immune Defic Syndr Hum Retrovirol 1997;15:341-345.
68. Smits AK, Goergen CA, Delaney JA, Williamson C, Mundy LM, Fraser VJ. Contraceptive use and pregnancy decision making among women with HIV. AIDS Patient Care and STDs 1999;13:739-746.
69. Cates W Jr. Use of contraception by HIV-infected women. IPPF Medical Bulletin 2001;35:February, 1-2.
70. Anderson JR. HIV and reproduction. In: Anderson JR (ed). A Guide to the Clinical Care of Women with HIV. Rockville MD: HIV/AIDS Bureau, Health Resources and Services Administration, 2001. Available online at http://www.hab.hrsa.gov/. Accessibility verified April 9, 2003.
71. Connor EM, Sperling RS, Gelber R, Kiselev P, Scott G, O'Sullivan MJ, VanDyke R, Bey M, Shearer W, Jacobson RL, Jimenez E, O'Neill E, Bazin B, Delfraissy J-E, Culnane M, Coombs R, Elkins M, Moye J, Stratton P, Balsley J, for the Pediatric AIDS CTG Protocol 076 Study Group. Reduction of maternal-infant transmission of human immunodeficiency virus type 1 with zidovudine treatment. N Engl J Med 1994;331:1173-1180.
72. Public Health Service Task Force recommendations for use of antiretroviral drugs in pregnant HIV-1-infected women for maternal health and interventions to reduce perinatal HIV-1 transmission in the United States. August 30, 2002. Available at http://aidsinfo.nih.gov. Accessibility verified April 9, 2003.
73. Fowler MG, Simonds RJ, Roongpisuthipong A. Update on perinatal HIV transmission. Pediatr Clin North Am 2000;47:21-38.
74. American College of Obstetricians and Gynecologists Committee Opinion. Scheduled cesarean delivery and the prevention of vertical transmission of HIV infection. Number 234, May 2000.
75. Simonds RJ, Steketee R, Nesheim S, Matheson P, Palumbo P, Alger L, Abrams EJ, Orloff S, Lindsay M, Bardaguez AD, Vink P, Byers R, Rogers M. Impact of zidovudine use on risk and risk factors for perinatal transmission of HIV. Perinatal AIDS Collaborative Transmission Studies. AIDS 1998;12:301-308.

76. Landesman SH, Kalish LA, Burns DN, Minkoff H, Fox HE, Zorrilla C, Garcia P, Fowler MG, Mofenson L, Tuomala R, for the Women and Infants Transmission Study. Obstetrical factors and the transmission of human immunodeficiency virus type 1 from mother to child. N Engl J Med 1996;334:1617-1623.

77. Bertolli J, St. Louis ME, Simmonds RJ, Nieburg P, Kamenga M, Brown C, Tarande M, Quinn T, Ou CY. Estimating the timing of mother-to-child transmission of human immunodeficiency virus in a breast-feeding population in Kinshasa, Zaire. J Infect Dis 1996;174:722-726.

78. Centers for Disease Control and Prevention, Garner JS, Hospital Infection Control Practices Advisory Committee. Guideline for isolation precautions in hospitals. Infect Control Hosp Epidemiol 1996;17:53-80, and Am J Infect Control 1996;24:24-52. Available online at http://www.cdc.gov/ncidod/hip/isolat/isolat/htm. Accessibility verified April 9, 2003.

79. Centers for Disease Control and Prevention. Surveillance of health care workers with HIV/AIDS, as of December 2001. Available online at http://www.cdc.gov. Accessibility verified April 9, 2003.

80. Gerberding JL, Prophylaxis for occupational exposure to HIV. Ann Intern Med 1996;125:497-501.

81. Centers for Disease Control and Prevention. Case-control study of HIV seroconversion in health-care workers after percutaneous exposure to HIV-infected blood— France, United Kingdom, and United States, January 1988-August 1994. MMWR 1995;44:929-933.

82. Centers for Disease Control and Prevention. Update: provisional public health service recommendations for chemoprophylaxis after occupational exposure to HIV. MMWR 1996;45:468-472.

83. Robert LM, Chamberland ME, Cleveland JL, Marcus R, Gooch BF, Srivastava PU, Culver DH, Jaffe HW, Marianos DW, Panlilio AL, Bell DM. Investigations of patients of health care workers infected with HIV. Ann Intern Med 1995;122:653-657.

Reproductive Tract Infections

Willard Cates, Jr., MD, MPH

- Reproductive tract infections (RTIs) are frequently encountered by reproductive health professionals. RTIs include both the traditional sexually transmitted infections (STIs) and also other common infections of the genital tract.

- RTIs have four serious health consequences:

  - Tubal occlusion leading to infertility and ectopic pregnancy

  - Pregnancy loss and neonatal morbidity caused by transmission of the infection to the infant during pregnancy and childbirth

  - Genital cancers

  - Enhanced transmission of the human immunodeficiency virus (HIV)

- Preventing RTIs and their consequences requires sexually active persons to adopt safer sexual behaviors and clinicians to diagnose and treat existing infections effectively.

- Assessing a client's risks for RTI can help both the client better select appropriate contraceptive methods and the clinician better diagnose and treat the client.

Healthy sexual relations and reproductive events should be free of infection.[1,2] However, preventing, diagnosing, and treating RTIs are growing more challenging, since an increasing number of people are infected with more severe infections.[3-5]

- Persistent viral infections, including the human immunodeficiency virus (HIV), herpes simplex virus (HSV), and hepatitis B virus (HBV) have afflicted millions of people with incurable diseases.

- Trichomonal and chlamydial infections are at high levels worldwide.

- Long-term consequences of pelvic inflammatory disease (PID) such as infertility, ectopic pregnancy, and chronic pain have increased.

- Neoplastic sequelae such as cervical cancer and hepatocellular carcinoma have been closely linked to some RTIs such as human papilloma virus (HPV) and HBV.

In *Contraceptive Technology*, the generic term RTI covers three types of infection: (1) sexually transmitted infections (STIs), (2) endogenous vaginal infections including bacterial vaginosis and candidiasis, and (3) iatrogenic infections associated with insertion of an intrauterine device (IUD) or induced abortion.

Preventing an infection is the most effective way to reduce the adverse consequences of RTIs. Diagnosing and treating a current infection in a timely manner can also prevent complications in the individual and interrupt transmission in the community. This chapter provides general background about RTI management in the reproductive health care setting.

MAGNITUDE AND RISKS OF RTIs

The number of people infected with RTIs or affected by their consequences is a major problem for our society.[3] The estimated total number of people newly infected each year with curable STIs is 15 million in the United States[5] and 340 million worldwide.[6] In the United States, the annual cost of pelvic inflammatory disease (PID) and its consequences is estimated to be $4.2 billion. Infertility caused by PID accounts for over $1 billion of health care costs and much emotional misery. Although deaths due to RTIs (primarily syphilis and PID) have declined over the past four decades, RTIs still cause almost one-third of reproductive mortality in the United States.

Individuals under age 25 account for a majority of RTI cases. Two-thirds of reported cases of gonorrhea and chlamydia occur in persons 24 years of age or younger.[7] Rates of chlamydia, gonorrhea, and PID are highest in adolescents and decline steadily as adults age. RTIs are concentrated in socio-geographic clusters, the so-called "core-populations." For example, persons of lower socioeconomic status are more likely to have RTIs than are persons of higher socioeconomic status.

Most RTIs show a "biological sexism." Compared with men, women suffer more severe long-term consequences, including PID, infertility, ectopic pregnancy, chronic pelvic pain, and cervical cancer. They are less likely to seek health care for infection because a higher proportion of their RTIs are asymptomatic or unrecognized as being serious.[1] Finally, due to the transmission dynamics of intercourse, women are more likely than men to acquire an STI from any single sexual encounter.

The probability that unprotected sexual intercourse will lead to an RTI or its consequences differs from the probability of unintended pregnancy (Table 8-1). The risk of pregnancy varies throughout the menstrual cycle. The risk of acquiring an RTI depends on (1) having intercourse with an infected person, (2) the transmissibility of the particular RTI, and (3) the gender of the infected person. For example, the risk of acquiring gonorrhea from a single sex act (where one partner is infectious) is approximately 25% for men and 50% for women.[8] The probability of suffering consequences from an RTI depends on whether or not the person received proper diagnosis and treatment.

One of the fundamental concepts underlying RTI risk is the "epidemiological synergy" between HIV and other RTIs.[9] Organisms that cause genital ulcers (HSV, syphilis, and chancroid) are most strongly correlated with the transmission and acquisition of HIV. Moreover, because immune dysfunction caused by HIV disease makes the ulcerative symptoms persist, these infections have a potentiating influence on each other. In addition, RTIs that produce vaginal or urethral discharge (such as gonorrhea, chlamydia, and trichomoniasis) have also been associated with higher levels of HIV infection. Because vaginal and urethral discharge are more common than genital ulcers, they account for a larger proportion of HIV spread. Always suspect HIV may be present in persons diagnosed with another RTI.

Table 8-1 Comparative risk of adverse consequences from coitus—RTI and unintended pregnancy

Unintended pregnancy/coital act[10]
17%-30% midcycle
< 1% during menses
Gonococcal transmission/coital act[8]
50% infected male, uninfected female
25% infected female, uninfected male
PID per woman infected with cervical gonorrhea[11]
40% if not treated
0% if promptly and adequately treated
Tubal infertility per PID episode[12]
8% after first episode
20% after second episode
40% after third or more episodes

RTI PREVENTION AND PERSONAL BEHAVIORS

Different individuals accept different levels of risk to satisfy personal needs. Not everyone will follow every safer sex recommendation but, with the proper knowledge, each person can make his or her own informed choices about reducing sexual risks. Just as with many other daily health decisions, each person will assess differently the factors affecting sexual choices. Thus, simplistic messages urging absolutist policies are ineffective.[13]

Preventive measures for avoiding transmission of RTIs are generally consistent with guidelines for reducing the risk of HIV infection. (See Chapter 7 on HIV/AIDS and Reproductive Health.) Risk-free options include having a mutually faithful relationship with an uninfected partner or completely abstaining from sexual activities that involve semen, blood, or other body fluids, or that allow for skin-to-skin contact. Examining a partner for lesions, discussing each new partner's previous sexual history, and avoiding partners who have had many previous sexual partners can augment other measures to prevent the transmission of RTIs. Educating patients about their bodies and teaching them to be active participants in their health care gives them more control over their reproductive health.

CONTRACEPTIVE CHOICE

Choice of contraception directly affects the risk of RTI (Table 8-2). Condoms reduce the risks of both bacterial and viral RTIs; the evidence is strongest for condom effectiveness against HIV and gonorrhea.[14] No recent data support spermicides' ability to prevent bacterial or viral infections, including HIV.[15] Diaphragms used with spermicides provide a barrier against cervical infection, but they have been associated with changes in vaginal flora and urinary tract infections. Although oral contraceptives are usually associated with an increase in chlamydia detected in the cervix, they protect against symptomatic PID, but not unrecognized endometritis.[16] IUDs are associated with a transient increased risk of PID in the first month after insertion, but have a strong record of safety even for HIV-infected women.[17]

Table 8-2 Effects of contraceptives on bacterial and viral RTI

Contraceptive Methods	Bacterial RTI	Viral RTI
Condoms	Protective	Protective
Spermicides	No evidence of protection	Not protective
Diaphragms	Protective against cervical infection Associated with vaginal anaerobic overgrowth	Protective against cervical neoplasia
Hormonal	Associated with increased cervical chlamydia Protective against symptomatic PID, but not unrecognized endometritis	Not protective
IUD	Associated with PID in first month after insertion	Not protective
Fertility Awareness	Not protective	Not protective

Source: Adapted from Cates and Padian (2000).[2]
See chapters on specific contraceptive methods for greater elaboration.

OTHER RISK BEHAVIORS

In addition to sexual activities, other practices have been linked to a risk of RTI. Routine douching for hygienic purposes has been associated with an increased risk of PID and ectopic pregnancy.[18] Postcoital washing or urination have been poorly studied, but appear to have little effect, if any, on reducing the risk of acquiring an RTI. Because postcoital urination could wash away bacteria that could cause cystitis, it was generally recommended for women susceptible to cystitis. However, clinical evidence has not supported this routine practice.[19]

Drug use influences the transmission of RTIs. Besides the blood-borne risks associated with needle-sharing (hepatitis B, HIV infection), using drugs such as crack cocaine has been associated with sexual behaviors that increase a person's risk of acquiring and transmitting many RTIs. Outbreaks of syphilis, antibiotic-resistant gonorrhea, and chancroid have been linked to crack-related sexual behaviors. Use of other drugs, especially alcohol binge drinking, also has been associated with risky sexual practices.

A SSESSMENT, DIAGNOSIS AND TREATMENT IN THE REPRODUCTIVE HEALTH CARE SETTING

Professionals in the fields of family planning and RTI have common reproductive health goals:

- Educating all patients about RTIs

- Providing diagnostic services that include risk assessment, RTI screening, and voluntary HIV testing

- Ensuring all persons diagnosed with an RTI get appropriate treatment, preferably before leaving the facility

- Counseling individuals about the need for simultaneous treatment for their sex partner(s)

- Assisting patients in choosing a contraceptive that will reduce their risk of acquiring an RTI

Risk assessment can help clinicians provide better contraceptive counseling and more cost-efficient RTI management. Risk assessment balances a variety of demographic, behavioral, and clinical information (other than laboratory test results) to assess the likelihood that persons are infected with an RTI or are at high risk of future infection and to counsel clients in selecting appropriate contraceptive methods. For example, an RTI risk assessment scale can help identify women who may be good candidates for barrier methods or inappropriate candidates for IUDs.[20]

With the emergence of HIV infection and its endpoint, acquired immunodeficiency syndrome (AIDS), clients need to be strongly counseled to use condoms for infection prevention, even in conjunction with other contraceptive methods for pregnancy prevention. While data are sparse on the effectiveness of dual protection approaches, condom counseling is becoming a mainstay for those advocating reproductive health.[21]

Laboratory diagnosis of most RTIs can be performed in nearly every reproductive health care setting.[22] For example, over the past decade, routine screening for chlamydia has been associated with a decreased prevalence of the infection among clients attending family planning clinics in several regions of the country. In addition, some family planning clinics have extended their range of services to male clients, including RTI diagnosis, treatment, and counseling. Finally, family planning staff have become more familiar with their local STI programs to help provide appropriate referrals.

STI partner notification is not part of the usual menu of services in reproductive health care clinics. However, an increasing number of counselors are being trained in this essential public health strategy. Going into the community to notify partners is probably most easily handled by the STI program.[23] Confidentiality is crucial, just as it is in all aspects of family planning and RTI care.

RTI DIAGNOSIS AND TREATMENT

Counseling patients with RTI requires an approach different than that generally used in family planning settings.[24] For couples trying to prevent unplanned pregnancies, counseling is typically non-directive to allow maximal opportunity for them to make an informed choice of the best contraceptive method. However, for patients who have RTIs, *directive* counseling is important to (1) prevent new infections; (2) increase adherence to treatment and follow-up; and (3) offer guidance on talking to partners about their RTI exposure. Patients must be made aware of both the potential serious consequences of RTIs and the behaviors that increase the likelihood of reinfection.

Education about infection and treatment. Make sure patients understand what infection they have, how it is transmitted, why it must be treated, and exactly when and how to take prescribed medication. Because unpleasant side effects from some medications may discourage patients from continuing treatment, discuss ways to minimize side effects. For example, doxycycline taken on an empty stomach may cause nausea that prompts the patient to stop taking the medication early. Advise a snack with medication.

Completion of treatment. Urge patients to finish their entire supply of medication even though their symptoms may diminish or disappear in a few days. Discontinuing antibiotics before the infection is completely cured can lead to recurrent infection and increase the likelihood that hard-to-cure strains of the pathogen may flourish. Advise patients to avoid intercourse until they complete the full course of therapy. After the infection is cured, urge the patient to use condoms to prevent repeated infection, especially if a woman wishes to have children in the future or continues to have intercourse with new partners.

Comfort. Provide patients with somatic and emotional comfort to enhance adherence with treatment. Treat nausea, pain, itching, or other physiologic discomforts symptomatically, if possible. Overcoming the psychosocial component of genital discomfort can be exceedingly important in RTI treatment. Remember, patients may be afraid or ashamed to ask a partner to seek treatment, embarrassed to admit their sexual practices, or concerned about confidentiality. Telling patients they have a sexually transmissible infection rather than "a disease" may help some people avoid feeling stigmatized.

Concurrent infections. Managing RTI requires that clinicians have a high index of suspicion. A patient will often have two or more RTIs concurrently. Be alert for symptoms that differ from those normally associated with the primary RTI infection. Treat all presumptive RTIs. For example, when a patient has gonorrhea, provide dual therapy for both gonorrhea and chlamydia—an approach that is epidemiologically indicated, cost-effective, and safe for the patient.

STI reporting. All states require the traditional "venereal diseases" (e.g., syphilis, gonorrhea, and chancroid) be reported to public health officials; many states have instituted reporting systems for specific STIs such as chlamydial infections and genital herpes. Nearly all states require HIV infection and AIDS be reported. Reporting of STI to public health authorities is not a breach of confidentiality; in fact, statutory protection of patients' names is a crucial part of STI control strategies. Accurate reporting of STI helps (1) identify trends in disease, (2) gain resources for high-prevalence communities, and (3) evaluate STI intervention efforts. Confer with STI control officials to ensure prompt and accurate reporting of the notifiable STIs.

Partner notification. Notify and treat sex partner(s) to prevent both reinfection of the patient and spread of disease through the community. Assist patients in notifying their partners by coaching them in partner notification techniques (patient referral) and using STI caseworkers (provider referral) to contact partners. An increasing number of family planning professionals are being trained in partner notification skills.

RTI DURING PREGNANCY

Question pregnant women and their sex partners about their risk of RTIs; counsel them about the possibility of transmitting an infection to their infant. Because of the severe effects RTIs may have on both the pregnancy and the developing fetus, assess whether the pregnant woman should be screened for infections with HIV, syphilis, hepatitis B, chlamydia, gonorrhea, bacterial vaginosis, and trichomoniasis (Tables 8-3 and 8-4). Encourage voluntary screening for HIV to detect infected women who could benefit from prophylactic antiretroviral therapy to reduce maternal-to-infant transmission. Routine screening for HPV is not recommended.

Management of specific RTIs is discussed in the Alphabetical Catalog of RTIs in this chapter. HIV and pregnancy is discussed in Chapter 7. For more complete information on RTIs in pregnant women, refer to Guidelines for Perinatal Care, jointly published by the American College of Obstetricians and Gynecologists and the American Academy of Pediatrics.[25]

Table 8-3 Risks of sexually transmitted bacterial organisms and syndromes in pregnancy and childbirth

Organism/Syndrome	Maternal Infection Rate (%)[1]	Infant Effects	Transmission Risk from Infected Mother	Prevention	Treatment of Mother, Neonate
Neisseria gonorrhoeae	1-30	Conjunctivitis, sepsis, meningitis	Approximately 30%	Screening; culture mother; apply ocular prophylaxis	Ceftriaxone
Chlamydia trachomatis	2-25	Conjunctivitis, pneumonia, bronchiolitis, otitis media	25%-50% conjunctivitis 5%-15% pneumonia	Screening in third trimester: culture mother, apply ocular prophylaxis	Amoxicillin Erythromycin
Treponema pallidum	0.01-15	Congenital syphilis, neonatal death	50%	Serologic screening in early and late pregnancy	Penicillin
Trichomonas vaginalis	10-35	Low birthweight, preterm delivery	N/A	Screening	Metronidazole
Bacterial vaginosis	10-35	Low birthweight, preterm delivery	N/A	Screening	Metronidazole Clindamycin

Source: Adapted from Cates (1995).

[1]Percentage of pregnant women with evidence of infection

Table 8-4 Risks of sexually transmitted viral organisms and syndromes in pregnancy and childbirth

Organism/Syndrome	Maternal Infection Rate (%)[1]	Infant Effects	Transmission Risk from Infected Mother	Prevention	Treatment of Mother, Neonate
Hepatitis B Virus	1-10	Hepatitis, cirrhosis	10%-90%	Active HBV immunization	Post-exposure passive HBV immunization
Herpes Simplex Virus	1-30	Disseminated, central nervous system, localized lesions	Recurrent: 3% at delivery; primary: 30% at delivery	Cesarean delivery if lesions present at delivery	Vidarabine Acyclovir
Human Papilloma Virus	10-60	Laryngeal papillomatosis	Rare	None	Surgical
Human Immunodeficiency Virus	0.01-40	Pediatric AIDS	27% without ART < 5% with ART	Pregnancy prevention; ART during pregnancy	Antiretrovirals (ART)

Source: Adapted from Cates (1995).

[1]Percentage of pregnant women with evidence of infection

RTI AND SEXUAL ASSAULT

In cases of sexual assault and abuse, clinicians must attend not only to physical and psychological trauma, but also the possibility of pregnancy or RTI. Any of the sexually transmissible infections, including HIV, can be acquired during a sexual assault. Some RTIs, such as gonorrhea or syphilis, are almost exclusively sexually transmitted and are therefore useful markers of assault in persons not previously sexually active.

To reduce the risk of pregnancy, emergency contraception can be used. (See Chapter 12 on Emergency Contraception.) To reduce the risk of RTI, the Centers for Disease Control and Prevention (CDC) recommends the following approach:[26]

Adult evaluation. If possible, initially evaluate the victim within 24 hours of the assault and take specimens to culture for N. gonorrhoeae and C. trachomatis. Examine microscopically for T. vaginalis and bacterial vaginosis (BV). Perform a pregnancy test, and keep a frozen serum sample for possible future testing. If treatment is not administered, schedule a repeat evaluation for 2 weeks later.

Presumptive treatment may be provided at the victim's request. While no regimen provides coverage against all potential pathogens, the following should be effective against the most frequent RTIs:

- Ceftriaxone 125 milligrams (mg) given intramuscularly (IM)

- Metronidazole 2 grams (g) given orally

- Azithromycin 1 g given orally

- Hepatitis B vaccination, first dose

- Post-exposure prophylaxis against HIV may also be considered (See Chapter 7 on HIV/AIDS and Reproductive Health) and

- Advise clients to use condoms until test results are reported.

Child evaluation. In general, identification of an STI in a child beyond the neonatal period suggests sexual abuse. However, unlike gonorrhea or syphilis, specific infections such as bacterial vaginosis (BV), genital mycoplasmas, and genital warts are not conclusive evidence of sexual abuse. Evaluation is essentially the same as described for adult victims, except culture specimens should be collected from the pharynx and rectum as well as from the vagina or urethra because the child's report of assault may not be complete. Presumptive treatment may be given at the family's request.

For more complete information regarding laboratory procedures, diagnosis, and treatment for sexual assault and abuse victims, refer to the 2002 Guidelines for Treatment of Sexually Transmitted Diseases.

ALPHABETICAL CATALOG OF REPRODUCTIVE TRACT INFECTIONS

ACQUIRED IMMUNODEFICIENCY SYNDROME (AIDS) and HIV (human immunodeficiency virus) infections are covered in Chapter 7.

ACUTE URETHRAL SYNDROME (dysuria-pyuria syndrome) can be caused by E. coli, C. trachomatis, N. gonorrhoeae, or other gram-negative bacteria.[27] Bacterial cystitis itself is not sexually transmitted per se; however, it is sexually-associated. "Honeymoon" cystitis is believed to be caused by friction against the urethra during sexual intercourse. The underlying etiology is mechanical, and coital movements help vaginal organisms ascend into the bladder. Use of the diaphragm with spermicides and spermicidally coated condoms have been associated with higher levels of acute urethral syndrome.[19]

Prevalence. Urinary tract infections are second in prevalence only to upper respiratory infections. Depending on the population studied, as many as 10% to 25% of reproductive-age women report dysuria during the previous year.

Symptoms. Painful, urgent, and frequent urination, as well as dyspareunia, characterizes this syndrome. Occasionally hematuria is the precipitating event for seeking clinical evaluation. Consider pyelonephritis if a patient's temperature exceeds 101° F or if costovertebral angle pain or tenderness are present.

Diagnosis. Women with $> 10^5$ organisms (coliform bacteria or other uropathogens) per milliliter (ml) of urine have bacterial cystitis; however, a smaller number of organisms may also cause symptoms. Women with dysuria, frequency, pyuria (10 white blood cells [WBCs] per 400x field on microscopic examination of urinary sediment), and a negative Gram stain of unspun urine have the acute urethral syndrome. A definitive diagnosis of the etiologic organism requires cultures of the urethra or urine. Dysuria may also be caused by vaginitis or genital herpes simplex virus infection.

Treatment. Acute urethral syndrome can be treated with a variety of antibiotics that achieve a high concentration in urine. Fluoroquinolones (e.g., ciprofloxacin 250 mg twice a day, OR ofloxacin 200 mg twice a day) can be effective. The length of therapy is dictated by clinical response, but 3 days is the usual course. Initial episodes of bacterial cystitis can be treated with appropriate single-dose therapy such as sulfamethoxazole 1.6 g plus trimethoprim 320 mg (Bactrim or Septra). However, higher cure rates are achieved with longer courses of therapy.

Potential complications. Left untreated, infections of the lower genito-urinary tract can ascend to the upper tract, leading to acute pyelonephritis, chronic pyelonephritis, and eventual kidney failure.

Behavioral messages to emphasize. Understand how to take any prescribed oral medications. Drink copious fluids to flush the genitourinary system. If C. trachomatis or N. gonorrhoeae organisms are isolated, refer sex partner(s) for examination. Return for evaluation 4 to 7 days after initiation of therapy.

BACTERIAL VAGINOSIS (BV) is a clinical syndrome in which several species of vaginal bacteria (including Gardnerella vaginalis, Mycoplasma hominis, and various anaerobes) replace the normal H2O2-producing lactobacillus species and cause vulvovaginitis symptoms. Bacterial vaginosis is a sexually associated condition, but is not usually considered a specific STI.[28] Treatment of the male partner has not been found to be effective in preventing the recurrence of BV.

Symptoms. Excessive or malodorous discharge is a common finding. Other signs or symptoms include erythema, edema, and pruritis of the external genitalia.

Diagnosis. The presumptive clinical criteria are typical clinical symptoms of vulvovaginitis, elevated vaginal pH (greater than 4.7), and identification of clue cells (small coccobacillary organisms associated with epithelial cells) in a saline wet mount or Gram stain of vaginal discharge. The diagnosis is further supported when a mixture of the vaginal discharge and 10% KOH liberates a fishy odor of volatile amines (Whiff test). Alternatively, a Gram stain of the vaginal discharge can reveal the relative absence of lactobacilli with replacement of other anaerobic organisms. Cultures for G. vaginalis, M. hominis, or Mobiluncus are not useful and are not recommended for diagnosing this syndrome.

Treatment. Only patients with symptomatic disease require treatment. The three recommended regimens are metronidazole, 500 mg orally twice daily for 7 days; OR clindamycin cream, 2%, one applicator full (5 g) intravaginally at bed time for 7 days; OR metronidazole gel, 0.75%, an applicator full (5 g) intravaginally two times a day for 5 days. Three alternatives are metronidazole 2 g orally in a single dose; oral clindamycin 300 mg two times a day for 7 days; OR clindamycin ovules 100 mg intravaginally at bedtime for 3 days. During the second and third trimester of pregnancy, oral metronidazole 250 mg three times a day for 7 days is the preferred treatment. Lower doses of medication are recommended during pregnancy because of the general desire to limit fetal exposure. Treatment is not recommended for asymptomatic carriers of G. vaginalis or male partners of women with this syndrome.

Potential complications. Secondary excoriation may occur. Recurrent infections are common. Bacterial vaginosis is associated with an increased risk of adverse pregnancy outcomes, including preterm delivery and low birthweight.

Behavioral messages to emphasize. Understand how to take or use any prescribed medications. Return if the problem is not cured or recurs. Avoid drinking alcohol until 24 hours after completing metronidazole therapy.

Screening for, and treatment of, BV before an induced abortion or a hysterectomy can reduce infectious complications.

CANDIDIASIS is caused by Candida albicans (and other Candida species), which are dimorphic fungi that grow as oval, budding yeast cells and as chains of cells (hyphae). Candida are normal flora of the skin and vagina and are not considered to be STIs. Treatment with antibiotics predisposes women to develop vulvovaginal candidiasis.

Symptoms. Clinical presentation varies from no signs or symptoms to erythema, edema, and pruritis of the external genitalia. Symptoms or signs alone do not distinguish the microbial etiology. Male sex partners may develop balanitis or cutaneous lesions on the penis.

Diagnosis. The presumptive criteria are typical clinical symptoms of vulvovaginitis and microscopic identification of yeast forms (budding cells) or hyphae in Gram stain or KOH wet-mount preparations of vaginal discharge. Candidiasis is definitively diagnosed when a vaginal culture is positive for C. albicans or other Candida species in a symptomatic woman. However, cultures are not recommended. Yeasts are part of the resident microflora of the vagina and anogenital skin. Cultures for Candida species may detect clinically insignificant infections, which should not be treated.

Treatment. Single dose oral fluconazole, 150 mg is a convenient therapy. In addition, many topical formulations provide effective candidiasis treatment. Examples include miconazole vaginal suppositories 200 mg intravaginally at bedtime for 3 days; OR miconazole 2% vaginal cream, one full applicator (5 g) intravaginally at bedtime for 3 days (and applied externally for vulvitis); OR clotrimazole vaginal tablets 100 mg intravaginally daily for 3 days; OR butoconazole cream, 2%, 5 g intravaginally for 3 days. A variety of other effective treatment regimens exist. In general, more severe infections may need treatment of longer duration. Over-the-counter preparations for intravaginal administration of miconazole, clotrimazole, and butaconazole are available.

Potential complications. Secondary excoriation may occur. Recurrent infections are common, particularly with antibiotic use or diabetes. Persistent candidiasis may indicate HIV infection.

Behavioral messages to emphasize. Understand how to take or use any prescribed medications. Return if the problem is not cured or recurs. Wear a sanitary pad to protect clothing. Change pads frequently. To reduce moisture in the area, avoid panty hose and non-cotton panties. Store suppositories in a refrigerator. Continue taking medicine even during your menstrual period.

CHANCROID is caused by Hemophilus ducreyi, a gram-negative bacillus with rounded ends commonly observed in small clusters along strands of mucus. On culture, the organism tends to form straight or tangled chains. Chancroid is implicated as potentiating HIV transmission.

Prevalence. Chancroid occurs more frequently in the developing than in the developed world. However, chancroid is endemic in selected areas of the United States, and specific chancroid outbreaks have occurred in settings where sex is exchanged for drugs or money.

Symptoms. Women are frequently asymptomatic. Usually a single painful ulcer, surrounded by erythematous edges, appears in men. Ulcers may be necrotic or severely erosive with a ragged serpiginous border. Painful inguinal lymphadenopathy presents in about half the cases and may rupture in 25% to 60% of cases. Ulcers usually occur on the coronal sulcus, glans, or shaft of the penis.

Diagnosis. A painful ulcer, particularly if accompanied by a unilateral bubo, suggests chancroid. Because other RTIs cause genital ulcers (principally syphilis and herpes), all ulcers should be examined with darkfield microscopy when adequate facilities exist. Serologic tests for syphilis and HIV should be performed. When the only organisms seen in a bubo aspirate or ulcer smear are arranged in chains or clumps along strands of mucus and they are morphologically similar to H. ducreyi, the diagnosis of chancroid is highly likely. The diagnosis is definitive when H. ducreyi is recovered by culture or appropriate selective media. Biopsy may be diagnostic but is not usually performed. PCR testing for H. ducreyi is now available.

Treatment. Azithromycin 1 g orally in a single dose OR ceftriaxone 250 mg IM in a single dose OR ciprofloxacin 500 mg orally twice a day for 3 days OR erythromycin base 500 mg orally four times a day for 7 days. Persons infected with HIV have higher rates of treatment failure with single-dose therapy. The susceptibility of H. ducreyi to this combination of antimicrobial agents varies throughout the world. Evaluate the results of therapy after a maximum of 7 days, and continue therapy until ulcers or lymph nodes have healed. Fluctuant lymph nodes should be aspirated through healthy, adjacent, normal skin. Incision and drainage or excision of nodes will delay healing and are contraindicated. Apply compresses to ulcers to remove necrotic material. All sex partners should be simultaneously treated.

Potential complications. Systemic spread is not known to occur. Lesions may become secondarily infected and necrotic. Buboes may rupture and suppurate, resulting in fistulae. Ulcers on the prepuce may cause paraphimosis or phimosis.

Behavioral messages to emphasize. Because genital ulcers can be a risk for HIV infection, get an HIV test at baseline treatment and again in 3 months. Refer sex partner(s) for examination as soon as possible. Return for evaluation 3 to 5 days after therapy begins and thereafter return weekly for evaluation until the infection is entirely healed. The prepuce should remain retracted during therapy, except in the presence of preputial edema. Use condoms to prevent future infections.

CHLAMYDIA is the common name for infections caused by Chlamydia trachomatis. Genital chlamydial infection is the leading cause of preventable infertility and ectopic pregnancy. Chlamydia is now the most commonly reported infectious disease in the United States. An estimated 3 million new cases occur annually.[5] Like viruses, chlamydiae are obligate intracellular parasites and can be isolated in the laboratory only by cell culture. Unlike viruses, C. trachomatis is susceptible to antibiotics. Because many chlamydial infections are asymptomatic and probably chronic, widespread screening is necessary to control this infection and its sequelae.[29-31] CDC recommends that all sexually-active women age 25 years or younger be screened annually for C. trachomatis. For further information about the syndromes caused by C. trachomatis, see the sections on Mucopurulent Cervicitis, Nongonococcal Urethritis, and Pelvic Inflammatory Disease (PID) in this chapter. The recommended regimens for all sites of uncomplicated chlamydial infection are azithromycin 1 g taken orally in a single dose OR doxycycline 100 mg orally twice a day for 7 days. Alternatives are ofloxacin 300 mg orally two times a day for 7 days OR levofloxacin 500 mg orally for 7 days OR erythromycin base 500 mg orally four times a day for 7 days OR erythromycin ethylsuccinate 800 mg orally four times a day for 7 days. During pregnancy, the recommended regimens are amoxicillin 500 mg orally three times daily for 7 days OR erythromycin base 500 mg orally four times daily for 7 days.

GENITAL HERPES is caused by herpes simplex virus (HSV) types 1 and 2 DNA viruses that cannot be distinguished clinically. HSV type 2 (HSV-2) is more common in genital disease.

Prevalence. Symptomatic primary (or initial) HSV infections affect an estimated 200,000 persons each year. Recurrent HSV infections are much more common. An estimated 45 million Americans are infected with genital HSV, though most infections are asymptomatic.[5,32] Persons without symptoms transmit most of the HSV infections.

Symptoms. Single or multiple vesicles, which are usually pruritic, can appear anywhere on the genitalia. Vesicles spontaneously rupture to form shallow ulcers that may be very painful. Lesions resolve spontaneously with minimal scarring. The first clinical occurrence is termed first episode infection (mean duration 12 days). Subsequent, usually milder, occurrences are termed recurrent infections (mean duration 4.5 days). The interval between clinical episodes is termed latency. Viral shedding from the cervix, vulva or penile skin occurs intermittently without clinical symptoms during latency. HSV-2 genital infections are more likely to recur than is HSV type 1 (HSV-1), thus identification of the type of infecting strain has prognostic value.

Diagnosis. When typical genital lesions are present or a pattern of recurrence has developed, suspect herpes infection. An HSV tissue culture demonstrates the characteristic cytopathic effect following inoculation of a specimen from the cervix, the urethra, or the base of a genital lesion. Several type-specific HSV serologic assays may help in the diagnosis of unrecognized infection, in management of sex partners of those with HSV, or, in pregnant women, to diagnose HSV susceptibility and/or recent infection.[33]

Treatment. No cure for HSV has been found; however, antiviral drugs have been helpful in reducing or suppressing symptoms. Oral administration is more effective than topical, both in treating clinically symptomatic episodes and in suppressing or reducing recurrent outbreaks. For clinical illness, oral acyclovir can be given in 400 mg doses three times a day OR in 200 mg capsules five times a day for 7 days (or until clinical resolution occurs). In addition, famciclovir 250 mg orally five times a day OR valacyclovir 1.0 g orally two times a day are recommended for first episode clinical illness. To prevent recurrences, acyclovir 400 mg orally twice a day, OR famciclovir 125 mg orally twice a day, OR valacyclovir 500 mg orally once a day have been used as daily suppressive therapy. Daily prophylaxis with valacyclovir by HSV-infected persons reduces the risk of transmission to uninfected partners. Intravenous regimens are used to treat uncommon disseminated forms of herpes infection requiring hospitalization. The new therapeutic agents offer more convenient dosing but are not more effective clinically than acyclovir. For persons infected with HIV, increased dosages and/or frequency is recommended.[26]

Potential complications. *Men and women*: HSV infection can cause neuralgia, meningitis, ascending myelitis, urethral strictures, and lymphatic suppuration. *Women:* Pregnancy loss and preterm delivery have been associated with HSV infections, usually in primary stages. *Neonates:* During vaginal delivery, virus from an active genital infection can cause neonatal herpes. This condition ranges in severity from clinically inapparent infections to local infections of the eyes, skin, or mucous membranes or to severely disseminated infection that may involve the central nervous system. Full-blown neonatal herpes has a high fatality rate, and survivors often have ocular or neurologic sequelae.

Behavioral messages to emphasize. Because both initial and recurrent lesions shed high concentrations of the virus, abstain from sexual activity while ulcers are present. The risk of HSV transmission also exists during asymptomatic intervals. Condoms offer some protection from HSV acquisition.[34] Prophylactic valacyclovir reduces HSV transmission risks.

The risk of transmission to the neonate from an infected mother is highest among women with primary herpes infection (the first time they have been infected with either HSV-1 or HSV-2) at the time of delivery, less with women with nonprimary first episode of the disease and lower among women with recurrent herpes. At the onset of labor, describe any symptoms and get examined for lesions. If you have no symptoms or signs, your infant may be delivered vaginally. Infants delivered through an infected birth canal should be cultured and followed carefully.

Genital herpes (and other diseases causing genital ulcers) have been associated with an increased risk of acquiring HIV infections. Evaluating asymptomatic partners has little value for preventing transmission of HSV.

GENITAL WARTS (Condyloma acuminata) are caused by several of the many types of human papilloma virus (HPV), a small, slowly growing DNA virus belonging to the papovavirus group. Types 6 and 11 usually cause the visible genital warts. Other HPV types in the genital region (16, 18, 31, 33, 35) are associated with vaginal, anal, and cervical dysplasia.

Prevalence. Genital warts account for more than 1 million physician office visits annually, making condyloma the most common symptomatic viral RTI in the United States. The most sensitive measures of HPV indicate up to 80% of all sexually active young women are infected with this virus.[35] Cases of condyloma have been correlated with earlier onset of sexual activity, multiple sex partners, and a higher frequency of casual relationships than in controls.

Symptoms. Single or multiple soft, fleshy, papillary or sessile, painless keratinized growths appear around the vulvovaginal area, penis, anus, urethra, or perineum. Women infected with condyloma may exhibit typical growths on the walls of the vagina or cervix and may be unaware of their existence. Regular genital self-examinations may be helpful in detecting such growths on the external genitalia of both women and men. From 60% to 90% of male partners of women with condyloma have HPV infection on the penis, although infection may not be visible to the naked eye.

Diagnosis. No evidence supports the use of HPV DNA tests in the routine diagnosis or management of visible genital warts.[35] A diagnosis is made from the typical clinical signs on the external genitalia. Colposcopy is valuable for diagnosing flat warts, which are difficult to see. Exclude the possible diagnosis of condylomata lata by obtaining a serologic test for syphilis. A biopsy is usually unnecessary but would be required to make a definitive diagnosis. When neoplasia is a possibility, take a biopsy of any atypical lesions or persistent warts before initiating therapy.

Treatment. Several different treatment regimens can be used, depending on client preference, available resources, and the experience of the health care provider. None of the currently available treatments is superior to others or are ideal for all patients. The currently available treatments for visible genital warts consist of two types: (1) patient-applied therapies and (2) provider-administered therapies.

Patient-applied therapies:

- *Podofilox* 0.5% solution or gel. Patients apply podofilox solution with a cotton swab, or a podofilox gel with a finger, to visible genital warts twice daily for 3 days, followed by 4 days of no therapy. This process may be repeated up to a total of four times. Podofilox should not be used during pregnancy.

- *Imiquimod* 5% cream. Patients should apply imiquimod cream with a finger, at bed time, 3 times a week, for up to 16 weeks. They should wash with mild soap and water after 6 to 10 hours. Imiquimod should not be used during pregnancy.

Provider-administered therapies:

- *Cryotherapy* with liquid nitrogen or cryoprobe. Repeat applications every 1 to 2 weeks.

- *Trichloroacetic acid (TCA) or bichloroacetic acid (BCA)* 80% to 90%. Apply a small amount to only the warts and allow to dry, at which time a white "frosting" develops. Repeat weekly as needed.

- *Podophyllin resin* 10% to 25% in tincture of benzoin. A small amount of podophyllin should be applied to each wart and allowed to air dry. Avoid normal tissue. Wash off thoroughly in 1 to 4 hours to reduce local irritation. Podophyllin should not be used during pregnancy and is not recommended for vaginal use.

- *Surgical removal.* Scissor or shaving excision, curette, or electrosurgery are possible.

HPV infection is a chronic condition even when asymptomatic. However, for most persons, it has a benign natural history. No therapy completely eradicates the virus. HPV has been demonstrated in adjacent tissue even after attempts to eliminate subclinical HPV by extensive laser vaporization of the anogenital area. The effect of genital wart treatment on HPV transmission and the natural history of HPV is unknown. Therefore, the goal of treatment is the temporary removal of visible genital warts and the amelioration of symptoms and signs, *not* the eradication of HPV.

Potential complications. Lesions may enlarge and destroy tissue. Giant condyloma, while histologically benign, may simulate carcinoma. In pregnancy, warts enlarge, are extremely vascular, and may obstruct the birth canal to necessitate a cesarean delivery. Neither routine HPV screening tests nor cesarean delivery for prevention of the transmission of HPV to the newborn is indicated. The perinatal transmission rate is unknown, although probably low. Persons with HIV disease can have rapidly growing genital warts. Women infected with HIV have an increased risk of progressive HPV-cervical disease.

Behavioral messages to emphasize. Return for regular treatment until lesions have resolved. Once warts have responded to therapy, no special follow-up is necessary. If you have anogenital warts, you are contagious to uninfected sex partners. Because most partners are probably already infected, examination of sex partners is not necessary.

To reduce risks of sequelae from cervical cancer, annual Pap smears are crucial for all women with documented HPV infection. HPV testing may be useful in triaging women with ASCUS pap smears. Smoking cessation will reduce the risk of HPV and neoplasia.

GONORRHEA is caused by Neisseria gonorrhoeae, a gram-negative diplococcus.

Prevalence. About 650,000 new cases of gonorrhea occur each year, making it the second most commonly reported infectious disease in the United States.

Symptoms. Symptomatic men usually have dysuria, increased frequency of urination, and purulent urethral discharge. An estimated one-fourth of infected men can be asymptomatic. Women may have abnormal vaginal discharge, abnormal menses, dysuria, or most commonly are asymptomatic. Pharyngeal gonorrhea can produce symptoms of pharyngitis.

Diagnosis. Presumptive diagnosis relies on microscopically identifying typical gram-negative intracellular diplococci on smear of urethral exudate (men) or endocervical material (women). Definitive diagnosis, especially in women, requires recovery of bacteria with typical colonial morphology, positive oxidase reaction, and typical Gram-stain morphology, grown on a selective culture medium. Ideally, all gonorrhea cases should be diagnosed by culture to facilitate antimicrobial susceptibility testing. However, increasing use of non-culture tests has increased the number of women tested. A definitive diagnosis by culture is required if the specimen is extragenital, from a child, or medico-legally important.

Treatment. In many areas of the United States about one-fourth of men and two-fifths of women with gonococcal infections also have a coexisting chlamydial infection. For this reason, use both a single-dose anti-gonococcal drug AND an anti-chlamydial regimen unless screening tests are negative. The recommended therapies for gonorrhea include cefixime 400 mg orally once; OR ceftriaxone 125 mg IM once; OR ciprofloxacin 500 mg orally once; OR ofloxacin 400 mg orally once; OR levofloxacin 250 mg orally once. For chlamydia, the recommended therapies are azithromycin 1 g orally in a single dose OR doxycycline 100 mg orally two times a day for 7 days. Treat patients with a history of oral-genital sex with a regimen effective against pharyngeal gonorrhea. Because of global resistance patterns, quinolones should not be used to treat infections that may have been acquired in Asia or the Pacific (including Hawaii).

Potential complications. Up to 40% of untreated women with cervical gonorrhea develop PID and are at risk for its sequelae (see the section on PID), including involuntary sterility and pelvic abscesses. Men are at risk for epididymitis, urethral stricture, and sterility. Newborns are at risk for ophthalmia neonatorum, scalp abscess at the site of fetal monitors, rhinitis, or anorectal infection. All infected untreated persons are at risk for disseminated gonococcal infection.

Behavioral messages to emphasize. Understand how to take any prescribed oral medications. Refer sex partner(s) for examination and treatment. Avoid sex until patient and partner(s) have been treated. Use condoms to prevent future infections.

GRANULOMA INGUINALE (Donovanosis) is caused by Calymmatobacterium granulomatis (formerly known as Donovania granulomatis), a bipolar, gram-negative bacterium (Donovan body) that in a crush preparation, appears in vacuolar compartments within histiocytes, white blood cells, or plasma cells.

Prevalence. Although one of the traditional venereal diseases, granuloma inguinale is rare in the United States. However, it is endemic in certain less developed countries including India, Papua New Guinea, Central Australia, and Southern Africa.

Symptoms. Initially, single or multiple subcutaneous nodules appear at the site of inoculation. Nodules erode to form granulomatous, heaped ulcers that are painless, bleed on contact, and enlarge slowly. Spread by autoinoculation is common.

Diagnosis. The typical clinical presentation is sufficient to suggest the diagnosis. Resolution of the lesions following specific antibiotic therapy supports the diagnosis. The patient's or partner's history of travel to endemic areas helps substantiate the clinical impression. A microscopic examination of biopsy specimens from the ulcer margin reveals the pathognomonic Donovan bodies. Tissue culture of C. granulomatis is not feasible.

Treatment. Recommended initial regimens are doxycycline 100 mg orally twice a day OR trimethoprim-sulfamethoxazole, 1 double-strength tablet twice a day until all lesions have completely healed (usually a minimum of 3 weeks). Alternatives are ciprofloxacin 750 mg orally twice a day OR erythromycin 500 mg orally four times a day OR azithromycin 1 mg orally once a week—all for at least 3 weeks.

Potential complications. Lesions may become secondarily infected. Fibrous, keloid-like formations may deform the genitalia. Pseudoelephantoid enlargement of the labia, penis, or scrotum occurs. Necrosis and destruction of the genitalia may result.

Behavioral messages to emphasize. Understand how to take prescribed oral medications. Return for evaluation 3 to 5 days after therapy begins. Assure examination of sex partner(s) as soon as possible. Return weekly or biweekly for evaluation until the infection is entirely healed.

HEPATITIS B is caused by hepatitis B virus (HBV), a DNA virus with multiple antigenic components.

Prevalence. In the United States, about 5% of the general population show evidence of past HBV infections. An estimated 120,000 new cases of HBV infection are transmitted sexually each year.[5] Heterosexual intercourse is now the predominant mode of HBV transmission.

Symptoms. Most HBV infections are not clinically apparent. When present, symptoms include a serum sickness-like prodrome (skin eruptions, urticaria, arthralgias, arthritis), lassitude, anorexia, nausea, vomiting, headache, fever, dark urine, jaundice, and moderate liver enlargement with tenderness.

Diagnosis. HBV infection is clinically indistinguishable from other forms of viral and other hepatitis. A patient with the typical clinical symptoms and exposure to a patient with definitive or presumed HBV infection may be presumed to have HBV infection. Serodiagnosis of HBV infection is the best method for clinicians to reach a definitive diagnosis. Positive results of the following tests are reliable:

- Hepatitis B surface antigen (HBsAg): Acute HBV infection or, with no acute disease exposure, the chronic carrier state (infectious)

- HBe antigen: More infectious than if just HBsAg-positive, because the virus is actively replicating

- Anti-HBsAg: Past infection with present immunity

- Anti-HB core antigen: Past or current infection

Treatment. No specific therapy exists. Provide supportive and symptomatic care. HBV is the only STI for which we have a vaccine. Vaccines made from recombinant genetic material are available. Specific vaccination and post-exposure prophylaxis strategies are of proven efficacy in preventing hepatitis B. Vaccinating all newborn infants and adolescents against hepatitis B is currently recommended. In addition, the Advisory Committee on Immunization Practices recommends HBV vaccination for all persons with recent STI and those who have a history of sexual activity with more than one partner in the previous 6 months. Subsidized HBV vaccine programs are available in many states through the hepatitis B coordinator.

Potential complications. Long-term sequelae include chronic, persistent, active hepatitis, cirrhosis, hepatocellular carcinoma, hepatic failure, and death. Rarely, the course may be fulminant with hepatic failure.

Behavioral messages to emphasize. HBV vaccination is strongly encouraged for all young, sexually active clients. The full three-vaccination regimen is necessary for maximum protection. Follow patients with hepatitis to see if they become HBsAg carriers and are capable of infecting others.

HUMAN PAPILLOMA VIRUS (HPV) See Genital Warts.

LYMPHOGRANULOMA VENEREUM (LGV) is caused by immunotypes L1, L2, or L3 of C. trachomatis.

Prevalence. LGV infections are more common than ordinarily believed. They are endemic in Asia and Africa but are rare in the United States.

Symptoms. The primary lesion of LGV is a 2 to 3 mm painless vesicle or nonindurated ulcer at the site of inoculation. Patients commonly fail to notice this primary lesion. Regional adenopathy follows a week to a month later and is the most common clinical symptom. A sensation of stiffness and aching in the groin, followed by swelling of the inguinal region, may be the first indications of infections for most patients. Adenopathy may subside spontaneously or proceed to the formation of abscesses that rupture to produce draining sinuses or fistulae.

Diagnosis. LGV is often diagnosed clinically and may be confused with chancroid because of the painful adenopathy. The LGV complement fixation test is sensitive; 80% of patients have a titer of 1:16 or higher. Levels of 1:64 are considered diagnostic. Because the sequelae of LGV are serious and preventable, do not withhold treatment pending laboratory confirmation. A definitive diagnosis requires isolating C. trachomatis from an appropriate specimen and confirming the isolate as an LGV immunotype. However, these laboratory diagnostic capabilities are not widely available.

Treatment. Give doxycycline 100 mg orally two times a day for 21 days OR erythromycin 500 mg orally four times a day for 21 days. Aspirate fluctuant lymph nodes as needed. Incision and drainage or excision of nodes will delay healing and are contraindicated.

Potential complications. Dissemination may occur with nephropathy, hepatomegaly, or phlebitis. Large polypoid swelling of the vulva (esthiomene), anal margin, or rectal mucosa may occur. The most common severe morbidity results from rectal involvement: perianal abscess and rectovaginal or other fistulae are early consequences, and rectal stricture may develop 1 to 10 years after infection.

Behavioral messages to emphasize. Understand how to take prescribed oral medications. Return for evaluation 3 to 5 days after therapy begins. Assure examination of sex partner(s) as soon as possible.

MOLLUSCUM CONTAGIOSUM is caused by molluscum contagiosum virus, the largest DNA virus of the poxvirus group.

Prevalence. As an RTI, molluscum contagiosum occurs infrequently, about 1 case for every 100 cases of gonorrhea. Outbreaks have been reported among groups at high risk for other RTIs.

Symptoms. Lesions are 1 to 5 mm, smooth, rounded, firm, shiny flesh-colored to pearly-white papules with characteristically umbilicated centers. They are most commonly seen on the trunk and anogenital region and are generally asymptomatic.

Diagnosis. Infection is usually diagnosed on the basis of the typical clinical presentation. Microscopic examination of lesions or lesion material reveals the pathognomonic molluscum inclusion bodies.

Treatment. Lesions may resolve spontaneously without scarring. However, they may be removed by curettage after cryoanesthesia. Treatment with caustic chemicals (podophyllin, trichloroacetic acid, silver nitrate) and cryotherapy (liquid nitrogen) have been successful. If every lesion is not extirpated, the condition may recur.

Potential complications. Secondary infection, usually with staphylococcus, may occur. Lesions rarely attain a size greater than 10 mm in diameter.

Behavioral messages to emphasize. Return for reexamination 1 month after treatment so any new lesions can be removed. Sex partner(s) should be examined.

MUCOPURULENT CERVICITIS (MPC) can be caused by C. trachomatis, N. gonorrhoeae, or possibly mycoplasmas.

Prevalence. Based on extrapolation from local studies, mucopurulent cervicitis (MPC) probably occurs more frequently than male urethritis. Up to 3 million cases per year may occur annually.

Symptoms. The mucopurulent discharge is exuded from the cervix. Often the patient does not recognize the discharge or may perceive it as normal vaginal discharge.

Diagnosis. Diagnosis is made by finding either mucopus on a swab of the endocervical secretions or friability (bleeding) on the first swabbing. In most cases of MPC, a microbial organism cannot be identified. A definitive etiologic diagnosis is made when either chlamydia or gonorrhea is isolated.

Treatment. The results of sensitive tests for C. trachomatis or N. gonorrhoeae should determine the need for treatment. Chlamydia is treated with azithromycin 1 g orally in a single dose OR doxycycline 100 mg orally twice a day for 7 days. The above section on Gonorrhea contains the range of recommended treatment regimens for this infection.

Potential complications. PID (with subsequent infertility) and pelvic abscesses may complicate infection. In addition, neonatal chlamydial infections, such as ophthalmia or pneumonia, may be acquired during delivery if the mother has an infected endocervix. If a pregnant woman is infected, she may be at risk for postpartum endometritis.

Behavioral messages to emphasize. If your infection involves C. trachomatis or N. gonorrhoeae, refer your sex partner(s) for examination and treatment. Avoid sex until you and your partner(s) are cured. Understand how to take prescribed oral medications. Return early if symptoms persist or recur. Use condoms to prevent future infections.

NONGONOCOCCAL URETHRITIS (NGU) is caused by Chlamydia trachomatis about 30% of the time. Other sexually transmissible agents, which cause 10% to 45% of NGU, include Ureaplasma urealyticum, Trichomonas vaginalis, and herpes simplex virus. The etiology of the remaining cases is unknown.

Prevalence. NGU appears more frequently than gonorrhea in both public STI clinics and private practices. More than 1 million cases annually are estimated to occur in men.

Symptoms. Men usually have dysuria, urinary frequency, and mucoid to purulent urethral discharge. Many men have asymptomatic infections.

Diagnosis. Men with typical clinical symptoms are presumed to have NGU when their gonorrhea tests are negative and they have either white blood cells (WBCs) on Gram stain of urethral discharge or sexual exposure to an agent known to cause NGU. Asymptomatic men with negative gonorrhea tests are also presumed to have NGU if > 5 WBCs per oil immersion field appear on an intraurethral smear. Chlamydia testing is strongly recommended for a specific diagnosis. Gonococcal and nongonococcal urethritis may coexist in the same patient.

Treatment. When the etiology is C. trachomatis, U. urealyticum, or unknown, the following treatment is recommended: azithromycin 1 g orally in a single dose OR doxycycline 100 mg orally twice daily for 7 days. Alternatives for patients who fail their first trial are erythromycin 500 mg orally four times a day for at least 7 days OR ofloxacin 300 mg orally twice a day for 7 days. For T. vaginalis or herpes simplex infections, see the sections of this chapter that deal specifically with these agents.

Potential complications. Urethral strictures or epididymitis may occur. If C. trachomatis is transmitted to female sex partners, the condition may result in mucopurulent cervicitis and PID. If C. trachomatis is transmitted to a pregnant woman, complications may include neonatal infections such as ophthalmia or pneumonia.

Behavioral messages to emphasize. Understand how to take any prescribed oral medications. If chlamydial infection is diagnosed, refer sex partner(s) for examination and treatment. Avoid sex until you and your partner(s) are cured. Use condoms to prevent future infections.

PELVIC INFLAMMATORY DISEASE (PID) can be caused by varying combinations of N. gonorrhoeae, C. trachomatis, anaerobic bacteria, facultative gram-negative rods (such as E. coli), Mycoplasma hominis, and a variety of other microbial agents. Clinical PID is usually of polymicrobial etiology. N. gonorrhoeae and C. trachomatis may cause antecedent inflammation, which makes the tubes susceptible to invasion by anaerobic organisms.

Prevalence. PID accounts for nearly 180,000 hospitalizations every year in the United States. More than 1 million episodes occur annually. Among American women of reproductive age, 1 in 7 reports having received treatment for PID.

Symptoms. Based on retrospective reports, many women with PID have atypical or no symptoms. Women may have pain and tenderness involving the lower abdomen, cervix, uterus, and adnexae, possibly combined with fever, chills, and elevated white blood cell (WBC) count and erythrocyte sedimentation rate (ESR). The condition is more likely if the patient has multiple sex partners, a history of PID, or is in the first 5 to 10 days of her menstrual cycle. More specific criteria, such as endometrial biopsy, magnetic resonance imaging or diagnostic laparoscopy, are warranted only in selected instances.

Diagnosis. Women who have the typical clinical symptoms are presumed to have PID if other serious conditions, such as acute appendicitis or ectopic pregnancy, can be excluded. The diagnosis of PID is often based on imprecise clinical findings.[36] Maintain a low threshold for diagnosing PID, because even mild or moderate PID has the potential for reproductive sequelae. Clinicians should use objective criteria to monitor response to antibiotics, especially if ambulatory treatment is given. Direct visualization of inflamed (edema, hyperemia, or tubal exudate) fallopian tube(s) during laparoscopy or laparotomy confirms the diagnosis of PID. Cultures of tubal exudate may help establish the microbiologic etiology.

Treatment. Because the causative organism is usually unknown at the time of the initial therapy, use treatment regimens that are active against the broadest possible range of pathogens. Antimicrobial coverage should include N. gonorrhoeae, C. trachomatis, anaerobes, Gram-negative facultative bacteria, and streptococci.

Hospitalization and inpatient care: Since hospitalization is no longer synonymous with parenteral therapy, the decision to hospitalize is based on the clinician's discretion. Consider hospitalizing patients with acute PID when (1) surgical emergencies, such as appendicitis and ectopic pregnancy, are not definitely excluded; (2) severe illness precludes outpatient management; (3) the woman is pregnant; (4) the woman is unable to follow or tolerate an outpatient regimen; or (5) the woman has failed to respond to outpatient therapy. Special consideration may be given to adolescents both to preserve their fertility and improve their adherence.

Combined drug therapy is recommended in all cases since the full bacterial etiology of PID is not clear and is generally polymicrobial.

Parenteral treatment: Two parenteral regimens are recommended for both inpatient and outpatient care:

- *Regimen A:* Either cefotetan 2.0 g IV every 12 hours, OR cefoxitin 2.0 g IV every 6 hours for at least 24 hours after the patient clinically improves PLUS doxycycline 100 mg orally or IV every 12 hours. Continue doxycycline 100 mg orally twice daily after discharge to complete at least 14 days of therapy.

- *Regimen B:* Clindamycin 900 mg, IV three times a day, PLUS gentamicin 2 mg per kilogram (kg) IV loading dose and maintenance 1.5 mg/kg IV every 8 hours. Continue oral therapy as above.

Oral treatment: Either of two oral regimens are recommended:

- *Regimen A:* Ofloxacin 400 mg twice daily OR levofloxacin 500 mg once daily with or without metronidazole 500 mg two times a day for 14 days.

- *Regimen B:* Ceftriaxone 250 mg IM; OR Cefoxitin 2.0 g IM along with probenecid 1.0 g orally PLUS doxycycline 100 mg taken orally twice daily for 14 days.

Potential complications. Potentially life-threatening complications include ectopic pregnancy and pelvic abscess. Other sequelae are involuntary infertility, recurrent or chronic PID, chronic abdominal pain, pelvic adhesions, premature hysterectomy, and depression.

Behavioral messages to emphasize. For outpatient therapy, return for evaluation 2 to 3 days after initiation of therapy. Return for further evaluation 4 days after completing therapy. Refer sex partner(s) for evaluation and treatment (up to half of sex partners of women with PID are infected but asymptomatic). Avoid sexual activity until the patient and her partner(s) are cured. Use condoms to prevent future infections. Understand how to take prescribed oral medications.

SYPHILIS is caused by Treponema pallidum, a spirochete with 6 to 14 regular spirals and characteristic motility.

Prevalence. Because of recent syphilis elimination efforts, primary and secondary syphilis currently are declining in the United States. Congenital syphilis is also on the wane. However, syphilis remains an important STI, with serious sequelae if not treated. Southeastern states have the highest rates of both syphilis and congenital syphilis.

Symptoms—

Primary: The classical chancre is a painless, indurated ulcer, located at the site of exposure. The differential diagnosis for all genital lesions should include syphilis.

Secondary: Patients may have a highly variable skin rash, mucous patches, condylomata lata (fleshy, moist tissue growths), lymphadenopathy, alopecia, or other signs.

Latent: Patients are without clinical signs of infection.

Diagnosis—

Primary: Patients have typical lesion(s) and either a positive darkfield exam; a fluorescent antibody technique in material from a chancre, regional lymph node, or other lesion; or their present serologic test for syphilis (STS) titer is at least fourfold greater than the last; or they have been exposed to syphilis within 90 days of lesion onset.

Secondary: Patients have the typical clinical presentation and a strongly reactive STS; condyloma lata will be darkfield positive.

Latent: Patients have serologic evidence of untreated syphilis without clinical signs.

Primary and secondary syphilis are definitively diagnosed by demonstrating T. pallidum with darkfield microscopy or fluorescent antibody technique. A definitive diagnosis of latent syphilis cannot be made under usual circumstances.

Treatment—

Primary, secondary, or early syphilis of less than 1 year duration: benzathine penicillin G 2.4 million units IM in a single dose.

Syphilis of indeterminate length or of more than 1 year duration: benzathine penicillin G 7.2 million units total; 2.4 million units IM, weekly, for 3 successive weeks.

Patients allergic to penicillin: Doxycycline 100 mg orally two times a day. [Note: Duration of therapy depends on the estimated duration of infection. If duration has been less than 1 year, treat the infection for 14 days; otherwise, treat for 28 days.]

Penicillin-allergic pregnant women or for doxycycline-intolerant patients only: Consult the 1998 Guidelines for Treatment of Sexually Transmitted Diseases.

Congenital syphilis or if the patient is simultaneously infected with syphilis and HIV: Refer to the 2002 Guidelines for Treatment of Sexually Transmitted Diseases.[26]

Potential complications. Late syphilis and congenital syphilis, both complications of early syphilis, are preventable with prompt diagnosis and treatment. Sequelae of late syphilis include neurosyphilis (general paresis, tabes dorsalis, and focal neurologic signs), cardiovascular syphilis (thoracic aortic aneurism, aortic insufficiency), and localized gumma formation.

Behavioral messages to emphasize. Because genital ulcers may be associated with HIV infection, get an HIV test. Return for follow-up syphilis serologies at 3 and 6 months for early syphilis, and at 6 and 12 months for late latent disease. HIV-positive patients should return 1, 2, 3, 6, 9, and 12 months after therapy; pregnant partners should be followed monthly. Understand how to take any prescribed oral medications. Refer sex partner(s) for evaluation and treatment. Avoid sexual activity until you and your partner(s) are cured. Use condoms to prevent future infections.

TRICHOMONIASIS is caused by Trichomonas vaginalis, a motile protozoan with an undulating membrane and four flagella.

Prevalence. Trichomoniasis is the most common curable STI in the United States and worldwide. Each year an estimated 3 million U.S. women become infected.

Symptoms. Excessive, frothy, diffuse, yellow-green vaginal discharge is common, although clinical presentation varies from no signs or symptoms to erythema, edema, and pruritis of the external genitalia. Dysuria and dyspareunia are also frequent. The type of symptoms or signs alone does not distinguish the microbial etiology. Male sex partners may develop urethritis, balanitis, or cutaneous lesions on the penis; however, the majority of males infected with T. vaginalis are asymptomatic.

Diagnosis. Trichomoniasis is diagnosed when a vaginal culture or fluorescent antibody is positive for T. vaginalis OR typical motile trichomonads are identified in a saline wet mount of vaginal discharge. Trichomonads found by Pap smear should be verified by examination of vaginal secretions.

Treatment. Metronidazole 2.0 g orally at one time. An alternative regimen is metronidazole 500 mg orally twice daily for 7 days. Metronidazole-resistant T. vaginalis, although uncommon, can occur. Most treatment failures respond to higher doses of therapy. Sex partners should be simultaneously treated with the same regimen as the index client.

Potential complications. Secondary excoriation may occur. Recurrent infections are common. Trichomoniasis has been associated with an increased risk of salpingitis, low birthweight, prematurity, and acquisition of HIV.

Behavioral messages to emphasize. Understand how to take or use prescribed medications. Return if the problem is not cured or recurs. Make sure sex partner(s) are treated. Use condoms to prevent future infections. Avoid drinking alcohol until 24 hours after completing metronidazole therapy.

REFERENCES

1. Tsui AO, Wasserheit JN, Haaga J, National Research Council (U.S.), Panel on Reproductive Health. Reproductive health in developing countries expanding dimensions, building solutions. Washington, DC: National Academy Press, 1997.
2. Cates W Jr, Padian NS. The interrelationship of reproductive health and sexually transmitted diseases. In: Goldman MBaHMC, (eds). Women and Health. San Diego, California: Academic Press, 2000: 381-389.
3. Eng TR, Butler WT, Committee on Prevention and Control of Sexually Transmitted Diseases, Institute of Medicine (U.S.), Division of Health Promotion and Disease Prevention. The hidden epidemic confronting sexually transmitted diseases. Washington, DC: National Academy Press, 1996.
4. Holmes KK, Mårdh PA, Sparling P.F. et al. (eds). Sexually transmitted diseases. Third edition. New York: McGraw-Hill, 1999.
5. Cates W Jr and the American Social Health Association Panel. Estimates of the incidence and prevalence of sexually transmitted diseases in the United States. Sex Transm Dis 1999; 26(4 Suppl):S2-7.
6. World Health Organization. Global prevalence and incidence of selected curable sexually transmitted infections: Overview and estimates. Geneva, Switzerland: WHO, 2001.
7. Mosure DJ, Berman S, Fine D, DeLisle S, Cates W Jr, Boring JR 3rd. Genital Chlamydia infections in sexually active female adolescents: do we really need to screen everyone? J Adolesc Health 1997; 20(1):6-13.
8. Anderson RM. Transmission dynamics of sexually transmitted infections. In: Holmes KK, et al. Sexually Transmitted Diseases. Third edition. New York: McGraw Hill, 1999: 25-37.
9. Fleming DT, Wasserheit JN. From epidemiologic synergy to public health policy and practice: The contribution of other sexually transmitted diseases to sexual transmission of HIV infection. Sex Transm Infect. New York: McGraw Hill, 1999: 25-37.
10. Trussell J, Kost K. Contraceptive failure in the United States: a critical review of the literature. Stud Fam Plann 1987; 18(5):237-283.
11. Platt R, Rice PA, McCormack WM. Risk of acquiring gonorrhea and prevalence of abnormal adnexal findings among women recently exposed to gonorrhea. JAMA 1983; 250(23):3205-3209.
12. Westrom L, Joesoef R, Reynolds G, Hagdu A, Thompson SE. Pelvic inflammatory disease and fertility. A cohort study of 1,844 women with laparoscopically verified disease and 657 control women with normal laparoscopic results. Sex Transm Dis 1992; 19(4):185-192.
13. Cates W Jr, Hinman AR. AIDS and absolutism—the demand for perfection in prevention [see comments]. N Engl J Med 1992; 327(7):492-494.
14. Cates W Jr. The NIH Condom Report: The glass is 90% full. Fam Plann Perspect 2001.
15. McCormack S, Hayes R, Lacey CJ, Johnson AM. Microbicides in HIV prevention. BMJ 2001; 322(7283):410-413.
16. Ness RB, Keder LM, Soper DE et al. Oral contraception and the recognition of endometritis. Am J Obstet Gynecol 1997; 176(3):580-585.
17. Grimes DA. Intrauterine device and upper-genital-tract infection. Lancet 2000; 356(9234):1013-1019.
18. Zhang J, Thomas AG, Leybovich E. Vaginal douching and adverse health effects: a meta-analysis. Am J Public Health 1997; 87(7):1207-1211.
19. Hooton TM, Scholes D, Hughes JP et al. A prospective study of risk factors for symptomatic urinary tract infection in young women. N Engl J Med 1996; 335(7):468-474.
20. Cates W Jr. A risk-assessment tool for integrated reproductive health services. Fam Plann Perspect 1997; 29(1):41-43.
21. Cates W Jr, Steiner MJ. Dual protection against unintended pregnancy and sexually transmitted infections: what is the best contraceptive approach? Sex Transm Dis 2002; 29:168-174.

22. Wentworth BB, Judson FN, Gilchrist MJR eds. Laboratory methods for the diagnosis of sexually transmitted diseases, second edition. Washington DC: American Public Health Association, 1991.
23. Rothenberg RB, Potterat JJ. Partner notification for sexually transmitted diseases and HIV infection. In: Holmes KK, Mårdh PA, Sparling P.F. *et al.* Sexually transmitted diseases. Third edition. New York: McGraw-Hill, 1999: 745-752.
24. Elwy AR, Hart GJ, Hawkes S, Petticrew M. Effectiveness of interventions to prevent sexually transmitted infections and human immunodeficiency virus in heterosexual men. Arch Int Med 2002; 162:1818-1830.
25. American College of Obstetrics and Gynecology and American Academy of Pediatrics. Guidelines for Perinatal Care, 4th edition. Washington, DC: American College of Obstetrics and Gynecology, and American Academy of Pediatrics, 1996.
26. Centers for Disease Control and Prevention. Guidelines for Treatment of Sexually Transmitted Diseases 2002. MMWR 2002; 51 (No. RR-6):1-78.
27. Stamm WE, Hooton TM. Management of urinary tract infections in adults. N Engl J Med 1993; 329(18):1328-1334.
28. Koumans EH, Kendrick JS. Preventing adverse sequelae of bacterial vaginosis: public health program and research agenda. CDC Bacterial Vaginosis Working Group. Sex Transm Dis 2001; 28(5):292-297.
29. Centers for Disease Control and Prevention. Recommendations for prevention and management of Chlamydia trachomatis infections. MMWR . 1993;43 (RR-12): 1-39.
30. Scholes D, Stergachis A, Heidrich FE, Andrilla H, Holmes KK, Stamm WE. Prevention of pelvic inflammatory disease by screening for cervical chlamydial infection. N Engl J Med 1996; 334(21):1362-1366.
31. Nelson HD, Helfand M. Screening for chlamydial infection. Am J Prev Med 2001; 20(3 Suppl):95-107.
32. Fleming DT, McQuillan GM, Johnson RE *et al.* Herpes simplex virus type 2 in the United States, 1976 to 1994. N Engl J Med 1997; 337(16):1105-1111.
33. Handsfield HH, Stone KM, Graber JM. Report of the Genital Herpes Prevention Consultant's Meeting, May 5-6, 1998. Atlanta, Georgia: Centers for Disease Control and Prevention, 1998.
34. Wald A, Langenberg AG, Link K *et al.* Effect of condoms on reducing the transmission of herpes simplex virus type 2 from men to women. JAMA 2001; 285(24): 3100-3106.
35. Division of STD Prevention. Prevention of genital HPV infection and sequelae: Report of an external consultants' meeting. Department of Health and Human Services, Atlanta: Centers for Disease Control and Prevention (CDC), 1999.
36. Kahn JG, Walker CK, Washington AE, Landers DV, Sweet RL. Diagnosing pelvic inflammatory disease. A comprehensive analysis and considerations for developing a new model. JAMA 1991; 266(18):2594-2604.

The Essentials of Contraception: Efficacy, Safety, and Personal Considerations

James Trussell, PhD

- Correct and consistent use of most contraceptive methods results in a low risk of pregnancy.
- Even a low annual risk of pregnancy implies a high cumulative risk of pregnancy during a lifetime of use. For example, an annual probability of pregnancy of 3% implies a 26% probability of pregnancy over 10 years.
- The simultaneous use of methods can dramatically lower the risk of pregnancy.
- Emergency contraception provides a last chance to prevent pregnancy after unprotected intercourse.
- Contraceptives pose little risk to a user's health, although personal risk factors should influence personal choice.
- Half of all pregnancies are unintended: 3 million each year.
- Contraception saves medical care dollars by preventing unintended pregnancy. Ironically, women typically must pay for contraception while insurers, who pay for the cost of unintended pregnancy, reap the benefits of contraceptive use.

Choosing a method of contraception is an important decision. A method that is not effective for an individual can lead to an unintended pregnancy. A method that is not safe for the user can create unfortunate medical consequences. A method that does not fit the individual's personal lifestyle is not likely to be used correctly or consistently. Individuals themselves must make the decision about the contraceptive method they use, taking into consideration the feelings and attitudes of their partners. The best method of contraception for an individual or couple is one that is safe and that will actually be used correctly and consistently.

Because most people will use a variety of contraceptive methods throughout their lives, they should be knowledgeable about various contraceptive methods. The patient's choice of a contraceptive method depends on several major factors: efficacy, safety, cost, noncontraceptive benefits, and personal considerations. Through counseling, you can help your patient choose the most suitable contraceptive method. You also can influence the user's motivation and ability to use the method correctly.[1] Encourage clients to educate themselves about the various methods available. Direct clients toward available literature. (See Chapter 11 on Reproductive Health Resources.)

Information on levels and trends in contraceptive use in the United States is based on the National Surveys of Family Growth (NSFG), periodic surveys conducted by the National Center for Health Statistics in which women ages 15 to 44 are interviewed about topics related to childbearing, family planning, and maternal and child health. Among the 60.2 million women of reproductive age (ages 15 to 44) in 1995, about 64% (38.6 million) were using some method of contraception, according to the 1995 NSFG. Among the 36% (21.6 million) who were not currently using a method, only about one-seventh were at risk of pregnancy. The remaining six-sevenths were not at risk because they had been sterilized for noncontraceptive reasons, were sterile, were trying to become pregnant, were pregnant, were interviewed within 2 months after the completion of a pregnancy, or were not having intercourse during the 3 months prior to the survey.[2]

Almost 93% of the women at risk were using a contraceptive method. Seven percent of all women at risk of unintended pregnancy did not use any contraceptive method. Today, the most popular contraceptive methods are female sterilization (10.7 million), oral contraceptive pills (10.4 million), male condoms (7.9 million), and male sterilization (4.2 million).[2] See Table 9-1 for information on contraceptive method use by age of woman.

Between 1988 and 1995, contraceptive method choices changed somewhat:[2,3]

- Male condom use increased from 13.2% to 18.9% among all women ages 15 to 44 at risk of pregnancy, generally because of the concern over acquired immune deficiency syndrome (AIDS) and sexually transmitted infections (STIs). Increases occurred in all age groups but were greatest among women ages 20 to 24 (from 12.9% to 24.0%) and women ages 25 to 29 (from 13.9% to 22.8%). Male condom use among women ages 15 to 19 increased from 26.7% to 29.7%.

- Pill use among all women ages 15 to 44 at risk declined slightly, from 27.7% to 24.9%. Pill use increased somewhat for women above age 30, but decreased among women below that age. Substantial declines among women ages 15 to 19 (from 47.1% to 35.4%) and 20 to 24 (from 59.8% to 47.6%) were compensated by use of two new methods, the implant and the injectable (used in 1995 by 10.1% and 9.0% of women ages 15 to 19 and 20 to 24, respectively).

Table 9-1 Percent and number of women at risk[1] and percent at risk currently using various methods from the 1995 National Survey of Family Growth

	Percent Using among Women at Risk[1]						
	15-44	15-19	20-24	25-29	30-34	35-39	40-44
Female sterilization	25.6	0.3	3.6	16.0	27.7	38.6	46.7
Pill	24.9	35.4	47.6	36.6	26.8	10.5	5.5
Male condom	18.9	29.7	24.0	22.8	17.3	15.9	11.5
Male sterilization	10.1	0.0	1.0	4.2	9.8	17.6	19.0
No method	7.5	19.3	8.6	6.4	5.7	5.6	6.7
Withdrawal	2.9	3.3	3.0	3.5	2.7	3.0	1.8
Injectable	2.7	7.9	5.6	3.9	1.7	1.0	0.3
Periodic abstinence	2.2	1.1	0.9	1.6	3.0	2.7	2.4
Natural family planning	0.3	0.0	0.1	0.3	0.4	0.5	0.3
Diaphragm	1.7	0.0	0.6	0.8	2.2	2.8	2.5
Implant	1.3	2.2	3.4	1.9	0.6	0.3	0.1
Spermicides	1.3	0.8	1.1	1.6	1.4	1.0	1.8
IUD	0.7	0.0	0.3	0.7	0.8	0.9	1.2
Other[2]	0.1	0.0	0.1	0.0	0.3	0.1	0.5
Female condom	0.0	0.0	0.1	0.0	0.0	0.0	0.0
	Number of Women in Cohort, Percent and Number at Risk[1]						
Number (millions) of Women	60.2	9.0	9.0	9.7	11.1	11.2	10.2
Percent at Risk[1]	69.4	36.9	69.4	74.0	77.1	77.2	76.6
Number (millions) at Risk[1]	41.8	3.3	6.3	7.2	8.5	8.7	7.8

Source: Abma et al. (1997),[2] Piccinino (1997).[4]

Notes:

[1] At risk = those who *either* are current contraceptive users *or* are nonusers who have had sex in the past three months and are not trying to become pregnant, are not pregnant, or were not interviewed within two months after the completion of a pregnancy and are not sterile. Percentages may not add to 100 due to rounding.

[2] Other methods = cervical cap, sponge, and other unspecified methods.

- Diaphragm use among all women ages 15 to 44 at risk declined from 5.2% to only 1.7%, with the biggest decline observed among women ages 30 to 34 (from 8.2% to 2.2%).

Actually, use of male condoms has increased more than these figures indicate, because some women are protected by dual methods. In the 1995 NSFG, women were asked to report all contraceptive methods used in the current month for any reason (for protection against either pregnancy or STIs). When more than one method was reported, only the most effective method is coded as the current method.[a] Concomitant use

[a] The NCHS hierarchy of effectiveness was established before the 1995 NSFG was conducted, and is not the same as that reported here in Table 9-2, which is based on the 1995 NSFG.

of male condoms and sterilization, hormonal contraception, intrauterine device (IUD), or diaphragm is coded in the NSFG as use of that other method, while concomitant use of male condoms and any contraceptive other than these methods is recoded as use of the male condom. When the data in Table 9-1 are recoded to capture all use of the male condom, the fraction using male condoms among all women at risk rises by 15%, from 18.9% to 21.6%. Increases are greatest among women ages 20 to 24 (a 28% increase, from 24.0% to 30.7%) and women ages 15 to 19 (a 25% increase, from 29.7% to 37.1%).[4]

The mix of methods shown in Table 9-1, including the 7.5% of women at risk who do not use any method, resulted in a staggering 3.04 million unintended pregnancies in 1994, the latest year for which data are available.[2,5,6] Nearly half (48.0%) of the 6.32 million pregnancies and nearly one-third (30.8% or 1.22 million) of the 3.95 million births were unintended.[2,6] Every night in the United States, about 10 million couples at risk of unintended pregnancy have intercourse; among these, about 27,000 experience a condom break or slip, and over 700,000 are not protected against pregnancy at all (see Table 9-1 and Chapter 31 on Contraceptive Efficacy).[2,7]

EFFICACY: "WILL IT WORK?"

"Is the condom really effective?"
"Which would be the most effective method for me?"
"Why did one magazine say diaphragms are 94% effective and another say they're 84% effective?"
"Can you still get pregnant if you take your pills every day on schedule?"

"Will it work?" is the question usually asked first and most frequently about any method of contraception.[8] Although this question cannot be answered with certainty for any particular couple, clinicians and counselors can try to help patients understand something of the difficulty of quantifying efficacy.

It is useful to distinguish between measures of contraceptive effectiveness and measures of the risk of pregnancy during contraceptive use. Many persons, including clinicians and clients, prefer positive rather than negative statements; instead of the negative statement that 20% of women using a method become accidentally pregnant during their first year of use, they prefer the alternative positive statement that the method is 80% effective. However, it does not follow that the method is 80% effective, because it is not true that 100% of these women would have become pregnant if they had not been using contraception. If 90% of these method users would have become pregnant had they used no method, then the use of the method reduced the number of accidental pregnancies from 90% to 20%, a reduction of 78%. In this sense, the method could be said to be 78% effective at reducing pregnancy in the first year. But if only 60% of these women would have become pregnant if they did not use contraception, then the method would be only 67% effective.[b] Because no study can ascertain the proportion of women who would have become pregnant had they not used the contraceptive method under investigation, it is simply not possible to measure effectiveness directly. Therefore, we focus attention entirely on pregnancy rates or probabilities of pregnancy during contraceptive use, which are directly measurable. However, we continue to use the term effectiveness in its loose everyday sense of how well a method works throughout this book, and we use the terms effectiveness and efficacy interchangeably. We also provide estimates of the proportion of women who would become pregnant if they did not use contraception, so that the reader may calculate rough effectiveness rates if they are needed.

THE RISK OF PREGNANCY DURING TYPICAL AND PERFECT USE

Four pieces of information about contraceptive efficacy would help couples to make an informed decision when choosing a contraceptive method:

- Pregnancy rates during *typical use* show how effective the different methods are during actual use (including inconsistent *or* incorrect use).
- Pregnancy rates during *perfect use* show how effective methods can be, where perfect use is defined as following the directions for use.
- Pregnancy rates during *imperfect use* show how ineffective methods will be if they are used incorrectly or inconsistently. Pregnancy rates can be computed separately for different categories of imperfect use to reveal which types of imperfect use are most risky.[9]
- The percentage of *perfect users* or percentage of months during which a method is used perfectly reveals how hard it is to use a method correctly and consistently.

The difference between pregnancy rates during *imperfect use* and pregnancy rates during *perfect use* reveals how forgiving of *imperfect use* a method is. The difference between pregnancy rates during *typical use* and pregnancy rates during *perfect use* reveals the consequences of *imperfect use*; this difference depends both on how unforgiving of *imperfect use* a method is and on how hard it is to use that method perfectly. Only the first two pieces of information are currently available. Our current understanding of the literature on contraceptive efficacy is summarized in Table 9-2.[10,11]

---

[b] Above, we have calculated effectiveness on an annual basis. Strictly, effectiveness is the proportionate reduction in the probability per cycle of conception c when no contraception is used. If this per-cycle probability is constant across women and over time, then the proportion conceiving in one year with no contraceptive method use is $1-(1-c)^{13}$. Therefore, if the annual probability of pregnancy is 90% then c=.162 and if the annual probability is 60% then c=.068. Using a contraceptive method with effectiveness e reduces the proportion becoming pregnant in one year to $1-\{1-c(1-e)\}^{13}$. Hence, in the first example, method effectiveness, strictly measured, is 90% and in the second example it is only 75%.

Table 9-2 Percentage of women experiencing an unintended pregnancy during the first year of typical use and the first year of perfect use of contraception and the percentage continuing use at the end of the first year. United States.

Method (1)	% of Women Experiencing an Unintended Pregnancy within the First Year of Use		% of Women Continuing Use at One Year[3] (4)
	Typical Use[1] (2)	Perfect Use[2] (3)	
No method[4]	85	85	
Spermicides[5]	29	18	42
Withdrawal	27	4	43
Periodic abstinence	25		51
Calendar		9	
Ovulation method		3	
Sympto-thermal[6]		2	
Post-ovulation		1	
Cap[7]			
Parous women	32	26	46
Nulliparous women	16	9	57
Sponge			
Parous women	32	20	46
Nulliparous women	16	9	57
Diaphragm[7]	16	6	57
Condom[8]			
Female (Reality)	21	5	49
Male	15	2	53
Combined pill and minipill	8	0.3	68
Evra patch	8	0.3	68
NuvaRing	8	0.3	68
Depo-Provera	3	0.3	56
Lunelle	3	0.05	56
IUD			
ParaGard (copper T)	0.8	0.6	78
Mirena (LNG-IUS)	0.1	0.1	81
Norplant and Norplant-2	0.05	0.05	84
Female sterilization	0.5	0.5	100
Male sterilization	0.15	0.10	100

Emergency Contraceptive Pills: Treatment initiated within 72 hours after unprotected intercourse reduces the risk of pregnancy by at least 75%.[9]
Lactational Amenorrhea Method: LAM is a highly effective, *temporary* method of contraception.[10]

(continued)

Table 9-2 Percentage of women experiencing an unintended pregnancy during the first year of typical use and the first year of perfect use of contraception and the percentage continuing use at the end of the first year. United States—*(cont'd)*

Source: See Chapter 31.

Notes:

1 Among *typical* couples who initiate use of a method (not necessarily for the first time), the percentage who experience an accidental pregnancy during the first year if they do not stop use for any other reason. Estimates of the probability of pregnancy during the first year of typical use for spermicides, withdrawal, periodic abstinence, the diaphragm, the male condom, the pill, and Depo-Provera are taken from the 1995 National Survey of Family Growth corrected for underreporting of abortion; see Chapter 31 for the derivation of estimates for the other methods.

2 Among couples who initiate use of a method (not necessarily for the first time) and who use it *perfectly* (both consistently and correctly), the percentage who experience an accidental pregnancy during the first year if they do not stop use for any other reason. See Chapter 31 for the derivation of the estimate for each method.

3 Among couples attempting to avoid pregnancy, the percentage who continue to use a method for 1 year.

4 The percentages becoming pregnant in columns (2) and (3) are based on data from populations where contraception is not used and from women who cease using contraception in order to become pregnant. Among such populations, about 89% become pregnant within 1 year. This estimate was lowered slightly (to 85%) to represent the percentage who would become pregnant within 1 year among women now relying on reversible methods of contraception if they abandoned contraception altogether.

5 Foams, creams, gels, vaginal suppositories, and vaginal film.

6 Cervical mucus (ovulation) method supplemented by calendar in the pre-ovulatory and basal body temperature in the post-ovulatory phases.

7 With spermicidal cream or jelly.

8 Without spermicides.

9 The treatment schedule is one dose within 120 hours after unprotected intercourse, and a second dose 12 hours after the first dose. Both doses of Plan B can be taken at the same time. Plan B (1 dose is 1 white pill) is the only dedicated product specifically marketed for emergency contraception. The Food and Drug Administration has in addition declared the following 18 brands of oral contraceptives to be safe and effective for emergency contraception: Ogestrel or Ovral (1 dose is 2 white pills), Alesse, Lessina, or Levlite, (1 dose is 5 pink pills), Levlen or Nordette (1 dose is 4 light-orange pills), Cryselle, Levora, Low-Ogestrel, or Lo/Ovral (1 dose is 4 white pills), Tri-Levlen or Triphasil (1 dose is 4 yellow pills), Portia, Seasonale, or Trivora (1 dose is 4 pink pills), Aviane (one dose is 5 orange pills), and Empresse (one dose is 4 orange pills).

10 However, to maintain effective protection against pregnancy, another method of contraception must be used as soon as menstruation resumes, the frequency or duration of breastfeeds is reduced, bottle feeds are introduced, or the baby reaches 6 months of age.

Typical use. In the second column, we provide estimates of the probabilities of pregnancy during the first year of typical use of each method in the United States. For most methods, these estimates were derived from the experience of women in the 1995 NSFG, so that the information pertains to nationally representative samples of users.[12] For the other methods, we based the estimates on evidence from surveys and clinical investigations. See Chapter 31 on Contraceptive Efficacy for more complete explanations and for tables summarizing the efficacy literature for each method.

Pregnancy rates during typical use reflect how effective methods are for the average person who does not always use methods correctly or consistently. Typical use does not imply that a contraceptive method was always used. In the NSFG and in most clinical trials, a woman is 'using' a contraceptive method if she considers herself to be using that method. So typical use of the condom could include actually using a condom only occasionally, and a woman could report that she is 'using' the pill even though her supplies ran out several months ago. In short, 'use'—which is identical to 'typical use'—is a very elastic concept that depends entirely on an individual woman's perception.

Perfect use. In the third column, we provide our best guess of the probabilities of *method* failure (pregnancy) during the first year of perfect use. A method is used perfectly when it is used consistently according to a specified set of rules. For many methods, perfect use requires use at every act of intercourse. Virtually all method failure rates reported in the literature have been calculated incorrectly and are too low (see the discussion of methodological pitfalls below). Hence, we cannot empirically justify our estimates except those for the ovulation method of periodic abstinence,[9] the cervical cap,[13,14] the diaphragm,[14] the sponge,[14] the male condom,[15,68,69] the female condom,[16] spermicides,[70] and methods for which there are extensive clinical trials with very low pregnancy rates. (See Chapter 31.) Even the estimates for the ovulation method of periodic abstinence, female condom, diaphragm, cervical cap, spermicides, and sponge are based on only one or two studies. Our hope is that our understanding of efficacy during perfect use for these and other methods will be enhanced by additional studies.

Continuation. The fourth column displays the first-year probabilities of continuing use. They are based on the same sources used to derive the estimates in the second column (typical use). (See Chapter 31.)

It is interesting to compare these estimates with pregnancy rates observed among women using isotretinoin, which is effective in treating severe acne but is also teratogenic. To minimize pregnancies among women undergoing treatment, the manufacturer and the U.S. Food and Drug Administration (FDA) implemented a pregnancy prevention program. Among 76,149 women who reported using contraception, 268 became pregnant, yielding a rate of 3.6 per 1,000 20-week courses of therapy;[17] this rate, if constant for a year, would be equivalent to an annual probability of pregnancy of 0.9%. The estimated annual probabilities of pregnancy were 0.8%, 2.1%, and 2.6% among women who reported using oral contraceptives, diaphragms, and condoms, respectively. Thus, women using diaphragms achieved lower rates of pregnancy than we estimate would occur during perfect use, and those using condoms and oral contraceptives experienced about the same pregnancy rates that would be expected during perfect use. Pregnancy rates for women using any of these three methods, however, were substantially below rates generally observed during typical use; this finding would appear to indicate that users' understanding of the teratogenic risks of isotretinoin substantially enhanced correct and consistent use. It is also possible that women in this study had lower than average fecundity (because acne is a marker for excess androgen production associated with anovulation[18]), that they lowered their coital frequency during treatment, or that they under-reported their number of pregnancies (and abortions).

SIMULTANEOUS USE OF METHODS

Using two methods at once dramatically lowers the risk of unintended pregnancy, provided they are used consistently. If one of the methods is a condom or vaginal barrier, protection from disease transmission is an added benefit. For example, the probabilities of pregnancy during the first year of perfect use of male condoms and spermicides are estimated to be 2% and 18%, respectively, in Table 9-2. It is reasonable to assume that during perfect use the contraceptive mechanisms of condoms and spermicides operate independently, since lack of independence during typical use would most likely be due to imperfect use (either use both methods or not use either). The annual probability of pregnancy during simultaneous perfect use of condoms and spermicides would be 0.2%, about the same as that achieved by the combined pill (0.3%) and LNG-IUS (0.1%) during perfect use.[19]

EFFICACY OVER TIME

We confine attention to the first-year probabilities of pregnancy solely because probabilities for longer durations are generally not available. There are three main points to remember about the effectiveness of contraceptive methods over time. First, the risk of pregnancy during either perfect or typical use of a method should remain constant over time *for an individual woman* with a specific partner (providing that her underlying fecundity and frequency of intercourse do not change). Second, in contrast, the risk of pregnancy during typical use of a method will decline over time *for a group of users*, primarily because those users prone to fail do so early, leaving a pool of more diligent contraceptive users or those who are relatively infertile or who have lower coital frequency. This decline will be far less pronounced among users of those methods with little or no scope for imperfect use. The risk of pregnancy during perfect use for a group of users should decline as well, but this decline will not be as pronounced as that during typical use, because only the relatively more fecund and those with higher coital frequency are selected out early. For these reasons, the probability of becoming pregnant during the first year of use of a contraceptive method will be higher than the probability of becoming pregnant during the second year of use. Third, probabilities of pregnancy are cumulative over time. Suppose that 15%, 12%, and 8% of women using a method experience a contraceptive failure during years 1, 2, and 3, respectively. The probability of not becoming pregnant within 3 years is calculated by multiplying the probabilities of *not becoming pregnant* for each of the 3 years: 0.85 times 0.88 times 0.92, which equals 0.69. Thus, the percentage becoming pregnant within 3 years is 31% (= 100% - 69%).

The lesson here is that the differences among probabilities of pregnancy for various methods will increase over time. For example, suppose that each year the typical proportion of women becoming pregnant while taking the pill is 8% and while using the diaphragm is 16%. Within 5 years, 34% of pill users and 58% of diaphragm users will become pregnant.

CONTRACEPTIVE FAILURES IN A LIFETIME

Data from the 1995 NSFG can be used to estimate age-specific contraceptive failure rates to produce a total lifetime contraceptive failure rate:

the number of contraceptive failures that the typical woman would experience in a lifetime if she used reversible methods of contraception continuously (except for the time spent pregnant after a contraceptive failure) from exact age 15 to exact age 45. This estimate is based on the standard synthetic-cohort assumption: that the typical woman uses at each age the same mix of methods observed at each age in the NSFG and experiences the same rate of contraceptive failure observed at that age. The typical woman who uses reversible methods of contraception continuously from age 15 to age 45 would experience 1.8 contraceptive failures. If we consider both reversible methods and sterilization, the typical woman would experience only 1.3 contraceptive failures from age 15 to age 45.[20]

FACTORS THAT INFLUENCE EFFICACY

Both you and your patients can better understand why the answer to the simple question "Will it work?" is such a complicated issue if you recall that many factors influence efficacy: (1) the inherent efficacy of the method when used correctly and consistently (perfect use) and the technical attributes of the method that facilitate or interfere with proper use, (2) characteristics of the user, and (3) competence and honesty of the investigator in planning and executing the study and in analyzing and reporting the results.

Inherent Efficacy

For some methods, such as sterilization, implants, and the copper-T IUD, the inherent efficacy is so high and proper and consistent use is so nearly guaranteed that extremely low pregnancy rates are found in all studies, and the range of reported pregnancy rates is quite narrow. For other methods such as the pill and injectable, inherent efficacy is high, but there is still room for potential misuse (forgetting to take pills or failure to return on time for injections), so that the second factor can contribute to a wider range of reported probabilities of pregnancy. In general, the studies of sterilization, injectable, implant, pill, patch, ring, and IUD use have been competently executed and analyzed. Studies of periodic abstinence, spermicides, and the barrier methods display a wide range of reported probabilities of pregnancy because the potential for misuse is high, the inherent efficacy is relatively low, and the competence of the investigators is mixed.

User Characteristics

Characteristics of the users can affect the pregnancy rate for any method under investigation, but the impact will be greatest when the pregnancy rates during typical use are highest, either because the method has less inherent efficacy or because it is hard to use consistently or correctly.

Imperfect use. The most important user characteristic is imperfect use of the method. Unfortunately, nearly all investigators who have attempted to calculate "method" and "user" failure rates have done so incorrectly. Investigators routinely separate the unintended pregnancies into two groups. By convention, pregnancies that occur during a month in which a method was used improperly are classified as user failures (even though, logically, a pregnancy might be due to failure of the method, if it was used correctly on some occasions and incorrectly on others), and all other pregnancies are classified as method failures. But investigators do not separate the exposure (the denominator in the calculation of failure rates) into these two groups.

For example, suppose that 2 method failures and 8 user failures occur during 100 women-years of exposure to the risk of pregnancy. Then the common calculation is that the user failure rate is 8% and the method failure rate is 2%; the sum of the two is the overall failure rate of 10%. By definition, however, method failures can occur only during perfect use and user failures cannot occur during perfect use. If there are 50 years of perfect use and 50 years of imperfect use in the total of 100 years of exposure, then the method failure rate would be 4% and the user failure rate would be 16%. The difference between the two rates (here 12%) provides a measure of how forgiving of imperfect use the method is. However, since investigators do not generally inquire about perfect use except when a pregnancy occurs, the proper calculations cannot be performed. The importance of perfect use is demonstrated in the few studies where the requisite information on quality of use was collected. For example, in a World Health Organization (WHO) study of the ovulation method of periodic abstinence, the proportion of women becoming pregnant among those who used the method perfectly during the first year was 3.1%, whereas the corresponding proportion failing during a year of imperfect use was 86.4%.[9] In a large clinical trial of the cervical cap conducted in Los Angeles, among the 5% of the sample who used the method perfectly, the fraction failing during the first year was 6.1%. Among the remaining 95% of the sample who at least on one occasion used the cap imperfectly, the first-year probability of pregnancy was nearly twice as high (11.9%).[13]

Frequency of intercourse. Among those who use a method consistently and correctly (perfect users), the most important user characteristic that determines the risk of pregnancy is frequency of intercourse. For example, in a study in which users were randomly assigned to either the diaphragm or the sponge, diaphragm users who had intercourse 4 or more times a week became pregnant in the first year twice as frequently as those who had intercourse fewer than 4 times a week.[21] In that clinical trial, among women who used the diaphragm at every act of intercourse, only 3.4% of those who had intercourse fewer than 3 times a week became pregnant in the first year, compared with 9.7% of those who had intercourse 3 or more times per week.[14]

Age. A woman's biological capacity to conceive and bear a child declines with age. This decline is likely to be pronounced among those who are routinely exposed to STIs such as chlamydia and gonorrhea. Among those not exposed, the decline is likely to be moderate until a woman reaches her late thirties.[22] Although many investigators have found that contraceptive failure rates decline with age,[23-26] this effect almost surely overstates the pure age effect because age in many studies primarily captures the effect of coital frequency, which declines both with age and with marital duration.[27] User characteristics such as race and income seem to be less important determinants of contraceptive failure.

Regular cycles. Women with regular cycles were 7.2 times as likely as were women with irregular cycles (one or more cycles < 17 days or > 43 days) to become pregnant while using the Reality female condom.[28]

Influence of the Investigator

The competence and honesty of the investigator also affect the published results. The errors committed by investigators range from simple arithmetical mistakes to outright fraud.[10] One well-documented instance of fraud involved the Dalkon shield. In a two-page article published in the *American Journal of Obstetrics and Gynecology*, a first-year probability of pregnancy of 1.1% was presented and the claim made that "only the combined type of oral contraceptive offers slightly greater protection."[29] It was not revealed by the researcher that some women had been instructed to use spermicides as an adjunctive method to reduce the risk of pregnancy, nor that he was part-owner of the Dalkon Corporation. Furthermore, he never subsequently revealed (except to the A.H. Robins Company, which bought the shield from the Dalkon Corporation but did not reveal this information either) that as the original trial matured, the first-year probability of pregnancy more than doubled.[30]

The system of drug testing in the United States, which demands that the company wishing to market a drug be responsible for conducting studies to assess its efficacy and safety, provides incentives for the unscrupulous to present less-than-honest results. Some actions that are not deliberately dishonest are, nevertheless, not discouraged by the incentives in the present system. For example, a woman who becomes pregnant may be discarded from a clinical trial if the researcher decides that she did not fit the protocols after all. Or one can be less than vigilant in trying to contact patients lost to follow-up (LFU). The standard assumption made at the time of analysis is that women who are LFU experience unintended pregnancy at the same rate as those who are observed. This assumption is probably innocuous when the proportion LFU is small. But in many studies the proportion LFU may be 20% or higher, so that what really happens to these women could drastically affect the estimate of the proportion becoming pregnant. Our strong suspicion is that women LFU are more likely to experience a contraceptive failure than are those who remain in the trial. For example, one study found that the pregnancy rate for calendar rhythm rose from 9.4 to 14.4 per 100 women-years of exposure as a result of resolution of cases LFU.[31]

The incentives to conduct research on contraceptive failure vary widely from method to method. Many studies of the pill and IUD exist because companies wishing to market them must conduct clinical trials to demonstrate their efficacy. In contrast, few studies of withdrawal exist because there is no financial reward for investigating this method. Moreover, researchers face differing incentives to report unfavorable results. The vasectomy literature is filled with short articles by clinicians who have performed 500 or 1,000 or 1,500 vasectomies. When they report pregnancies (curiously, pregnancy is seldom mentioned in discussions of vasectomy "failures," which focus on the continued presence of sperm in the ejaculate), their pregnancy rates are invariably low. Surgeons with high pregnancy rates simply do not write articles calling attention to their poor surgical skills. Likewise, drug companies do not commonly publicize their failures. Even if investigators prepared reports describing failures, journal editors would not be likely to publish them.

Methodological Pitfalls

Several methodological pitfalls can snare investigators. One of the most common is a misleading measure of contraceptive failure called the Pearl-index, which is obtained by dividing the number of unintended pregnancies by the number of years of exposure to the risk of unintended pregnancy contributed by all women in the study. This measure can be misleading when one wishes to compare pregnancy rates obtained from studies with different average amounts of exposure. The likelihood of pregnancy declines over time because those most likely to become pregnant do so at earlier durations of contraceptive use and exit from observation. Those still using contraception after long durations are unlikely to become pregnant, so that an investigator could (wittingly or unwittingly) drive the reported pregnancy rate toward zero by running the trial "forever." Two investigators using the NSFG could obtain Pearl-index pregnancy rates of 7.5 and 4.4 per 100 women-years of exposure for the condom.[32] One (who got 4.4) allowed each woman to contribute a maximum of 5 years of exposure while the other (who got 7.5) allowed each woman to contribute only 1 year. Which investigator is incorrect? Neither. The two rates are simply not comparable. As discussed in Chapter 30 on Dynamics of Reproductive Behavior and Population Growth, life-table measures of contraceptive failure are easy to interpret and control for the distorting effects of varying durations of use. Another problem occurs when deciding which pregnancies to count. Most studies count only the pregnancies observed and reported by the women. If, on the other hand, a pregnancy test were administered every month, the number of pregnancies (and hence the pregnancy rate) would increase because early fetal losses not observed by the woman would be added to the number of observed pregnancies. Such routine pregnancy testing in the more recent contraceptive trials has resulted in higher pregnancy rates than would otherwise have been obtained and makes the results not comparable to those from other trials. Other, more technical, errors that have biased reported results are discussed elsewhere.[10,33,34]

GOALS FOR TEACHING EFFICACY

Keep these thoughts in mind when counseling about contraceptive efficacy:

1. **What matters most is correct and consistent use.** For example, an 8% probability of pregnancy during the first year for typical use of the pill will not protect the careless user. The 16% probability of pregnancy during the first year of typical diaphragm use need not discourage a careful and disciplined woman who has infrequent intercourse from using a diaphragm.

2. **Make sure your staff provides consistent and correct information.** One study of the information provided by family planning staff indicated that providers tended to give the lowest reported probabilities of pregnancy for pills and IUDs, probabilities of pregnancy during typical use for diaphragms and spermicides, and higher-than-typical probabilities of pregnancy for condoms.[35] Thus, family planning providers may extensively bias their patient education in favor of methods they provide most frequently. Condoms and withdrawal get an undeserved low efficacy score within many family planning clinics and offices. You can avoid unintentional bias by deciding carefully what pregnancy rates your clinic or staff members are going to use.

3. **Technology fails people just as people fail technology.** Patients are sometimes told that unintended pregnancies are their own fault because they did not use their method correctly or carefully. Contraceptive methods are imperfect and can fail even the most diligent user.

4. **Using two methods at once dramatically lowers the risk of unintended pregnancy**, provided they are used consistently. If one of the methods is a condom, protection from disease transmission is an added benefit.

5. **Emergency contraception provides a last chance to prevent pregnancy after unprotected intercourse.** Emergency contraceptive pills (ECPs) are an especially important second method for those relying on condoms, in cases of breakage or slippage, for those who do not actually use their ongoing method for whatever reason, and those who are forced to have unprotected intercourse.

6. **Methods that protect a person for a long time** (sterilization, implants, IUDs, and long-acting injections) **tend to be associated with lower pregnancy rates**, primarily because they allow little scope for user error.

SAFETY: "WILL IT HURT ME?"

"I smoke. Won't the pill give me a heart attack?"
"Could the IUD puncture my womb?"
"Will I be able to get pregnant after stopping my method?"

In general, contraception poses few serious health risks to users. Moreover, the safety considerations of contraceptive methods are not as great as those of pregnancy-related complications. Unplanned and unwanted pregnancies place women at risk unnecessarily. Women in many developing countries will experience an even greater advantage in using contraceptive methods, especially in comparison to pregnancy-related mortality. Nonetheless, some contraceptive methods pose potential risk to the user.

- The method itself may have inherent dangers: death, hospitalization, surgery, medical side effects, infections, loss of reproductive capacity, or pain.

- Pregnancy itself is associated with risk: a woman must assess both the likelihood of contraceptive failure and the dangers that a pregnancy would pose.

- Future fertility may be influenced by choice of a contraceptive method.

MAJOR HEALTH RISKS

When it comes to the most serious outcome of all—death—the absolute level of risk is extraordinarily low for most women. Table 9-3 puts into perspective some of the risks of everyday life in the United States.[36-42] Although the information in this table should not be used to dismiss the concerns of a woman who is worried about pills, abortion, or tampons, it may help her compare these risks with other risks she voluntarily faces in her life.

Other major health risks are not only uncommon, they are most likely to occur in women who have underlying medical conditions that may be influenced by hormonal contraception:

Cardiovascular disease. The pill has been associated with an increased risk of myocardial infarction and stroke. About 1.5 deaths per year in 100,000 nonsmoking users under the age of 45 have been attributable to use of the pill.[39] Risk increases with age because risk factors such as hypertension, thromboembolic disease, diabetes, and a sedentary lifestyle increase with age. Smoking definitely increases this risk, especially in women over age 35 who smoke more than 25 cigarettes a day.

Cancer. The pill appears to protect users against cancers of the endometrium and ovary.[43] The net effect of pill use on cancer is negligible.[43] The association between cancer of the breast and cervix and the use of the pill remains under scrutiny.

Table 9-3 Voluntary risks in perspective

Activity	Chance of Death in a Year
Risks per year for men and women of all ages who participate in:	
Motorcycling	1 in 1,000
Automobile driving	1 in 5,900
Power boating	1 in 5,900
Rock climbing	1 in 7,200
Playing football	1 in 25,000
Canoeing	1 in 100,000
Risks per year for women aged 15 to 44 years:	
Using tampons	1 in 350,000
Risks for women preventing pregnancy:	
Using oral contraceptives (per year)	
Nonsmoker	1 in 66,700
aged less than 35	1 in 200,000
aged 35-44	1 in 28,600
Heavy smoker (25 or more cigarettes per day)	1 in 1,700
aged less than 35	1 in 5,300
aged 35-44	1 in 700
Using IUDs (per year)	1 in 10,000,000
Using diaphragm, condom, or spermicides	None
Using fertility awareness methods	None
Undergoing sterilization:	
Laparoscopic tubal ligation	1 in 38,500
Hysterectomy	1 in 1,600
Vasectomy	1 in 1,000,000
Risk per pregnancy from continuing pregnancy beyond 20 weeks	1 in 10,000
Risk from terminating pregnancy:	
Legal abortion	
Before 9 weeks	1 in 262,800
Between 9 and 12 weeks	1 in 100,100
Between 13 and 15 weeks	1 in 34,400
After 15 weeks	1 in 10,200

Sources: Cates (1980),[36] Dinman (1980),[37] Escobedo, et al. (1989),[38] Harlap, Kost and Forrest (1991),[39] Koonin, et al. (1997),[40] Lawson, et al. (1994),[41] Lee (1981).[42]

- Women face a slightly increased risk (about 20% higher) for having breast cancer diagnosed while they are using oral contraceptives and for 10 years after stopping use. Cancers diagnosed in these women are less advanced clinically than those diagnosed in women of the same age who have never used oral contraceptives.[44] The increased risk is apparent soon after exposure but does not increase with exposure and does not persist beyond ten years after exposure ceases. These patterns are not typical for a carcinogenic agent but could be consistent with promotion of already existing tumors or with earlier diagnosis of breast cancer in women who have used the pill.

- The incidence of cervical cancer is increased in women using oral contraceptives, particularly long-term users.[45-47] Cervical cancer risk is strongly linked to infection with human papilloma virus (HPV).[48] It is possible that pill use could affect cervical cancer directly, or indirectly by altering susceptibility to infection with HPV. Epidemiological studies indicate that this excess risk persists after adjustment for potential confounding factors such as cigarette smoking, age at first intercourse, number of sexual partners, sexual behavior of male partners, and pap smear screening history.[49] Barrier methods used in conjunction with spermicides decrease the user's risk of cervical cancer.[50]

FUTURE FERTILITY

An important issue in helping a couple evaluate safety as they choose a contraceptive method may be their future childbearing aspirations. Several important considerations may help to protect the future fertility of patients:

- **Abstinence** from vaginal intercourse is the single most effective and risk-free means of protecting future fertility.
- **Pregnancy** and the outcomes of pregnancy carry risks to future fertility. About 20% of women undergo surgical (cesarean) delivery, which involves an increased risk of infection that could result in permanent tubal damage. Postpartum infection can also occur after vaginal delivery.
- **Oral contraceptives and other hormonal methods** do not provide protection against STIs, which can cause pelvic inflammatory disease (PID) and lead to infertility. When STI risk is a concern, avoiding intercourse, or using condoms correctly and consistently, is essential for preserving future fertility.
- **Mechanical and chemical barriers** reduce the risk of PID and of ectopic pregnancy, with the greatest risk reduction for those using a combination of both.[51]
- **The IUD** does not protect against STIs. Women in recent IUD clinical trials who are presumed to have been at low risk of STIs have had no increased risk of PID, except in the first few weeks following IUD insertion.[52]

- **Sterilization** must be considered permanent. It does not protect against STIs.

SIDE EFFECTS

Often, the minor side effects of contraceptive methods, in addition to the more serious complications, influence whether an individual selects a certain method. "What physical changes will I undergo?" "Will I be annoyed by spotting, cramping, or the sensation or messiness of using a given method?" Do not dismiss the important role that side effects play when an individual must repeatedly assess whether to continue using a method or whether to use it consistently.

Side effects can be hormonally, chemically, or mechanically induced. Headaches and depression can be side effects of hormonal methods. Menstrual changes such as spotting and decreased or increased bleeding can be caused by hormonal methods and IUDs. Physical sensations such as decreased penile sensitivity, pressure on pelvic walls, or uterine cramping may be caused by mechanical methods. Other mechanically-induced side effects include perforation of the uterus during IUD insertion and vaginal trauma from vaginal barrier methods. Use of a diaphragm and spermicide is associated with an increased risk of urinary tract infection (UTI). The causal mechanism was long thought to be mechanical but is now believed to be the effect of spermicides on vaginal bacterial flora. Nonoxynol-9 use results in replacement of normal lactobacilli in the vagina by anaerobic organisms.[53-55] Other chemically-induced side effects include allergic reactions to latex and to copper.

With the great majority of these side effects, instruction and patient education can help users accept and understand what is happening. The appearance of side effects that are not serious is not a medical reason to preclude use of a method.

SAFETY TERMINOLOGY

Most methods of contraception are extremely safe. However, some women have medical conditions that increase their risks of complications. Identifying these women is one of the key roles played by health care providers. Most of the serious pill and IUD problems could be minimized by (1) avoiding methods for which medical precautions are present and (2) teaching the user to recognize the early danger signals for serious complications.

Throughout this book, except where explicitly stated otherwise, the authors adopt the medical eligibility criteria established by the WHO.[56] The conditions affecting eligibility for using each contraceptive method are classified under one of the following four categories:

1. A condition for which there is no restriction for the use of the contraceptive method.

2. A condition where the advantages of using the method generally outweigh the theoretical or proven risks.

3. A condition where the theoretical or proven risks usually outweigh the advantages of using the method.

4. A condition which represents an unacceptable health risk if the contraceptive method is used.

Categories 1 and 4 are self-explanatory. Category 2 indicates the method can generally be used, but careful follow-up may be required. However, providing a method to a woman with a condition classified as category 3 requires careful clinical judgment and access to clinical services; for such a woman, the severity of the condition and the availability, practicality, and acceptability of alternative methods should be taken into account. For a condition classified as category 3, use of that method is not usually recommended unless more appropriate methods are not available or acceptable. Careful follow-up will be required.[56]

GOALS FOR TEACHING SAFETY

1. **Try to educate the patient about misconceptions.** People who are afraid do not respond well to rational persuasions. Many patients hold certain opinions about contraceptive methods— that the pill is very dangerous even to healthy, nonsmoking young women or that injectables lead to permanent sterility. If you see that you are getting nowhere, stop. Help each client select a method that can be used correctly and consistently without fear.

2. **Make sure that you and your staff know all about the major side effects** of contraceptive methods, such as the relation between pill use and blood clots or reproductive cancers. Give accurate information.

3. **Tell patients what they need to know** even if they do not ask. Patients do not always ask the questions they need answered.

4. **Compare risks of using contraception with pregnancy risks.** In general, the risks of pregnancy, abortion, and delivery are far greater than those for using a contraceptive method.

5. **Help patients make a contraceptive method choice that will protect them from both pregnancy and STIs.** Safety concerns often overlap with worries about infections. With the exception of abstinence, currently available methods that protect best against infection are not those that provide greatest protection against pregnancy. Conversely, the most highly effective methods of contraception provide *no* protection against infection. Therefore, highly effective protection against both risks requires use of two methods. Even "abstinence" has different rules for protection against pregnancy and protection against infection: oral and anal intercourse can result in STI transmission but not in pregnancy.

6. **Teach patients the danger signals** of the method they select. If a danger signal does appear, the informed user can quickly seek help.

NONCONTRACEPTIVE BENEFITS

Although the noncontraceptive benefits provided by certain methods are not generally the major determinant for selecting a contraceptive method, they certainly can help patients decide between two or more suitable methods. (See Table 9-4.)

Reducing the user's risk of STIs may weigh as heavily as preventing pregnancy. Any sexually active person who may be at risk of acquiring infection with HIV, HPV, gonorrhea, syphilis, chlamydia, herpes, or other STIs should consider condoms.[57]

Fertility awareness methods educate women about their menstrual physiology. This knowledge can also help couples achieve a planned pregnancy.

Mirena (LNG-IUS) markedly reduces menstrual blood loss and pain, has a very low ectopic pregnancy rate, and reduces risk of PID and endometritis.[58] It can be used to treat menorrhagia and to induce regression of endometrial hyperplasia or uterine fibroids. In addition, it may provide a new way of adding progestin in hormone replacement therapy.

Combined oral contraceptives protect against PID, cancers of the ovary and endometrium, recurrent ovarian cysts, and benign breast cysts and fibroadenomas.[39] Some protect against acne, a key concern among youth. As women who have suffered menstrual cramps and discomforts can attest, the pill eases their discomforts. The pill also provides relief from perimenopausal symptoms. All these benefits presumably accrue to users of the Evra patch, NuvaRing, and Lunelle.

Make it a practice to tell your patients about the noncontraceptive benefits of the various methods. If patients have additional reasons for using the contraceptive method, their motivation to use the method correctly and consistently will probably be improved.

PERSONAL CONSIDERATIONS

A typical woman in the United States spends about 39 years—almost half of her lifespan of 80 years—at potential biological risk of pregnancy, during the time from menarche (at age 12.6) to natural menopause (at age 51.3).[59,60] What matters most to a woman when she considers a contraceptive method will ordinarily change over the course of her reproductive lifespan. Different reproductive stages are associated with distinct fertility goals and sexual behaviors (Table 9-5).[61] From menarche to first birth, the primary fertility goal is to postpone pregnancy and birth. Between the first birth and the time when a woman intends to have no more children, the primary goal is to space pregnancies leading to births. Between the time when a woman intends to have no more children and menopause, the goal is to cease childbearing altogether. The biggest demands on a contraceptive method are generated during the period between first intercourse and first birth, when the typical woman may have several sexual partners with periods of high coital frequency; the typical woman may attach great importance to preventing pregnancy and STIs and to a method's reversibility and ease of use. In the last stage of her reproductive lifespan, from the time when a woman intends to have no more children to menopause, the most important factor is a method's efficacy at preventing pregnancy.

Table 9-4 Major methods of contraception and some related safety concerns, side effects, and noncontraceptive benefits

Method	Dangers	Side Effects	Noncontraceptive Benefits
Combined hormonal contraception (pill, and presumably Evra patch, NuvaRing, and Lunelle)	Cardiovascular complications (stroke, heart attack, blood clots, high blood pressure), depression, hepatic adenomas, possible increased risk of breast and cervical cancers	Nausea, headaches, dizziness, spotting, weight gain, breast tenderness, chloasma	Decreases menstrual pain, PMS, and blood loss; protects against symptomatic PID, some cancers (ovarian, endometrial) and some benign tumors (leiomyomata, benign breast masses), and ovarian cysts; reduces acne
Minipill	May avoid some dangers of combined hormonal contraceptives	Less nausea than with combined pills	Lactation not disturbed
IUD	PID post insertion, uterine perforation, anemia	Menstrual cramping, spotting, increased bleeding	None known except progestin-releasing IUDs, which decrease menstrual blood loss and pain
Male condom	Anaphylactic reaction to latex	Decreased sensation, allergy to latex, loss of spontaneity	Protects against STIs, including HIV; delays premature ejaculation
Female condom	None known	Aesthetically unappealing and awkward to use for some	Protects against STIs
Norplant and Norplant-2	Infection at implant site, complicated removals, depression	Tenderness at site, menstrual changes, hair loss, weight gain	Lactation not disturbed; may decrease menstrual cramps, pain, and blood loss
Depo-Provera	Depression, allergic reactions, pathologic weight gain, possible bone loss	Menstrual changes, weight gain, headaches, adverse effects on lipids	Lactation not disturbed; reduces risk of seizures; may protect against ovarian and endometrial cancers
Sterilization	Infection; anesthetic complications; if pregnancy occurs after tubal sterilization, high risk that it will be ectopic	Pain at surgical site, psychological reactions, subsequent regret that the procedure was performed	Tubal sterilization reduces risk of ovarian cancer and may protect against PID
Abstinence	None known		Prevents STIs, including HIV, if anal and oral intercourse are avoided as well
Diaphragm, Cap, Sponge	Vaginal and urinary tract infections, toxic shock syndrome	Pelvic pressure, vaginal irritation, vaginal discharge if left in too long, allergy	
Spermicides	Vaginal and urinary tract infections	Vaginal irritation, allergy	
Lactational Amenorrhea Method (LAM)	Increased risk of HIV transmission to infant if mother HIV+	Mastitis from staphylococcal infection	Provides excellent nutrition for infants under 6 months old

Table 9-5 The stages of reproductive life

	Adolescents/Young Adults		Later Reproductive Years	
	Menarche to First Intercourse	First Intercourse to First Birth	First Birth to Intend No More Children	Intend No More Children to Menopause
Fertility goals				
Births	postpone	postpone	space	stop
Ability to have children	preserve	preserve	preserve	irrelevant
Sexual behavior				
Number of partners	none	multiple?	one?	one?
Coital frequency	zero	moderate to high	moderate	moderate to low
Coital predictability	low	moderate to high	high	high
Importance of method characteristics				
Pregnancy prevention		high	moderate	high
PID prevention		high	moderate	low
Not coitus-linked		high	low	moderate
Reversibility		high	high	low
Most common methods				
Most common		pill	pill	sterilization
Next most common		condom	condom	pill, condom

Source: Forrest (1993).[61]

More than half the entire reproductive lifespan—20.4 years or 53% of the reproductive span of 38.7 years—is spent trying to avoid further childbearing, in the stage from the time when a woman intends to have no more children to menopause (Figure 9-1).[59,60] The typical woman accomplishes this goal via female or male sterilization. A further 13.4 years or 35% of the reproductive span, from menarche to the first birth, is characterized by no desire to become pregnant. Thus, of a total reproductive span of 38.7 years during which a woman is potentially biologically at risk of conception, only 4.9 years (13% of the total), from the first birth to the time when a woman intends to have no more children, is characterized by any desire to become pregnant. Even this figure is exaggerated since a great fraction of this stage is spent in the pregnant or lactating state or trying to postpone the next pregnancy.

The best method of contraception for patients is one that will be in harmony with their wishes, fears, preferences, and lifestyle. Specific questions can help clients determine whether or not a contraceptive method under consideration is a realistic choice (Table 9-6). These questions may

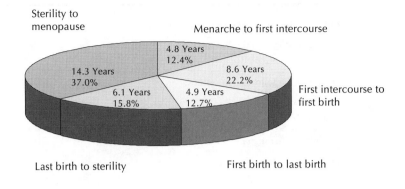

Sterility to menopause

Menarche to first intercourse

4.8 Years 12.4%

14.3 Years 37.0%

8.6 Years 22.2%

6.1 Years 15.8%

4.9 Years 12.7%

First intercourse to first birth

Last birth to sterility

First birth to last birth

Source: AGI (2000),59 Finer and Darroch (2001).[60]

Figure 9-1 Time spent in the stages of reproductive life

be used exactly as is or they may be adapted without permission. "Don't know" answers point to a need for more thinking, more introspection, or more information. "Yes" answers may mean users might not like or be successful with the method. Most individuals will have a few "yes" answers. If they have more than a few "yes" responses, they may want to talk to their physician, counselor, partner, or friend. Talking it over can help them to decide whether to use this method, or how to use it so it will really be effective for them.

Cost and cost-effectiveness of contraceptive methods. Tell every woman in advance what her ongoing expenses will be. Table 9-7 shows typical costs of providing methods in private and public sector settings.[7,62] Currently, these contraceptive method costs are generally not borne by third-party payers. With private insurers, contraceptive coverage varies dramatically. Virtually all cover surgical sterilization. Some provide broad coverage for all methods, but most do not, leaving the individual to pay for contraception herself.[63] The public sector generally provides broader coverage than private payers although payment levels often are low, perhaps low enough to limit access.[64] If cost will impose a major hardship, then offer an alternative contraceptive method or a means of obtaining the desired contraceptive method less expensively.

The costs of providing contraceptive methods represent only part of the medical care dollars associated with use of contraception. To these must be added the net costs of treating side effects and the costs of unintended pregnancies resulting from a method or user failure. Unintended pregnancies

Table 9-6 Contraceptive method comfort and confidence scale

Method of contraception you are considering using: _____

Length of time you used this method in the past: _____

Answer YES or NO to the following questions:	YES	NO
1. Have I had problems using this method before?		
2. Have I ever become pregnant while using this method?		
3. Am I afraid of using this method?		
4. Would I really rather not use this method?		
5. Will I have trouble remembering to use this method?		
6. Will I have trouble using this method correctly?		
7. Do I still have unanswered questions about this method?		
8. Does this method make menstrual periods longer or more painful?		
9. Does this method cost more than I can afford?		
10. Could this method cause me to have serious complications?		
11. Am I opposed to this method because of any religious or moral beliefs?		
12. Is my partner opposed to this method?		
13. Am I using this method without my partner's knowledge?		
14. Will using this method embarrass my partner?		
15. Will using this method embarrass me?		
16. Will I or my partner enjoy intercourse less because of this method?		
17. If this method interrupts lovemaking, will I avoid using it?		
18. Has a nurse or doctor ever told me NOT to use this method?		
19. Is there anything about my personality that could lead me to use this method incorrectly?		
20. Am I at any risk of being exposed to HIV (the AIDS virus) or other sexually transmitted infections if I use this method?		

Total number of YES answers: _____

Most individuals will have a few "yes" answers. "Yes" answers mean that potential problems may arise. If you have more than a few "yes" responses, you may want to talk with your physician, counselor, partner, or friend to help you decide whether to use this method or how to use it so that it will really be effective for you. In general, the more "yes" answers you have, the less likely you are to use this method consistently and correctly at every act of intercourse.

Table 9-7   Unit costs for contraceptive methods and associated services

Method	Unit Cost $	
	Managed Care Setting	Public Provider Setting
Tubal ligation[a]	2466.80	1190.00
Vasectomy[a]	755.70	353.28
Oral contraceptives		
Drug	21.00/cycle	17.70/cycle
Office visit[a]	38.00	16.56
Implant		
Drug[a]	365.00	365.00
Insertion[a]	333.00	47.96
Removal	100.00	79.64
Injectable contraceptive		
Drug	30.00/quarter	30.00/quarter
Office visit	38.00/quarter	16.56/quarter
Progesterone-T IUD		
Device	82.00/year	82.00/year
Insertion	207.00/year	62.42/year
Removal	70.00/year	10.80/year
Copper-T IUD		
Device[a]	184.00	109.00
Insertion[a]	207.00	62.42
Removal	70.00	10.80
Diaphragm[b]		
Device	18.00/3 years	15.00/3 years
Office visit (device fitting)	38.00	15.59
Spermicidal jelly (12 uses)	12.00	8.75
Male condom[b]	1.00	0.33
Female condom[b]	3.66	1.25
Sponge[b]	1.50	0.83
Spermicides (12 uses)[b]	12.00	8.75
Cervical cap[b]		
Device	31.00/3 years	19.00/3 years
Office visit (device fitting)[a]	38.00	15.59
Spermicidal jelly (12 uses)	12.00	8.75
Withdrawal	0.00	0.00
Periodic abstinence	0.00	0.00
No method	0.00	0.00

Source: Trussell, et al. (1995),[62] Smith (1993).[7]

Notes:

[a] First year only.

[b] Method costs in Figures 9-2 and 9-3 were calculated based on 83 acts of intercourse per year among sexually active women aged 18-49 (unpublished tabulations from the 1989, 1990, 1991, and 1993 General Social Surveys, Smith 1993).

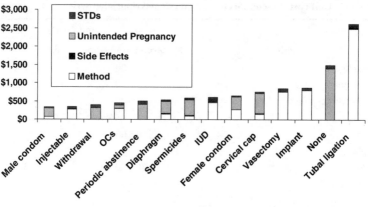

Source: Trussell, Koenig, Stewart and Darroch (1997).[65]

Figure 9-2 One-year costs associated with contraceptive method use in the private sector

result in births, induced abortions, spontaneous abortions, or ectopic pregnancies. The cost of a typical unintended pregnancy is high: $1,651 in the private sector and $778 in a publicly funded program.[65] The total costs of using different methods are compared with the costs of using no method in the private sector over periods of 1 year in Figure 9-2[65] and 5 years in Figure 9-3.[65] Four points emerge from examination of these figures.

- Use of any method of contraception is very cost-effective when compared with use of no method.

- Because unintended pregnancy is so expensive, those highly effective methods with high costs of acquisition actually save the most money; in particular, the long-term methods (sterilization, the implant, and the copper-T IUD) become especially cost-effective for longer durations of use.

- Method costs (Table 9-7) are misleading indications of the total costs.

- The net costs of treating side-effects and STIs are a minuscule fraction of total costs.

The same conclusions emerge for publicly funded programs. Cost-savings for the less effective methods would increase substantially if they were used correctly and consistently at every act of intercourse. For an individual couple, methods that will be most cost-effective are those that would be used correctly and consistently.

Emergency contraceptive pills (ECPs) are cost-effective whether they are provided when the emergency arises or provided in advance to be used as needed. A single treatment after unprotected intercourse saves $142 ($54) when combined ECPs and $119 ($29) when progestin-only

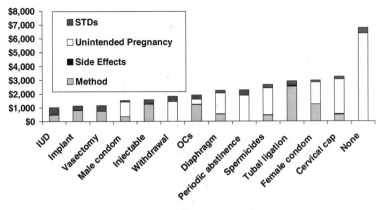

Source: Trussell, Koenig, Stewart and Darroch (1997).[65]

Figure 9-3 Five-year costs associated with contraceptive method use in the private sector

ECPs are used in a private sector (public payer) setting. The copper-T IUD is not cost-effective as an emergency contraceptive alone but savings quickly exceed costs as use continues.[66] Advance provision of emergency contraceptive pills to women using barrier contraceptives, spermicides, withdrawal, or periodic abstinence results in annual cost savings ranging from $96 to $193 in private sector setting; cost-savings in the public sector are lower, but advance provision of ECPs is still cost effective.[65] By reducing unintended pregnancies, more extensive use of emergency contraception could save considerable medical and social costs.

Pattern of sexual activity. In choosing their contraceptive method, women and men should consider their number of partners and their frequency of intercourse.

The number of partners affects the risk of STIs. In more obvious cases, the individual will have more than one partner at any given time. Less obvious are the individuals who practice serial monogamy. That is, they have only one partner at a time; however, the relationships are not permanent, so at the end of one relationship, the individual will move on to a new partner. Indeed, having more than one partner in a lifetime is the norm, and it is not uncommon for unmarried men and women to have more than 1 partner per year. (See Chapter 2 on Sexuality and Reproductive Health.) The barrier methods that would most protect individuals from STIs require commitment, understanding, and assertiveness on behalf of the client. The practitioner recommending the use of male or female condoms must be prepared to take the time required to discuss risks, encourage behavioral change, and teach skills.

The frequency of intercourse also has bearing on a person's contraceptive method choice. For example, the woman who has infrequent intercourse may not wish to use a method that requires daily medication or continuous exposure to possible side effects posed by hormonal methods or IUDs. On the other hand, infrequent intercourse may also indicate that a client is at risk of intercourse at unpredictable times. These clients may need skills in "expecting the unexpected."

Pattern of childbearing. Couples should choose their contraceptive method based on the number of children they desire and the timing of those births. For example, couples who plan on having a few children or having children early in their reproductive life cycle may have more flexible requirements about the spacing before and between pregnancies and may be more willing to risk a mistimed, but not unwanted, pregnancy. Such flexibility may mean that contraceptive method choices would not be limited to those with highest efficacy.

On the other hand, the couples who want only one child or want to delay childbearing until the woman is in her late 30s or early 40s may be less willing to choose any but the most highly effective methods. Among these couples, the reversible long-term methods may be more appealing than they would be for couples for whom a several-year span of protection is not an absolute necessity.

Access to medical care. Some people in our society have difficulty gaining access to the health care system: they do not understand the system or cannot afford it or find that it shuns them. Others may find their access hampered by too long a wait at the clinic. Studies in other nations have shown that access has great bearing on contraceptive method compliance and choice.[67] Presumably, the degree of access can also influence women in the United States. Access can be eased for all clients by providing a full year's supply of contraceptives. While many clinicians do provide 13 cycles of pills, for example, most do not offer sufficient quantities of condoms.

Intimate partner violence. Women at risk of intimate partner violence probably cannot rely on their partners to use withdrawal or a male condom. A non-coitally dependent or a female-controlled coital method would probably be a better choice.

GOALS FOR TEACHING ABOUT PERSONAL CONSIDERATIONS

Key concepts for discussing and teaching about contraceptive method choice and personal considerations include these:

1. **The patient decides which personal considerations matter.** Only the potential user can weigh all the elements for personal choice, and the clinician will not be able to predict what matters. Privacy? Lubrication? Light periods? What big sister uses? Do not guess; ask.

2. **It is a long way from the exam room to the bedroom.** We offer methods as medicines in a clinical setting, and then our

patients go home and use them in a sexual setting, be it a bedroom, motel room, car seat, or tent. Remember to help your patient think through the sexual aspects of contraception.

3. **Give patients permission to make a second (or third) contraceptive method choice.** They may not like the first method at all and will need to know it is acceptable to come back and try something else. Besides, it is always good to know how to use several methods.

4. **Encourage your patients to talk about contraceptive issues with their partners.** How can one person decide if a method of contraception will be compatible with a couple's personal and sexual styles? Help your clients practice discussing contraception with their partners if this is new territory for them.

5. **Personal considerations are likely to change over time.** Teenagers and 35-year-olds will use different criteria as they evaluate their contraceptive method choices. Encourage patients to rethink their contraceptive method needs as life and sex and bodies change over time.

6. **Teach patients a wise and cautious approach to sexual activity.** All sexually active people need to know the risk factors for STIs and HIV infection. Moreover, they need to know how to avoid those risk factors.

SUGGESTED READING

Brown SS, Eisenberg L. The best intentions: unintended pregnancy and the well-being of children and families. Washington DC: National Academy Press, 1995.

Harrison PF, Rosenfield A. Contraceptive research and development: looking to the future. Washington DC: National Academy Press, 1996.

REFERENCES

1. Gallen M, Lettenmaier C. Counseling makes a difference. Popul Rep 1987;15, Series J(35).
2. Abma JC, Chandra A, Mosher WD, Peterson LS, Piccinino LJ. Fertility, family planning, and women's health: new data from the 1995 National Survey of Family Growth. Vital Health Stat 1997;Series 23, Number 19.
3. Trussell J, Vaughan B. Selected results concerning sexual behavior and contraceptive use from the 1988 National Survey of Family Growth and the 1988 National Survey of Adolescent Males. Working Paper #91-12. Princeton NJ: Office of Population Research, Princeton University, 1991.
4. Piccinino LJ. Personal communication to James Trussell, March 24, 1997.
5. Henshaw SK. Unintended pregnancy in the United States. Fam Plann Perspect 1998;30:24-29, 46.
6. Ventura SJ, Martin JA, Matthews TJ, Clarke SC. Advance report of final natality statistics, 1994. Mon Vital Stat Rep 1996;44(11-Suppl).
7. Smith TW. Personal communication to James Trussell, December 13, 1993.
8. Grady WR, Klepinger DH, Nelson-Wally A. Contraceptive characteristics: the perceptions and priorities of men and women. Fam Plann Perspect 1999;31:168-175.

9. Trussell J, Grummer-Strawn L. Contraceptive failure of the ovulation method of periodic abstinence. Fam Plann Perspect 1990;22:65-75.
10. Trussell J, Kost K. Contraceptive failure in the United States: a critical review of the literature. Stud Fam Plann 1987;18:237-283.
11. Trussell J, Hatcher RA, Cates W, Stewart FH, Kost K. Contraceptive failure in the United States: an update. Stud Fam Plann 1990b;21:51-54.
12. Fu H, Darroch JE, Haas T, Ranjit N. Contraceptive failure rates: new estimates from the 1995 National Survey of Family Growth. Fam Plann Perspect 1999; 31:56-63.
13. Richwald GA, Greenland S, Gerber MM, Potik R, Kersey L, Comas MA. Effectiveness of the cavity-rim cervical cap: results of a large clinical study. Obstet Gynecol 1989;74:143-148.
14. Trussell J, Strickler J, Vaughan B. Contraceptive efficacy of the diaphragm, the sponge and the cervical cap. Fam Plann Perspect 1993;25:100-105, 135.
15. Frezieres RG, Walsh TL, Nelson AL, Clark VA, Coulson AH. Evaluation of the efficacy of a polyurethane condom: results from a randomized controlled clinical trial. Fam Plann Perspect 1999;31:81-87.
16. Farr G, Gabelnick H, Sturgen K, Dorflinger L. Contraceptive efficacy and acceptability of the female condom. Am J Public Health 1994;84:1960-1964.
17. Mitchell AA, Van Bennekom CM, Louik C. A pregnancy-prevention program in women of childbearing age receiving isotretinoin. N Engl J Med 1995;333:101-106.
18. Speroff L, Glass RH, Kase NG. Clinical gynecologic endocrinology and infertility (Sixth Edition). Baltimore MD: Williams and Wilkins, 1999.
19. Kestelman P, Trussell J. Efficacy of the simultaneous use of condoms and spermicides. Fam Plann Perspect 1991;23:226-227, 232.
20. Trussell J, Vaughan B. Contraceptive failure, method-related discontinuation and resumption of use: results from the 1995 National Survey of Family Growth. Fam Plann Perspect 1999;31:64-72, 93.
21. McIntyre SL, Higgins JE. Parity and use-effectiveness with the contraceptive sponge. Am J Obstet Gynecol 1986;155:796-801.
22. Menken J, Trussell J, Larsen U. Age and infertility. Science 1986;233:1389-1394.
23. Grady WR, Hayward MD, Yagi J. Contraceptive failure in the United States: estimates from the 1982 National Survey of Family Growth. Fam Plann Perspect 1986;18:200-209.
24. Schirm AL, Trussell J, Menken J, Grady WR. Contraceptive failure in the United States: the impact of social, economic, and demographic factors. Fam Plann Perspect 1982;14:68-75.
25. Sivin I, Schmidt F. Effectiveness of IUDs: a review. Contraception 1987;36:55-84.
26. Vessey M, Lawless M, Yeates D. Efficacy of different contraceptive methods. Lancet 1982;1:841-842.
27. Trussell J, Westoff CF. Contraceptive practice and trends in coital frequency. Fam Plann Perspect 1980;12:246-249.
28. Steiner MJ, Hertz-Picciotto I, Raymond E, Trussell J, Wheeless A, Schoenbach V. Influence of cycle variability and coital frequency on the risk of pregnancy. Contraception 1999;60:137-143.
29. Davis HJ. The shield intrauterine device. A superior modern contraceptive. Am J Obstet Gynecol 1970;106:455-456.
30. Mintz M. At any cost: corporate greed, women, and the Dalkon shield. New York NY: Pantheon Books, 1985.
31. Tietze C, Poliakoff SR, Rock J. The clinical effectiveness of the rhythm method of contraception. Fertil Steril 1951;2:444-450.
32. Trussell J, Menken J. Life table analysis of contraceptive failure. In: Hermalin AI, Entwisle B (eds). The role of surveys in the analysis of family planning programs. Liege, Belgium: Ordina Editions, 1982:537-571.
33. Trussell J. Methodological pitfalls in the analysis of contraceptive failure. Stat Med 1991;10:201-220.
34. Trussell J, Hatcher RA, Cates W, Stewart FH, Kost K. A guide to interpreting contraceptive efficacy studies. Obstet Gynecol 1990a;76:558-567.

35. Trussell TJ, Faden R, Hatcher RA. Efficacy information in contraceptive counseling: those little white lies. Am J Public Health 1976;66:761-767.
36. Cates W. Putting the risks in perspective. Contraceptive Technology Update 1980;1:111.
37. Dinman BD. The reality and acceptance of risk. JAMA 1980;244:1226-1228.
38. Escobedo LG, Peterson HB, Grubb GS, Franks AL. Case-fatality rates for tubal sterilization in U.S. hospitals, 1979-1980. Am J Obstet Gynecol 1989;160:147-150.
39. Harlap S, Kost K, Forrest JD. Preventing pregnancy, protecting health: a new look at birth control choices in the United States. New York NY: The Alan Guttmacher Institute, 1991.
40. Koonin LM, MacKay AP, Berg CJ, Atrash HK, Smith JC. Pregnancy-related mortality surveillance—United States, 1987-1990. MMWR 1997;46(SS-4):17-36.
41. Lawson HW, Frye A, Atrash HK, Smith JC, Schulman HB, Ramick M. Abortion mortality, United States, 1972 through 1987. Am J Obstet Gynecol 1994;171:1365-1372.
42. Lee BW. Risk assessment. JAMA 1981;246:1196-1197.
43. Schlesselman JJ. Net effect of oral contraceptive use on the risk of cancer in women in the United States. Obstet Gynecol 1995;85:793-801.
44. Collaborative Group on Hormonal Factors in Breast Cancer. Breast cancer and hormonal contraceptives: collaborative reanalysis of individual data on 53,297 women with breast cancer and 100,239 women without breast cancer from 54 epidemiological studies. Lancet 1996;347:1713-1727.
45. Thomas DB, Ray RM, The World Health Organization Collaborative Study of Neoplasia and Steroid Contraceptives. Oral contraceptives and invasive adenocarcinomas and adenosquamous carcinomas of the uterine cervix. Am J Epidemiol 1996;144:281-289.
46. WHO Collaborative Study of Neoplasia and Steroid Contraceptives. Invasive squamous-cell cervical carcinoma and combined oral contraceptives: results from a multinational study. Int J Cancer 1993;55:228-236.
47. Zondervan KT, Carpenter LM, Painter R, Vessey MP. Oral contraceptives and cervical cancer—further findings from the Oxford Family Planning Association contraceptive study. Br J Cancer 1996;73:1291-1297.
48. Bosch FX, Manos MM, Muñoz N, Sherman M, Jansen AM, Peto J, Schiffman MH, Moreno V, Kurman R, Shah KV, International Biological Study on Cervical Cancer (IBSCC) Study Group. Prevalence of human papillomavirus in cervical cancer: a worldwide perspective. J Natl Cancer Inst 1995;87:796-802.
49. Brinton LA. Oral contraceptives and cervical neoplasia. Contraception 1991; 43:581-595.
50. Coker AL, Hulka BS, McCann MF, Walton LA. Barrier methods of contraception and cervical intraepithelial neoplasia. Contraception 1992;45:1-10.
51. Cates W. Contraceptive choice, sexually transmitted diseases, HIV infection, and future fecundity. J Br Fertil Society 1996;1:18-22.
52. Farley TMM, Rosenberg MJ, Rowe PJ, Chen J-H, Meirik O. Intrauterine devices and pelvic inflammatory disease: an international perspective. Lancet 1992;339:785-788.
53. Fihn SD, Boyko EJ, Normand EH, Chen C-L, Grafton JR, Hunt M, Yarbro P, Scholes D, Stergachis A. Association between use of spermicide-coated condoms and *Escherichia coli* urinary tract infection in young women. Am J Epidemiol 1996;144:512-520.
54. Hooton TM, Scholes D, Hughes JP, Winter C, Roberts PL, Stapleton AE, Stergachis A, Stamm WE. A prospective study of risk factors for symptomatic urinary tract infection in young women. N Engl J Med 1996;335:468-474.
55. Fihn SD, Boyko EJ, Chen CL, Normand EH, Yarbro P, Scholes D. Use of spermicide-coated condoms and other risk factors for urinary tract infection caused by Staphylococcus saprophyticus. Arch Intern Med 1998;158:281-287.
56. Improving access to quality care in family planning. Medical eligibility criteria for contraceptive use. Second edition. Geneva, Switzerland: World Health Organization, 2000. WHO/RHR/00.2.

57. Feldblum PJ, Morrison CS, Roddy RE, Cates W. The effectiveness of barrier methods of contraception in preventing the spread of HIV. AIDS 1995;9(Suppl A):S85-S93.
58. Luukkainen T, Toivonen J. Levonorgestrel-releasing IUD as a method of contraception with therapeutic properties. Contraception 1995;52:269-276.
59. The Alan Guttmacher Institute. Fulfilling the promise: public policy and U.S. family planning clinics. New York, NY: The Alan Guttmacher Institute, 2000.
60. Finer LB, Darroch JE. Special tabulations of the 1995 National Survey of Family Growth. New York, NY: The Alan Guttmacher Institute, 2001.
61. Forrest JD. Timing of reproductive life stages. Obstet Gynecol 1993;82:105-110.
62. Trussell J, Leveque JA, Koenig JD, London R, Borden S, Henneberry J, LaGuardia KD, Stewart F, Wilson TG, Wysocki S, Strauss M. The economic value of contraception: a comparison of 15 methods. Am J Public Health 1995;85:494-503.
63. Alan Guttmacher Institute (AGI). Uneven and unequal: insurance coverage and reproductive health services. New York NY: The Alan Guttmacher Institute, 1994.
64. Sollom T, Gold RB, Saul R. Public funding for contraceptive, sterilization and abortion services, 1994. Fam Plann Perspect 1996;28:166-173.
65. Trussell J, Koenig J, Stewart F, Darroch JE. Medical care cost savings from adolescent contraceptive use. Fam Plann Perspect 1997;29:248-255, 295.
66. Trussell J, Koenig J, Ellertson C, Stewart F. Emergency contraception: a cost-effective approach to preventing unintended pregnancy. Am J Public Health 1997; 87:932-937.
67. Tsui AO, Ochoa LH. Service proximity as a determinant of contraceptive behaviour: evidence from cross-national studies of survey data. In: Philips JF, Ross JA (eds). Family planning programmes and fertility. Oxford, England: Clarendon Press, 1992:222-256.
68. Walsh TL, Frezieres RG, Peacock K, Nelson AL, Clark VA, Bernstein L. Evaluation of the efficacy of a nonlatex condom: results from a randomized, controlled clinical trial. Perspect Sex Reprod Health 2003;35:79-86.
69. Steiner MJ, Dominik R, Rountree RW, Nanda K, Dorflinger LJ. Contraceptive effectiveness of a polyurethane condom and a latex condom: a randomized controlled trial. Obster Gynecol 2003;101:539-547.
70. Raymond EG, Chen PL, Luoto J. Contraceptive effectiveness and safety of five nonoxynol-9 spermicides: a randomized trial. Ostet Gynecol 2004;103:430-439.

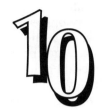

Education and Counseling

Felicia Guest, MPH, CHES

- Daily choices about personal risks exert a powerful influence on health. No caregiver task is more important than helping patients change their personal behavior to reduce health risks.

- People change behaviors more often as a result of new skills than of new knowledge. Teaching new skills to patients is most helpful when the caregiver matches the intervention to the patient's own readiness to change.

- Sex, relationships, pregnancy, and health are subjects loaded with emotional content. Attending to this emotional content is essential if we are to help patients learn new information, acquire new skills, and change behavior patterns.

- Informed consent is an educational process, not a piece of paper. The consent form documents the educational process.

FACTORS INFLUENCING EDUCATION AND COUNSELING

Meaningful discussion between a patient and her provider is critical to good health care delivery. The provider role is to create a safe environment for discussing feelings and needs, to coax insight out of a discussion, and to clarify options and choices for the patient. Few people innately possess these skills; you may need training to master them. Patient characteristics—age, cultural background, literacy, emotional state, and readiness for behavior change—influence the encounter as well. The specific goals of both patient and care giver, the time available for the encounter, and the need for a formal informed consent process will all influence education and counseling.

In this chapter, *education* refers to the exchange of factual information, and *counseling* refers to discussion that responds to emotions, as the provider elicits, recognizes, and normalizes patient feelings so that learning and behavior change can move forward.

AGE AND DEVELOPMENT

Patients may seek reproductive health care as children, adolescents, or adults. Cognitive and emotional capacities are strongly influenced by age. Developmentally, children move through early, middle, and late adolescence as they approach adulthood,[1] and educational strategies for one stage may be wrong for another. Young adolescents (age 11 to 13 or so) are still quite childlike, and older adolescents (age 17 or older) may have many adult characteristics. You may have only moments to ascertain whether a 14-year-old patient is more like a child or like an adult.

A substantial portion of patients making their first visit for reproductive care are in middle adolescence, about age 14 or 15. The stage can be distinctly characterized:

- Concrete thinking, especially under stress
- Intense peer involvement around certain issues
- Idealized and romanticized first-love relationships

You can help by taking into account their special needs. For example, be respectful of concrete thinking by asking, "Exactly where would you keep your pills? What do you do every day that can remind you to take your pill?" Use the peer involvement issue. Ask, for example, "Do you have any friends who use pills? What do they say about them?" About romance you might say, "I know it's hard to imagine that Mike could have any infections that would hurt you, but it happens sometimes. I'd like to help you stay safe. Love doesn't protect anybody from infection!"

Young people often experiment with sex, alcohol, and drugs, and may need counseling about these activities. In raising these sensitive issues, you may find it helpful to ask open-ended questions and target those questions to a third person rather than asking too directly about the young person herself: "Lots of young people I've talked with have told me how drinking or using drugs sometimes happens before they have sex with their partner. How have alcohol or other drugs affected your sexual behavior?"[2]

Stressful lives can retard cognitive and emotional growth,[1] so assess developmental status by what patients say and do more than by their chronological age.

The ability to plan ahead is a skill developed later in adolescence, usually about age 17 or older. All methods of contraception require at least some ability to plan ahead and are therefore incompatible with the developmental skills of early and middle adolescence. To be successful at reducing their risks of pregnancy and reproductive tract infection (RTI), these young people will need to practice new skills with you. Adolescents may need your help making decisions about whom to date, understanding what kinds of characteristics to look for—and avoid—in a potential partner. See Table 10-1 for ideas on picking a partner. For further insight into counseling young people, see "Compassionate Counseling for Adolescents" and Table 10-2, Collected wisdom on education and counseling, in this chapter.

Table 10-1   Counseling guide on "How to Pick a Partner"

How To Pick A Partner

Never, ever, date anyone charming — a hottie or a player!
Remember, people get that way through practice!

-- Felicia H. Stewart, MD

- **Don't even think about it**

  Involved in crime

  Needle drug user, even once

  Wants you to use drugs (rohypnol, ecstasy)

  Violent

- **You deserve better**

  More than two or three years older or younger than you

  Dated *lots* of people in the past

  Doesn't listen to you

  Doesn't want you to have other friends

  Uses and/or wants your money

  Lies, blaming, bossy

  Pressures you to have sex

  Wants you to have a baby and you're not ready

- **This could work!**

  Appeals to you

  Listens to you

  Respects your wishes

  Never, ever scares you

  Has plans and goals compatible with yours

But what if he or she isn't in the "this could work" category,
and you are in love anyway?

- *Love isn't supposed to hurt*

- *Love isn't supposed to be incompatible with the rest of your life*

- *Love is supposed to bring out the best in you*

Source: Felicia Guest, 2003

COMPASSIONATE COUNSELING FOR ADOLESCENTS

Sharon Schnare, CNM, MSN, FNP

THE SILENT ADOLESCENT

Young people have the right to be silent and keep their feelings and views safe from adult intrusion. Often the most profound communication has no words. Occasionally you may feel frustrated that a silent adolescent seemed to get little from a clinical encounter, only to have the adolescent return, ready to share, at a later date. Set a fertile atmosphere for the relationship to grow.

Begin a clinical encounter by sharing general concerns of other adolescents. "Other young women and men have concerns and questions about having sex, masturbation, and contraception. Perhaps you can identify with these issues. I am here to talk to you about these or other issues you have questions about." If the adolescent remains quiet, consider choosing a topic of common concern: "Other young women have shared concerns about feeling pressured to have sex, and some are not sure how they feel about using contraception. One young woman, a little older than you, told me she was afraid her boyfriend would find another girlfriend if she didn't have sex with him. She told me she really loved him and didn't want to lose him, but she was also hurt that he didn't love her enough to respect her feelings. I asked her how she planned to solve this dilemma and this is what she told me . . ." (If your patients have not shared their solutions with you, then begin asking how they or their friends have solved sensitive situations.)

ANSWERING ADOLESCENT QUESTIONS

Be flexible with adolescent patients and respond to their "need to know right now." Adolescents need to know there is a person who will be honest and non-biased about sex. When adolescents are especially anxious about a situation, ask what concerns them most about the matter, or ask what they think would worry a friend about the topic. This technique can help elucidate a hidden agenda or an unspoken conflict.

Help the adolescent understand how information empowers us all. For example, "You now know a lot about contraception and especially about condoms. You can be a great teacher to your friends. What's the most important piece of information you can see yourself telling your friends about?"

SECRETS

Some adolescents may be struggling with sexual orientation. Never assume a sexual partner is of the opposite sex. Be aware of support and counseling available in your community for gay, lesbian, and bisexual adolescents.

Be vigilant in assessing for factors that suggest a possible history of molestation or abuse: first intercourse before age 14; a series of men (unrelated or related) living in the home; poor school performance; sexual acting out; running away from home; exchanging sex for money, food, or shelter; somatization and dissociation; substance abuse by the adolescent or family member; and cervical dysplasia in a woman younger than 25.

THE 14-YEAR-OLD WHO WANTS TO HAVE A BABY

Many adolescents fantasize about "a baby of my own." Adolescents need to share these longings and ambivalent feelings, and to hear from their caregiver that these feelings are normal and shared by women the world over. Once adolescents express their desire to have a baby, they can give up their denial and discuss their feelings without shame, guilt, or fear. A young woman is then free to take control, rather than to let pregnancy "just happen." Ambivalence can result in not using contraception or using it inconsistently.

You can clarify her perspective and demonstrate your willingness to hear her view of the issue simply by asking "What do you think would be the best thing about having a baby?" Knowing you have genuinely listened to her, she in turn may be able to listen to the disadvantages of having a baby at such a young age.

Having a pregnancy is one of the most seductive ways for adolescents to feel grown up. A potent question to ask an adolescent is, "What will this baby need from you?" Sit quietly and wait for the question to ripen. Help the adolescent imagine the baby in a cradle across the room, and slowly begin: "The baby will need to be kept warm, to be fed and changed and vaccinated and to go to the doctor or clinic for checkups, to be kept safe and loved and never to be left alone." At this point, the adolescent may begin to see that it will not be her needs that are met by having a baby, because the baby has many, many needs beyond her own.

When an adolescent seems determined to become or remain pregnant, punitive or parental finger-wagging may simply reinforce her determination. Discuss the need to take preconceptual folic acid and vitamins and to make nutritional and behavioral changes (such as avoiding tobacco and alcohol and sexually transmitted infections). Ask the adolescent who will help her care for the baby and what her living situation will be like. Generally she will tell you she plans to live with her mother, who will also help her care for the baby. React to her plan positively. "That's great that you have talked with your mother about this, and that she is willing to help support you and your baby and also to help take care of your baby." The adolescent may look uncomfortable. "Well, I haven't talked with her yet." Respond with concern. "I see. I wonder how fair your mother will feel you are being, by not talking about your plans with her first? What if she promised a friend that you would care for her baby every day after school but didn't ask you first?" Adolescents can be wonderful moral warriors when it comes to injustices or unfairness, so use this quality to help her see it is unfair to expect her parent to support her and a baby without asking her first.

Remember that children generally meet the expectations society sets out for them, and these expectations sometimes seem to conflict:

- Yes, have our grandchildren . . .but not now.

- Yes, be popular and attractive to boys, especially older boys . . . but don't get sexually involved.

- Yes, society values women's bodies as sexual objects, especially young women's bodies . . .but your self-concept shouldn't be influenced by media images.

If we as health-care providers, family members, and adult models do not fill in the picture of what an authentic human being is, the unhealthy images will prevail.

Personal and Cultural Values

The values and ideas learned at home during childhood strongly influence each person. Cultures and families vary widely in many characteristics that influence reproductive lives. Learn the personal values and beliefs of the cultural groups represented in your patient population:[3]

- What is the ideal family size?
- Who makes sexual decisions?
- What is the desirable marriage age?
- How is same-gender sexuality regarded and handled?
- How does the patient understand the causation of illness?
- Who are the highly respected healers? Medical doctors? Neighborhood lay healers? Lay midwives?
- What is safe to tell the caregiver?
- Is the general communication style direct or indirect? Formal or informal?

You can gain insight into cultural values by asking questions such as, "In your family, what do people say is the right age to get married?"

Balance an understanding of each patient's unique personality with an awareness of and respect for influential cultural values and characteristics. A study of interventions to teach young black women social skills to reduce sexual risk taking found that programs sensitive to gender and cultural values can enhance consistent condom use more effectively than other types of interventions.[4] For example, young women can attend weekly group sessions to discuss positive attributes of being a black woman and identify personal role models among black women.

Culturally competent communication skill begins with an awareness of how we are defined by our own culture. For example, many clinics use an appointment system (based on Western European cultural values about the importance of punctuality) while serving a patient population that may not share that cultural value (such as a Latino[a] community where being hospitable to a drop-in visitor may be more important than getting to the clinic on time). In such settings, an appointment system can set up a no-win situation that frustrates everyone.

Remember that persons one or two generations removed from the immigration experience have already assimilated into the prevailing culture. In isolated communities with little exposure to other groups, strong cultural influences tend to persist. There is tremendous diversity within all cultural groups, so be careful not to stereotype individual patients.

Literacy

Successful education and counseling use communication styles with which patients are comfortable and familiar. Perhaps the most common error is using print materials with patients who do not customarily read.

A good screening question might be, "How many newspapers and magazines do you read in a typical week?"[5]

The 94 million illiterate and marginally literate adult Americans feel deep shame about their lack of reading skill and also have grave difficulties following medical instructions.[6,7] If in your judgment print materials are appropriate, match the readability of materials to the reading skill of the patient population. College students can usually read at almost any level. For other groups, aim for a seventh-grade reading level, the U.S. average. Use a tool such as the SMOG formula to determine the reading grade level of your materials.[8,9] The SMOG formula is a quick way to get an approximate idea of reading difficulty. A good place to start assessing reading level is with your contraceptive consent forms, because they tend to be quite difficult to read.

SMOG FORMULA FOR READING LEVEL

When the text has at least 30 sentences:

1. Count three sets of 10 sentences each, one near the beginning, one in the middle, and one near the end.

2. Circle all words with three or more syllables, including repetitions of the same word. Total all circled words in the 30 sentences.

3. Find the nearest perfect square to your total. (Examples: total is 98, use 100; total is 51, use 49.) Take the square root. (Examples: 100 is 10; 49 is 7.)

4. Add 3 to your square root for the reading grade level. (Examples: 10 plus 3 = thirteenth grade; 7 plus 3 = tenth grade.)

When the text has fewer than 30 sentences:

1. Count all words in the text with three or more syllables. Next count the total number of sentences. Then divide to find the average number of long words per sentence. (Example: 40 circled words divided by 20 sentences = an average of 2 per sentence.)

2. Multiply your average number of long words per sentence by the number of sentences short of 30. (Example: 2 times 10 = 20.)

3. Add your answer to your total number of long words, find the square root, and then add 3.

   (Example: 20 plus 40 = 60. Nearest perfect square is 64. Square root is 8. 8 plus 3 = eleventh grade.)

The grade level tells you that two-thirds of the U.S. students in that grade could read the sample with 100% comprehension. The standard error of prediction is 1.5 grades in either direction. The most important strategies for lowering reading levels are to use short words and short sentences.[10]

EMOTIONAL STATE

Intense feelings of anger, anxiety, fear, disappointment, elation, or even being in love must be acknowledged and discussed before effective patient education can begin. "Yes, you are pregnant, and here are your options" is callous as well as ineffective. "Yes, you are pregnant. Can you tell me how this news feels to you?" gets off to a better start. People who learn their test for human immunodeficiency virus (HIV) is positive often say they remember nothing the counselor said after hearing the word "positive." Take extra time to explore feelings before beginning the educational process. Also, making an emotional connection with the patient may increase the likelihood that the patient will want to come back.

Adolescents relieved at receiving negative pregnancy test results may be an especially at-risk group of patients for prevention skills intervention. In one study, about 1 in 4 pregnant adolescents age 17 and younger had a previous clinic-based negative test result.[11]

COUNSELING TO SUPPORT BEHAVIOR CHANGE[2]

Even when behavior change is good for one's health, it can look like a risky, costly, even frightening undertaking. While behavior changes such as abstaining from sex or using condoms may have the positive effect of reducing infections and unintended pregnancy, from the patient's perspective they may also have potential negative effects on relationships or on self esteem and identity.

Much of the health education and counseling designed to support behavior change is grounded in the theory that behavior change is incremental, and that interventions must be tailored to the patient's particular position along a continuum of change. Perhaps the most thoroughly studied model was developed in psychotherapy and smoking cessation research,[12,13] where scientists describe sequential steps along a behavior-change continuum. Other interventions use models that include key elements of a number of accepted behavior-change theories.

A model that has been used to train HIV counselors[14] describes the process of change and provides intervention strategies using these key points:

- *Knowledge and awareness* come first. Behavior change begins in understanding the consequences of a behavior. Health educators can respond at this stage with facts and role model stories.

- Knowledge and awareness are not enough. *Significance to self*, or ownership of the new knowledge and awareness, is critical for progressing to action. "This consequence doesn't just happen to other people; it can happen to me." Respond by assisting patients with personal goal-setting: "What do you want your life to be like in three years?" Ask questions to raise awareness of the impact of behavior on those goals. "How would having a baby affect those goals?" While helping the patient to relate contraception and safer sex to achieving those goals, respect and attend to the feelings that are expressed, verbally and nonverbally, regarding the difficulty of change.

- *Self-efficacy* determines the ability to use new knowledge and insights. Unless the patient sees herself or himself as *able* to change and *able* to be in control of a situation, she or he may not be able to act on the new insights. People who have low levels of self-efficacy feel helpless to change. Your support as a caregiver, with praise for any steps taken toward better health behaviors, and expressions of respect for the patient as a person who is able to change, can facilitate the undertaking of personal change.

- From the patient's perspective, the status quo has both pros and cons, just as healthier behavior does. Be careful not to short-change the pros of the status quo (such as sexual risk taking) or the cons of the healthier behavior, because they matter greatly to the patient. For example, beginning condom use could carry these actual or potential cons: loss of an important relationship, loss of self-esteem from being in a relationship, loss of economic support from a partner, and even risk of personal violence. Each patient undertakes a *cost-benefit analysis*, so take care to address all the costs and all the benefits.

- Change requires more than new knowledge. It requires new skills. This *capacity-building* must include help from you in communicating with a sexual partner and coping with both the patient's and the partner's fears and discomforts. If you have five minutes to teach condom skills, take one minute to teach the how-to's of using a condom, but take four minutes to role-play how to discuss condoms with a partner.

- Behavior change is rarely like flicking an on-and-off switch. Usually it takes a series of *provisional tries* at new behavior. Help by framing all attempts as successes, not failures, and by assisting with course corrections, boosting self-efficacy, offering empathetic understanding, and praising efforts to change.

Patients may or may not seek or achieve behavior change. However, health educators can and must be adept at change, matching our interventions to patients' needs. In counseling, one or two questions ("What are you doing to protect yourself from accidental pregnancy?" "When would you like to become pregnant?") can help focus your efforts so that the limited time available for education can be used effectively and take into account the patient's readiness for new behaviors.

TIME CONSIDERATIONS

Because it is extremely rare to have all the time you and your patient need for talking, use contracting in the beginning of an encounter. Contracting makes clear from the outset what your priorities are for the time together, makes clear approximately how much time is available to

Table 10-2 Collected wisdom on education and counseling

Education

- **The learner learns from what the learner does, not from what the teacher does.** Involve patients in their own education, encouraging them to touch and handle medicines and supplies, repeat instructions in their own words, and practice anticipated conversations with partner or parent.

- **Limit take-home messages to about three.** Give your messages careful priority ranking and don't overload patients with data.

- **Honor the patient's agenda.** Allow time for patients to discuss their questions and concerns. There will almost certainly be questions you haven't thought of.

- **Evaluate patient learning.** You don't know what patients have learned until you hear what they say.

- **People learn best in an environment that feels safe and calm.** A person on the way to a medical exam rarely feels safe and calm. Allow time after the exam for more education, and invite callbacks later on.

- **Teens and adults may need different styles of education.** Learn about the cognitive and emotional developmental stages so you can frame your education to fit the patient.

Counseling

- **Listening is helpful. Almost always. All by itself.** Sometimes patients need to be heard and understood more than they need anything else.

- **With the exception of life-threatening emergencies, avoid making decisions for the patient.** You will almost certainly do harm, sooner or later, if you are authoritative. The best response to "What do you think I should do?" is, "What do you think? I'll help you sort out all your choices, and then we will look at the pros and cons for each choice."

- **Avoid thinking in "me" vs. "them" terms.** The successful counselor cherishes the common human ground shared with each patient.

- **Not all people are able to be "compliant."** When you and your patients are face to face, be honest, direct, and hold them accountable for their actions. Once they leave your office, let it go.

- **Denial and anger are common, normal responses to trouble.** Reflect and discuss these feelings when you encounter them in patients. Anger is usually a sane, healthy response to feelings of vulnerability and loss of control. Denial can be given up by the denier, but cannot be forcibly taken away by the counselor.

- **Be open to the broad variety of healthy, effective human coping styles.** Your way will almost never be the only way. People solve their own problems.

- **Assume nothing.** Discipline yourself to forestall labeling or stereotyping. Accept your patient where she or he is right now.

- **The patient knows what she or he wants from you.** Just ask! "Tell me how we can help you today," or "What do you most want to get out of this visit?"

- **Respect the patient's right to privacy.** Acknowledge the right to withhold personal information with a comment such as, "You don't have to tell me anything you don't want to. [Pause] The more you're able to tell me, the more helpful I can be to you." Be careful that you don't promise more confidentiality than you can deliver. Say something like, "Just about everything a patient tells me is absolutely private. If someone lets me know that something is happening that could put her in danger, that could hurt her, I must and will do whatever I can to be sure that she is protected."

Source: Collected from educators and counselors in reproductive health care, 1970–2003, with special thanks to Joan Mogul Garrity and Terry Beresford.

talk, and encourages the patient to raise issues that are uppermost in her or his mind. For example, contracting with a first-time family planning patient might sound like this: "We have about 15 minutes to talk today, Linda. I will tell you about what we have to offer you here, and I'll ask you some questions about your health. What do you most want to talk about in our time together?"

When education and counseling issues are unfinished and more time is not immediately available, the following options can help:

- Schedule a return visit if possible for the patient.
- Schedule a telephone appointment for more discussion.
- Refer to a hotline or Internet site for specific issues such as HIV or abuse. (For ideas, see Chapter 11, Reproductive Health Resources.)
- Offer print material if the patient reads comfortably.
- Refer to another source of care, such as a prenatal clinic, mental health counselor, or substance abuse treatment center.

Table 10-2 distills some of the collected wisdom of reproductive health educators and counselors over the past three decades.

INFORMED CONSENT

Inform all patients about their complete range of options and allow them to choose freely. Once patients choose a course of action, give full disclosure about their choice. Only when these two steps have been completed can the patient provide an informed and documented consent to care.[15] Help patients view informed choice and informed consent not as legal paperwork but as a serious process for ensuring voluntary, clearly understood medical care, beginning with the tone the caregiver sets as educator. Remember that you do not truly know what patients have learned until you hear them rephrase the information in their own words. This specialized aspect of patient education is the highest priority of all educational tasks in the health care setting.

Because contraceptive methods and medications are usually initiated at the request of a healthy person who has no traditional medical indications for treatment, informed choice and consent can sometimes be overlooked; however, informed choice and consent in family planning and reproductive health have three bases: ethical, pragmatic, and legal. Ethically, people have a right to thorough information about products or procedures that can affect health and a right to decide what is done to their bodies. Pragmatically, people are more likely to use their contraceptive method safely and effectively or undergo a medical procedure when they freely choose and thoroughly understand it. Legally, you must provide adequate information to help patients reach a reasonable and informed decision about contraceptive options, medications, procedures, and devices.

Legals standards for informed consent can vary, but often depend on the "reasonable person" standard. Did the patient receive all the information that a reasonable person would need to make a sound decision and a truly informed choice and consent? Did the patient truly understand? It is your responsibility to ensure that patients sufficiently understand all reasonable alternatives and to determine whether the patient is competent to consent to the chosen medication, device, or procedure.

Federal regulations for informed consent to sterilization[16] provide helpful guidance to the contraceptive field in general for information that constitutes informed consent. According to these Department of Health and Human Services regulations, informed consent comprises seven basic elements. The word to remember is "BRAIDED":

Benefits of the method

Risks of the method (all major risks, all common minor risks, and related uncertainties and unanswered questions); be sure to include consequences of method failure

Alternatives to the method (including abstinence and no method)

Inquiries about the method are the patient's right and responsibility

Decision to withdraw from using the method without penalty is the patient's right at any time

Explanation of the method is owed the patient, in a format that is understandable to the patient

Documentation that the caregiver has ensured understanding of each of the preceding six points, usually by use of a consent form

A voluntary decision—free from any coercion—is paramount. Although documentation is essential, a written consent form with a signature is not enough. It may also be helpful to document what print, audiovisual, or electronic aids you used to inform the patient.

COMPETENCE TO CONSENT

These are the basic criteria for competence to consent:

- Is the patient capable of understanding the proposed treatment, alternatives, and risks?
- Is the patient capable of making rational decisions?

In some situations, the patient's competence is difficult to evaluate. A very young teen, a person with a developmental disability, an intoxicated person, and a mentally ill person are examples of such patients. If you have any doubt regarding a patient's competence to consent, consult with other professionals to determine the appropriate course of action. Be sure to document your consultation in the patient's record.

EDUCATIONAL CONSIDERATIONS FOR CONSENT

Adults and adolescents best learn, and make considered decisions, under the following circumstances:

- In the absence of threat
- When information seems relevant
- When teaching takes cultural factors into account[17]
- When the learning process is interactive
- When having a chance to ask and receive answers to questions
- With time to digest, and room for insight

Provide audiotaped consent forms (in appropriate languages) for illiterate, marginally literate, and visually impaired patients, so they can learn by listening. Write consent forms at a manageable reading level, about grade seven or eight. Evaluate learning and comprehension by having patients *say in their own words* what they have learned.

CONSENT FORMS

A number of family planning programs view the consent form as an important piece of patient education literature and give each patient a copy to keep. This practice is entirely consistent with the philosophy of full disclosure, so consider using consent forms that include all the BRAIDED elements in simple language. Be sure to stress warning signs for serious complications on consent forms, especially for IUDs and hormonal methods.

REFERENCES

1. Hofmann AD. Adolescent growth and development. In: Hofmann AD, Greydanus D (eds). Adolescent medicine, 3rd ed. Stamford CT: Appleton & Lange, 1997.
2. Garrity JM. Personal communication, August 2001.
3. Randall-David E. Culturally competent HIV counseling and education. Rockville MD: National Hemophilia Program, 1994.
4. DiClemente RJ, Wingood GM. A randomized controlled trial of an HIV sexual risk-reduction intervention for young African-American women. JAMA 1995;274:1271-1276.
5. Wells JA, Sell RL. Learning AIDS: 1991 supplement: a special report on readability, literacy, and the HIV epidemic. New York: American Foundation for AIDS Research, 1991.
6. Baker DW, Parker RM, Williams MV, Pitkin K, Parikh NS, Coates W, Imara M. The health care experience of patients with low literacy. Arch Fam Med 1996;5:329-334.
7. Parikh NS, Parker RM, Nurss JR, Baker DW, Williams MV. Shame and health literacy: the unspoken connection. Patient Educ Couns 1996;27:33-39.
8. McLaughlin GH. SMOG grading—a new readability formula. J of Reading 1969;12:639-646.
9. Meade CD, Smith CF. Readability formulas: cautions and criteria. Patient Educ Couns 1991;17:153-158.
10. Manning D. Writing readable health messages. Pub Health Rep 1981;96:464-465.
11. Zabin LS, Emerson MR, Ringers PA, Sedivy V. Adolescents with negative pregnancy test results: an accessible at-risk group. JAMA 1996;275:113-117.
12. Prochaska JO, DiClemente CC, Norcross JC. In search of how people change. Am Psychologist 1992;47:1102-1114.
13. Prochaska JO, Norcross JC, DiClemente CC. Changing for good. New York: William Morrow, 1994, 38-50.
14. Garrity JM, Jones SJ. HIV prevention counseling: A training program. Atlanta GA: Centers for Disease Control and Prevention, 1993.

15. Upadhyay UD. Informed choice in family planning: helping people decide. Population Reprts 2001; Series J (No. 50):1-39.
16. U.S. Food and Drug Administration. Sterilization of persons in federally assisted family planning projects. Federal Register 1978;43:52146-52175.
17. Gostin LO. Informed consent, cultural sensitivity, and respect for persons. JAMA 1995;274:844-845.

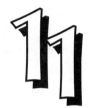

Reproductive Health Resources

Tara Shochet, MPH
James Trussell, PhD

Keeping current on reproductive health issues and finding answers to your and your patients' questions are more easily accomplished if you have on hand an array of resources and materials. This chapter presents some selected reproductive health resources that colleagues have brought to our attention.

Several organizations have a wealth of helpful and quality resources (Tables 11-1 and 11-2). The authors of Contraceptive Technology are developing a website to supplement some of the information in the current edition of the book; please consult www.contraceptivetechnology.org. Materials from the Association of Reproductive Health Professionals, Family Health International, and any branch of the federal government are not copyrighted and may be reproduced.

Table 11-1 Reproductive health organizations

American College Health Association	1-410-859-1500	www.acha.org
American College of Obstetrics and Gynecology	1-202-638-5577	www.acog.com
American Medical Women's Association	1-703-838-0500	www.amwa-doc.org
American Social Health Association	1-919-361-8400	www.ashastd.org
American Society for Reproductive Medicine	1-205-978-5000	www.asrm.org
Association of Reproductive Health Professionals	1-202-466-3825	www.arhp.org
National Abortion Federation	1-202-667-5881	www.prochoice.org
National Association of Nurse Practitioners in Women's Health	1-202-543-9693	www.npwh.org
Planned Parenthood Federation of America	1-212-261-4300	www.ppfa.org
Program for Appropriate Technology in Health	1-206-285-3500	www.path.org
Sexuality Information and Education Council of the United States	1-212-819-9770	www.siecus.org

Table 11-2 Research and advocacy organizations

Advocates for Youth	1-202-419-3420	www.advocatesforyouth.org
Alan Guttmacher Institute	1-212-248-1111	www.guttmacher.org
Center for Reproductive Rights	1-917-637-3600	www.reproductiverights.org
Contraceptive Research and Development	1-703-524-4744	www.conrad.org
Education Training Research Associates	1-831-438-4060	www.etr.org
Family Health International	1-919-544-7040	www.fhi.org
Ibis Reproductive Health	1-617-349-0040	www.ibisreproductive health.org
International Center for Research on Women	1-202-797-0007	www.icrw.org
International Planned Parenthood Federation	011-44-0-20-7487-7900	www.ippf.org
JHPIEGO (an affiliate of Johns Hopkins University)	1-410-537-1800	www.jhpiego.org
NARAL Pro-Choice America	1-202-973-3000	www.naral.org
National Organization for Women	1-202-628-8669	www.now.org
Pathfinder International	1-617-924-7200	www.pathfind.org
POPLINE (database of journal abstracts)	1-410-659-6300	db.jhuccp.org/popinform/basic.html
The Population Council	1-212-339-0500	www.popcouncil.org
Population Reference Bureau	1-202-483-1100	www.prb.org
Population Services International	1-202-785-0072	www.psi.org
Reproductive Health Technologies Project	1-202-557-3417	www.rhtp.org
World Health Organization	011-41-22-791-21-11	www.who.int

PRINT AND MULTIMEDIA MATERIALS
PROFESSIONAL EDUCATION

- *Guide to Clinical Preventive Services: Report of the United States Preventive Services Task Force.* How effective are the various periodic screening evaluations? This compendium details the quality of the research and the strength of the recommendations for performing Papanicolaou smears, conducting breast examinations, measuring blood pressure, counseling about sexually transmitted infections, and performing numerous other measures on patients of diverse age and risk groups. Available at www.ahrq.gov/clinic/cps3dix.htm or from Lippincott Williams & Wilkins at bookstores or at www.lww.com.

- *2002 Guidelines for Treatment of Sexually Transmitted Diseases.* The latest recommendations on preventing and treating sexually transmitted infections, by the Centers for Disease Control and Prevention. View guidelines at www.cdc.gov/std/treatment/ or order a copy at 1-888-232-3228.

- *Selected Practice Recommendations for Contraceptive Use.* This document provides selected practice recommendations based on the best available evidence and is intended to be used by policy-makers, program managers, and the scientific community. It aims to provide guidance to national family planning/reproductive health programs in the preparation of guidelines for service delivery of contraceptives. Available from the World Health Organization at www.who.int/reproductive-health/publications/rhr_02_7/index.htm.

- *Medical Eligibility Criteria for Contraceptive Use.* This book sets out detailed criteria for determining whether individual family planning clients are medically eligible to use, or continue using, a particular contraceptive method. This new edition incorporates all new available evidence on the safety and use of contraceptives, including the relationship between contraception and HIV risk. These medical eligibility criteria were developed to help national family planning programs update their policies and practices in line with the latest scientific knowledge. Available from the World Health Organization at www.who.int/reproductive-health/publications/RHR_00_2_medical_eligibility_criteria_second_edition/.

- *Clinical Gynecologic Endocrinology and Infertility*, 6th edition, by Speroff, Glass, and Kase. Available from Lippincott Williams & Wilkins at bookstores or at www.lww.com.

- *American College of Obstetricians and Gynecologists (ACOG) Practice Bulletin on Emergency Contraception.* March 2001. To order single copies, call 1-202-863-2518 and request Practice Bulletin #25.

- Contraceptive Technology slide sets. The Contraceptive Technology and Reproductive Health series covers topics such as injectables, lactational amenorrhea, postpartum contraception, and intrauterine devices. The sets include teaching modules with narrative, slides, audience handouts, references, and reprints of scientific articles. Available from Family Health International at 1-919-544-7040 or www.fhi.org.

- Annotated bibliographies of print materials. SIECUS (Sexuality Information and Education Council of the U.S.) offers a lengthy list of topics for which it has compiled annotated reference lists. Sexuality topics range from sexual abuse to sexual activities when you have disabilities, are in adolescence or middle and later ages; religion and spirituality and sexuality; and gay and lesbian issues.

Available from the Publications Department at 1-212-819-9770 or www.siecus.org.

- "Emergency Contraception" provider resource packet. Prepared by the Program for Appropriate Technology in Health (PATH), the packet includes sample patient brochures, fact sheets, office poster, and a provider manual with prescribing information and sample protocols. Available from Planned Parenthood Federation of America at 1-800-669-0156.

- Emergency contraception "Train-the-Trainer" slide sets. PowerPoint presentation on emergency contraception can be downloaded from the Association of Reproductive Health Professionals' website at www.arhp.org/ec.

- *Early Medical Abortion: Issues for Practice.* This monograph summarizes information about early abortion, including steps needed for early identification of pregnancy, an overview of early abortion methods, advice on how to establish medical abortion services, and a list of useful resources. Copies can be ordered from University of California, San Francisco at reprohealth.ucsf.edu.

- *The Best Intentions: Unintended Pregnancy and the Well-being of Children and Families.* This book details the causes, consequences, and costs of unintended pregnancy. The reference list is extensive. Available from the National Academy Press at book stores, by calling 1-800-624-6242, or online at www.nap.edu.

- *Dubious Conceptions: The Politics of Teenage Pregnancy* by Luker. One of the most articulate treatises on teenagers and pregnancy, the book takes an empathetic, myth-busting approach. Available from Harvard University Press at bookstores or at www.hup. harvard.edu.

- *Perspectives on Sexual and Reproductive Health* (formerly, *Family Planning Perspectives*). This peer-reviewed journal offers the latest policy-relevant, widely referenced research and analysis on reproductive health in the United States and other developed countries. Read updates and digests of research in the field, special reports and forums on timely topics, and original research and analysis in every issue. Available at www.guttmacher.org/journals.

- *The Guttmacher Report on Public Policy.* This publication analyzes reproductive health policy-making in Washington and state capitals across the country. This bimonthly review relates state to national and international developments and highlights all aspects of reproductive health policy. Available at www.guttmacher. org/journals.

- *State Policies in Brief* by The Alan Guttmacher Institute (AGI). This series of fact sheets provides information on key issues affecting reproductive health and rights in the United States. They are updated monthly by AGI's policy analysts to reflect the most recent legislative, administrative, and judicial actions. Each edition provides background on the issue, state-by-state policy breakdowns, and information on where to go to learn more. State Policies in Brief are available in PDF format at AGI's web site at www.guttmacher.org/pubs/spib.html.

- "News Providers Can Use." In concise and clear language, this quarterly e-mail newsletter identifies key questions of interest in family planning and reproductive health, summarizes recent AGI research and policy analyses that address these questions, puts new findings in a programmatic context and provides links to more detailed information. To sign up, type your e-mail address into the green-labeled "subscribe" box at www.guttmacher.org/listserv/#3.

- "AGI Update." Keep current with the latest AGI research and policy analyses before you receive them in print. Subscribe to this electronic mailing list to receive previews of upcoming publications, as well as links to background information to help you place new developments in context. To sign up, type your e-mail address into the blue-labeled "subscribe" box at www.guttmacher.org/listserv.

- *Kaisernetwork.org.* This Internet service provides three daily online reports: the Kaiser Daily Reproductive Health Report, the Kaiser Daily HIV/AIDS Report, and the Kaiser Daily Health Policy Report. Each provides summaries of current news stories plus maintains a fully searchable archive. To read the reports or sign up to receive them via email, visit www.kaisernetwork.org/daily_reports/rep_index.cfm.

- *The Program Archive on Sexuality, Health & Adolescence.* PASHA is a collection of pregnancy and STI prevention programs that have been selected for their demonstrated effectiveness in changing behavior among teens. Each program comes with all the necessary materials for program implementation. Find out more at www.socio.com/pasha.htm.

- Educational materials. Many companies provide a wide range of health education materials ranging from anatomical models and flip charts to videotapes and pamphlets. A few favorites: Health Education Services (www.hes.org), NASCO (www.nascofa.com), and WRS Group (www.wrsgroup.com).

PATIENT EDUCATION

- Flip charts and leader's guides. Educate your patients with these exceptionally illustrated flip charts on "Birth Control," "Reproductive Anatomy and Physiology," "HIV/AIDS," and "Sexually Transmitted Diseases." Available from ETR Associates at 1-800-321-4407 or www.etr.org.

- *Project Wise*, Project Inform's program on HIV/AIDS, provides information on research, treatment and advocacy for women. Project Wise publishes a newsletter three times a year (available online or by mail), and offers fact sheets (in English and Spanish) and articles about women and HIV. Available at www.projectinform. org/pub/ww_index.html.

- "Now What Do I Do?" Designed to help parents communicate with pre-teens, these materials help answer the tough questions. Available from SIECUS at 1-212-819-9770 or www.siecus.org.

- *Beyond the Big Talk: Every Parent's Guide to Raising Sexually Healthy Teens, From Middle School to College* by Haffner. For parents of teenagers. Available from Newmarket Press in bookstores or at www.newmarketpress.com.

PHARMACEUTICAL HOUSE RESOURCES

Almost every contraceptive has a patient package insert. Some provide excellent information. Some are easier to read than others. All are free. Pharmaceutical houses are generally responsive to inquiries about educational materials for providers or patients (Table 11-3).

Table 11-3 Pharmaceutical company websites and toll-free phone numbers

Allendale Pharmaceuticals: sponge	1-888-343-4499	www.todaysponge.com
Ansell Healthcare: condoms		www.ansell.com
Apothecus: VCF	1-800-227-2393	www.apothecus.com
Barr Pharmaceuticals Plan B ECP	1-800-330-1271	www.go2planb.com
Berlex Laboratories: OCs, progestin IUD	1-888-237-5394	www.berlex.com
Bristol-Myers Squibb Company: OCs, ERT	1-800-321-1335	www.bms.com
Church & Dwight: condoms	1-800-833-9532	www.churchdwight.com
Danco Laboratories: mifepristone	1-877-432-7596	www.earlyoptionpill.com
GlaxoSmithKline: antivirals, antibiotics	1-800-722-9292	www.gsk.com
Mayer Laboratories: condoms, female condoms	1-800-426-6366	www.mayerlabs.com
Okamoto: condoms	1-800-283-7546	www.okamotousa.com
Organon: OCs, vaginal ring	1-800-631-1253	www.organon.com
Ortho-McNeil Pharmaceutical: OCs, patch, diaphragm, IUD	1-800-542-5365	www.ortho-mcneil.com
Parke Davis (Pfizer): OCs	1-800-223-0432	www.pfizer.com
Pharmacia (Pfizer): injectables, ERT	1-800-323-4204	www.pfizer.com
Smart Practice: non-allergenic gloves	1-800-522-0800	www.smartpractice.com
3M Pharmaceuticals: wart treatment, BV treatment	1-800-328-0255	www.3m.com/us/healthcare
Watson Pharmaceuticals: OCs	1-800-272-5525	www.watsonpharm.com
Wyeth Ayerst: OCs	1-800-777-6180	www.wyeth.com

TELEPHONE HOTLINES AND WEBSITES

Numerous organizations have set up hotlines and websites for providers and patients (Tables 11-4 and 11-5). Remember that while the Internet offers myriad resources for both professionals and patients, health and medical sites are not peer-reviewed, and clinical decisions should not be based on information found on line.

Table 11-4 Hotlines and websites

Topic	Organization	Hotline	Website
Abortion	Abortion Clinics OnLine		www.gynpages.com
	Ibis Reproductive Health		www.medication abortions.org
	NARAL Pro-Choice America		www.naral.org
	National Abortion Federation	1-877-4ProChoice	www.prochoice.org
Adoption	Adopt a Special Kid-America	1-888-680-7349	www.adoptaspecial kid.org
	Adoptive Families	1-800-372-3300	www.adoptive families.com
AIDS *(see HIV/AIDS)*			
AIDS Advocacy	Gay Men's Health Crisis	1-800-AIDS-NYC	www.gmhc.org
	Mother's Voices		www.mvoicesfl.org
	Project Inform	1-800-822-7422	www.projinf.org
Alcoholism	Alcoholics Anonymous		www.aa.org
	Al-Anon & Alateen Family Groups	1-888-4AL-ANON	www.al-anon.org
	American Council on Alcoholism		www.aca-usa.org
	Children of Alcoholics Foundation		www.coaf.org
	Co-dependents Anonymous		www.codependents.org
	National Organization on Fetal Alcohol Syndrome	1-800-66-NOFAS	www.nofas.org
Anxiety *(see also Depression)*	Anxiety Disorders Association of America		www.adaa.org
	Freedom from Fear	1-888-442-2022	www.freedomfrom fear.org
	NIMH Panic Disorder Information Line	1-800-64-PANIC	www.nimh.nih.gov/ anxiety/upd.cfm
Breast Cancer *(see also Cancer)*	National Alliance of Breast Cancer Organizations	1-888-80-NABCO	www.nabco.org
	Reach to Recovery (mastectomy patients)	1-800-ACS-2345	www.cancer.org
	Y-Me National Breast Cancer Organization	1-800-221-2141	www.y-me.org

(continued)

Table 11-4 Hotlines and websites—*(cont'd)*

Topic	Organization	Hotline	Website
Breastfeeding	International Lactation Consultant Association		www.ilca.org
	La Leche League International	1-800-LA-LECHE	www.lalecheleague.org
	The Linkages Project		www.linkagesproject.org
Cancer *(see also specific cancers)*	American Cancer Society	1-800-ACS-2345	www.cancer.org
	Candlelighters Childhood Cancer Foundation	1-800-366-2223	www.candlelighters.org
	National Cancer Institute's Cancer Information	1-800-4-CANCER	cancer.gov/ cancerinformation
Child Abuse	Childhelp USA National Child Abuse Hotline	1-800-4-A-CHILD	www.childhelpusa.org
	KidsPeace National Center for Kids Overcoming Crisis	1-800-334-4KID	www.kidspeace.org
	National Center for Missing & Exploited Children	1-800-THE-LOST	www.ncmec.org
	Prevent Child Abuse America		www.preventchild abuse.org
Contraception	Association of Reproductive Health Professionals		http://www.arhp.org/ patienteducation
	EngenderHealth		www.engender health.org
	Planned Parenthood Federation of America	1-800-230-PLAN	www.ppfa.org
	World Health Organization		www.who.int/health_ topics/contraception/ en/
Depression	Depression and Bipolar Support Alliance	1-800-826-3632	www.ndmda.org
	National Foundation for Depressive Illness	1-800-248-4344	www.depression.org
Domestic Violence	Family Violence Prevention Fund (for clinicians)		endabuse.org/programs /healthcare
	Family Violence Prevention Fund (for women)		endabuse.org
	National Domestic Violence Hotline	1-800-799-SAFE	www.ndvh.org
	National Resource Center on Domestic Violence	1-800-537-2238	
Drug Abuse	Alcohol & Drug Helpline	1-800-821-4357	
	Narcotics Anonymous World Services		www.na.org
Eating Disorders	National Association of Anorexia Nervosa and Associated Disorders	1-847-831-3438	www.altrue.net/site/ anadweb/
	National Eating Disorders Association	1-800-931-2237	www.nationaleating disorders.org

(continued)

Table 11-4 Hotlines and websites—*(cont'd)*

Topic	Organization	Hotline	Website
Emergency Contraception	Emergency Contraception Website & Hotline	1-888-NOT-2-LATE	not-2-late.com
	Planned Parenthood Federation of America	1-800-230-PLAN	www.ppfa.org/ec
Endometriosis	Endometriosis Association	1-800-992-ENDO	www.Endometriosis Assn.org
Family/ parenting	American Academy of Family Physicians	1-800-274-AAFP	www.aafp.org
	American Academy of Pediatrics	1-800-433-9016	www.aap.org
Fitness	Aerobics and Fitness Association of America	1-800-225-AFAA	www.afaa.com
Headaches	National Headache Foundation	1-800-843-2256	www.headaches.org
Hepatitis	Hepatitis B Coalition		www.immunize.org
Herpes	National Herpes Hotline (ASHA)	1-919-361-8488	www.ashastd.org
HIV/AIDS	AIDSinfo	1-800-HIV-0440	www.aidsinfo.nih.gov/
	AIDS Research Information Center		www.critpath.org/aric/
	American Red Cross		www.redcross.org/ services/hss/hivaids
	CDC National HIV/AIDS Hotline	1-800-342-AIDS	www.cdc.gov/hiv/ pubs/facts.htm
	International AIDS Society-USA		www.iasusa.org
	Spanish CDC National HIV/AIDS Hotline	1-800-344-7432	www.ashastd.org/ nah/sida
	UNAIDS		www.unaids.org
HIV/AIDS *(for health care professionals)*	National HIV/AIDS Clinicians' Consultation Center		www.ucsf.edu/hivcntr
	Warmline for clinical consultation	1-800-933-3413	
	Post-Exposure Prophylaxis Hotline	1-888-HIV-4911	
Hospice	National Hospice and Palliative Care Organization	1-800-658-8898	www.nhpco.org
	National Hospice Foundation		hospiceinfo.org
HPV	National HPV and Cervical Cancer Prevention Hotline	1-919-361-4848	www.ashastd.org
Hypertension	American Heart Association	1-800-AHA-USA-1	www.americanheart.org
Infertility	Resolve National Infertility Helpline	1-888-623-0744	www.resolve.org
Interstitial Cystitis	Interstitial Cystitis Association	1-800-HELP-ICA	www.ichelp.org

(continued)

Table 11-4   Hotlines and websites—*(cont'd)*

Topic	Organization	Hotline	Website
Lactational Amenorrhea Method	The Linkages Project		www.linkages project.org
Menopause	North American Menopause Society		www.menopause.org
Microbicides	Alliance for Microbicide Development		www.microbicide.org
Natural Family Planning	FertilityUK		www.fertilityUK.org
Osteoporosis	National Osteoporosis Foundation	1-800-223-9994	www.nof.org
Ovarian Cancer *(see also Cancer)*	Roswell Park Cancer Institute	1-800-OVARIAN	www.roswellpark.org
Overweight	American Heart Association	1-800-AHA-USA-1	www.americanheart.org
	Take Off Pounds Sensibly (TOPS)	1-800-932-8677	www.tops.org
Pregnancy, crisis *(see also Adoption)*	America's Pregnancy Helpline	1-888-672-2296	www.thehelpline.org
Pregnancy, delivery and postpartum	Bradley Method	1-800-4-A-BIRTH	www.bradleybirth.com
	Depression After Delivery, Inc.	1-800-944-4773	www.depressionafter delivery.com
	Lamaze International	1-800-368-4404	www.lamaze.org
	Postpartum Support International	1-805-967-7636	www.chss.iup.edu/ postpartum
Premenstrual Syndrome	PMS Access	1-800-222-4PMS	www.womenshealth. com/hotline.html
Q & A	Go Ask Alice		www.goaskalice. columbia.edu
Reproductive Health	Managing Contraception		www.managing contraception.com
	Reproductive Health ReproLine		www.reproline.jhu.edu
Sexual Assault	Rape Abuse & Incest National Network	1-800-656-HOPE	www.rainn.org
Sexually Transmitted Infections	American Social Health Association	1-800-227-8922	www.ashastd.org
	CDC Sexually Transmitted Disease Hotline	1-800-342-AIDS	www.cdc.gov/nchstp/ dstd/dstdp.html
	Spanish CDC Sexually Transmitted Disease Hotline	1-800-344-7432	www.ashastd.org/ nah/sida
Smoking	American Cancer Society	1-800-ACS-2345	www.cancer.org
	American Lung Association	1-800-586-4872	www.lungusa.org

(continued)

Table 11-4 Hotlines and websites—*(cont'd)*

Topic	Organization	Hotline	Website
Teens	Teenwire		www.teenwire.com
Urinary Incontinence	National Association for Continence	1-800-BLADDER	www.nafc.org
Vulvodynia	National Vulvodynia Association		www.nva.org
Women's Health	Office on Women's Health (DHHS)		www.4women.gov
Youth At-Risk	The Bureau for At-Risk Youth	1-800-99-YOUTH	www.at-risk.com

Table 11-5 Online resource lists

Webpages with Active Links to Many Other Websites	
Ardent Media Inc	www.ardentmediainc.com
CDC National Prevention Network	cdcnpin.org
Contraceptive Technology	www.contraceptivetechnology.org
Department of Health and Human Services	www.healthfinder.gov
Johns Hopkins Center for Communication Programs	www.jhuccp.org/info/netlinks.php
MedWeb at Emory University	www.medweb.emory.edu/medweb
Princeton University	ec.princeton.edu/info/contrac.html

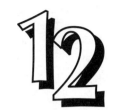

Emergency Contraception

Felicia Stewart, MD
James Trussell, PhD
Paul F.A. Van Look, MD, PhD, FRCOG

- Emergency use of oral contraceptive pills containing levonorgestrel alone reduces the risk of pregnancy after unprotected intercourse by 89%. If a levonorgestrel only product is not available, pills containing a combination of ethinyl estradiol and either norgestrel or levonorgestrel can be provided to reduce the risk by 75%. Emergency insertion of a copper-releasing IUD reduces the risk of pregnancy by as much as 99%.

- There are no medical contraindications to treatment with emergency contraceptive pills (ECPs), except pregnancy. If a woman is already pregnant, treatment is ineffective.

- Providing information about emergency contraception, treatment when needed, and advance prescription for women who want to have ECPs on hand have become accepted "standards of care" in the United States.

- In the United States, emergency contraception could potentially prevent as many as 1.5 million unintended pregnancies—about half of the estimated 3 million unintended pregnancies that occur annually.

Given the chance, most women would prefer to prevent an unplanned pregnancy rather than decide what to do once one occurs. In some instances, unintended pregnancy is entirely unexpected, such as when a woman conceives while wearing an IUD or following sterilization. Often, however, unintended pregnancies occur after contraceptive failure that was recognized at the time it occurred. Typical examples of such situations include breakage or slippage of a barrier method, missing hormonal contraceptive pills during risky days of the cycle, being too late for a contraceptive injection, or erring in practicing coitus interruptus or abstinence. In these instances, as well as in all situations in which sexual intercourse was unprotected, including rape, emergency contraception offers a second chance to avoid unintended pregnancy.

Table 12-1 Twenty OCs that can be used for emergency contraception in the United States[a]

Brand	Company	Pills per Dose[b]	Ethinyl Estradiol per Dose (µg)	Levonorgestrel per Dose (mg)[c]
Plan-B	Barr	1 white pill	0	0.75
Ogestrel	Watson	2 white pills	100	0.50
Ovral	Wyeth-Ayerst	2 white pills	100	0.50
Cryselle	Barr	4 white pills	120	0.60
Levora	Watson	4 white pills	120	0.60
Lo/Ovral	Wyeth-Ayerst	4 white pills	120	0.60
Low-Ogestrel	Watson	4 white pills	120	0.60
Levlen	Berlex	4 light-orange pills	120	0.60
Nordette	Wyeth-Ayerst	4 light-orange pills	120	0.60
Portia	Barr	4 pink pills	120	0.60
Seasonale	Barr	4 pink pills	120	0.60
Trivora	Watson	4 pink pills	120	0.50
Tri-Levlen	Berlex	4 yellow pills	120	0.50
Triphasil	Wyeth-Ayerst	4 yellow pills	120	0.50
Enpresse	Barr	4 orange pills	120	0.50
Alesse	Wyeth-Ayerst	5 pink pills	100	0.50
Lessina	Barr	5 pink pills	100	0.50
Levlite	Berlex	5 pink pills	100	0.50
Aviane	Barr	5 orange pills	100	0.50
Ovrette	Wyeth-Ayerst	20 yellow pills	0	0.75

Notes:

[a] Plan-B is the only dedicated product specifically marketed for emergency contraception. Alesse, Aviane, Cryselle, Enpresse, Lessina, Levlen, Levlite, Levora, Lo/Ovral, Low-Ogestrel, Nordette, Ogestrel, Ovral, Portia, Seasonale, Tri-Levlen, Triphasil, and Trivora have been declared safe and effective for use as ECPs by the U.S. Food and Drug Administration. Outside the United States, more than 20 emergency contraceptive products are specifically packaged, labeled, and marketed. For example, Gedeon Richter and HRA Pharma are marketing in many countries the levonorgestrel-only products Postinor-2 and NorLevo, respectively, each consisting of a two-pill strip with each pill containing 0.75 mg levonorgestrel. NorLevo became available over-the-counter without a prescription in Norway in October 2000 and in Sweden in late 2001.

[b] The treatment schedule is one dose within 120 hours after unprotected intercourse, and another dose 12 hours later. However, recent research has found that both doses of Plan B can be taken at the same time.

[c] The progestin in Cryselle, Lo/Ovral, Low-Ogestrel, Ogestrel, Ovral, and Ovrette is norgestrel, which contains two isomers, only one of which (levonorgestrel) is bioactive; the amount of norgestrel in each tablet is twice the amount of levonorgestrel.

Emergency contraceptives are methods women can use after intercourse to prevent pregnancy.[1] Two dedicated emergency contraceptive products have been approved by the FDA for use in the U.S.:

- Plan B, containing two tablets of levonorgestrel (750 mcg) was approved in 1999.

- Preven, containing two doses of ethinyl estradiol (100 mcg) combined with levonorgestrel (500 mcg) was approved in 1998 but withdrawn from the market in 2004.

Other options include use of the following:

- Ordinary birth control pill products containing ethinyl estradiol and either norgestrel or levonorgestrel (See Table 12-1)
- Progestin-only minipills, to provide a hormone dose comparable to the regimen in a dedicated product (see Table 12-1)
- Insertion of a copper-releasing intrauterine device (IUD) within 5 days

Oral regimens (called ECPs, for emergency contraceptive pills) involve one or two doses. Treatment should be initiated as soon as possible after unprotected intercourse, and definitely within 120 hours. When using a two-dose regimen, the second dose should be taken 12 hours after the first. To describe these methods, terms such as "postcoital" contraception and "morning-after" pills are not recommended because they may be misleading: treatment can be initiated sooner than the morning after or later—as long as 120 hours (5 days) after intercourse.

HISTORY

Use of high-dose postcoital estrogen began in the 1960s as a treatment for rape victims.[2,3] The combined estrogen-progestin (Yuzpe) regimen was introduced in the 1970s[4,5] and soon replaced the high-dose estrogen approach. Postcoital insertion of a copper-releasing IUD for emergency contraception was first reported in 1976. Safety for emergency use of pills containing norethindrone has been documented in one study which found an efficacy slightly lower than that for levonorgestrel pills,[6] but no published studies are available for pills containing other progestins such as gestodene or etonorgestrel; such pills should not be used in routine practice.

Pills containing progestin alone have also been used for intermittent contraception in China,[7] and tablets containing 750 mcg levonorgestrel were marketed for this purpose in several countries under the trade name Postinor. Although this approach has proven to be unsuitable for ongoing postcoital use because of its low efficacy,[8] single or infrequent use for emergency contraception is effective. Before 1999, when the levonorgestrel emergency contraceptive product was approved by the U.S. Food and Drug Administration (FDA), no single levonorgestrel tablet of similar hormone content was available in the United States. Providing an equivalent dose using available progestin-only birth control pills required 20 Ovrette tablets for each ECP dose of 750 mcg levonorgestrel (each Ovrette tablet contains 75 mcg norgestrel, equivalent to 37.5 mcg levonorgestrel).

In the future, antiprogestins may be another option for emergency contraception. This family of compounds, which includes mifepristone (Mifeprex, also known as RU 486), blocks the effects of progesterone by binding to its receptors. Antiprogestin effects prevent or stop ovulation and disrupt luteal phase events and endometrial development, depending on whether the drug is administered before or after ovulation.[9] A single 10 milligram (mg) dose of mifepristone, initiated within 120 hours after unprotected intercourse,[10-12] is highly effective in preventing pregnancy. Further, mifepristone causes less nausea and vomiting and fewer side effects than does the Yuzpe regimen.[10,13,14]

Older methods for emergency contraception, no longer recommended, include high-dose estrogen or danazol. Treatment with diethylstilbestrol (DES), 25 mg to 50 mg, or ethinyl estradiol, 5 mg to 10 mg, given daily for 5 days provides efficacy similar to the Yuzpe method,[15,16] but with a high incidence of nausea. Studies of danazol, an androgenic and progestogenic steroid, were initially promising[17] but this approach was abandoned when a subsequent study found an unacceptably low efficacy.[14]

FUTURE POTENTIAL FOR EMERGENCY CONTRACEPTIVE USE

Wider use of emergency contraception could prevent a substantial proportion of the millions of unplanned pregnancies that occur every year. Emergency contraception is also highly cost-effective. Compared to the health care costs for unintended pregnancies that would otherwise occur, ECP treatment provided to one woman results in a net saving of $54 (Medicaid) to $124 (managed care).[18] Educate women about this option during routine visits, provide information materials, provide a prescription or pills in advance for later use if needed, and make certain that office telephone and appointment procedures call for prompt response to any request for emergency contraceptive help.

That many hospital emergency departments do not provide emergency contraceptive services to women who have been raped is a tragic example of neglected preventive health care.[19] Legal precedent also indicates that this failure constitutes inadequate care, and confers to a woman in this situation the standing to sue the hospital.[20] Of the 683,000 rapes identified by the 1992 National Women's Study, only 17% of the women involved received medical care within the first week, and only half of these women recalled being counseled about the possibility of pregnancy. As many as 22,000 pregnancies resulting annually from rape could be prevented by appropriate care. In addition, such care could provide testing and prophylaxis for sexually transmitted infection (STI).[21]

One concern often voiced about making ECPs more widely available is that women who know they can use ECPs might become less diligent with their ongoing contraceptive method. If used as a sole method, repeated ECP therapy would be far less effective than most other contraceptive methods. For a typical woman who used combined ECPs repeatedly as her sole method for a year, the risk of pregnancy would exceed 35%; if she used progestin-only ECPs, she would still have a 20% chance of pregnancy. Therefore, repeated ECP use would not be a rational contraceptive strategy. Also, side effects such as nausea and vomiting that are quite common with combined ECP use are likely to dissuade women from adopting ECP as a principal strategy. Even if ECP availability did adversely affect regular contraceptive use, however, women are nevertheless entitled to know about all contraceptive options and make decisions themselves about method use.[22]

Research evidence so far reported indicates that making ECPs more readily available does not increase women's likelihood of engaging in unprotected sex[23-25] and that women rarely rely on ECPs as their sole contraceptive method.[26] In a recent study considering the effect of advance ECP provision, participants receiving emergency contraception supplies in advance were three times as likely to use ECPs when needed, but they did not report higher frequencies of unprotected sex.[24]

Many policy initiatives have been undertaken to encourage greater awareness and use of emergency contraception. In 1997, when providing emergency contraception involved evidence-based use of tablets from oral contraceptive pill packets for a non-approved indication, the U.S. Food and Drug Administration (FDA) reviewed relevant research and published the following statement in the Federal Register:[27]

> "Summary: The Food and Drug Administration (FDA) is announcing that the Commissioner of Food and Drugs (the Commissioner) has concluded that certain combined oral contraceptives containing ethinyl estradiol and norgestrel or levonorgestrel are safe and effective for use as postcoital emergency contraception. . . . The Commissioner bases this conclusion on FDA's review of the published literature concerning this use, FDA's knowledge of the safety of combined oral contraceptives as currently labeled, and on the unanimous conclusion that these regimens are safe and effective made by the agency's Advisory Committee for Reproductive Health Drugs at its June 28, 1996 meeting."

This action provides reassurance for providers about using ordinary oral contraceptive products containing ethinyl estradiol and either norgestrel or levonorgestrel for this unlabeled indication. In 1996, an American College of Obstetricians and Gynecologists (ACOG) Practice Pattern detailed the use of emergency oral contraception,[28] and in 2001 an ACOG Practice Bulletin updated information about emergency contraception and recommended that clinicians consider giving an advance prescription for emergency contraception at the time of a routine gynecologic visit.[29]

Clinical guidelines that include emergency contraception options have been released by the International Planned Parenthood Federation,[30] by the Royal College of Obstetricians and Gynaecologists;[31] and by the World Health Organization (WHO) for its Essential Drugs List.[32] In its clinical standards and guidelines, Planned Parenthood Federation of America now includes advance provision of ECPs for later use (adopted in 1996) or a prescription given over the telephone (adopted in 1998). Family planning clinics in the federally funded Title X program received explicit authorization to provide emergency contraceptive treatment in April 1997.[33] The feasibility of providing emergency contraceptives as a service to members of a large HMO (Health Maintenance Organization) was documented in a demonstration project involving more than 100 providers at Kaiser Permanente medical offices in San Diego.[34] An innovative program in the State of Washington has shown that pharmacists can effectively provide emergency contraceptives directly to patients.[35] A similar pharmacist program began in California in 2002, and was adopted in the United Kingdom in January, 2001.[36] Practical steps such as these to increase timely access may be of special importance for teen women. Young women have high rates of unintended pregnancy and are likely to face significant financial and confidentiality obstacles in obtaining services.[37]

The importance of timely access underlay the decision in France in 1999 to make ECPs available from pharmacists and in 2000 to provide ECPs free to young women who need treatment. Norway and Sweden changed ECP status from prescription to over-the-counter in 2000 and 2001, respectively. Levonorgestrel-only ECPs are also available from pharmacists in Alaska, California, Hawaii, Maine, New Mexico, Washington State, Albania, Belgium, Benin, Cameroon, some provinces in Canada, Congo, Denmark, Estonia, Finland, France, Gabon, Guinea, Guinea-Bissau, India, Israel, Nigeria, Israel, Ivory Coast, Latvia, Madagascar, Mali, Mauritania, Mauritius, Namibia, New Zealand, Nigeria, Portugal, Senegal, South Africa, Sri Lanka, Switzerland, Tunisia, Uganda, and the United Kingdom. Changing ECPs from prescription to OTC in the U.S. has been recommended by respected reproductive health leaders[38,39] and endorsed by many professional organizations including the American College of Obstetricians and Gynecologists (ACOG) and the American Medical Association (AMA).[39] In December 2003, an FDA advisory committee voted 23 to 4 to approve Plan B OTC.

MECHANISM OF ACTION
EMERGENCY CONTRACEPTIVE PILLS

There are many steps in the process of reproduction that potentially could be affected by emergency contraception:[40]

- Follicle maturation, egg maturation and the ovulatory process
- Sperm migration and function
- Fertilization
- Zygote, morula, and blastocyst development, and transport in the fallopian tube and uterine cavity
- Development of receptive uterine lining
- Maintenance of necessary hormone levels by the corpus luteum

The effect of treatment depends on when in the woman's cycle emergency contraception is used. During the pre-ovulatory phase of the cycle, steps in follicle maturation, egg maturation, and the ovulatory process can be altered. After ovulation, there is an interval of approximately 7 days during which the remaining steps above occur. If these steps are successful, implantation starts at about the 7th day after ovulation. Implantation is, by definition, the criterion for the beginning of pregnancy (National Institutes of Health, the Food and Drug Administration, and the American College of Obstetricians and Gynecologists).[41,42] If these steps are not successful, pregnancy is prevented.

When given before ovulation, both progestin-only and estrogen-progestin combination ECPs can disrupt normal follicular development and maturation, resulting in anovulation or delayed ovulation with a deficient luteal function.[40,43-46,88-90] In contrast, when treatment is administered after ovulation has occurred and fertilization may have taken place, whatever effectiveness the treatment has cannot depend on disruption of ovulation. Some studies have shown histologic or biochemical alterations in the endometrium after treatment with the combination estrogen-progestin regimen, leading to the conclusion that combined ECPs may act by impairing endometrial receptivity to implantation of a fertilized egg.[43,47-49] However, other studies found no such effects on the endometrium.[45,50,51,89,90] Additional possible mechanisms include interference with corpus luteum function; alteration of cervical mucus resulting in trapping of sperm or impaired sperm function; alteration in the tubal transport of sperm, egg, or embryo; and direct inhibition of fertilization.[40,52,91] One study documented impaired sperm migration and function after postcoital administration of 0.4 mg levonorgestrel,[53] but no clinical data exist regarding tubal transport or inhibition of fertilization. Nevertheless, statistical evidence on the effectiveness of ECPs suggests that in a small percentage of cases there must be a mechanism of action other than delaying or preventing ovulation.[54] To make an informed choice, women who are concerned about the mechanism of action need to know that ECPs—like all regular hormonal contraceptives including the birth control pill, the implant Norplant, the injectable Depo-Provera,[55] and even breastfeeding (see Chapter 23 on Postpartum Contraception and Lactation)—may prevent pregnancy by delaying or inhibiting ovulation, inhibiting fertilization, or inhibiting implantation of a fertilized egg. Analysis of ECP effectiveness in relation to the timing of intercourse and treatment in relation to cycle day found that effectiveness was substantially higher when intercourse and treatment occurred before ovulation, and concluded that inhibition of implantation is unlikely to be the primary mechanism of action for this contraceptive method.[56]

COPPER-RELEASING IUDS

When used as a regular method of contraception, copper-releasing IUDs act primarily to prevent fertilization. Copper IUD use for emergency contraception may involve the same mechanism in some cases. Emergency insertion of a copper-IUD, however, is significantly more effective than use of ECPs, reducing the risk of pregnancy following unprotected intercourse by as much as 99%.[57,58] This very high level of effectiveness implies that emergency insertion of a copper-IUD must also be able to prevent pregnancy after fertilization. (See Chapter 21 on Intrauterine Devices.)

EFFECTIVENESS

Use of ECPs containing progestin only (levonorgestrel, 750 mcg in each dose) reduces the risk of pregnancy by 89%;[59] use of ECPs containing combined estrogen-progestin (ethinyl estradiol 100 mcg and levonorgestrel 500 mcg in each dose) reduces the risk of pregnancy by about 75%.[60,61] These statements do not mean that 12% to 25% of women using ECPs will become pregnant. Rather, if 100 women had unprotected intercourse once during the second or third week of their cycle and were not treated with ECPs, about 8 would become pregnant. Following treatment with ECPs, only 1 or 2 women would become pregnant, a 75% to 89% reduction.

Over 9,400 postcoital insertions of copper-bearing IUDs are known to have been carried out since the practice was introduced in 1976. With only 10 failures, this approach probably has a pregnancy rate no higher than 0.2%.[57,58] The effectiveness of using a levonorgestrel-releasing IUD (LNg-20) for emergency contraception has not been studied and is not recommended.

Because emergency contraception is used only once or infrequently, traditional measures of contraceptive effectiveness, such as the life-table pregnancy rate, are not applicable. One way to measure effectiveness is the treatment failure rate: the number of pregnancies that occur in 100 treatment cycles. After ECP treatment, pregnancy rates typically range from 0.5% to 2.5%.[62] A treatment failure rate of 1.0% does not mean, however, that the method was 99.0% effective. Actual efficacy is much lower because most of the women would not have become pregnant even without treatment. Even at the most fertile interval of the menstrual cycle (beginning 6 days before ovulation and ending the day after ovulation), the pregnancy risk is only 10% to 30%. Before and after that interval, pregnancy is unlikely.[63] (See Chapter 27 on Impaired Fertility.)

Treatment failure rates in studies are strongly influenced by the specific day of the cycle that the women in the study had unprotected intercourse. For this reason, failure rates of different studies cannot be meaningfully compared. A study in which all the women were treated after exposure to unprotected intercourse during the fertile phase of the cycle is bound to find a higher failure rate than a study in which women were treated irrespective of the day of the cycle they had unprotected intercourse.

Comparing the number of pregnancies observed in a study with the number that would have been expected without treatment is therefore a more appropriate way of measuring efficacy. The expected number of pregnancies is computed by multiplying the number of women having unprotected intercourse at each day of the cycle by the probability of conception for that day.

Any estimate of risk reduction is dependent on the underlying accuracy of the "expected" risk rates—in this case, the likelihood of pregnancy by cycle day in the absence of treatment. Unfortunately, research evidence about pregnancy likelihood is limited. Likelihood is also very sensitive to the characteristics of the population studied[64] since fecundity is affected by many factors (for example, age, previous gynecologic and obstetrical history) including some that are not directly observable (such as unrecognized damage to Fallopian tubes from asymptomatic infection).

A large study by WHO found that increasing delay between unprotected intercourse and the initiation of treatment was associated with decreasing efficacy (see Figure 12-1).[65,66] This finding suggests that ECPs should be initiated as soon after unprotected intercourse as is possible. When taking the second dose 12 hours later would be difficult, however, the timing of the second dose might be altered. For example, a woman who took her first dose at 3 p.m. immediately following the discovery of a burst condom might delay taking the second dose until 7 a.m. The goal should be to make the therapy as user-friendly as possible.[67] New research does indicate, however, that in the case of combined estrogen-progestin ECPs, the second dose appears to increase efficacy of the therapy and so should not be skipped.[6]

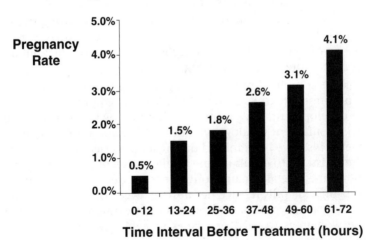

Source: Piaggio, von Hertzen, Grimes and Van Look (1999).[66]

Figure 12-1   Impact of delay in treatment on ECP effectiveness

It is biologically implausible that efficacy would abruptly plummet to zero after 72 hours.[68] Moreover, new research directly investigating the effectiveness beyond 72 hours suggests that both progestin-only and combined estrogen-progestin ECPs are effective when taken 73–120 hours after unprotected intercourse.[12,69,70] Therefore, clinical protocols that deny treatment beyond 72 hours are unnecessarily restrictive, particularly if the alternative of emergency insertion of a copper-IUD is not immediately available or appropriate. In the case of progestin-only ECPs, new evidence suggests that providing both doses (1,500 mcg levonorgestrel) at the same time is as effective as taking two doses 12 hours apart,[12,71] but does not increase the risk of side effects.[12]

ADVANTAGES AND INDICATIONS

Emergency contraceptives are the only methods a couple can use to prevent pregnancy after unprotected sexual intercourse or after a contraceptive "accident." Emergency contraception also is an essential part of treatment, and standard of care, following sexual assault for women who were not protected by an effective contraceptive method when the assault occurred.[72] Emergency contraception may be an appropriate option in the following circumstances:[73]

- No contraceptive was used when intercourse took place.
- A male condom slipped, broke, or leaked.
- A woman's female condom, diaphragm or cervical cap was inserted incorrectly, dislodged during intercourse, was removed too early, or was found to be torn.
- A woman missed too many pills at the wrong time:
  — 2 or more combined oral contraceptive pills during the first week of a pill pack
  — 5 or more pills during the second or third week of a pill pack
  — 2 or more days late starting a new pill pack

  Because combined pills act by suppressing ovulation, the risk of conception occurs some days after the missed pills when follicular development, freed from the inhibition by the oral contraceptive, is sufficient to allow ovulation. Ovulation is unlikely if only a few pills have been missed during a pill cycle. Advise a woman who misses 2 to 4 pills during the last week of a pill pack simply to resume pill taking and continue for 3 weeks with no break so the "missed" pills replace her normal "week off." (Note: no matter how many pills have been missed, treatment is reasonable if the woman is worried or wishes to avoid even a small risk of pregnancy.)
- A woman who does have menstrual cycles missed 1 or more progestin-only pills or is 3 or more hours late taking a pill. In contrast to combined pills, progestin-only pills do not consistently suppress ovulation, and the risk of pregnancy after missing progestin-only pills is greater and more immediate than is the case with missed combined pills.

- A woman is more than 7 days late in getting a monthly contraceptive injection.
- A woman is more than 14 days late in getting a 3-month progestin-only contraceptive injection, or the date or type of the previous injection is unknown.
- A woman was 2 or more days late starting a new vaginal ring cycle.
- A woman was 2 or more days late starting a new patch cycle.
- A female condom was inserted or removed incorrectly leading to spillage of semen, or the penis was inserted mistakenly between the female condom and the vaginal wall resulting in intravaginal ejaculation.
- The couple erred in practicing coitus interruptus (ejaculation in vagina or on external genitalia).
- The couple erred in practicing periodic abstinence (sexual intercourse on a fertile day of the cycle).
- An IUD was partially or totally expelled or has been removed 7 days or less after the last act of intercourse.
- A woman was exposed to a possible teratogen such as retinoic acid or a cytotoxic drug when she was not protected by effective contraception.

Because it provides extremely high emergency contraceptive efficacy for at least 5 days after intercourse, the IUD may be an especially useful option for women who present 4 or 5 days after unprotected intercourse. It may also be a good choice for the woman who wishes to continue using an IUD as her long-term method of contraception.

DISADVANTAGES AND CAUTIONS
SIDE EFFECTS—HORMONAL METHODS

Nausea and vomiting. Following treatment with combined estrogen-progestin ECPs, nausea occurs in about 50% of women, and vomiting in about 20%. These side effects are about half as common following treatment with progestin-only ECPs.[65] Other reported complaints include fatigue, breast tenderness, headache, abdominal pain, and dizziness. Side effects subside within a day or two after treatment is completed. Routine use of the anti-nausea medication meclizine 1 hour before the first ECP dose may help reduce nausea and vomiting.[74]

There is no research to indicate whether it is necessary to repeat the ECP dose if the woman vomits within 2 hours after taking ECPs. Some practitioners take the view that a replacement dose should be given orally, or in the opinion of some, vaginally to prevent the tablets from being vomited a second time. Other providers, believing that nausea and vomiting are evidence of an estrogen-mediated effect on the central nervous system and thus of absorption of the drugs, conclude that a replacement dose is not necessary unless an ECP tablet is visible in the vomitus.

Ectopic pregnancy. No evidence suggests that ECP treatment is associated with an increased risk of ectopic pregnancy. However, no studies have focused specifically on this issue and ectopic pregnancy can occur following ECP treatment.[75,76] This possibility must be kept in mind whenever a treatment failure occurs.

Menstrual changes. ECPs can cause spotting or change the amount, duration, and timing of the next menstrual period. In most cases this effect is minor, and menstruation occurs a few days earlier or later than expected. If the delay in the onset of the menstrual period is greater than 7 days, consider the possibility of pregnancy. Menstrual cycle changes following progestin-only emergency treatment are similar to those seen after the combined estrogen-progestin regimen.[65]

SIDE EFFECTS—COPPER-RELEASING IUD

Side effects after emergency insertion of an IUD are similar to those seen after routine insertion at other times and include abdominal discomfort and vaginal bleeding or spotting. (See Chapter 21 on Intrauterine Devices.)

CAUTIONS

There are no evidence-based medical contraindications to the use of ECPs, with the exception of pregnancy.[28,29,77,78] The reason ECPs should not be used in pregnancy is not because they are thought to be harmful, but because they are ineffective. The advantages of ECP use generally outweigh the theoretical risks even for women who have one or more contraindications to the ongoing use of combined oral contraceptives, such as a history of heart disease, acute focal migraine, or severe liver disease. Use of progestin-only emergency treatment, however, may be preferable to use of combined estrogen and progestin ECPs for a woman who has a history of thromboembolic disease and wishes to be treated.

Few adverse events have been reported for women using emergency contraception. The Committee on Safety of Medicines in the United Kingdom reviewed all problems reported during the first 13 years of use of the combination estrogen-progestin ECP product available there (PC4) and found 61 pregnancies, 3 cases of venous thrombosis (including one death) and 3 cerebrovascular disorder cases among 4 million uses. The Committee further concluded that none of the 6 serious cases could be definitely linked to ECP use because of the significant time delay in their onset.[52]

In the United States, the labeling for Plan B includes three contraindications: pregnancy, hypersensitivity to any component of the product, or undiagnosed abnormal genital bleeding.

Women who are fully breastfeeding and amenorrheic have little risk of pregnancy during the first 6 weeks postpartum. Thereafter, initiation of progestin-only oral contraceptives is recommended without caution,[78] and use of progestin-only ECPs is not contraindicated.[59] Progestin from pills taken by the mother does appear at low levels in breast milk (1–6% of the maternal serum level), but no adverse effects on the quality or quantity of milk, or on the infant, have been identified.[59] Ongoing use of contraceptive pills containing estrogen is recommended only with caution for breastfeeding women from 6 weeks through 6 months postpartum. During this interval, if emergency contraception is needed, use of a progestin-only option may be preferable to a combined estrogen and progestin product.

Medication for epilepsy such as phenytoin, or for treatment of tuberculosis (rifampin) could theoretically reduce the effectiveness of ECPs. Whether treatment effectiveness with combined or progestin-only ECPs is actually reduced, however, is not known. No significant interactions have been found with concurrent use of other antibiotics.[59]

Eligibility criteria and contraindications for emergency insertion of an IUD are the same as for insertion at other times. (See Chapter 21.) A particular concern is the risk of pelvic inflammatory disease, particularly in women requesting emergency contraception after unprotected intercourse with a new sexual partner and in victims of sexual assault, when the risk of STI may be high.

PROVIDING EMERGENCY CONTRACEPTION

If progestin-only ECPs are immediately available, providing this option is preferable to providing combined estrogen-progestin ECP treatment. There is evidence that the progestin-only option is more effective and that the incidence of nausea and vomiting is significantly lower.[65] Availability, however, is an important consideration, because treatment may be most effective when initiated promptly.[79]

About half of the women who request emergency contraception have not used contraception, 35% experienced a problem with a condom or other barrier method, and the remaining 10% experienced failed coitus interruptus, were raped, or missed oral contraceptive pills (Table 12-2). Although women who request emergency contraception come from all age groups and walks of life, the typical user is young (15 to 25 years of age), single, and nulliparous.

Although pregnancy can result from intercourse only during the fertile phase of the cycle, any woman requesting emergency contraception after unprotected intercourse should be offered treatment unless there are sound medical grounds for not doing so. For example, a woman may present more than 72 hours (the currently labeled time window for ECPs) after unprotected intercourse. In this case, offering ECPs should be considered:

Table 12-2 Reasons for requesting emergency contraception, selected studies

		Reason		
Reference	Number	No Method Used	Barrier Method Failed	Other[a]
Tully, 1983[83]	511	52%	34%	14%
Hoffmann, 1983[84]	737	46%	43%	11%
Bagshaw et. al., 1988[85]	1,200	57%	32%	11%
Kane et. al., 1989[86]	909	67%	25%	8%
Roberts et. al., 1995[87]	596	45%	48%	7%
Total	3,953	**55%**	**35%**	**10%**

Notes:

[a] Missed pill(s), vomiting of pills, failed coitus interruptus, rape, etc.

treatment effectiveness through 120 hours has been documented.[12,69,70] Unless the woman is already pregnant and has a positive pregnancy test, it is also illogical to withhold treatment in situations involving more than one unprotected coital exposure or exposure on a low-risk day. In reviewing the cycle day when exposure occurred, you may determine whether the risk of pregnancy is likely to be high or low, but what matters most is how the woman feels about her risk, no matter whether it is likely to be high or low. Also, it is important to remember that determining pregnancy risk is not always straightforward. The risk is low except for the 5 days just before ovulation and on the day of ovulation (see Figure 12-2, graph 1).[80] The problem is that neither the woman nor her clinician is likely to know for sure which day ovulation occurs. What will be known is menstrual period dates. Plotting pregnancy probability versus menstrual period dates (see Figure 12-2, graph 2) shows that late (or early) ovulation is common enough that pregnancy risk is above 1% beginning as early as cycle day 7 and continuing until at least day 39.[80]

COUNSELING

In counseling women who seek emergency contraceptive treatment, remember this is often a difficult and stressful situation. Be respectful of the woman and responsive to her needs. Explain reporting requirements for statutory rape if applicable, and otherwise reassure the woman that all information will be kept confidential. Be as supportive as possible of the woman's choices and refrain from making judgmental comments or indicating disapproval through body language or facial expressions. Supportive attitudes will help improve compliance and set the stage for effective follow-up counseling about regular contraceptive use and prevention of STI.[81]

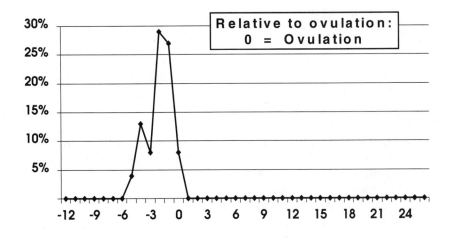

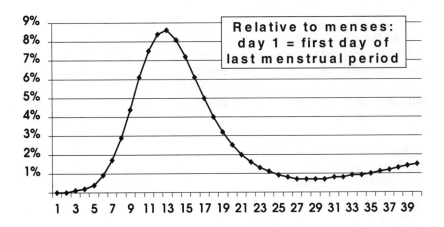

Source: adapted from Wilcox et al. (2001).[80]

Figure 12-2 Pregnancy probability by cycle day

After unprotected intercourse, some women may feel particularly anxious about becoming pregnant and missing the 120-hour window of opportunity for ECPs. They may feel embarrassed about failing to use regular contraception effectively. Rape survivors will feel traumatized. Women may be very concerned about possible infection, especially in cases of rape. Counsel women and provide STI diagnostic services (or referrals) and information about preventive measures. Women must understand that emergency contraception offers no protection against STIs, including infection with the human immunodeficiency virus (HIV). Additional emergency treatment measures may be needed. (See Chapter 7 on HIV/AIDS and Reproductive Health and Chapter 8 on Reproductive Tract Infections.)

Women who would not plan to have an abortion in case of treatment failure can be reassured that pregnancies occurring despite treatment do not have an increased risk of adverse outcome.

OTHER ISSUES

Frequent use. Emphasize that ECPs are for emergency use only. They are not recommended for routine use because they are less effective than regular contraceptives. (Note: Although not recommended, repeated ECP use is not known to pose health risks to users and concern about risk is not a logical reason for denying women access to treatment.)

Use after 72 hours. Although most studies of ECP treatment have specified treatment within 72 hours, more recent studies have demonstrated efficacy of giving ECPs up to 120 hours after unprotected intercourse.[12,69,70]

Use after multiple acts of unprotected intercourse. If more than 120 hours have elapsed since the time of the first unprotected exposure, ECPs may be less effective in preventing pregnancy that resulted from the first exposure. Providing ECPs, however, would not be expected to disrupt or harm subsequent pregnancy development and would reduce the risk that pregnancy would result from later exposures that did occur within the preceding 120 hours.

Ongoing contraception refused. Women requesting emergency contraception should be offered information and services for regular contraception. Not all of them, however, will want contraceptive counseling. Thus, while counseling about regular contraceptives is recommended, it should not be a prerequisite for providing emergency treatment. If the reason for requesting emergency contraception is that the regular contraceptive method failed, discuss the reasons for failure and how it can be prevented in the future.

BEFORE PROVIDING EMERGENCY CONTRACEPTIVE TREATMENT

Exclude the possibility that a woman may already be pregnant: assess the date of the last menstrual period and whether it was normal. Establish the time of the first episode of unprotected intercourse to determine whether a pregnancy test before treatment may be indicated, and assess the time of the most recent episode of unprotected intercourse to ensure she is within the treatment time frame (120 hours for ECPs or insertion of a copper-releasing IUD). Ask if the woman is currently using a regular method of contraception. This question can be a good starting point for a discussion of regular contraceptive use and how to use methods correctly.

Make certain the woman does not want to become pregnant and understands there is still a chance of pregnancy even after treatment. Describe common side effects. Advance counseling about possible side effects helps women know what to expect and may lead to greater tolerance. If the patient will be using a combined estrogen-progestin ECP option, provide meclizine or another anti-nausea medication or recommend an over-the-counter product to be taken 1 hour before starting ECP treatment (see Table 12-3).

Table 12-3 Anti-nausea treatment options

Drug	Dose	Timing of Administration
Non-prescription Drugs		
Meclizine hydrochloride (Dramamine II, Bonine)	One or two 25 mg tablets	1 hour before first ECP dose; repeat if needed in 24 hours
Diphenhydramine Hydrochloride (Benadryl)	One or two 25 mg tablets	1 hour before first ECP dose; repeat as needed every 4-6 hours
Dimenhydrinate (Dramamine)	One or two 50 mg tablets or 4-8 teaspoons liquid	30 minutes to 1 hour before first ECP dose; repeat as needed every 4–6 hours
Cyclizine hydrochloride (Marezine)	One 50 mg tablet	30 minutes before first ECP dose; repeat as needed every 4–6 hours
Prescription Drugs		
Meclizine hydrochloride (Antivert)	One or two 25 mg tablets	1 hour before first ECP dose; repeat if needed in 24 hours
Trimethobenzamide hydrochloride (Tigan)	One 250 mg tablet or 200 mg suppository	1 hour before first ECP dose; repeat as needed every 6–8 hours
Promethazine hydrochloride (Phenergan)	One 25 mg tablet or suppository	30 minutes to 1 hour before first ECP dose; repeat as needed every 8–12 hours

Source: Wells et al. (1997) with permission.[77]

A pregnancy test may be helpful if there is some doubt about whether she is already pregnant from intercourse in the past (more than 1 week earlier). If the test is positive, ECP treatment will not be effective. A negative test, however, *does not mean* that ECPs are unnecessary. Rather, this is the situation when ECPs *can* work to reduce the risk of pregnancy. Unless there is a doubt about pregnancy from intercourse more than 1 week ago, it makes more sense to use a pregnancy test only after the next period fails to come on time.[82]

Make sure the woman understands that ECPs will not protect her from pregnancy if she engages in unprotected intercourse in the days or weeks following treatment. This is a common misperception. If the woman wishes to use combined oral contraceptives as an ongoing method, she can take one oral contraceptive tablet the day after emergency treatment is completed and then continue with daily pills, as if the ECP treatment days had been the beginning of a new pill cycle. If the woman does not want to continue using oral contraceptives, but needs contraceptive protection, she can begin a 1-month or 3-month injectable, the vaginal contraceptive ring, or patches immediately after ECP treatment or she can use a barrier method, such as condoms, for the remainder of her cycle. A different contraceptive method such as an IUD can be initiated at the beginning of her next cycle (see Table 12-4).

Table 12-4 Initiating ongoing contraception after ECP use

Because ECPs can delay ovulation, a woman could be at risk of pregnancy in the first few days after treatment. Women should use an effective method of contraception for the remainder of the treatment cycle and thereafter.

Method	When to Initiate
Condom	Can be used immediately
Diaphragm	Can be used immediately
Spermicide	Can be used immediately
Oral Contraceptive (OC)	Initiate a new pack, either according to manufacturer's instructions after beginning the next menstrual cycle, or begin taking one OC tablet daily the day after ECP treatment is completed. Women using Levlen, Levora, Lo/Ovral, Low-Ogestrel, Nordette, or Portia for emergency contraception can continue taking one pill per day from the same pack. Women using other brands can begin a new pack the day after ECP treatment is completed.
Progestin-only Minipills (POP)	Initiate a new pack, either according to manufacturer's instructions after beginning the next menstrual cycle, or begin taking one POP tablet daily the day after ECP treatment is completed. Use condoms in addition to POPs for the first 2 days of the POP pack. Be sure to have a pregnancy test if you do not have a menstrual period within the first three weeks after taking ECPs.
One-Month Injectable	Initiate the day after ECP treatment is completed or within 7 days of beginning the next menstrual period*
Vaginal Ring Contraception	Initiate the day after ECP treatment is completed or within 5 days of beginning the next menstrual period; use condoms along with the ring for the first 2 days
Contraceptive Patch	Initiate the day after ECP treatment is completed or within 5 days of beginning the next menstrual period; use condoms along with the patch for the first 2 days
Three-Month Injectable	Initiate the day after ECP treatment is completed or within 7 days of beginning the next menstrual period*
Implants	Initiate within 7 days of beginning the next menstrual period
Intrauterine Device (IUD)	Initiate during the next menstrual period (If the patient intends to use an IUD for ongoing contraception, consider inserting a copper-releasing IUD for emergency contraception treatment.)
Fertility Awareness	Initiate after onset of the next normal menstrual period and after the patient has been trained in using the method
Sterilization	Perform the operation any time after beginning the next menstrual period

Source: adapted from Wells et al. (1997) with permission.[77]

* If a woman goes to a clinician for ECPs, she can get the injectable at that time.

EMERGENCY CONTRACEPTION TREATMENT REGIMENS

Emergency contraceptive pills. For maximum effectiveness, ECP treatment should be started as soon as possible after unprotected intercourse, and within 120 hours. Progestin-only ECP treatment (two tablets of 750 mcg levonorgestrel taken together as one dose) is more effective and causes significantly less nausea and vomiting than does treatment with combined estrogen-progestin ECP options (100–120 mcg ethinyl estradiol and 500–600 mcg levonorgestrel in each dose).

Combined estrogen-progestin treatment involves two doses taken 12 hours apart. If necessary, timing for the second dose can be adjusted to avoid a middle of the night dose. Drugs and doses are shown in Table 12-1.

Intrauterine devices. The copper-bearing IUD as an emergency contraceptive method can be inserted up to 5 days after ovulation. Thus, if a woman had unprotected intercourse 3 days before the day ovulation is estimated to have occurred in that cycle, the IUD could, in principle, be inserted up to 8 days after the intercourse. Most family planning providers, however, limit insertion to the first 5 days after intercourse because it is difficult to estimate reliably the day of ovulation. If emergency IUD insertion is planned, but cannot be carried out immediately, provide ECP treatment when the woman is initially evaluated. Even if the ECP effectiveness is not optimal because of an interval longer than 72 hours since unprotected intercourse, it may help reduce pregnancy risk. If IUD insertion is subsequently not feasible, or does not occur, the patient will at least have had the possible benefit of ECP treatment.

AFTER PROVIDING EMERGENCY CONTRACEPTIVE TREATMENT

If the woman has already adopted a method of contraception for regular use and wishes to continue using this method, no follow-up is needed unless she does not have a normal menstrual period within 3 weeks, suspects she may be pregnant, or has other reasons for concern. If a follow-up appointment is indicated, be sure to record information about the woman's menstrual periods and any other bleeding she has experienced to verify that she is not pregnant. If there is any doubt, perform a pregnancy test. Also, review her contraceptive options as appropriate and provide a method if she has not already initiated one.

If emergency contraception has failed and the woman is pregnant, advise her of the possible options and provide appropriate referral information. If she decides to continue the pregnancy, reassure her there is no evidence of any teratogenic effect following the use of ECPs. Pregnancy following emergency insertion of a copper IUD should be managed the same way as IUD-associated pregnancy following routine insertion (see Chapter 21).

ESTABLISHING EMERGENCY CONTRACEPTIVE SERVICES

Additional information and materials that may be of help in establishing emergency contraception services are available from the following sources:

- Information about emergency contraception method options and access to the U.S. directory of providers via internet: http://www.NOT-2-LATE.com, or http://ec.princeton.edu.
- Toll-free telephone information about method options and referral to providers listed in the directory nearest the caller's telephone area code: call 1-888-NOT-2-LATE.
- Information about enrolling as a provider in the U.S. directory: http://ec.princeton.edu/questions/ecsignup.html.
- Copy of the Food and Drug Administration Federal Register notice regarding emergency contraception: request document number 0265 at 1-800-342-2722.
- *Emergency Contraceptive Pills: Common Legal Questions about Prescribing, Dispensing, Repackaging, and Advertising*: order from the Center for Reproductive Rights, 120 Wall Street, New York, NY 10005.
- Information for pharmacists interested in provision of emergency contraception through collaborative practice agreements, and CME accredited, on-line self-instruction: American Pharmaceutical Association, 2215 Constitution Avenue NW, Washington, D.C. 20037-2985; 1-800-237-APhA; http://www.aphanet.org.
- Resource Packet for Health Care Providers and Programme Managers (in English and Spanish): Consortium for Emergency Contraception: order from Consortium Coordinator, P.O. Box 13950, Research Triangle Park, Durham, NC 27709; email: cecinfo@fhi.org.

∎NSTRUCTIONS FOR USING EMERGENCY CONTRACEPTION

Instructions for women who have emergency insertion of an IUD are the same as for IUD insertion at other times (see Chapter 21 on Intrauterine Devices).

Women provided with ECPs should receive medication labeling that identifies the specific product prescribed and the number of tablets needed for each dose (see Table 12-1). The following instructions can be given to women to ensure correct use. For progestin-only ECP treatment, omit the anti-nausea medication instruction.

1. **If you are taking progestin-only ECPs, swallow the two tablets as one dose as soon as possible within 120 hours after unprotected sex. Do not take any extra pills.** More pills will not decrease the risk of pregnancy any further.

2. **If you are taking combined estrogen-progestin ECPs, swallow the first dose as soon as possible within 120 hours after unprotected sex. Do not take any extra pills.** More pills will not decrease the risk of pregnancy any further but may increase the risk of nausea, possibly causing you to vomit.

   Swallow the second dose 12 hours after taking the first dose. If necessary, you can delay the second dose by a few hours to avoid having to take your second dose in the middle of the night.

   Take anti-nausea medication 1 hour before the first dose. About one-half of women who use combined ECPs have temporary nausea. It is usually mild and should stop in a day or so. If you vomit within 2 hours after taking a dose, call your clinician. You may need to repeat a dose.

3. **If your period does not start within 3 weeks, see your clinician for an exam and pregnancy test.** Your next period may start a few days earlier or later than usual. If you think you may be pregnant, see your clinician at once, whether or not you plan to continue the pregnancy.

4. **Do not have unprotected intercourse in the days or weeks following treatment.** ECPs will not protect you from pregnancy if you do so. Continue or start taking normal birth control pills, one tablet daily, or use a vaginal ring, contraceptive patches, or a barrier method such as a condom for the remainder of your cycle. After your menstrual period, continue using pills, patches, rings, or condoms, or begin another method of contraception.

5. As soon as you possibly can, **begin using a method of birth control** you will be able to use on an ongoing basis. Emergency contraceptive pills **are not as effective** as other forms of contraception. They are meant for one-time, emergency protection. Discuss with your clinician which method may suit you best and when you can start it.

REFERENCES

1. Anonymous. Consensus statement on emergency contraception. Contraception 1995;52(4):211-213.
2. Morris JM, Van Wagenen G. Compounds interfering with ovum implantation and development. 3. The role of estrogens. Am J Obstet Gynecol 1966;96(6):804-815.
3. Van Look PF, von Hertzen H. Emergency contraception. BMJ 1993;49(1):158-170.
4. Yuzpe AA, Lancee WJ. Ethinylestradiol and dl-norgestrel as a postcoital contraceptive. Fertil Steril 1977;28(9):932-936.
5. Yuzpe AA, Smith RP, Rademaker AW. A multicenter clinical investigation employing ethinyl estradiol combined with dl-norgestrel as postcoital contraceptive agent. Fertil Steril 1982;37(4):508-513.
6. Ellertson C, Webb A, Blanchard K, et al. Modifying the Yuzpe regimen of emergency contraception: A multi-center randomized, controlled trial. Obstet Gynecol 2003;101(6):1160-1167.

7. Lei H, Hu Z-Y. The mechanisms of action of vacation pills. In: Chang C, Griffin D, Woolman A, eds. Recent advances in fertility regulation: proceedings of a Symposium organized by the Ministry of Public Health of the People's Republic of China, and the World Health Organization's Special Programme of Research, Development and Research Training in Human Reproduction: Beijing, 2-5 September, 1980. Geneva: Atar; 1981.

8. Task Force on Post-Ovulatory Methods for Fertility Regulation. Efficacy and side effects of immediate postcoital levonorgestrel used repeatedly for contraception. Contraception 2000;61(5):303-308.

9. Van Look PF, von Hertzen H. Clinical uses of antiprogestogens. Hum Reprod Update 1995;1(1):19-34.

10. Van Look F. Emergency contraception: the Cinderella of family planning. In: Rodríguez-Armas O, Hédon B, Daya S, eds. Infertility and contraception: a textbook for clinical practice. New York: Parthenon; 1998:238.

11. Task Force on Postovulatory Methods of Fertility Regulation. Comparison of three single doses of mifepristone as emergency contraception: a randomised trial. Lancet 1999;353(9154):697-702.

12. von Hertzen H, Piaggio G, Ding J, et al. Low dose mifepristone and two regimens of levonorgestrel for emergency contraception: a WHO multicentre randomised trial. Lancet 2002;360(9348):1803-1810.

13. Glasier A, Thong KJ, Dewar M, Mackie M, Baird DT. Mifepristone (RU 486) compared with high-dose estrogen and progestogen for emergency postcoital contraception. N Engl J Med 1992;327(15):1041-1044.

14. Webb AM, Russell J, Elstein M. Comparison of Yuzpe regimen, danazol, and mifepristone (RU486) in oral postcoital contraception. BMJ (Clinical Research Ed.) 1992;305(6859):927-931.

15. Morris JM, Van Wagenen G. Postcoital oral contraception. In: Hankinson R, Kleinman R, Esckstein P, Romero H, eds. Proceedings of the Eighth International Conference of the International Planned Parenthood Federation, April 9-15, 1967. Santiago, Chile and London: International Planned Parenthood Federation; 1967.

16. Van Look F. Postcoital contraception: a cover-up story. In: Diczfalusy E, Bygdeman M, eds. Fertility regulation today and tomorrow. Vol 36. New York: Raven Press; 1987.

17. Zuliani G, Colombo UF, Molla R. Hormonal postcoital contraception with an ethinylestradiol-norgestrel combination and two danazol regimens. Europ J Obstet Gynecol Reprod Biology 1990;37(3):253-260.

18. Trussell J, Koenig J, Ellertson C, Stewart F. Preventing unintended pregnancy: the cost-effectiveness of three methods of emergency contraception. Am J Publ Health 1997;87(6):932-937.

19. Smugar SS, Spina BJ, Merz JF. Informed consent for emergency contraception: variability in hospital care of rape victims. Am J Publ Health 2000;90(9):1372-1376.

20. Goldenring JM, Allred G. Post-rape care in hospital emergency rooms. Am J Publ Health 2001;91(8):1169-1170.

21. Stewart FH, Trussell J. Prevention of pregnancy resulting from rape: a neglected preventive health measure. Am J Prevent Med 2000;19(4):228-229.

22. Shelton JD. Repeat emergency contraception: facing our fears. Contraception 2002;66(1):15-17.

23. Glasier A, Baird D. The effects of self-administering emergency contraception. N Engl J Med 1998;339(1):1-4.

24. Raine T, Harper C, Leon K, Darney P. Emergency contraception: advance provision in a young, high-risk clinic population. Obstet Gynecol 2000;96(1):1-7.

25. Ellertson C, Ambardekar S, Hedley A, Coyaji K, Trussell J, Blanchard K. Emergency contraception: randomized comparison of advance provision and information only. Obstet Gynecol 2001;98(4):570-575.

26. Kosunen E, Sihvo S, Hemminki E. Knowledge and use of hormonal emergency contraception in Finland. Contraception 1997;55(3):153-157.

27. Food and Drug Administration. Prescription drug products; certain combined oral contraceptives for use as postcoital emergency contraception: Food and Drug Administration; 1997. Report Number 62.
28. ACOG. Emergency oral contraception. Washington DC: The American College of Obstetricians and Gynecologists; 1996. ACOG Practice Patterns #3.
29. ACOG. Emergency oral contraception. Washington DC: American College of Obstetricians and Gynecologists; 2001. Report Number 25.
30. International Planned Parenthood Federation (IPPF). IMAP statement on emergency contraception. IPPF Medical Bulletin. 2000;34(3).
31. Kubba A, Wilkinson C. Emergency contraception update. Br J Fam Plann 1998; 23(4):135-137.
32. World Health Organization. The use of essential drugs. Model list of essential drugs (eleventh list). Ninth report of the WHO Expert Committee. Geneva: World Health Organization, 2000. (WHO Technical Report Series No. 895).
33. Kring T. Emergency contraception. Washington DC: Department of Health and Human Services, Office of Population Affairs; 1997. Report Number 97-2.
34. Beckman LJ, Harvey SM, Sherman CA, Petitti DB. Changes in providers' views and practices about emergency contraception with education. Obstet Gynecol 2001;97(6):942-946.
35. Downing D. Helping pharmacists determine their role in emergency contraception. U.S. Pharmacist 2000;supplement.
36. Harrison-Woolrych M, Howe J, Smith C. Improving access to emergency contraception. BMJ (Clinical Research Ed.) 2001;322(7280):186-187.
37. Gold MA. Prescribing and managing oral contraceptive pills and emergency contraception for adolescents. Pediatr Clin N Am 1999;46(4):695-718.
38. Grimes DA. Emergency contraception and fire extinguishers: a prevention paradox. Am J Obstet Gynecol 2002;187(6):1536-1538.
39. Grimes DA, Raymond EG, Scott Jones B. Emergency contraception over-the-counter: the medical and legal imperatives. Obstet Gynecol 2001;98(1):151-155.
40. Croxatto HB, Devoto L, Durand M, et al. Mechanism of action of hormonal preparations used for emergency contraception: a review of the literature. Contraception 2001;63(3):111-121.
41. ACOG. Obstetric-gynecologic terminology, with section on neonatology and glossary of congenital anomalies. Philadelphia, Pa: F.A. Davis Company; 1972.
42. OPRR. Protection of Human Subjects: OPRR; March 8 1983. Report Number 45CFR 46.
43. Ling WY, Robichaud A, Zayid I, Wrixon W, MacLeod SC. Mode of action of DL-norgestrel and ethinylestradiol combination in postcoital contraception. Fertil Steril 1979;32(3):297-302.
44. Rowlands S, Kubba AA, Guillebaud J, Bounds W. A possible mechanism of action of danazol and an ethinylestradiol/norgestrel combination used as postcoital contraceptive agents. Contraception 1986;33(6):539-545.
45. Swahn ML, Westlund P, Johannisson E, Bygdeman M. Effect of post-coital contraceptive methods on the endometrium and the menstrual cycle. Acta Obstetricia et Gynecologica Scandinavica 1996;75(8):738-744.
46. Hapangama D, Glasier AF, Baird DT. The effects of peri-ovulatory administration of levonorgestrel on the menstrual cycle. Contraception 2001;63(3):123-129.
47. Yuzpe AA, Thurlow HJ, Ramzy I, Leyshon JI. Post coital contraception—A pilot study. J Reprod Med 1974;13(2):53-58.
48. Ling WY, Wrixon W, Zayid I, Acorn T, Popat R, Wilson E. Mode of action of dl-norgestrel and ethinylestradiol combination in postcoital contraception. II. Effect of postovulatory administration on ovarian function and endometrium. Fertil Steril 1983;39:292-297.
49. Kubba AA, White JO, Guillebaud J, Elder MG. The biochemistry of human endometrium after two regimens of postcoital contraception: a dl-norgestrel/ethinylestradiol combination or danazol. Fertil Steril 1986;45(4):512-516.

50. Taskin O, Brown RW, Young DC, Poindexter AN, Wiehle RD. High doses of oral contraceptives do not alter endometrial alpha 1 and alpha v beta 3 integrins in the late implantation window. Fert Steril 1994;61(5):850-855.
51. Raymond EG, Lovely LP, Chen-Mok M, Seppälä M, Kurman RJ, Lessey BA. Effect of the Yuzpe regimen of emergency contraception on markers of endometrial receptivity. Hum Reprod 2000;15(11):2351-2355.
52. Glasier A. Emergency postcoital contraception. N Engl J Med 1997;337(15):1058-1064.
53. Kesseru E, Garmendia F, Westphal N, Parada J. The hormonal and peripheral effects of d-norgestrel in postcoital contraception. Contraception 1974;10(4):411-424.
54. Trussell J, Raymond EG. Statistical evidence about the mechanism of action of the Yuzpe regimen of emergency contraception. Obstet Gynecol 1999;93(5 Pt 2):872-876.
55. ACOG. Statement on contraceptive methods. Washington DC: The American College of Obstetricians and Gynecologists; July 1998.
56. Trussell J, Ellertson C, Dorflinger L. Effectiveness of the Yuzpe regimen of emergency contraception by cycle day of intercourse: implications for mechanism of action. Contraception 2003;67(3):167-171.
57. Trussell J, Ellertson C. Efficacy of emergency contraception. Fertility Control Reviews 1995;4:8–11.
58. Zhou L, Xiao B. Emergency contraception with Multiload Cu-375 SL IUD: a multicenter clinical trial. Contraception 2001;64(2):107-112.
59. Women's Capital Corporation. Plan B package insert: information for providers and clients. Washington DC: Women's Capital Corporation; 1999.
60. Trussell J, Rodríguez G, Ellertson C. New estimates of the effectiveness of the Yuzpe regimen of emergency contraception. Contraception 1998;57(6):363-369.
61. Trussell J, Rodríguez G, Ellertson C. Updated estimates of the effectiveness of the Yuzpe regimen of emergency contraception. Contraception 1999;59(3):147-151.
62. Trussell J, Ellertson C, Rodríguez G. The Yuzpe regimen of emergency contraception: how long after the morning after? Obstet Gynecol 1996;88(1):150-154.
63. Wilcox AJ, Weinberg CR, Baird DD. Timing of sexual intercourse in relation to ovulation. Effects on the probability of conception, survival of the pregnancy, and sex of the baby. N Engl J Med 1995;333(23):1517-1521.
64. Trussell J, Ellertson C, von Hertzen H, et al. Estimating the effectiveness of emergency contraceptive pills. Contraception 2003;67(4):259-265.
65. Task Force on Postovulatory Methods of Fertility Regulation. Randomised controlled trial of levonorgestrel versus the Yuzpe regimen of combined oral contraceptives for emergency contraception. Lancet 1998;352(9126):428-433.
66. Piaggio G, von Hertzen H, Grimes DA, Van Look PF. Timing of emergency contraception with levonorgestrel or the Yuzpe regimen. Task Force on Postovulatory Methods of Fertility Regulation. Lancet. 1999;353(9154):721.
67. Webb A. Emergency contraception. Fertility Control Review 1995;4:3-7.
68. Grou F, Rodrigues I. The morning-after pill--how long after? Am J Obstet Gynecol 1994;171(6):1529-1534.
69. Rodrigues I, Grou F, Joly J. Effectiveness of emergency contraceptive pills between 72 and 120 hours after unprotected sexual intercourse. Am J Obstet Gynecol 2001;184(4):531-537.
70. Ellertson C EM, Evans M, Ferden S, Leadbetter C, Spears A, Johnstone K, Trussell J. Extending the time limit for starting the Yuzpe regimen of emergency contraception to 120 hours. Obstet Gynecol 2003;101:1168-1171.
71. Arowojolu AO, Okewole IA, Adekunle AO. Comparative evaluation of the effectiveness and safety of two regimens of levonorgestrel for emergency contraception in Nigerians. Contraception 2002;66(4):269-273.
72. Feldhaus KM. A 21st-century challenge: improving the care of the sexual assault victim. Ann Emerg Med 2002;39(6):653-655.
73. WHO. Selected Practice Recommendations for Contraceptive Use. Geneva: WHO; 2002.

74. Raymond EG, Creinin MD, Barnhart KT, Lovvorn AE, Rountree RW, Trussell J. Meclizine for prevention of nausea associated with use of emergency contraceptive pills: a randomized trial. Obstet Gynecol 2000;95(2):271-277.
75. Nielsen CL, Miller L. Ectopic gestation following emergency contraceptive pill administration. Contraception 2000;62(5):275-276.
76. Sheffer-Mimouni G. Ectopic pregnancies following emergency levonorgestrel contraception. Contraception 2003;67:267-269.
77. Wells E, Crook B, Muller N. Emergency contraception: a resource manual for providers. Seattle: Program for Appropriate Technology in Health; 1997.
78. WHO. Improving access to quality care in family planning. Medical eligibility criteria for contraceptive use. Geneva: World Health Organization; 2000.
79. Ellertson C, Blanchard K, Webb A, Bigrigg A, Haskell S. Emergency contraception. Lancet 1998;352(9138):1477.
80. Wilcox AJ, Dunson DB, Weinberg CR, Trussell J, Baird DD. Likelihood of conception with a single act of intercourse: providing benchmark rates for assessment of post-coital contraceptives. Contraception 2001;63(4):211-215.
81. Consortium for Emergency Contraception. Emergency contraceptive pills. A resource packet for health care providers and programme managers: Welcome Md: Consortium for Emergency Contraception; 1996.
82. Grimes DA, Raymond EG. Bundling a pregnancy test with the Yuzpe regimen of emergency contraception. Obstet Gynecol 1999;94(3):471-473.
83. Tully B. Post-coital contraception--a study. Br J Fam Plann 1983;8:119-124.
84. Hoffmann K. Postcoital contraception: experiences with ethinyloestradiol/norgestrel and levonorgestrel only. In: Harrison R, Bonnar J, Thompson W, eds. Fertil Steril. The proceedings of the XIth World Congress on Fertility and Sterility, Dublin, June 1983, held under the auspices of the International Federation of Fertility Societies. Lancaster UK: MTP Press; 1983.
85. Bagshaw SN, Edwards D, Tucker AK. Ethinyl oestradiol and D-norgestrel is an effective emergency postcoital contraceptive: a report of its use in 1,200 patients in a family planning clinic. Austral NZ J Obstet Gynaecol 1988;28(2):137-140.
86. Kane LA, Sparrow MJ. Postcoital contraception: a family planning study. NZ Med 1989;102(865):151-153.
87. Roberts RN, Moohan JM, McNeil S, Lyons MS. Audit of an emergency contraception service. Br J Fam Plann 1995;21:22-25.

LATE REFERENCES

88. Croxatto HB, Fuentalba B, Brache V, Salvatierra AM, Alvarez F, Massai R, Cochon L, Faundes A. Effects of the Yuzpe regimen, given during the follicular phase, on ovarian function. Contraception 2002;65:121-128.
89. Durand M, del Carmen Cravioto M, Raymond EG, Durán-Sánchez O, De la Luz Cruz-Hinojosa L, Castell-Rodriguez A, Schiavon R, Larrea F. On the mechanisms of action of short-term levonorgestrel administration in emergency contraception. Contraception 2001;64:227-234.
90. Marions L, Hultenby K, Lindell I, Sun X, Ståbi B, Gemzell Danielsson K. Emergency contraception with mifepristone and levonorgestrel: mechanism of action. Obstet Gynecol 2002;100:65-71.
91. Ling WY, Wrixon W, Acorn T, Wilson E, Collins J. Mode of action of dl-norgestrel and ethinylestradiol combination in postcoital contraception. III. Effect of preovulatory administration following the luteinizing hormone surge on ovarian steroidogenesis. Fertil Steril 1983;40:631-636.

Abstinence and the Range of Sexual Expression

Deborah Kowal, MA, PA

- Abstinence can be primary or secondary. Primary abstainers have not had a sexual experience with another person. Secondary abstainers are sexually experienced persons who become sexually inactive.
- Abstinence, or celibacy, may be voluntary or involuntary. Many abstainers engage in other forms of sexual intimacy.
- The care provider's role is one of support: encouraging the use of abstinence when it is chosen or, when it is involuntary, counseling about relationships or other forms of sexual expression.

Historically, sexual abstinence has probably been the single most important factor in curtailing human fertility.[1] In the United States of the 21st century, however, there is a lack of consensus about what abstinence does, and does not, entail.[2] Some people define abstinence as refraining from all sexual behavior, including masturbation. Some people define abstinence as refraining from sexual behavior involving genital contact. Others define it as refraining from penetrative sexual practices. Still others would offer different definitions.

Asking clients what they define as abstinence is an important question with clinical implications. In a study of high-school students who consider themselves virgins, 30% had engaged in heterosexual masturbation of or by a partner, 9% had engaged in fellatio with ejaculation, and 10% had engaged in cunnilingus.[3] More than half (59%) of college undergraduates in another study responded that oral-genital contact did not constitute having "had sex" with a partner, and 19% said the same about penile-anal intercourse.[4]

While allowing that individuals have personal definitions regarding what is meant by abstinence, the authors of *Contraceptive Technology* use situational definitions. For purposes of contraception, abstinence is defined as refraining from penile-vaginal intercourse. For purposes of protection from sexually transmitted infections (STIs), abstinence is defined as refraining from those acts that permit exposure to infectious lesions or secretions.

Abstinence can be primary or secondary. Primary abstainers have never had sexual intercourse with another person. Secondary abstainers are sexually experienced but for various reasons are no longer engaging in behaviors they consider as "having sex."

Primary abstinence is not uncommon among young persons. Among never-married adolescent men age 15 to 19 years, 45% report never having had sexual intercourse.[5] Among adolescent women age 15 to 19 years, half report never having had voluntary sexual intercourse since menarche, according to the 1995 National Survey of Family Growth (NSFG).[6] After the teen years, the percentage of women who have not had sexual intercourse drops dramatically to 12% and below (Table 13-1).

Table 13-1 Percentage of women age 15-44 who report having had no sexual intercourse in the 3 months prior to NSFG interview, 1995

	Age						
	15–44	15–19	20–24	25–29	30–34	35–39	40–44
No Intercourse in 3 Months Before Interview	17.1	56.9	18.9	9.9	7.6	7.6	8.2
Never had intercourse	10.9	49.8	12.1	4.2	2.7	1.4	1.4
Has had intercourse but not in 3 months before interview	6.2	7.1	6.8	5.7	4.9	6.2	6.8

Source: Abma et al. (1997).

About 17% of women age 15 to 44 years reported that they had not had sexual intercourse in the 3 months prior to the interview. Of these women, 11% had never had sexual intercourse and 6% had reported having had no sexual intercourse in those 3 months.[6] Whether these latter women deliberately chose to abstain, merely had a brief lapse in a relationship, or had other reasons for not having had sexual intercourse is not known.

At a number of times throughout their lives, people of all ages may become abstinent. For those who deliberately choose to abstain, your role as care provider is to support the choice of abstinence and to teach negotiation and planning skills for using abstinence effectively and safely. For those who reluctantly choose to abstain, it is important that they see abstinence as normal, common, and acceptable—and reversible.

In some cases, abstinence is involuntary.[7] These individuals may require help if they feel abstinence stems from a dysfunction. They may abstain for a range of reasons:

- Unhappiness with a relationship, or an estranged relationship
- Fear of sexually transmitted infection
- Increased age
- Presence of preschoolers
- Poor health, illness, or injury
- Pregnancy or recent childbirth

Counsel patients who abstain, whether voluntarily or involuntarily, that they are still sexual human beings, and explore with them the range of sexual expression (see next section). Because opportunities may arise for having sex and because resolve may weaken, educate all abstemious persons about the other methods of contraception and safer sex available to them, including the following:

- Effective over-the-counter products
- Prescription methods
- Emergency contraception options
- Safer-sex practices

THE RANGE OF SEXUAL EXPRESSION

Although abstinence has become associated with saying "no," viewed from another perspective, abstinence can mean saying "yes" to a number of other sexual activities. For some people, only penile penetration of the vagina equals intercourse. Most people, however, have a more expansive view of sexual expression, and other activities give them pleasure and meaning. Holding hands, kissing, massage, solo masturbation, mutual masturbation, dancing, oral-genital sex, fantasy, and erotic books and movies all fit along the sexual continuum, as do many other activities. Taste, smell, vision, and hearing may matter as much as touch for erotic pleasure. All human beings need touching—for nurture, for solace, for communication, for simple affection. Most human beings enjoy erotic touching as well, a specialized language of sexual gratification and more intimate forms of affection.

INDICATIONS FOR ABSTINENCE OR OTHER FORMS OF SEXUAL EXPRESSION

Consider discussing abstinence even with patients who currently engage in intercourse and other sexual behaviors. At some point in their lives, they may choose to become abstinent, removing themselves at least for a while from the health risks of intercourse. You can help people learn that the door between abstinence and sexual activity opens in both directions.

Contraception. When the only goal of abstinence is to avoid unwanted pregnancy, then all forms of sexual expression are available to a couple except for penis-in-vagina intercourse.

STI protection. When a goal of abstinence is to avoid STIs, then not only penile-vaginal, but also oral-genital sex, anal intercourse, and other practices that expose the partner to pre-ejaculatory fluid, semen, cervical-vaginal secretions, or blood must be reconsidered. Some couples avoid these practices altogether, and others use condoms, latex dams, or other barriers to inhibit body fluid transmission during these practices. The care provider's role is to offer factual, explicit guidance on safer-sex options. (See Chapter 7 on HIV/AIDS and Reproductive Health.)

Lack of partner. Patients may be abstinent if they lack a partner or their partner becomes celibate, for any number of reasons. The care provider can give these individuals permission to engage in auto-gratification or, if needed, refer them for counseling if they are dissatisfied with their celibacy.

Medical reasons. Some situations in which insertive sex may be ill-advised and alternatives recommended include the following:

- Known or suspected STI (also avoid other sexual practices that transmit pre-ejaculatory fluid, semen, cervical-vaginal secretions, and blood)
- Post-operative pain or tenderness, such as from episiotomy, hemorrhoidectomy, vasectomy, and other procedures
- Pelvic, vaginal, or urinary tract infection
- Gastrointestinal illness or infection
- Dyspareunia or other pelvic pain
- Undiagnosed postcoital bleeding
- Late third trimester of pregnancy, postpartum, or postabortion
- Postmyocardial infarction
- Certain disabling physical conditions
- Known or suspected allergic sensitization to a partner's semen

Sex therapy. Therapy for a variety of sexual problems may include exploration of avenues of sexual gratification other than intercourse. Temporarily forbidding intercourse takes performance pressure off couples struggling with erection difficulty, orgasm difficulty, or rapid ejaculation. (See Chapter 2 on Sexuality and Reproductive Health.)

INSTRUCTIONS FOR USING ABSTINENCE FOR CONTRACEPTION OR STI PROTECTION

1. Decide what you want to do about sex at a time when you feel clearheaded, sober, and good about yourself. If you have a partner,

decide together at a time when you feel close to each other but not sexual. For example, try talking while you take a walk and hold hands.

2. Decide in advance what sexual activities you will say "yes" to and discuss these with your partner.

3. Tell your partner, very clearly and in advance—not at the last minute—what activities you will not do.

4. Avoid high-pressure sexual situations; do not get drunk or high.

5. If you say "no," say it so it is clear that you mean it.

6. Learn more about your body and how to keep it healthy.

7. Learn about contraception and safer sex, so you will be ready if you change your mind. Always keep condoms on hand.

8. Refrain from intercourse if you do not have a contraceptive method available. Learn about emergency contraception in case you have intercourse when you did not expect it. If your health care provider does not provide emergency contraception, call 1-888-NOT-2-LATE for a listing of emergency contraception providers in your area.

Emergency Contraceptive Pills: Treatment initiated within 72 hours after unprotected intercourse reduces the risk of pregnancy by at least 75%.

REFERENCES

1. Hajnal J. European marriage patterns in perspective. In: Glass DV, Eversley DEC (eds). Population in history: essays in historical demography. London: Aldine, 1986:101.
2. Remez L. Oral sex among adolescents: is it sex or is it abstinence? Fam Plann Perspect 2000;32:298-304.
3. Schuster MA, Bell RM, Kanouse DE. The sexual practices of adolescent virgins: genital sexual activities of high school students who have never had vaginal intercourse. Am J Publ Health 1996:86:1570-1576.
4. Sanders SA, Reinisch JM. Would you say you "had sex" if ...? JAMA 1999;281:275-277.
5. Sonenstein FL, Pleck JH, Ku L, Lindberg LD, Turner CF. Changes in sexual behavior and contraception among adolescent males: 1988 and 1995. Unpublished manuscript. Washington DC: The Urban Institute, 1997.
6. Abma JC, Chandra A, Mosher WD, Peterson LS, Piccinino LJ. Fertility, family planning, and women's health: new data from the 1995 National Survey of Family Growth. Vital Health Stat 1997;Series 23, Number 19.
7. Donnelly D, Burgess E, Anderson S, Davis R, Dillard J. Involuntary celibacy: a life course analysis. J Sex Research 2001;38:159-169.

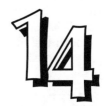

Coitus Interruptus (Withdrawal)

Deborah Kowal, MA, PA

- Coitus interruptus does not eliminate the risk of sexually transmitted infections (STIs): the pre-ejaculate can contain HIV-infected cells, and lesions or ulcers on the genitals can transmit pathogens.
- Although popularly considered an ineffective method, coitus interruptus provides efficacy similar to that of barrier methods of contraception.

Coitus interruptus, or the withdrawal method, was a natural response to the discovery that ejaculation into the vagina caused pregnancy.[1] The method was probably widely practiced throughout history, playing a predominant role in fertility declines occurring prior to the advent of the pill. Although the 1995 National Survey of Family Growth (NSFG), the most recent published, reports the prevalence of coitus interruptus is only 2.9%,[2] figures this low are probably a marked underestimate.[3] For example, single women may rely on the method more frequently than do married women who frequently tend to be the survey subjects. In addition, respondents may not regard coitus interruptus as a legitimate method and therefore fail to note its use.

Withdrawal is more commonly reported among high school students. In 1997, 13% of sexually active high school students who completed the national Youth Risk Behavior Survey (YRBS) reported using withdrawal to prevent pregnancy during their last intercourse.[4] Use of withdrawal as a contraceptive method dropped significantly since 1991, when 18% reported use. In an earlier study, it appeared that adolescents who hold negative views about oral contraceptives may view withdrawal as an alternative to pill use.[5]

MECHANISM OF ACTION

Coitus interruptus prevents fertilization by preventing the contact between spermatozoa and the ovum. The couple may have penile-vaginal intercourse until ejaculation is impending, at which time the male partner withdraws his penis from the vagina and away from the external genitalia of the female partner. The man must rely on his own sensations to determine when he is about to ejaculate. The pre-ejaculate, which is usually released just prior to full ejaculation, goes unnoticed by both the man and the woman during the course of intercourse and so is not a sign that ejaculation is about to occur.

EFFECTIVENESS

Although coitus interruptus has often been criticized as an ineffective method, it probably confers a level of contraceptive protection similar to that provided by barrier methods. Effectiveness depends largely on the man's ability to withdraw prior to ejaculation. How effective the method would be if used consistently and correctly is highly uncertain. Our best guess is that the probability of pregnancy among perfect users would be about 4% in the initial year of use (Table 14-1). Among typical users, the probability of pregnancy would be about 27% during the first year of use.

As with other methods, withdrawal's efficacy in preventing pregnancy probably depends not only on characteristics of the method, but also on characteristics of the user. Women who are younger and who are married are less likely to experience an accidental pregnancy during the first two years of use.[6] It may be that certain cultural factors influence how successful a woman may be in using withdrawal. A recent study found that Hispanic women were less likely to experience accidental pregnancy than were black or white women.[6] Men who are less experienced with using the method or who have difficulty in foretelling when ejaculation will occur could have a greater risk of failure.

Table 14-1 First-year probability of pregnancy* for withdrawal, chance, condoms, and pills

| Method | % of Women Experiencing an Unintended Pregnancy Within the First Year of Use | | % of Women Continuing at 1 Year |
	Typical Use (%)	Perfect Use (%)	
Chance	85	85	
Condoms (male)	15	2	53
Pill	8	0.3	68
Withdrawal	27	4	43

* See Table 9-2 for first-year probability of pregnancy for all methods.

Emergency Contraceptive Pills: Treatment initiated within 72 hours after unprotected intercourse reduces the risk of pregnancy by at least 75%. (See Chapter 12 for more information.)

ADVANTAGES AND INDICATIONS

As a method of contraception, withdrawal has several distinct advantages. It costs nothing, requires no devices, involves no chemicals, and is available in any situation. Some couples may select withdrawal as their method because it requires no physical examination or contact with a clinic or pharmacy.[3] Practicing coitus interruptus causes no medical side effects. Couples who cannot or do not wish to use other contraceptive methods and who can accept the potential for unintended pregnancy may find withdrawal an acceptable alternative. It is a back-up contraceptive that is always available.

DISADVANTAGES AND CAUTIONS

The method is unforgiving of incorrect or inconsistent use, leading to a probability of pregnancy in typical users that is substantially higher than the rates for hormonal methods or intrauterine devices (IUDs). One reason for contraceptive failure may be a lack of the self-control demanded by the method. With impending orgasm, men (and women) experience a mild to extreme clouding of consciousness during which coital movement becomes involuntary.[7] The man may feel the urge to achieve deeper penetration at the time of impending orgasm and may not withdraw in sufficient time to avoid depositing semen in his partner's vagina or on her external genitalia. In addition, some men have difficulty foretelling when they will ejaculate. For some couples, interruption of the excitement or plateau phase of the sexual response cycle may diminish pleasure.

Withdrawal does not completely protect couples from exposure to sexually transmitted infections, because not all pathogens are limited to seminal fluid. Surface lesions, such as those from herpes genitalis or human papilloma virus, may be actively infective. In one prospective study, the condom failed to protect some users against gonorrhea because they were exposed to infectious secretions before the condom was used.[8]

SPECIAL ISSUES

Studies of stable couples in which the man was infected with human immunodeficiency virus (HIV) and the woman was not demonstrate that coitus interruptus may reduce the risk of infection somewhat better than unprotected intercourse with ejaculation. Coitus interruptus cut the HIV conversion rate of women by half in one study,[9] and by a larger percentage in another study.[10] Because these studies examined only stable heterosexual couples, the findings may not hold true for women with several HIV-infected partners.

Coitus interruptus probably decreases HIV exposure by reducing the amount of semen that enters the woman's vagina. However, the seminal fluid that emerges from the penis prior to ejaculation may contain some

HIV.[11-13] Although coitus interruptus may be less likely to transmit HIV than intercourse with ejaculation, women have become infected while their partners consistently practiced withdrawal. Coitus interruptus has not been studied as a way to reduce HIV transmission from woman to man.

Some concern exists that the pre-ejaculate fluid may carry sperm into the vagina. In itself, the pre-ejaculate, a lubricating secretion produced by the Littre or Cowper's glands, contains no sperm. Two studies examining the pre-ejaculate for the presence of spermatozoa found none.[12,13] However, a previous ejaculation may have left some sperm hidden within the folds of the urethral lining. In examinations of the pre-ejaculate in one small study,[14] the pre-ejaculate was free of spermatozoa in all of 11 HIV-seronegative men and 4 of 12 seropositive men. Although the 8 samples containing spermatozoa revealed only small clumps of a few hundred sperm, these could theoretically pose a risk of fertilization. In all likelihood, the spermatozoa left from a previous ejaculation could be washed out with the force of a normal urination; however, this remains unstudied.

INSTRUCTIONS FOR USING COITUS INTERRUPTUS

1. Before intercourse, the man should urinate and wipe off the tip of his penis to remove any sperm remaining from a previous ejaculation.

2. When he feels he is about to ejaculate, the man should withdraw his penis from his partner's vagina, making sure that ejaculation occurs away from his partner's genitalia.

3. Withdrawal is not a good contraceptive method under the following conditions:
   - The man cannot predictably withdraw prior to ejaculation.
   - The man intends to have repeated orgasms, which may cause the pre-ejaculate to contain spermatozoa.

4. Withdrawal does not effectively protect against sexually transmitted infections (STIs), including infection with the human immunodeficiency virus (HIV). Abstinence or use of latex or plastic condoms provide better protection.

5. Withdrawal is a considerably better method of contraception than no method at all.

6. As a couple, learn what options are available for postcoital protection should any ejaculate come in contact with the vagina. Try to have a supply of contraceptive foam or some type of spermicide available in case of unintentional ejaculation in or near the woman's vagina. Despite the seeming optimism of this suggestion, it is probably too late to stop some sperm from swimming up into the

uterus. If you think you may have been exposed to a risk of pregnancy, contact your clinician about emergency contraception. (You can also call the toll-free number 1-888-NOT-2-LATE [1-888-668-2528] for a listing of emergency contraception providers near you.)

REFERENCES

1. Robertson W. An illustrated history of contraception. Park Ridge NJ: Parthenon Publishing Group, 1990.
2. Abma JC, Chandra A, Mosher WD, Peterson LS, Piccinino LJ. Fertility, family planning, and women's health: new data from the 1995 National Survey of Family Growth. Vital Health Stat 1997;Series 23, Number 19.
3. Rogow D, Horowitz S. Withdrawal: a review of the literature and an agenda for research. Stud Fam Plann 1995;26:140-153.
4. Everett SA, Warren CW, Santelli JS, Kann L, Collins JL, Kolbe LJ. Use of birth control pills, condoms, and withdrawal among U.S. high school students. J Adolesc Health 2000;27:112-118.
5. Moore PJ, Adler NE, Kegeles SM. Adolescents and the contraceptive pill: the impact of beliefs on intentions and use. Obstet Gynecol 1996;88:48S-56S.
6. Ranjit N, Bankole A, Darroch J, Singh, S. Contraceptive failure in the first two years of use: differences across socioeconomic subgroups. Fam Plann Perspect 2001;33:19-27.
7. Kinsey AC, Pomeroy WB, Martin CE, Gebhard PH. Sexual behavior in the human female. Philadelphia PA: W.B. Saunders Co., 1953.
8. Darrow WW. Condom use and use-effectiveness in high-risk populations. Sex Transm Dis 1989;16:157-160.
9. Musicco M, Nicolosi A, Saracco A, Lazzarin A (for the Italian Study Group on HIV Heterosexual Transmission). The role of contraceptive practices in HIV sexual transmission from man to woman. In: Nicolosi A (ed). HIV epidemiology: models and methods. New York: Raven Press, Ltd., 1994:121-135.
10. DiVincenzi I (for the European Study Group). A longitudinal study of human immunodeficiency virus transmission by heterosexual partners. N Engl J Med 1994;331:341-346.
11. Howe JE, Minkoff HL, Duerr AC. Contraceptives and HIV. AIDS 1994;8:861-871.
12. Ilaria G, Jacobs JL, Polsky B, Koll B, Baron P, MacLow C, Armstrong D, Schlegel PN. Detection of HIV-1 DNA sequences in pre-ejaculatory fluid [Letter]. Lancet 1992;340:1469.
13. Zukerman Z, Weiss DB, Orvieto R. Does preejaculatory penile secretion originating from Cowper's gland contain sperm? J Assist Reprod Genet 2003;20:157-159.
14. Pudney J, Oneta M, Mayer K, Seage G, Anderson D. Pre-ejaculatory fluid as potential vector for sexual transmission of HIV-1 [Letter]. Lancet 1992;340:1470.

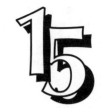

Fertility Awareness-Based Methods

Victoria H. Jennings, PhD
Marcos Arevalo, MD, MPH
Deborah Kowal, MA, PA

- Fertility awareness helps couples understand how to avoid pregnancy or how to become pregnant.
- Regardless of whether they use family planning, or which method they use, every woman and man will find value in learning fertility awareness.

Fertility Awareness-Based (FAB) methods of family planning depend on identifying the "fertile window," or the days each menstrual cycle when intercourse is most likely to result in a pregnancy. Some FAB methods may simply involve a woman's understanding which days of her cycle she is most likely to be fertile and keeping track of her cycle days. To use other FAB methods, she observes, records, and interprets her body's fertility signs.

To avoid pregnancy, couples can either use a barrier method or not have intercourse during the fertile time. If couples use barrier methods, they are using fertility awareness-combined methods (FACM). If they abstain, they are using natural family planning (NFP).

MECHANISM OF ACTION

FAB methods of family planning use one or more indicators to identify the beginning and end of the fertile time during the menstrual cycle. They are effective when they are used correctly. However, they are not effective when used incorrectly because, with incorrect use, unprotected intercourse takes place when the woman is potentially fertile.

In most women, ovulation usually occurs near the middle of the cycle.[1] The fertile window of the menstrual cycle lasts for only about 6 days: the 5 days preceding ovulation and the day of ovulation (this is related to the lifespan of the gametes).[2,3] In cycles that range between 26 and 32 days long (approximately 80% of cycles), the fertile window is highly likely to fall within cycle days 8 to 19.[4]

Two FAB methods, the Standard Days Method™ (SDM™) and the Calendar Rhythm Method (CRM), involve counting the days in the menstrual cycle. SDM requires only that the woman know which day of her menstrual cycle she is on and that she consider herself potentially fertile on days 8 through 19. CRM not only involves counting cycle days, but it also requires that the woman have a record of the length of her last several menstrual cycles, identify the longest and shortest of these cycles, and perform a mathematical calculation to identify the probable days of fertility during the current cycle. While survey results show that, in many countries, a significant number of couples state that they are using the CRM,[5] most have little understanding of how to use it and are simply abstaining from intercourse on a few days of the woman's cycle when they believe (often erroneously) that she is most likely to become pregnant. It appears that "calendar rhythm" has become a generic term for occasional abstinence.

Other FAB methods, such as the Ovulation Method or the Symptothermal Method, involve actual observation of fertile signs such as changes in characteristics of cervical secretions, or changes in basal body temperature (BBT). Changes in these signs are caused by fluctuations in circulating hormone levels during the cycle. Women who use these methods identify the start of the fertile time by observing cervical secretions. To identify the end of the fertile time, women can observe their cervical secretions as well as monitor the change in their BBT.

EFFECTIVENESS

Successful use of FAB methods depends on (1) the accuracy of the method in identifying the woman's actual fertile window, (2) a woman's/couple's ability to correctly identify the fertile time, and (3) their ability to follow the instructions of the method they are using—that is, to use a barrier method or avoid intercourse on the days the method identifies as fertile.

Among perfect users of FAB methods (i.e., those who correctly and consistently use a barrier method or avoid intercourse during the fertile time), the percentage of women experiencing an unintended pregnancy during the first year of use ranges from 2% to 5%, depending on the method. In typical use (i.e., correct and consistent use during some cycles, but incorrect or inconsistent use during others), pregnancy rates are higher (see Table 15-1). (See Chapter 31 on Contraceptive Efficacy.)

Table 15-1 First-year probability of pregnancy* for women using no method, a FAB method, and barrier methods

| Method | % of Women Experiencing an Unintended Pregnancy Within the First Year of Use | |
	Typical Use	Perfect Use
No Method	85	85
Periodic Abstinence	25	
Standard Days Method	12	5
Ovulation Method	22	3
Symptothermal	13–20	2
Condom (male)	15	2
Spermicides	29	18

* See Table 9-2 for first-year probability pregnancy rates for all methods.

Ovulation method. The first-year probability of pregnancy for methods based on using only cervical secretions to identify the beginning and end of the fertile time is about 3% among perfect users and 22% among typical users.[6,7] Most efficacy studies of the OM do not enroll women in the study until they have completed 3 cycles of use, and most use providers with extensive training and experience with the method.

Symptothermal method. The first-year probability of pregnancy among couples who use two or more fertility indicators (usually cervical secretions and BBT, but others such as cervix position or a calendar calculation may also be used as a "double check" to identify the start and end of the fertile time) are about 2% to 3% among perfect users and as high as 13% to 20% among typical users.[8] As with the OM studies, most efficacy studies of the Symptothermal Method (STM) include women with at least three cycles of use and involve experienced providers.

Calendar rhythm method. Estimates of pregnancy rates for the Calendar Rhythm Method (CRM) vary widely, partially because the estimates come from flawed studies. One relatively recent comparative study reported a first-year pregnancy rate of 5% with correct use.[9] The probability of pregnancy during the first year of typical use of the CRM is estimated to be about 13%,[10] but no well-designed prospective studies have been conducted.

Standard Days Method. The first-year probability of pregnancy for women using the SDM is about 5% if the method is used correctly. During typical use, the probability of pregnancy is 12%.[11] In contrast to most efficacy studies of other FAB methods, the efficacy study of the SDM on which these percentages are based included women from their first cycle of method use. Providers who taught the women how to use the SDM received 2 to 3 days training in the method and had no prior experience with the SDM.

COST

The cost of FAB methods depends on the materials and supplies used and the amount of time required to provide the method. Since no technologically sophisticated materials are required and tools for monitoring a woman's menstrual cycles entail minimal expense, FAB methods are relatively low cost. Some programs offer training without any charge to the client, while others charge a nominal fee. The amount of time required to learn how to use FAB methods depends on the method and on the woman. The SDM requires a single teaching session, usually lasting less than a half hour. Methods that rely on observation of fertility signs require significantly more time. A woman who is younger and normally cycling generally has fertility signs that are easier to interpret than does a woman who has just discontinued taking oral contraceptives, is breast-feeding, or is approaching menopause. The cost would vary accordingly.

If a couple uses a barrier method during the fertile time, there are additional costs for obtaining and resupplying the barrier and, as appropriate, spermicides.

ADVANTAGES AND INDICATIONS

Fertility awareness is important for all women and men, regardless of which family planning method they use or whether they choose to use family planning at all. Fertility awareness increases the users' knowledge of their reproductive potential and enhances self-reliance. Some couples like the active involvement of the male partner. Fertility awareness information can be used for a number of purposes:

To avoid pregnancy. For maximum effectiveness, couples should abstain from intercourse or use a barrier method during the entire fertile time.

To conceive. Couples have intercourse on days the woman is potentially fertile. Depending on the method used, these may include days 8 to 19 of the cycle, or the days she observes cervical secretions. Conception is most likely to occur within 1 to 2 days of ovulation.[2]

To detect pregnancy. A postovulatory temperature rise (see the section on Basal Body Temperature Charting) sustained for 18 or more days is an excellent early indicator that pregnancy is underway.

To detect impaired fertility. Charting fertility signs costs relatively little and can aid in diagnosing and treating fertility problems due to infrequent or absent ovulation. Women who do not ovulate tend to have a meandering BBT pattern throughout the cycle, rather than the typical pattern (lower in the first part and higher in the second).

To detect a need for medical attention. Changes in cervical secretions, abdominal pain, and other signs may indicate the need for medical attention. (See Chapter 8 on Reproductive Tract Infections.)

DISADVANTAGES AND CAUTIONS

FAB methods produce no side effects. Like other methods except some barrier methods, however, they offer no protection against sexually transmitted infections (STIs), including infection with the human immunodeficiency virus (HIV). Also, lack of the male partner's cooperation will be a distinct obstacle for women who wish to practice abstinence or use an alternative method during the fertile time. Certain conditions may make FAB more difficult to use and require more extensive counseling and follow-up:

- Recent childbirth
- Current breastfeeding
- Recent menarche
- Recent discontinuation of hormonal contraceptive methods
- Approaching menopause

FAB methods are not recommended for women with the following difficulties:

- Irregular cycles (Standard Days Method)
- Inability to interpret their fertility signs correctly (Ovulation Method, Symptothermal Method)
- Persistent reproductive tract infections that affect the signs of fertility (Ovulation Method, Symptothermal Method)

SPECIAL ISSUES

Safety

Because unintended pregnancies among couples who use FAB methods usually result from having intercourse at the beginning or end of the fertile time, concerns have been raised about the risk of birth defects or poor pregnancy outcomes due to aged ovum or sperm. A prospective study showed no significant differences in rates of spontaneous abortion, low birthweight, or preterm birth among women who had an unintended pregnancy while using a FAB method compared with women who had intended pregnancies.[12] However, women with a history of spontaneous abortion had a greater chance of having a spontaneous abortion when conception occurred very early or late in the fertile time (23% versus 10% to 15%). Furthermore, fertilization involving aging gametes is not associated with major birth defects and Down's syndrome.[13] Reassure your clients that NFP does not pose a threat to the health of mothers and their offspring. However, to reduce their risk of pregnancy loss, counsel women with a history of spontaneous abortion to time intercourse as close as possible to ovulation if they are attempting to conceive.

Sex selection

A study of about 1,000 births showed no association between timing of conception and the sex ratio at birth.[14] These results do not substantiate claims that couples can select the sex of their child by timing intercourse.

PROVIDING FERTILITY AWARENESS-BASED METHODS

To use FAB methods, couples must adjust their sexual behavior according to their fertility intentions. Users of NFP will need to abstain from intercourse for about 10 to 14 days of the woman's menstrual cycle, depending on her cycle length and the method used. Users of FACM will need to use a barrier method on fertile days. Successful use of these methods therefore requires a couple be able to communicate effectively with each other about sexual matters.

The Institute for Reproductive Health at Georgetown University estimates it takes just a few minutes for a woman to learn that she should consider herself fertile on days 8 to 19 of her cycle and to keep track of her cycle days. Counseling may be needed to provide the support necessary to help her use the method correctly. Most couples using other FAB methods need an instructor's help to learn how to observe, record, and interpret the woman's fertility signs and patterns. The National Health Service in Great Britain estimates it takes 4 to 6 hours to teach a woman fertility awareness skills, including charting fertility signs and identifying the fertile time.[15] This estimate includes initial classes and follow-up until the woman can use the method without assistance.

INSTRUCTIONS FOR USING FERTILITY AWARENESS-BASED METHODS

CALENDAR RHYTHM METHOD

The CRM is rarely taught by programs and thus is not described here in detail. To use this method, you will need to follow these steps:

1. Keep a record of your past 6 to 12 menstrual cycle lengths.

2. Find the longest and shortest of your past menstrual cycles.

3. Subtract 18 from the number of days in your shortest cycle to find the first fertile day in your current cycle.

4. Subtract 11 from the number of days in your longest cycle to find the last fertile day in your current cycle.

5. **For contraception.** From the first through the last days identified as fertile, you should use a barrier method or avoid intercourse if you do not want to become pregnant.

6. **For conception.** Have intercourse on the days identified as fertile.

7. Update the calculation every cycle to determine your fertile days.

CycleBeads

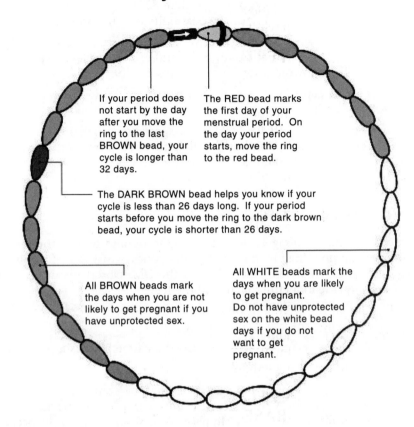

If your period does not start by the day after you move the ring to the last BROWN bead, your cycle is longer than 32 days.

The RED bead marks the first day of your menstrual period. On the day your period starts, move the ring to the red bead.

The DARK BROWN bead helps you know if your cycle is less than 26 days long. If your period starts before you move the ring to the dark brown bead, your cycle is shorter than 26 days.

All WHITE beads mark the days when you are likely to get pregnant. Do not have unprotected sex on the white bead days if you do not want to get pregnant.

All BROWN beads mark the days when you are not likely to get pregnant if you have unprotected sex.

Figure 15-1 CycleBeads for Standard Days method

STANDARD DAYS METHOD

The SDM is most appropriate for women who usually have cycles between 26 and 32 days long. To use the SDM, you will need to count the days of your menstrual cycle, starting with the day your menstrual bleeding begins.

1. Count the first day of your menstrual bleeding as day 1.

2. Continue counting every day.

3. On days 1 to 7, you can have unprotected intercourse.

4. On days 8 to 19, you should use a barrier method or avoid intercourse if you do not want to become pregnant.

5. From day 20 through the end of your cycle, you can have unprotected intercourse.

6. The SDM works best for women who have cycles between 26 and 32 days long. If you have more than one cycle in one year that is shorter than 26 days or longer than 32 days, you should contact your provider to discuss the possibility of using another method.

7. **For contraception.** Have unprotected intercourse only on days 1 to 7 and from day 20 until the end of your cycle. Use a barrier method or avoid intercourse on days 8 to 19.

8. **For conception.** Have unprotected intercourse on days 8-19 of your cycle.

Most women who use the SDM use a specially-designed color-coded string of beads called CycleBeads™ to help them keep track of their cycle days. See Figure 15-1 for an illustration of the CycleBeads and instructions for use.

OVULATION METHOD

Cervical mucus changes signal the beginning and end of the fertile time, even among those who have irregular cycles. Assistance of a trained instructor is necessary for correct use of the OM. Observe your cervical secretions by 'the look, the touch, and the feel':

1. *Look* at the secretions on your panties, fingers, or toilet paper to determine color and consistency.

2. *Touch* the secretions to determine their stretch and slipperiness.

3. *Feel* how wet the sensation is at your vulva.

When they first appear, the secretions may be scant but sticky and thick with a cloudy or whitish color. Highly fertile secretions are abundant, clear, stretchy, wet, and slippery. Ovulation most likely occurs within 1 day before, during, or 1 day after the last day of abundant, clear, stretchy, slippery cervical secretions. When you are observing your cervical secretions, do not douche, because it can wash out the secretions, making it very difficult to notice changes.

Use your cervical secretions to identify the beginning and end of the fertile time:

1. Observe your cervical secretions every day, beginning the day after your menstrual bleeding has stopped, and record them daily on a special chart (Figure 15-2). To help you avoid confusing cervical secretions with semen and normal sexual lubrication, some counselors advise complete sexual abstinence throughout the first cycle. Alternatively, you can use a condom.

2. Check secretions each time before and after you urinate by wiping (front to back) with tissue paper. Note and record the color and appearance (yellow, white, clear, or cloudy) and consistency (thick, sticky, or stretchy) of the secretions, and how they feel

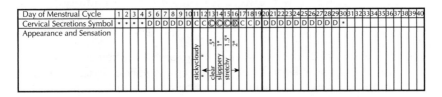

Day of Menstrual Cycle	1	2	3	4	5	6	7	8	9	10	11	12	13	14	15	16	17	18	19	20	21	22	23	24	25	26	27	28	29	30	31	32	33	34	35	36	37	38	39	40
Cervical Secretions Symbol	•	•	•	•	D	D	D	D	D	D	C	C	C	C	C	C	C	C	D	D	D	D	D	D	D	D	D	D	•											
Appearance and Sensation																																								

Figure 15-2 Cervical secretion variations during a model menstrual cycle

(dry, wet, or slippery). Record how much they stretch when pulled between your thumb and index finger. Also, note and chart the sensations of dryness, moistness, or wetness at your vulva. Always record the 'most fertile' observations you see during the day.

3. **For contraception.** Check for secretions as soon as your menses ends. (Some counselors recommend avoiding intercourse or using a barrier method during menses because it is difficult to detect secretions when they are mixed with menstrual blood.) You can have sexual intercourse on preovulatory days if no secretions are present. (Some counselors recommend abstaining the next day and night following intercourse to allow time for bodily fluids to drain out of your body so you will not confuse semen and arousal fluids with cervical secretions. The following day, check your cervical secretions.) The fertile time begins when cervical secretions are first observed until 4 days past the peak day (the last day of clear, stretchy, slippery secretions).

4. **For conception.** Have intercourse when cervical secretions are present. The probability of conception is greatest when the secretions are abundant, clear, stretchy, and slippery.

5. Most women need help in the first few cycles to interpret their cervical secretion patterns and charts to determine the fertile time.

SYMPTOTHERMAL METHOD

Some couples prefer to observe more than one indicator of the woman's fertility. Most couples who use a combined or symptothermal approach use cervical secretions and BBT to identify the fertile time. The BBT, the temperature of the body at rest, is lower in the first part of the cycle, rises to a higher level beginning around the time of ovulation, and remains at the higher level for the rest of the cycle. By taking her temperature when she first wakes in the morning and recording her temperature on a chart each day of her menstrual cycle, a woman can retrospectively identify whether she has ovulated and, thus, calculate the end of her fertile time.

To use the STM, follow the steps for the OM and, in addition, take and record your BBT as follows to determine the postovulatory infertile time:

1. Take your BBT every morning at the same time before getting out of bed (after at least 3 hours of sleep). A special calibrated thermometer makes temperature reading easier. Take the BBT orally, rectally, or vaginally, but take it at the same site each day so changes in BBT can be detected accurately.

2. Record your BBT readings daily on a chart (Figure 15-3). Connect the dots for each day so a line connects dots from day 2 to day 3, and so on.

3. Your temperature will probably rise at least 0.4 degrees F° around the time of ovulation and remain elevated until the next menses begins. Your actual temperature and maximum temperature are not important, just the rise over the baseline (preovulatory) temperatures.

4. If you have 3 days of continuous temperature rise following 6 lower temperatures, you have ovulated and your postovulatory infertile time has begun. To see the baseline and rise clearly on the chart, draw a line just above (0.1 degree line) the lower (preovulatory) temperatures. When you record 3 continuous temperatures above this line and the last temperature is 0.4 degrees higher than this line, your postovulatory infertile time has begun.

5. If you cannot detect a sustained rise in BBT, you may not have ovulated in that cycle. A true postovulatory BBT rise usually persists 10 days or longer.

6. Some women notice a temperature drop about 12 to 24 hours before it begins to rise after ovulation, whereas others have no drop in temperature at all. A drop in your BBT probably means ovulation will occur the next day.

7. **For contraception.** Rely on your cervical secretions to identify the beginning of your fertile time. Your BBT can help you identify the end of your fertile time. You should use a barrier method or not have intercourse during the fertile time if you do not want to become pregnant.

8. **For conception.** It is not possible to predict fertile days using BBT. By the time the rise is detected, you are probably in the infertile phase of your menstrual cycle and have missed the opportunity to become pregnant. To conceive, you should rely on your cervical secretions.

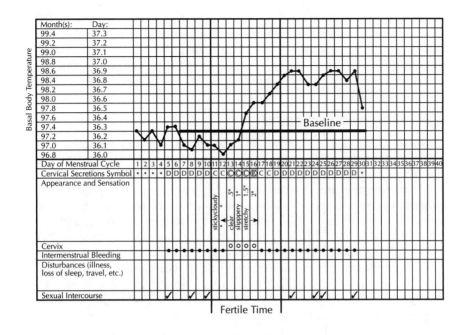

Figure 15-3 Symptothermal variations during a model menstrual cycle

FAB Methods in Development

Home Test Kits for Ovulation Prediction and Detection

Most research on home test kits for ovulation prediction and detection has focused on helping women with fertility problems, but several kits recently have been developed to detect the fertile window of the menstrual cycle for contraceptive purposes. These include mini-microscopes (PG53, PC 2000, and Maybe Baby) that identify the fertile days based on salivary or cervical mucus ferning; temperature computers (Babycomp/Ladycomp, Bioself 2000, and Cyclotest 2 Plus) that measure BBT and cycle length history; and hormone computers (Persona) that identify fertile days by measuring hormone profiles in urine. A recent study compared the probable failure rates for women using these kits and women using the Symptothermal method.[16] High failure rates were projected with use of mini-microscopes. The Symptothermal method was most accurate in detecting the actual fertile phase, as identified by daily LH measurements and ultrasound, followed by the temperature computers; the hormone computers were somewhat less accurate. In another comparative study, the Clearplan Easy Fertility Monitor underestimated the fertile phase, and the Ovulation Method overestimated the actual fertile phase.[17] Home test kits cost between $50 and $500, plus supplies. Additional efficacy studies are needed before they can be recommended for pregnancy prevention.

A hydration detection device, which monitors the variations in the water content of cervical secretions with a tampon-shaped probe that contains a tiny light sensor, is being developed by researchers at Duke University. The device measures the increase in the percentage of water in cervical secretions as ovulation approaches, and the decrease in hydration right after ovulation occurs.[17]

Simple Observation Method

Another method, the TwoDay method, also has been developed. Unlike the Symptothermal and Ovulation methods, which require the woman to observe and determine the consistency and appearance of cervical secretions, the TwoDay method is based only on presence or absence of cervical secretions. To use this method, the woman asks herself two questions every day of her cycle: Do I have secretions today?, and Did I have secretions yesterday? If she had secretions of any type either "today" or "yesterday," she should consider herself fertile. Results of trials in several countries suggest that the method is acceptable to women and as effective as other FAB methods when used correctly.[18,19]

REFERENCES

1. Lamprecht VM, Grummer-Strawn L. Development of new formulas to identify the fertile time of the menstrual cycle. Contraception 1996;54:339-343.
2. Wilcox AJ, Weinberg CR, Baird DD. Timing of sexual intercourse in relation to ovulation. N Engl J Med 1995; 333:1517-1521.
3. Wilcox AJ. Dunson D, Baird DB. The timing of the "fertile window" in the menstrual cycle:day specific estimates from a prospective study. BMJ 2000,321:1259-62.
4. Arévalo M, Sinai I, Jennings V. A Fixed Formula to Define the Fertile Window of the Menstrual Cycle as the Basis of a Simple Method of Natural Family Planning, Contraception, 2000; 60:357-360.
5. Chey, Cleland JG, Ali MM. Periodic abstinence in developing countries: an assessment of failure rates and consequences. Contraception 2004; 69(1):15-21.
6. Trussell J, Grummer-Strawn L. Contraceptive failure of the ovulation method of periodic abstinence. Fam Plann Perspect 1990;22:65-75.
7. World Health Organization. A prospective multicentre trial of the ovulation method of natural family planning. II. The effectiveness phase. Fertil Steril 1981; 36:591-598.
8. Frank-Herrmann P, Freundl G, Baur S, Bremme M, Doring GK, Godehardt EAJ, Sottong U. Effectiveness and acceptability of the symptothermal method of natural family planning in Germany. Am J Obstet Gynecol 1991; 165:2052-2054.
9. Dicker D, Wachsman T, Feldbergt D. The vaginal contraception diaphragm and the condom: a evaluation and comparison of two barrier methods with the rhythm method. Contraception 1989; 40:497-503.
10. Kambic RT, Lamprecht V. Calendar rhythm efficacy: a review. Adv Contracept 1996;12:123-128.
11. Arévalo M, Jennings V, Sinai I. Efficacy of the Standard Days Method of Family Planning, Contraception, 2002;65:333-338.
12. Gray RH, Simpson JL, Kambic RT, Queenan JT, Mena P, Perez A, Barbato M. Timing of conception and the risk of spontaneous abortion among pregnancies occurring during use of natural family planning. Am J Obstet Gynecol 1995; 172:1567-1572.
13. Simpson JL, Gray R, Perez A, Mena P, Queenan JT, Barbato M, Pardo F, Kambic R, Jennings V. Fertilization involving aging gametes, major birth defects and Down's syndrome. Lancet 2002;359:1670-1671.

14. Gray RH, Simpson JL, Bitto AC, Queenan JT, Chuanjun L. Sex Ratio associated in timing of insemination and length of the follicular phase in planned and unplanned pregnancies during use of NFP. Hum Reprod 1998;13(5):1397-1400.
15. Clubb EM, Pyper CM, Knight J. A pilot study on teaching natural family planning in general practice. Natural family planning: current knowledge and new strategies for the 1990s, Part II 1992:130-132.
16. Freundl G, Godehardt E, Kern PA, Frank-Hermann P, Koubenec HJ, Gnoth C. Estimated maximum failure rates of cycle monitors using daily conception probabilities in the menstrual cycle. Human Reproduction 2003;18(12):2628-2633.
17. Fehring R, Raviele K, Schneider M. A comparison of the fertile phase as determined by the Clearplan Easy Fertility Monitor and self-assessment of cervical mucus. Contraception 2003;69(1):9-14.
18. Sinai I, Arevalo M, Jennings V. The TwoDay Algorithm: A New Algorithm to Identify the Fertile Time of the Menstrual Cycle. Contraception 1999;60(2):65-70.
19. Arevalo M, Jennings V, Sinai I. Efficacy of the TwoDay Method. Fertility and Sterility 2004 (in press).

Male Condoms

Lee Warner, PhD, MPH
Robert A. Hatcher, MD, MPH
Markus J. Steiner, PhD

- When used consistently and correctly, latex or synthetic male and female condoms can prevent pregnancy and many sexually transmitted infections (STIs), including infection with human immunodeficiency virus (HIV).

- Condoms are inexpensive, available without a prescription, and easy to use.

- By preventing STIs and their long-term sequelae, condoms help protect future fertility.

- Clients potentially at risk for STI should be encouraged to use condoms even if they already rely on oral contraceptives, implants, injectables, intrauterine devices (IUDs), fertility awareness, spermicides, or sterilization (including hysterectomy) for contraception.

The condom remains the most widely available and popular male contraceptive method in the United States. According to the 1995 National Survey of Family Growth (NSFG), more than 9 million reproductive-age women in the United States reported using condoms for contraception or protection from sexually transmitted infections (STIs).[1] Among women using any contraceptive, 20% reported current use of male condoms for prevention of pregnancy.[1] Condom use continues to be an important part of public health efforts to prevent new cases of infection with human immunodeficiency virus (HIV) as well as other STIs.

In the year following the 1986 U.S. Surgeon General's report, which stated that latex condoms should be used to prevent AIDS, condom sales, the best indicator of condom use, rose by 20%.[2] Consumers now purchase more than 440 million condoms per year.[3] Between 1988 and 1995, the percentage of reproductive-age women who reported using male condoms for contraception increased nearly 50%, from 13% to 19%, with marked increases reported by women ages 20 to 29. Among adolescent women ages 15 to 19, condom use rose slightly from 27% to 30%. Increases in condom use have also been reported among both male and female adolescents, based on results from nationally representative surveys.[1,4,5]

MECHANISM OF ACTION

The male condom, a thin sheath placed over the glans and shaft of the penis, acts as a physical barrier. The condom prevents pregnancy by blocking the passage of semen and is most effective when used from "start to finish" during every act of intercourse. Among barrier contraceptive methods, the condom provides the most protection of the genital tract and is thus the most effective method for reducing the risk of STIs.[6,7]

A sheath worn over the penis can be traced as far back as 1350 B.C., when Egyptian men wore decorative covers for their penises. In 1564 A.D., Fallopius first described linen sheaths used to protect against syphilis.[8] Protective sheaths were made from dried animal intestines in the 18th century, when they were first given the name "condom," presumably after inventor Colonel Cundum.[8] With the advent of vulcanized rubber in 1843 came the mass production of condoms made from natural rubber latex.[9] In the 1990s, manufacturers also began to use synthetic materials (e.g., polyurethane) to develop new condom options.

CONDOM OPTIONS

Most commercially available condoms are manufactured from natural rubber latex ("rubber" condoms). A small proportion are made from the intestinal caecum of lambs ("natural skin," "natural membrane," or "lambskin" condoms). Natural membrane condoms may not offer the same level of protection against STIs as natural rubber latex condoms, however. Unlike latex condoms, natural membrane condoms contain small pores that may permit the passage of viruses, including hepatitis B virus, herpes simplex virus, and HIV,[10] and are recommended for contraceptive use only.

A similarly small proportion of condoms are now manufactured from polyurethane and other synthetic materials. These new synthethic condoms are more resistant to deterioration than those manufactured from natural rubber latex, may provide a less constricting fit, and may enhance sensitivity. Unlike latex condoms, condoms made from synthetic materials are generally compatible with oil-based lubricants.[11] Synthetic condoms have not been well studied for protection against STIs but are believed to provide protection similar to that of natural rubber latex condoms.

As of August 2003, five synthetic condoms had been cleared by the U.S. Food and Drug Administration (FDA) for persons sensitive to natural rubber latex and were commercially available: two Avanti condoms (Durex

Consumer Products), Trojan Supra (ARMKEL), eZ·on (Mayer Laboratories), and the Reality female condom (The Female Health Company). (A detailed discussion of the female condom can be found in Chapter 18 on Vaginal Barriers.) A number of additional synthetic condoms have been cleared by the FDA and may be marketed in the United States in the coming years. See Table 16-1 for a comparison of condom types.

Table 16-1 Characteristics of latex, natural membrane, and synthetic condoms

Type	Latex	Natural Membrane	Synthetic
Material	Natural rubber	Lamb caecum	Polyurethane*
Lubricant use	Water-based only	Any	Any
Cost	Low	Moderate	Moderate/high
Prevention of Pregnancy	Yes	Yes	Yes
Prevention of STIs and HIV	Yes	No	Likely

Source: Modified from Contraceptive Technology Update (March, 1995).
* Other synthetic condoms may become available soon.

SPERMICIDAL CONDOMS

Condoms lubricated with a small amount of the spermicide, nonoxynol-9 (N-9), ranging in concentration from 1% to 12%,[12] have been available in the United States since 1983. There is no evidence to suggest that spermicidal condoms are more effective than condoms without spermicide despite their higher cost and shorter shelf-life.[13,14]

There has been recent concern about genital ulceration and irritation resulting from high-frequency use of vaginal spermicidal products containing N-9 and the potential for facilitating transmission of STIs including HIV.[15,16] (See Chapter 18 on Vaginal Barriers.) Spermicidal condoms lubricated with N-9, however, deliver much lower doses of N-9 than separately applied vaginal spermicides, and are probably less likely to cause significant genital ulceration or irritation. These condoms may still cause adverse effects in some users. One study, for example, found that use of spermicide-coated condoms was associated with a significantly increased risk of urinary tract infections among young women.[17] While condoms lubricated with or without spermicide are appropriate for most clients,[16] there is currently a move away from the use of N-9 products altogether, and the future availability of spermicidal condoms is unclear.

EFFECTIVENESS AGAINST PREGNANCY

Method failure of the male condom resulting in unintended pregnancy is uncommon, estimated to occur in about 2% of couples using condoms consistently and correctly during the first year of use (Table 16-2). A summary of studies of contraceptive failure for the male condom, as well as a detailed discussion of the estimates used to derive these rates, can be found in Chapter 31 on Contraceptive Efficacy.

The 2% probability of pregnancy during a year of perfect use of the male condom does not mean that 2 of every 100 condoms used will result in unintended pregnancy. What this means is that only 2 of 100 couples who use condoms perfectly for 1 year will experience an unintended pregnancy. If each couple had intercourse at the average coital frequency for U.S. women of 83 acts per year,[18] then the 100 couples would have had intercourse a combined total of 8,300 times over the course of a year. Two pregnancies resulting from 8,300 acts of condom use (or about one pregnancy per 4,150 acts of intercourse) is a remarkably low pregnancy rate (0.02%) when calculated on a per-condom basis.

Table 16-2 First year probability of pregnancy* for couples using condoms, withdrawal, diaphragm, and pill

Method	% of Women Experiencing an Unintended Pregnancy Within the First Year of Use		% of Women Continuing Use at One Year
	Typical Use	Perfect Use	
Withdrawal	27	4	43
Diaphragm	16	6	57
Condom			
Male	15	2	53
Female (Reality)	21	5	49
Pill	8	0.3	68

* See Table 9-2 for first-year probability of pregnancy for all methods.

Emergency Contraceptive Pills: Treatment initiated within 72 hours after unprotected intercourse reduces the risk of pregnancy by at least 75%. (See Chapter 12 for more information.)

However, couples vary widely in their ability to use condoms consistently and correctly. Among those using condoms for contraception, about 15% will experience an unintended pregnancy during the first year of typical use. The marked difference between the condom's probability of pregnancy during typical use and during perfect use generally reflects errors in use, most notably the failure of couples to use condoms during every act of sexual intercourse. Several user behaviors, described later, likely contribute to the risk of unintended pregnancy and the transmission of infection despite condom use. Detailed instructions for proper condom use are provided at the end of this chapter.

CONDOM TESTING

Since 1976, condoms have been regulated as medical devices by the U.S. Food and Drug Administration (FDA). Manufacturers are required to test each lot of condoms according to voluntary performance standards established by the American Society for Testing and Materials (ASTM) and International Standards Organization (ISO).[19] As new technologies and testing procedures develop, these standards undergo periodic review.

Every condom manufactured in the United States is tested electronically for holes and weak spots before it is released for sale. Samples of condoms from each lot that pass electronic testing then undergo a series of standardized laboratory tests for leakage, strength, dimensional requirements, and package integrity. For example, in the freedom-from-holes test, randomly selected condoms are filled with 300 ml of water and visually examined for holes. Moisture detected on the outside of the condom confirms that a hole exists, and the condom is rejected. The Acceptable Quality Limit (AQL) for the freedom-from-holes test has been recently lowered from 0.40 to 0.25, resulting in a higher level of confidence in the product. In the air-burst test adopted by ASTM in 1994, samples of condoms are inflated until they burst. The volume and pressure at the burst are recorded, and must comply with a 1.5 AQL. Dimensional requirements vary depending on the size and design of the condom. However, all condoms must comply with a minimum width and thickness. If the sample condoms fail any of these tests, the entire lot is rejected and destroyed to prevent access to the public. Imported condoms are required to comply with the same performance requirements as domestic condoms and should be equally safe.

COST

The condom is among the most inexpensive and cost-effective contraceptives, especially considering the added protection against STIs and HIV. In a 1999 Consumer Reports survey, high-quality latex condoms ranged in price from $0.27 to $1.09 per unit.[20] There is no evidence to suggest that less expensive condoms indicate lower quality. Based on the average coital frequency for U.S. women,[18] and an average cost of 50 cents per condom,[21] the cost to a couple using condoms with every act of intercourse amounts to about $40 annually. Although few men complain that condoms cost too much, cost may be a barrier to condom acquisition and use for some persons at risk for STIs.[22] Non-profit facilities may purchase latex condoms in bulk at reduced cost to encourage distribution to family planning or STI clients (often from less than 5 cents to 10 cents per condom). Both natural membrane condoms and synthetic condoms are considerably more expensive than latex condoms.[20]

ADVANTAGES AND INDICATIONS

Condom use offers several noncontraceptive benefits. Emphasize that the condom can be fun for both partners when it is made a part of sexual intercourse.

1. **Protection against STIs.** When used consistently and correctly, condoms should effectively reduce the risk of many STIs, including HIV.

2. **Prevention of infertility.** By preventing STIs and their long-term sequelae, condoms protect fertility. (See Chapter 27 on Impaired Fertility.)

3. **Accessibility.** Usage does not require medical examination, prescription, or fitting. Condoms can be obtained from many sources, including drug stores, grocery stores, family planning and STI clinics, vending machines, gas stations, bars, and mail-order services.

4. **Low cost.** Condoms are available at low cost in both the private and public sectors. Users can often obtain condoms for free from publicly funded programs.

5. **Male participation.** Condom use allows men to participate actively in contraception and protection from infection.

6. **Hygiene.** Postcoital leakage of semen from the vagina or anus, a bothersome aftermath for some persons, is avoided by using condoms.

7. **Prevention of sperm allergy.** Women are occasionally allergic to the sperm or semen of their partner to the extent that they have urticarial and anaphylactic reactions. In some infertile couples, the woman's body produces antibodies to her partner's sperm; use of condoms for 3 to 6 months may prevent the release of sperm antigens into the vagina.

8. **Personal concerns.** Men or women who do not wish to have the penis in direct contact with the mouth, vagina, or anus may find condom use preferable.

9. **Portability.** Condoms can be easily and discretely carried by men or women.

10. **Minimal side effects.** Because condoms are non-hormonal, they cause few medical problems among users. The most frequent side effect is most likely latex sensitivity; men or women with this condition can be directed to use synthetic condoms if STIs are of concern.

PROTECTION AGAINST STIS AND HIV

Latex or synthetic condom use reduces the risk of many bacterial and viral STIs. When placed on the penis before any genital contact, the condom prevents direct contact with semen; genital lesions on the shaft of the penis; and penile, vaginal, or anal discharges. Condoms should thus effectively prevent STIs that are transmitted primarily through genital secretions (e.g., gonorrhea, chlamydia, trichomoniasis, hepatitis B infection and HIV infection). Condoms should also provide some protection against STIs that are transmitted primarily through skin-to-skin contact (e.g., herpes simplex virus-2, human papilloma virus (HPV), syphilis, and chancroid) when lesions, ulcers, or shedding occur in areas covered by the condom.[7,23] In vitro laboratory studies show latex condoms provide a highly effective mechanical barrier to a wide range of bacterial and viral STIs (12) including HIV.[24,25]

Clinical studies have shown latex condoms to be highly effective against HIV infection,[26,27] the most serious STI, and should be promoted to sexually active clients at risk for STI for this reason alone. Studies of heterosexual couples with discordant HIV status (where one partner is infected and the other is not) offer compelling evidence of the effectiveness of consistent condom use against HIV infection. Two recent meta-analyses of these studies estimate that consistent condom use reduces the risk of HIV transmission by approximately 90%.[28,29]

Clinical studies of effectiveness against most other STIs suggest more variable protection for condoms; however, interpretation of these studies is complicated by methodologic limitations in study design that would tend to underestimate the true protective effect of condoms.[7,26,30–36] Nevertheless, numerous clinical studies suggest condoms can reduce the risk of a wide variety of STIs in addition to HIV infection, including gonorrhea, chlamydia, trichomoniasis, syphilis, and genital herpes.[37–49]

Condom Use During Anal and Oral Intercourse

Latex and synthetic condoms can also be used during anogenital and orogenital intercourse to prevent STIs. The risk of HIV transmission during anal intercourse can be reduced with the use of latex or synthetic condoms, although the FDA has not approved the use of condoms for this purpose in the United States.[50] The use of a thicker condom or two condoms simultaneously, or the application of an adequate amount of lubricant appropriate for the condom type, may help minimize the risk of breakage during anal intercourse. HIV can be transmitted orally,[51–56] and mouth-to-penis contact (fellatio) and mouth-to-vulva contact (cunnilingus) can also transmit other bacterial and viral pathogens. Unlubricated, scented, or flavored latex or synthetic condoms are recommended for use during fellatio. Household plastic wrap can be used during cunnilingus and anilingus, although it has not been manufactured, intended, or cleared by the FDA for medical applications. Household plastic wrap offers many advantages for persons having oral intercourse in that it is safe, cheap, widely available, conducts heat, and is large enough to cover large areas. Although research on barrier properties of household plastic wrap against viral transmission is extremely limited, one study found it effectively blocked the passage of herpes simplex virus,[57] which is comparable in size to HIV. Dental dams (or oral dams) and condoms adapted to form a barrier sheet have also been proposed as barriers for cunnilingus; however, their limited size may allow potentially infectious fluids to roll onto adjacent tissues, and these products also have not been evaluated or cleared by the FDA for this use.

DISADVANTAGES AND CAUTIONS

Male condom use does have disadvantages that may cause men and women to use them inconsistently or not at all. Many of the barriers to condom use can likely be overcome with practice and experience. Encourage men or women to try different brands of condoms and lubricants until they find one most suitable for them.

1. **Sensitivity.** Many men and their partners complain that condoms reduce sensitivity. Men can try different types of condoms and add lubricant to the outside of the condom to increase sensation.

2. **Spontaneity.** Some men and their partners dislike interrupting foreplay to put on the condom.[117] One solution may be for the partner to put the condom on the penis as part of foreplay.

3. **Problems with erection.** Some men cannot consistently maintain an erection during condom use, so condom use becomes impossible. To help overcome this obstacle, couples may integrate condom use into foreplay. Female condom use may be appropriate in some cases.

4. **Embarrassment.** Some men and women may be embarrassed to obtain condoms from a drug-store shelf or a family planning or STI clinic. Others may be embarrassed to suggest or initiate using condoms because they perceive condom use implies a lack of trust or intimacy. Counsel clients about their embarrassment and teach clients about condoms and how to negotiate their use. Include clients' partners in these discussions when possible.

5. **Coitus dependence.** Some men and their partners may find it inconvenient to use a condom with every act of intercourse.

6. **Lack of cooperation.** In some instances, men will not accept responsibility for contraception or prevention of infection, thus making male condom use impossible. Encourage clients whose partners are resistant to condom use to communicate their concerns to their partners and teach them the skills necessary to negotiate condom use.

7. **Latex allergy.** Some men and women, especially health care workers repeatedly exposed to latex, may be allergic or sensitive to latex and thus unable to use latex condoms. Synthetic condoms are excellent alternatives. (See the section on Managing Problems and Follow-Up.)

PROVIDING CONDOMS

COUNSELING

While men perceive several advantages to condom use (e.g., peace of mind, ease of use, and prolonging of sex[12,58]), men also express concern that condoms reduce sensation, decrease spontaneity, interfere with erection, make intercourse unnatural, and imply a lack of trust between partners.[59-64] Such concerns likely affect men's decisions to use condoms consistently during intercourse. (See the sections on Advantages and Indications and Disadvantages and Cautions.) All clients should understand when to use condoms, how to use condoms most effectively, how to discuss condom use with their partner(s), and how to integrate condom use into intercourse:

STI protection. Recommend condoms to at-risk clients using contraceptive methods that offer little or no protection against STIs or HIV. At-risk clients using another method (oral contraceptives, implants, injectables, IUDs, fertility awareness, spermicides, or sterilization) or who have had hysterectomies should be strongly and frequently encouraged to use condoms. Although women using these methods are generally believed to be less likely to use condoms for prevention of infection,[65] one study found consistent condom use increased among STI clinic clients following an intervention to promote condoms, regardless of their contraceptive method at enrollment.[66]

Emphasize the need for condom use during all sexual activities that can transmit STIs and HIV. Recommend that clients use a new condom for each act of anal, vaginal, or oral intercourse when any risk of infection exists.[13] (See the section on Effectiveness Against STIs and HIV).

Dual method use. Encourage clients to use a condom plus another contraceptive, which may dramatically reduce the risk of both pregnancy and STI.[67] Clients potentially at risk for STI who appear amenable to this strategy should be encouraged to use multiple methods of contraception. Use caution when recommending dual method use to clients, however, since simultaneous use of multiple methods can be overly complicated for some couples, who may instead opt to use no method of contraception at all. Follow the client's lead and perhaps suggest a brief trial period of dual method use. If this proves difficult for the client, consider recommending consistent and correct use of condoms alone to provide adequate protection against both pregnancy and infection. Emergency contraception can be used as a back-up method against pregnancy in case a condom breaks, falls off, or is not used.

Tailored counseling. Adapt counseling messages on condom use to each client's needs. Clients may have formed their own attitudes about condom use and may have had varying experiences with condoms. Tailor the counseling session to each client's risk factors, abilities, needs, and readiness to change.[68] Many clinicians use behavioral change models[69] to assess the ability of their clients to use condoms consistently and to guide the content of the counseling session, a process that makes effective use of time.[70] (See Chapter 10 on Education and Counseling.)

Personal benefits. Make sure clients understand how condom use benefits them personally. Explain that condoms protect future fertility by preventing long-term sequelae of STIs. (See Chapter 8 on Reproductive Tract Infections.) Strongly encourage pregnant women at high risk for STIs to use condoms to protect their fetus, their partner(s), and themselves.

Partner negotiation. Teach clients how to negotiate condom use with partners. Many clients may have contemplated using condoms but may be uncomfortable suggesting condom use to their partners. Teach clients how to negotiate condom use with their partner(s) and help clients develop replies they can use when a partner objects to condoms[71-73] (Table 16-3). Assess the likelihood of a partner's negative reaction to the suggestion of condom use; some clients fear that they will be abused or abandoned if they insist on using condoms. Counsel or refer as appropriate if you detect battering or other forms of abuse.

Table 16-3 Dialogues for negotiating condom use with sex partners

Objection	Response
Sensation	
"I won't feel as much if I have a condom on."	"You won't feel anything if you don't have a condom on."
"It doesn't feel good."	"I think it's really sexy when a guy uses a condom. It shows he cares. What if I put it on for you?"
	"I'd feel better"
Availability	
"I don't have one."	"I do, and it's ribbed for your pleasure."
Disease prevention	
"If you trusted me, you wouldn't ask me to use one."	"I trust that you're telling me the truth, the best you can. But with some STIs, you can't tell if you have them just by looking. Let's be safe and use condoms."
"You won't catch anything from me."	"If you love me, respect my health."
	"Condoms protect. Love doesn't."
Spontaneity	
"It will interrupt sex."	"Let me put it on you. You'll love it."
	"I'll wait."
"It spoils the mood."	"It puts me in the mood."
	"Not if I help."
	"We could always go to a movie."

Adapted from California Office of AIDS, Grieco (1987), and Sapsis (1996).

Effective use. Make sure clients understand how to use condoms effectively. Emphasize that condoms are most effective when used correctly during every act of intercourse. Assessing condom use among clients is a two-tiered process. First ask clients how often they are using condoms (e.g., always, most of the time, sometimes, never). Then, to recognize potential misuse, ask clients to explain (and perhaps demonstrate on an appropriate model of a penis) how they use condoms. (See the section on Minimizing User Errors and on Instructions for Condom Use.) Encourage clients to use condoms consistently and correctly with every act of anal, vaginal, and oral intercourse.

Suitability. Encourage clients who experience problems using condoms to try different brands, until they find one most suitable for them. Ask clients what does not work about using condoms and offer to help them select a condom most suitable to their needs. Remember that all condoms are not the same, and clients will undoubtedly find some condoms more acceptable than others. Some clinics now provide a variety of condoms to clients, including male and female condoms. Although cost is often the primary factor when deciding which condom to distribute in the clinic, many condom brands are similarly priced when purchased in bulk.

Practice. Encourage clients to practice using condoms. Many problems that occur during condom use can be attributed to inexperience[74] and can be overcome with practice. Users who have had negative experiences with condoms may be at risk of discontinuing condom use altogether;[75] encourage them to continue practicing with condoms. When providing instruction on how to use condoms, have the client unroll a condom onto a model of a penis or similarly shaped object, both with eyes open and then again in the dark. Men can also practice using condoms during masturbation, either while alone or with a partner. Condom use during masturbation may provide men with visible proof that they can successfully ejaculate while wearing a condom.

Provision of condoms. Provide each client a large number of condoms at low or no cost. Providing clients with a few condoms is only a short-term solution for clients who find the health care system inaccessible or who find it embarrassing to return repeatedly for condoms.

CONDOM PREFERENCES

More than 100 brands of condoms are available in the United States. Condoms are available in a wide variety of shapes, sizes, colors, and thicknesses, as well as with or without lubricants or spermicides, and with or without reservoir-tip or nipple-ends. Condoms can be straight-sided or tapered toward the closed end, textured (e.g., ribbed) or smooth, solid-colored or nearly transparent, and odorless or scented or flavored. Most condoms are about 7 inches (180 mm) long, 2 inches (52 mm) wide, and .003 inches (.08 mm) thick. More comprehensive listings of the names and characteristics of available condoms can be found in the 17th revised edition of Contraceptive Technology and in two recent articles from Consumer Reports.[20,59]

Recent attention has focused on the characteristics that men, women, and their partners seek when choosing a condom. In a Consumer Reports survey of self-selected readers, lubrication and the reservoir tip were named as the two most important condom features. Some men also preferred natural membrane condoms because they reported more sensitivity with these condoms.[12] In the more representative National Survey of Men, those surveyed preferred condoms that stayed on during sex, were easy to put on, and contained the right amount of lubrication. Few men considered color, ribbing, or cost when purchasing condoms (Table 16-4).[61]

Table 16-4 Characteristics men seek when selecting a condom, 1991 National Survey of Men

Characteristic	% of Men Agreeing
Stays on	58
Easy to put on	57
Right amount of lubrication	54
Easy to obtain	47
Reservoir tip	43
Thin, greater sensation	42
Spermicidal	33
No unpleasant odor	32
Partner likes it	27
Low cost	18
Ribbing	13
Color	7

Source: Grady et al. (1993).

MINIMIZING USER ERROR

Condoms should be highly effective at preventing pregnancy and STIs when used consistently and correctly. Condom effectiveness depends heavily on the skill level and experience of the user.[61,62,74,76–78] Many problems that occur during condom use and present risk of pregnancy or infection are user-related and can be minimized with appropriate counseling and practice.[30,79]

Common problems with condoms that facilitate exposure to STIs and pregnancy include:

- **Failure to use condoms with every act of intercourse.** Nonuse of condoms, rather than poor condom quality or other condom-related problems, is the most common error resulting in risk of pregnancy or STI.[80] *Thus, the highest priority for any STI/HIV or pregnancy prevention program should be to address factors that lead to nonuse of condoms.*

- **Failure to use condoms throughout intercourse.** Some men put condoms on after starting intercourse or remove condoms before ejaculating, practices that expose men and their partners to risks of pregnancy or STIs.[30,81,82] In one study, men and women who acquired gonorrhea despite condom use failed to put the condom on before starting intercourse.[83] Encourage clients to use condoms every time from "start to finish."

- **Condom breakage.** Although users often fear the condom will break or fall off during use,[12,58] these events rarely occur during proper use and tend to be concentrated among a small proportion of users.[74,76] In prospective studies, condoms break generally about 2% of the time during intercourse or withdrawal during vaginal intercourse.[76,85–89] Breakage rates during anal intercourse are similar.[90–93] Not all condom breaks are equally risky. Many condom breaks occur before intercourse[74,78,94,95] and thus pose no risk of pregnancy or infection if a new condom is used.[78] *Thus, advise users to have several condoms available in case a condom is torn or put on incorrectly, or repeated intercourse is desired.*

- **Condom slippage.** Condoms completely fall off the penis in about 2% of acts of vaginal intercourse according to results from prospective studies.[76,85–87,89] Data on rates of complete slippage during anal intercourse, although very limited, appear to range more widely.[92,96] Condoms may also slip down partially during intercourse without falling off, which could pose risk for STIs that are transmitted primarily through skin-to-skin contact (e.g., herpes simplex virus-2, HPV, syphilis, and chancroid). Unfortunately, since very few studies distinguish partial from complete slippage, the degree to which slippage increases the risk of pregnancy or STIs due to semen leakage or exposure to genital lesions is unknown.

- **Poor withdrawal technique.** Although slippage during withdrawal, normally considered user error, may be prevented if the condom's rim is held against the base of the erect penis soon after ejaculation, one study found only 71% of men held the rim during withdrawal and only 50% withdrew immediately after ejaculation.[62]

- **Incorrect placement of the condom on the penis.** Condoms may tear if clients are not careful when removing the condom from the package, test condoms for holes by filling them with air or water, or unroll condoms before putting them on.[62,95,97] Some men accidentally place the condom inside-out on the penis and then flip the condom over and use it for intercourse,[30,81] a practice that may expose their partner to pre-ejaculatory fluid or infectious penile secretions resulting in STI acquisition. Although pregnancy is unlikely to result from exposure to pre-ejaculate, HIV and STI pathogens have been detected in the pre-ejaculatory fluid of infected men.[98,99] Whether the amount of HIV in pre-ejaculate is sufficient to cause infection has not been established.

- **Improper lubricant use with latex condoms.** Unlike water-based lubricants (e.g., K-Y Jelly), oil-based lubricants (e.g., petroleum jelly, baby oil, and hand lotions) reduce latex condom integrity[84] and facilitate breakage.[78] (Table 16-5). Some clients use oil-based products as condom lubricants, mistaking them for water-based lubricants because they readily wash off with water. Because vaginal medications (e.g., for yeast infections) often contain oil-based ingredients that can damage latex condoms, clients who are using or prescribed these medications should be advised to remain abstinent, use synthetic condoms, or use other contraceptives until the medication is fully completed and the infection is cured. Oil-based products may be safely used as lubricants with polyurethane condoms, although they may not be compatible with all synthetic condoms.

Table 16-5 Examples of lubricant products that should and should not be used with natural rubber latex condoms[a]

Safe	Not safe
Egg whites	Baby oil
Glycerine	Cold creams
Saliva	Edible oils (olive, peanut, corn, sunflower)
Silicone	Hand and body lotions
Spermicides in silicone or water-based lubricants	Massage oil
	Petroleum jelly
Water	Rubbing alcohol
Water-based lubricants (e.g., K-Y Jelly, Astroglide)	Suntan oil and lotions
	Vegetable or mineral oil
	Vaginal yeast infection medications in cream or suppository form

[a] All lubricants, including oil-based products, may be used with polyurethane condoms.

PROMOTION AMONG ADOLESCENTS

Despite their increasing popularity, condom promotion programs may be difficult to implement in some settings. Among the most controversial questions are whether adolescents, who may be too embarrassed to purchase or otherwise obtain condoms, should be able to obtain condoms and contraceptive counseling through schools.[100] Although schools can be an important source of information on STIs and HIV for adolescents,[101] only 2% of public high schools make condoms available to students as of the mid-1990s.[102] Surveys of high school students suggest students obtain condoms when they are made available through schools.[103,104] Most evidence to date suggests condom education and availability programs do not hasten the onset or frequency of sexual activity among students.[105]

A need clearly exists for increased condom promotion among sexually active adolescents, given that many youth engage in behaviors that place them at increased risk of STIs,[4] including HIV, and that adolescents account for approximately one-fourth of all new STIs.[106] Three million new cases of STIs are diagnosed among adolescents each year.[101] Additionally, recent national surveys of high school students indicate that approximately half of high school students have sexual intercourse. Despite increases in condom use in recent years, only 51% of females and 63% of males report using a condom at last intercourse,[4] a figure that is insufficient to reduce unintended pregnancy and STI.[105]

Given the small proportion of schools that make condoms available to students, new approaches to condom promotion are needed, ideally before the onset of sexual activity. Access, availability, confidentiality, cost, and perception of peer norms supportive of condom use may all be important determinants of use among adolescents.[101,105] Parents and providers can also play an important role in condom promotion to adolescents. One study found that adolescents who discussed condom use with their parents prior to initiating sexual activity were more likely to use condoms at first intercourse as well as subsequently.[107] Facilitate parent-adolescent discussions about condom use by providing parents with information on condoms and sexual behavior among adolescents.[103]

MANAGING PROBLEMS AND FOLLOW-UP

Persons sensitive or allergic to natural rubber latex may experience irritation, allergic contact dermatitis, or systemic anaphylactic symptoms when exposed to latex-containing products.[108,109] While only 1% of the U.S. population are believed to be allergic to latex,[110] the prevalence of latex sensitivity is much higher among health care workers (17 to 25%[111]) who have repeated exposure to latex-containing medical devices (e.g., surgical and examination gloves, catheters, intubation tubes, anesthesia masks, and dental dams).[109,112] Proteins in the latex appear to be the primary source of allergic reactions.[112]

The FDA has recommended that all patients be questioned for potential latex allergy. Ask whether the client experiences itching, rash, or wheezing after wearing latex gloves or inflating a balloon.[112] From a family planning and STI prevention standpoint, the implications of latex allergy also extend to the use of condoms.[113] If you suspect a client has generalized latex sensitivity, consider recommending synthetic condoms and refer the client for allergy skin testing.[111] While latex condom use is contraindicated for clients with general latex sensitivity, both synthetic and natural membrane condoms can be recommended for prevention of pregnancy, but only synthetic condoms should be recommended for prevention of STIs, including HIV.

Allergic reactions that occur only after exposure to latex condoms and not after exposure to other latex-containing products may be attributable to brand-specific condom attributes such as spermicides, lubricants, perfumes, local anesthetics, or other chemical agents added during the manufacturing process.[114] Advise clients to try different brands of latex and synthetic condoms. In any case, clients should immediately contact their health care provider for follow-up if they or their partner(s) experience a severe allergic reaction while using latex condoms or spermicides. Additional information on latex allergies can also be obtained from the American Latex Allergy Association (see www.latexallergyresources.org).

INSTRUCTIONS FOR USING CONDOMS

Use latex or synthetic condoms when you have any concern about reproductive tract infections, including infection with the human immunodeficiency virus (HIV). When used consistently and correctly, condoms also provide good protection against unintended pregnancy. Instructions for condom use are often overcomplicated and may have no scientific basis.[115] There are three important things to remember when using condoms:

Three Key Instructions for Condom Use

1. Use a new condom with every act of intercourse, if you think there is any risk of pregnancy or sexually transmissible infections (STI).

2. Before penetration, carefully unroll the condom onto the erect penis, all the way to the base.

3. During withdrawal of the penis after ejaculation (while the penis is still erect), hold the rim of the condom against the base of the penis.

BEFORE INTERCOURSE

1. Have on hand an adequate supply of latex or synthetic condoms and water-based lubricant if you think you may need to use a condom, even if you plan to use another contraceptive. Have extra condoms available in case the first is damaged, torn before use, or put on incorrectly. You will need a new condom if you have repeated intercourse.

2. Discuss condom use with your partner before you have intercourse.

AT TIME OF INTERCOURSE

1. Open the condom package carefully to avoid damaging it with fingernails, teeth, or other sharp objects.

2. Put on the condom before the penis comes in contact with the partner's mouth, anus, or vagina. If the penis is uncircumcised, pull the foreskin back before putting on the condom. Keep the condom on the penis until after intercourse or ejaculation.

3. Unroll the condom a short distance to make sure the condom is being unrolled in the right direction. The rolled ring should be on the outside. Then hold the tip of the condom and unroll it down to the base of the erect penis. If the condom does not unroll easily, you probably put it on inside-out. Discard the condom and begin with a new one, because flipping it over and using it could expose your partner to infectious organisms contained in the pre-ejaculate.

4. Adequate lubrication is important. For latex condoms, use only water-based lubricants like water, lubricating jellies (e.g., K-Y Jelly), or spermicidal lubricants, jellies, foam, or suppositories. Avoid oil-based lubricants like cold cream, mineral oil, cooking oil, petroleum jelly, body lotions, massage oil, or baby oil that can damage latex condoms (see Table 16-5). While oil-based products may be safely used as lubricants with polyurethane condoms, they are not necessarily compatible with all synthetic condoms.

5. If the condom breaks or falls off during intercourse but before ejaculation, stop and put on a new condom. A new condom can also be used when you have prolonged intercourse or different types of intercourse within a single session (e.g., vaginal and anal).

AFTER INTERCOURSE

1. Soon after ejaculation, withdraw the penis while it is still erect. Hold the condom firmly against the base of the penis to prevent slippage and leakage of semen.

2. Check the condom for visible damage such as holes, then wrap it in tissue and discard. Do not flush condoms down the toilet.

3. If the condom breaks, falls off, leaks, or is not used, the following may help:

   a. Discuss the possibility of pregnancy or infection with your partner and contact your health care provider as soon as you can. Do not douche. Emergency contraception may be used to prevent pregnancy if started within 72 hours of having unprotected intercourse. Call 1-888-NOT-2-LATE to learn more about emergency contraceptives and to obtain phone numbers of providers of emergency contraception nearest to you, or obtain this information from the World Wide Web at http://ec.princeton.edu. (See Chapter 12 on Emergency Contraception.)

b. Gently wash the penis, vulva, anus, and adjacent areas with soap and water immediately after intercourse to help reduce the risk of acquiring an STI.[43] Then insert an applicator full of spermicide into the vagina as soon as possible.

REPEATED INTERCOURSE

1. Use a new condom from "start to finish" with each act of anal, vaginal, or oral intercourse. Do not reuse condoms.

TAKING CARE OF SUPPLIES

1. Store condoms in a cool and dry place out of direct sunlight (excessive heat will weaken latex). Latex condoms can probably be stored in a wallet for up to 1 month when kept away from heat and sunlight.[116]

2. Check the expiration or manufacture date on the box or individual package of condoms. Expiration dates are marked as "Exp"; otherwise, the date is the manufacture date (MFG). Latex condoms should not be used beyond their expiration date or more than 5 years after the manufacturing date. Latex condoms lubricated with spermicide should probably be used within 2 years of the manufacture date. Condoms in damaged packages or that show obvious signs of deterioration (e.g., brittleness, stickiness, or discoloration) should not be used regardless of their expiration date.

REFERENCES

1. Abma JC, Chandra A, Mosher WD, Peterson LS, Piccinino LJ. Fertility, family planning, and women's health: new data from the 1995 National Survey of Family Growth. Vital Health Stat 1997;Series 23, Number 9.
2. Moran JS, Janes HR, Peterman TA, Stone KM. Increase in condom sales following AIDS education and publicity, United States. Am J Public Health 1990;80:607-608.
3. Personal communication from Ted Conley to Markus Steiner, February 12, 2002.
4. Centers for Disease Control and Prevention. Trends in sexual risk behaviors among high school students – United States, 1991-1997. MMWR 1998;47:749-752.
5. Sonenstein FL, Ku L, Lindberg LD, Turner CF, Pleck JH. Changes in sexual behavior and condom use among teenaged males: 1988 to 1995. Am J Public Health 1998;88:956-959.
6. Stone, KM. HIV, other STDs, and barriers. In: Mauck CK, Cordero M, Gabelnick HL, Spieler JM, Rivera R (eds). Barrier contraceptives: current status and future prospects. New York: Wiley-Liss, Inc., 1994.
7. Stone KM, Thomas E, Timyan J. Barrier methods for the prevention of sexually transmitted diseases. In: Holmes KK, Sparling PF, Mardh P-A, eds. Sexually Transmitted Diseases 1998, 3rd ed., McGraw-Hill, New York.
8. Valdiserri RO. Cum hastis sic clypeatis: the turbulent history of the condom. Bull NY Acad Med 1988;64:237-245.
9. Murphy JS. The condom industry in the United States, 1990. Jefferson NC: McFarland & Company, Inc., Publishers, 1990.
10. Cates W, Stone KM. Family planning, sexually transmissible infections and contraceptive choice: a literature update D Part I. Fam Plann Perspect 1992;24:75-84.

11. Rosenberg MJ, Waugh MS, Solomon HM, Lyszkowski ADL. The male polyurethane condom: a review of current knowledge. Contraception 1996;53:141-146.
12. Consumers Union. Can you rely on condoms? Consum Rep 1989;March:135-142.
13. Centers for Disease Control and Prevention. 1998 Guidelines for Treatment of Sexually Transmitted Diseases. MMWR 1998;47(RR-01).
14. Roddy RE, Cordero M, Ryan KA, Figueroa J. A randomized controlled trial comparing nonoxynol-9 lubricated condoms with silicone lubricated condoms for prophylaxis. Sex Transm Inf 1998;74:116-199.
15. van Damme L. Advances in topical microbicides. Presented at the XIII International AIDS Conference, July 9-14, 2000, Durban, South Africa.
16. Centers for Disease Control and Prevention. CDC statement on study results of products containing nonoxynol-9. MMWR 2000;49:717-718. August 4, 2000.
17. Fihn SD, Boyko EJ, Normand EH, Chen CL, Grafton JR, Hunt M, et al. Association between use of spermicide-coated condoms and Escherichia coli urinary tract infection in young women. Am J Epidemiol 1996;144:512-520.
18. Trussell J, Leveque JA, Koenig JD, London R, Borden S, Henneberry J, et al. The economic value of contraception: a comparison of 15 methods. Am J Publ Health 1995;85:494-503.
19. ASTM (American Society for Testing Materials). Annual book of ASTM standards: Easton MD: ASTM: section 9, rubber. Volume 09.02 Rubber products; standard specifications for rubber contraceptives (male condoms-D3492). West Conshohocken, PA: American Society for Testing Materials, 1996.
20. Consumer's Union. Condoms get better: tests of 30 models show far fewer failures than in past years. Consumer Reports 1999; June.
21. Liskin L, Wharton C, Blackburn R, Kestelman P. Condoms: now more than ever. Pop Rep 1990;8(Series H).
22. Cohen D, Scribner R, Bedimo R, Farley TA. Cost as a barrier to condom use: the evidence for condom subsidies in the United States. Am J Publ Health 1999;89:567-568.
23. Wasserheit JN, Valdiserri RO, Wood RW. Assessment of STD/HIV prevention programs in the United States: national, local, and community perspectives. In: Holmes KK, Sparling PF, Mardh P-A, eds. Sexually Transmitted Diseases 1998, 3rd ed., McGraw-Hill, New York.
24. Carey RF, Herman WA, Retta SM, Rinaldi JE, Herman BA, Athey TW. Effectiveness of latex condoms as a barrier to human immunodeficiency virus-sized particles under conditions of simulated use. Sex Transm Dis 1992;19:230-234.
25. Lytle CD, Routson LB, Seaborn GB, Dixon LG, Bushar HF, Cyr WH. An in vitro evaluation of condoms as barriers to a small virus. Sex Transm Dis 1997;24:161-164.
26. National Institute of Allergy and Infectious Disease. Workshop Summary: Scientific Evidence on Condom Effectiveness for Sexually Transmitted Disease (STD) Prevention. July, 2001.
27. Cates W Jr. The NIH condom report: the glass is 90% full. Family Plann Perspect 2001; 33(5):231-233.
28. Davis KR, Weller SC. The effectiveness of condoms in reducing heterosexual transmission of HIV. Fam Plann Perspect 1999; 31:272-279.
29. Pinkerton SD, Abramson PR. Effectiveness of condoms in preventing HIV transmission. Soc Sci Med 1997; 44:1303-1312.
30. Warner L, Clay-Warner J, Boles J, Williamson J. Assessing correct condom use: implications for evaluating condom use effectiveness. Sex Transm Dis 1998; 25:273-277.
31. Peterman TA, Lin LS, Newman DR, Kamb ML, Bolan G, et al. Does measured behavior reflect STD risk? An analysis of data from a randomized controlled behavioral intervention study. Sex Transm Dis 2000;27:446-451.
32. Feldblum PJ, Morrison CS, Roddy RE, Cates W Jr. The effectiveness of barrier methods of contraception in preventing the spread of HIV. AIDS 1995;9(suppl A):585-593.

33. Warner DL, Hatcher RA. A meta-analysis of condom effectiveness in reducing sexually transmitted HIV. Soc Sci Med 1994;38:1169-1170.
34. Weir, SS, Feldblum PJ. Condom use to prevent incident STDs [letter]. Sex Transm Dis 1996;23:76-77.
35. Turner CF, Miller HG. Zenilman's anomaly reconsidered: fallible reports, ceteris paribus, and other hypotheses. Sex Transm Dis 1997;24:522-527.
36. Warner L, Newman DR, Austin HA, Kamb ML, Douglas JM Jr., Malotte CK, et al. Condom effectiveness for reducing transmission of gonorrhea and chlamydia: the importance of assessing partner infection status. Am J Epidemiol 2004; 159:242-251.
37. Barlow D. The condom and gonorrhoea. Lancet 1977; 222:811-812.
38. Ramstedt K, Forssman L, Giesecke J, Granath F. Risk factors for Chlamydia trachomatis in 6810 young women attending family planning clinics. Int J STD AIDS 1992;3:117-122.
39. Upchurch DM, Brady WE, Reichart CA, Hook EW III. Behavioral contributions to acquisition of gonorrhea in patients attending an inner-city sexually transmitted disease clinic. J Infect Dis 1990;161:938-941.
40. Fennema JSA, van Ameijden EJC, Coutinho RA, van Den Hoek A. Clinical sexually transmitted diseases among human immunodeficiency virus-infected and noninfected drug-using prostitutes. Associated factors and interpretation of trends, 1986 to 1994. Sex Transm Dis 1997; 24:363-371.
41. Levine WC, Revollo R, Kaune V, Vega J, Tinajeras F, Garnica, et al. Decline in sexually transmitted disease prevalence in female Bolivian sex workers: impact of an HIV prevention project. AIDS 1998;12:1899-1906.
42. Wald A, Langenberg AG, Link K, Izu AE, Ashley R, Warren T, et al. Effect of condoms on reducing the trans- mission of herpes simplex virus type 2 from men to women. JAMA 2001;285:3100-3106.
43. Hooper RR, Reynolds GH, Jones OG, Zaidi A, Wiesner PJ, Latimer KP, et al. Cohort study of venereal disease. I: the risk of gonorrhea transmission from infected women to men. Am J Epidemiol 1978;108:136-144.
44. Joesoef MR, Linnan M, Barakbah Y, Idajadi A, Kambodji Schulz K. Patterns of sexually transmitted diseases in female sex workers in Surabaya, Indonesia. Int J STD AIDS 1997;8:576-580.
45. Cates W Jr., Holmes KK. Re: condom efficacy against gonorrhea and nongonococcal urethritis. Am J Epidemiol 1996;143:843-844.
46. Pemberton J, McCann JS, Mahony JDH, Mackenzie G, Dougan H, Hay I. Sociomedical characteristics of patients attending a V.D. clinic and the circumstances of infection. Br J Vener Dis 1972; 48:391-396.
47. Sanchez J, Gutuzzo E, Escamilla J. Sexually transmitted infections in female sex workers: reduced by condom use but not by a limited periodic examination program. Sex Transm Dis 1998;25:82-89.
48. Zenilman JM, Weisman CS, Rompalo AM, Ellish N, Upchurch DM, Hook EW 3rd, et al. Condom use to prevent incident STDs: the validity of self-reported condom use. Sex Transm Dis 1995;22:15-21.
49. Schwartz MA, Lafferty WE, Hughes JP, Handsfield HH. Risk factors for urethritis in heterosexual men. Sex Transm Dis 1997;24:449-455.
50. Silverman BG, Gross TP. Use and effectiveness of condoms during anal intercourse. Sex Transm Dis 1997;24:11-17.
51. Keet IPM, Van Lent NA, Sandfort TGM, Coutinho RA, Van Griensven GJP. Orogenital sex and the transmission of HIV among homosexual men. AIDS 1992;6:223-226.
52. Lifson AR, O'Malley PM, Hessol NA, Buchbinder SP, Cannon L, Rutherford GW. HIV seroconversion in two homosexual men after receptive oral intercourse with ejaculation: implications for counseling concerning safe sexual practices. Am J Publ Health 1990;80:1509-1511.
53. Rozenbaum W, Gharakhanian S, Cardon B, Duval E, Coulaud JP. HIV transmission by oral sex. Lancet 1988;1:1395.

54. Schacker T, Collier AC, Hughes J, Shea T, Corey L. Clinical and epidemiologic features of primary HIV infection. Ann Intern Med 1996;125:257-264.
55. Spitzer PG, Weiner NJ. Transmission of HIV infection from a woman to a man by oral sex. N Engl J Med 1989;320:251.
56. Hawkins DA. Oral sex and HIV transmission. Sex Transm Infect 2001;77:307-308.
57. Garland SM, Newnan DM, de Crespigny LC. Plastic wrap for ultrasound transducers. J Ultrasound Med 1989;8:661-663.
58. Grady WR, Klepinger DH, Billy JOG, Tanfer K, Condom characteristics: the perceptions and preferences of men in the United States. Fam Plann Perspect 1993;25;67-73.
59. Consumer's Union. How reliable are condoms? Consumer Reports 1995; May:320-325.
60. Forrest JD, Singh S. The sexual and reproductive behavior of American women, 1982-1988. Fam Plann Perspect 1990;22:206-214.
61. Grady WR, Klepinger DH, Billy JOG, Tanfer K. Condom characteristics: the perceptions and preferences of men in the United States. Fam Plann Perspect 1993;25:67-73.
62. Warner DL, Hatcher RA, Boles J, Goldsmith J. Practices and patterns of condom usage for prevention of infection and pregnancy among male university students (Session PS-12). Proceeding of the Eleventh Annual National Preventive Medicine Meeting. March 1994.
63. Weinstock HS, Lindan C, Bolan G, Kegeles SM, Hearst N. Factors associated with condom use in a high-risk heterosexual population. Sex Transm Dis 1993;20:14-20.
64. Williamson NE, Joanis C. Acceptability of barrier methods for prevention of unwanted pregnancy and infection. In: Mauck CK, Cordero M, Gabelnick HL, Spieler JM, Rivera R (eds). Barrier contraceptives: current status and future prospects. New York: Wiley-Liss, Inc., 1994.
65. Anderson JE, Brackbill R, Mosher WD. Condom use for disease prevention among unmarried U.S. women. Fam Plann Perspect 1996;28:25-28,39.
66. Centers for Disease Control and Prevention. Contraceptive practices before and after an intervention promoting condom use to prevent HIV infection and other sexually transmitted diseases among women, selected U.S. sites, 1993-1995. MMWR 1997;46:373-377.
67. Cates W Jr., Steiner MJ. Dual protection against unintended pregnancy and sexually transmitted infections: What is the best contraceptive approach? Sex Transm Dis 2002;29:168-174.
68. Centers for Disease Control and Prevention. Revised Guidelines for HIV Counseling, Testing and Referral. MMWR 2001;50 (RR-19):1-58.
69. Prochaska JO, Norcross JC, DiClemente CC. Changing for good. New York: Avon Books, 1994.
70. Contraceptive Technology Update. Can't get patients to use condoms? Try mix of staging and counseling. Contraceptive Technology Update 1997;18:1-12.
71. California Office of AIDS. Condom comebacks: what to say when your partner doesn't want to use a condom. California AIDS Clearinghouse and California Office of AIDS, publication date unknown.
72. Grieco A. Cutting the risks for STDs. Med Aspects Hum Sex 1987;21:70-84.
73. Sapsis K. Putting theory into practice: tools for change. January, 1996.
74. Steiner M, Piedrahita C, Glover L, Joanis C. Can condom users likely to experience condom failure be identified? Fam Plann Perspect 1993;25:220-223,226.
75. Norris AE, Ford K. Associations between condom experiences and beliefs, intentions, and use in a sample of urban, low-income, African-American and Hispanic youth. AIDS Educ Prev 1994;6:27-39.
76. Albert AE, Warner DL, Hatcher RA, Trussell J, Bennett C. Condom use among female commercial sex workers in Nevada's legal brothels. Am J Publ Health 1995;85:1514-1520.
77. Centers for Disease Control and Prevention. Update: barrier protection against HIV infection and other sexually transmitted diseases. MMWR 1993;42:589-591, 597.

78. Steiner M, Trussell J, Glover L, Joanis C, Spruyt A, Dorflinger L. Standardized protocols for condom breakage and slippage trials: a proposal. Am J Publ Health 1994;84:1897-1900.
79. Spruyt A, Steiner MJ, Joanis C, Glover LH, Piedrahita C, Alvarado, et al. Identifying condom users at risk of breakage and slippage: findings from three international sites. Am J Public Health 1998;88:239-244.
80. Steiner MJ, Cates W Jr, Warner L. The real problems with male condoms is nonuse. Sex Trans Dis 1999;26:459-461.
81. Fishbein M, Pequegnat W. Evaluating AIDS prevention interventions using behavioral and biological outcome measures. Sex Transm Dis 2000;37:101-110.
82. Mertz KJ, Finelli L, Levine WL, et al. Gonorrhea in male adolescents and young adults in Newark, New Jersey. Sex Transm Dis 2000;27:201-207.
83. Darrow W. Condom use and use-effectiveness in high-risk populations. Sex Transm Dis 1989;16:157-160.
84. Voeller B, Coulson A, Bernstein GS, Nakamura R. Mineral oil lubricants cause rapid deterioration of latex condoms. Contraception 1989;39:95-101.
85. Cook L, Nanda K, Taylor D. Randomized crossover trial comparing the eZ·on plastic condom and a latex condom. Contraception 2001;63:25-31.
86. Macaluso M, Kelaghan J, Artz L, Austin H, Fleenor M, Hook EW 3rd, et al. Mechanical failure of the latex condom in a cohort of women at high STD risk. Sex Transm Dis 1999;26:450-458.
87. Frezieres RG, Walsh T, Nelson AL, Clark VA, Coulson AH. Breakage and acceptability of a polyurethane condom: a randomized controlled study. Fam Plan Perspect 1999;30:73-78.
88. Nelson A, Frezieres R, Walsh T, Berstein L, Clark V. Phase II/III contraceptive efficacy trial comparing male latex condoms and a male non-latex condom - final report, NIH contract No1-HD-7-3275: National Institute of Health, unpublished paper; 2001.
89. Frezieres RG, Walsh TL. Acceptability evaluation of a natural rubber latex, a polyurethane, and a new non-latex condom. Contraception 2000; 61:369-377.
90. Silverman BG, Gross TP. Use and effectiveness of condoms during anal intercourse. Sex Transm Dis 1997;24:11-17.
91. Buchbinder SP, Douglas JM, McKirnan DJ, Judson FN, Katz MH, MacQueen KM. Feasibility of human immunodeficiency virus vaccine trials in homosexual men in the United States: risk behavior, seroincidence, and willingness to participate. J Infect Dis 1996;174:954-961.
92. Wigersma L, Oud R. Safety and acceptability of condoms for use by homosexual men as a prophylactic against transmission of HIV during anogenital sexual intercourse. BMJ 1987;295:94.
93. Richters J, Donovan B, Gerofi J, Watson L. Low condom breakage rate in commercial sex [letter]. Lancet 1988;2:1487-1488. Correction by John Gerofi in personal communication to Philip Kestelman, July 1989.
94. Trussell J, Warner DL, Hatcher RA. Condom performance during vaginal intercourse: comparison of Trojan-Enz and Tactylon condoms. Contraception 1992;45:11-19.
95. Trussell J, Warner DL, Hatcher RA. Condom slippage and breakage rates. Fam Plann Perspect 1992;24:20-23.
96. Golombok S, Sheldon J. Evaluation of a thicker condom for use as a prophylactic against HIV transmission. AIDS Educ Prev 1994;6:454-458.
97. Family Health International. How human use affects condom breakage. Network 1991;12:10-14.
98. Ilaria G, Jacobs JL, Polsky B, Koll B, Baron P, Maclow C, Armstrong D. Detection of HIV-1 DNA sequences in pre-ejaculatory fluid. Lancet 1992;340:1469.
99. Pudney J, Oneta M, Mayer K, Searge G (III), Anderson D. Pre-ejaculatory fluid as potential vector for sexual transmission of HIV-1. Lancet 1992;340:1470.
100. Mahler K. Condom availability in the schools: lessons from the courtroom. Fam Plann Perspect 1996;28:75-77.

101. Institute of Medicine. The hidden epidemic: confronting sexually transmissible infections. In: Eng TR, Butler WT (eds). Washington DC: National Academy Press, 1997.
102. Kirby DB, Brown NL. Condom availability programs in U.S. schools. Fam Plann Perspect 1996;28:196-202.
103. Kirby DB, Miller KS, Whitaker DJ. Predictors of mother-adolescent discussions about condoms: implications for providers who serve youth. Pediatrics 2001;108:1-7.
104. Schuster MA, Bell RM, Berry SH, Kanouse DE. Impact of a high school condom availability program on sexual attitudes and behaviors. Fam Plann Perspect 1998;30:67-72, 88.
105. American Academy of Pediatrics. Condom use by adolescents. Pediatrics 2001;107:1463-1469.
106. ASHA. Sexually transmitted diseases in America: how many cases and at what cost? Kaiser Family Foundation, December 1998.
107. Miller KS, Levin ML, Whitaker DJ, Xu X. Patterns of condom use among adolescents: the impact of mother-adolescent communication. Am J Publ Health 1998;88:1542-1544.
108. Anglia and Oxford Regional Health Authority. Latex allergy: implications for patients and health care workers. Bandolier 1994;7:1-3.
109. Zaza S, Reeder JM, Charles LE, Jarvis WR. Latex sensitivity among perioperative nurses. AORN 1994;60:806-812.
110. Sprouls LS. When latex gloves aren't a perfect fit: reactions, sensitivity plague 12 percent of HCWs. Dental Teamwork 1992;November-December:28-31.
111. Yassin MS, Lierl MB, Fischer TJ, O'Brien KO, Cross J, Steinmetz C. Latex allergy in hospital employees. Ann Allergy 1994;72:245-249.
112. Food and Drug Administration. Allergic reactions to latex-containing medical devices [press release]. Rockville MD; Food and Drug Administration, March 29, 1991.
113. Fisher AA. Condom dermatitis in either partner. Cutis 1987;39:284-285.
114. Hamann CP, Kick SA. Update: immediate and delayed hypersensitivity to natural rubber latex. Cutis 1993;52:307-311.
115. Mindel A. Condoms. First ed. London: BMJ Publishing Group, 2000.
116. Glasser G, Hatcher RA. The effect on condom integrity of carrying a condom in a wallet for three months [abstract]. Proceedings of the American College of Obstetricians and Gynecologists District IV Conference, November 1992. San Juan PR.

LATE REFERENCE

117. Warner L, Steiner MJ. Condom access does not ensure condom use: you've got to be putting me on. Sex Transm Inf 2002; 78:225.

Vaginal Spermicides

Willard Cates Jr., MD, MPH
Elizabeth G. Raymond, MD, MPH

- Spermicides are simple, free of systemic side effects, and available without prescription. They can be used intermittently with little advance planning.
- Spermicides are an integral component of vaginal barrier methods (diaphragm, sponge, and cap).
- Spermicides provide little, if any, protection against transmission of STIs.
- Spermicides do not protect against HIV.
- Frequent (≥2/day) spermicide use may cause tissue irritation that theoretically could increase susceptibility to HIV.

Spermicide products can be purchased without prescription in pharmacies and supermarkets. They can be used alone, with a vaginal barrier method, or as an adjunct to any of the other contraceptive methods for added protection against pregnancy.

MECHANISM OF ACTION

Spermicidal preparations consist of two components:
- Formulation (gel, foam, cream, film, suppository, or tablet), also called a carrier or base
- Chemical that kills the sperm in different doses and concentrations

For some products, the formulation helps disperse the spermicide. In the case of viscous gel and foam, the formulation itself may provide both lubrication and an additional barrier effect. Nonoxynol-9 (N-9), the active chemical agent in spermicide products available in the United States, is a surfactant that destroys the sperm cell membrane. Other surfactant products, including octoxynol, menfegol, and benzalkonium chloride, are widely used in other parts of the world. Because of the current emphasis on developing microbicides for female-initiated methods to prevent HIV/STIs, more than 20 chemical barrier methods are in various stages of development and evaluation.[1,2] Some have contraceptive properties, while some do not.

Gels and creams. Gels, creams, and foam are commonly marketed for use with a diaphragm, but they can also be used alone. One application delivers 52.5 mg to 150 mg of spermicide, depending on the product: the spermicide concentration ranges from 8% to 12.5% in foam and from 2% to 4% in gels and creams.

Suppositories. Spermicide suppositories can be used alone or with a condom. Suppositories have a spermicide concentration of 3% to 5% and provide 100 mg to 125 mg of spermicide. Adequate time between insertion and intercourse (10 to 15 minutes depending on the product) is essential for the spermicide to dissolve and disperse. Incomplete dissolution of the suppository may reduce its contraceptive efficacy and may cause an uncomfortable gritty sensation or friction for the woman or the man.

Film. N-9 film can be used alone or with barriers. Each paper-thin sheet of film has a spermicide concentration of 28% and contains 72 mg to 100 mg of N-9. The sheet must be inserted on or near the cervix at least 15 minutes before intercourse to allow time for the sheet to melt and disperse. Placing film on the tip of the penis for insertion is not recommended; the film will not have adequate time to dissolve, and it may not be properly placed so as to cover the cervical os.

Spermicidal condoms. Latex condoms coated with N-9 have been available in the United States since 1983. (See Chapter 16 on Male Condoms.) However, no evidence to date shows that male condoms pre-lubricated with spermicide offer any contraceptive benefit versus condoms alone or condoms with non-spermicidal lubricant.

EFFECTIVENESS

Reported pregnancy rates among typical users cover a wide range, from less than 5% to more than 50% in the first year of use. Most published clinical trials of spermicide used alone do not meet modern standards for study design and analysis; thus, we must be cautious when comparing the contraceptive effectiveness of spermicides with that of other contraceptive methods.

A randomized trial of nonoxynol-9 film and foaming tablets found high unintended pregnancy rates for both products—25% and 28% pregnant in six months, respectively.[3] The population studied was young (58% younger than 25 years) and had frequent coitus (71% more than 10 acts per month). A more recent randomized trial of five nonoxynol-9 spermicide products conducted in the United States showed somewhat lower pregnancy rates, from 10% to 22% in 6 months. In this trial, a gel containing 52.5 mg of nonoxynol-9 was less effective at preventing pregnancy than gels containing 100 or 150 mg. However, no difference was found between a gel, a film, and a suppository each containing 100 mg of nonoxynol-9.[4]

The effectiveness of spermicides, like any barrier method, depends largely on consistent and correct use. For spermicide to be effective, manufacturers recommend that it be placed correctly in the vagina no longer than 1 hour before intercourse. The spermicide gel, tablet, suppository, or film needs to make contact with the cervix, which for most women is deep in the vagina. Suppositories, foaming tablets, and films require adequate time for dissolution and dispersion.

A method's characteristics (timing, degree of lubricating effect, or required delay for suppository or film to melt) may influence a woman's ability to use the spermicide effectively. A woman is most likely to succeed with a method that is compatible with her sexual routines.

Using a physical and a chemical barrier method together increases contraceptive efficacy. For example, diaphragm users have a lower risk of pregnancy when they also use a spermicide. (See Chapter 9 on Essentials of Contraception.) Likewise, using emergency contraception to back up spermicides in situations of incorrect or non-use will increase effectiveness.

Douching is not a reliable contraceptive, even when a spermicide is in the douching solution, because sperm enter the cervical canal soon after ejaculation. A woman who has used a vaginal spermicide for contraception should not douche until at least 6 hours after sexual intercourse to avoid washing away the spermicide prematurely.

COST

Film and suppositories can be purchased for less than $1.00 per dose. Retail prices for foams and gels range from $10 to $15 per multidose container. The more frequently a woman uses spermicide for intercourse, the greater her cost.

ADVANTAGES AND INDICATIONS

Spermicides are a short-term contraceptive option and may be a reasonable long-term choice for couples who use them consistently.

1. Spermicides can be purchased over-the-counter and do not require the user to seek medical consultation.

2. A male partner need not be involved in the decision to initiate the use of spermicides.

3. Spermicides can be kept available for immediate protection, for those who have intercourse infrequently or after long intervals.

4. Spermicides are a simple back-up option for a woman who is waiting to start oral contraceptives or have an intrauterine device

(IUD) inserted, forgets two or more pills, runs out of pills, or suspects her IUD has been expelled, or who is breastfeeding.

5. Spermicides can be used to augment the effectiveness of fertility awareness methods.

PROTECTION AGAINST STIS AND HIV

Our currently-available spermicides containing nonoxynol-9 are ineffective as microbicides.[5] In the laboratory, N-9 is lethal to organisms that cause gonorrhea, genital herpes, trichomoniasis, syphilis, and acquired immune deficiency syndrome (AIDS).[6] However, activity in the test tube does not mean spermicides can provide reliable protection in actual use. Findings from human studies on the effectiveness and the safety of N-9 have not lived up to hopes.[7,8]

The optimal study designs are randomized controlled trials (RCT), also referred to as level I scientific evidence. (See Chapter 1 on Expanding Perspectives on Reproductive Health.) Because both randomization and masking help eliminate behavioral and other differences among the study populations being compared, bias and confounding are eliminated or greatly reduced.[9] The highest-quality RCTs have studied three different formulations containing N-9—a gel,[10–14] the film,[8,15] and the sponge.[16] In the aggregate, these studies have shown that N-9 spermicide used alone has minimal, if any, impact on preventing bacterial reproductive tract infections. The users' risk of acquiring gonorrhea, chlamydia, trichomoniasis, or bacterial vaginosis formed no consistent pattern of protection or harm and the 95% confidence intervals could not rule out chance.

In addition, evidence indicates that N-9 provides no protection against HIV.[8,12,13,16] Thus, do not recommend the use of spermicide alone to prevent HIV. Furthermore, frequent use (more than 2 times per day) of spermicides causes higher levels of vulvovaginal epithelial disruption,[17] which theoretically could increase susceptibility to HIV. (See Chapter 7 on HIV/AIDS and Reproductive Health.)

We have a critical need for female-initiated methods to prevent STIs, including HIV. While male condoms provide protection against most STIs,[18] their use is low among many couples. Methods women can use autonomously may improve levels of protection because of better adherence. However, the lengthy research required for developing and testing new microbicidal products means these methods are years away.[1,19]

D ISADVANTAGES AND CAUTIONS

Spermicides are not a reasonable contraceptive choice in the following circumstances:

- Allergy or sensitivity to the spermicidal agent or to ingredients in the base.

- Inability to learn correct insertion technique.
- Abnormal vaginal anatomy (such as vaginal septum, prolapsed uterus, or double cervix) that interferes with appropriate placement or retention of spermicide.
- If STI/HIV exposure is likely, situations that would involve frequent use, e.g., 2 times or more a day.
- Recurrent urinary tract infections.

Irritation. Temporary skin irritation involving the vulva, vagina, or penis caused by either local toxicity or allergy is the most common problem associated with spermicide use. When an allergy is suspected, suggest the client try another contraceptive method. Vaginal epithelial disruption has been associated with frequent use (twice a day or more).[17,20] However, epithelial disruption does not always cause noticeable symptoms, and symptoms do not necessarily indicate tissue harm. If any signs of irritation are found, advise the client to use spermicides less frequently or to discontinue their use.

Common dislikes. In a study of film and suppositories, the main complaints were messiness, having to wait before coitus, having to touch the genitals, and excessive lubrication.[3] Some couples find the taste of spermicide unpleasant when they engage in oral-genital sex. Occasionally, women find the effervescence of foaming vaginal suppositories is unpleasant.

Yeast vaginitis. Use of a diaphragm with spermicide can also increase vaginal colonization with Candida species. However, use of spermicides alone have not been associated with higher rates of vaginal candidiasis.[11,13]

Bacterial vaginosis. Spermicide use can encourage selective colonization of the vagina with anaerobic bacteria and uropathogens relatively resistant to N-9. However, clinical studies have not shown N-9 increases BV.

Urinary Tract Infection. Higher rates of urinary tract infection have been reported among women who use spermicide with either diaphragms or male condoms.[21] The N-9 effect on vaginal flora, interacting with barrier methods, may play a role in the UTI risk.

Systemic effects. No serious adverse reactions to the spermicide products now marketed in the United States have been reported. In 1980, an advisory panel for the U.S. Food and Drug Administration (FDA), reviewing published information and information from manufacturers, approved them as safe and effective. However, toxicology studies to determine the degree of vaginal absorption and to detect possible systemic effects are limited.

Spermicide use and pregnancy. Several early studies reported possible adverse associations between spermicide exposure and birth defects; however, serious methodologic problems invalidate their conclusions.[22] Subsequent research has found no link between adverse fetal effects and spermicide use.[23,24] Thus, no apparent causal association exists between spermicide use and fetal defects.

PROVIDING SPERMICIDES

Spermicides are currently available over the counter. When providing spermicides in a clinical setting, reinforce instructions for proper use and remind users about common errors that can lead to unintended pregnancy. (See the section on Instructions for Using Spermicides). Counsel users about emergency contraception as a back-up. Warn women who have abnormalities of vaginal anatomy (such as a septate vagina or a severe uterine prolapse), which may interfere with proper spermicide placement, that spermicide use may not be effective for them.

Correct and consistent use of spermicides determine contraceptive effectiveness.[25] In one study, women have found the N-9 film and gel formulations preferable to suppositories.[26] Men have found spermicides to be at least as acceptable as women have. Encouraging men to suggest spermicide use or at least to cooperate with their partner's desire to use spermicides could be a helpful approach for increasing spermicide effectiveness.

MANAGING PROBLEMS AND FOLLOW-UP

Spermicide use does not require any special follow-up. Women who experience irritation may seek care. If symptoms persist more than a day or two after the patient discontinues using spermicides, evaluate the underlying factors, such as STI exposure, yeast vaginitis, or bacterial vaginosis. Changing to an alternative product with a different formulation or changing to a less concentrated product may help.

Ask about spermicide use (including condoms lubricated with spermicide) when evaluating a woman with recurrent urinary tract infections. Switching to another contraceptive strategy may help in managing recurrent UTIs.

INSTRUCTIONS FOR USING SPERMICIDES

1. Use spermicide every time you have intercourse. Be sure spermicide is in place before your partner's penis enters your vagina.

2. If you have problems with vaginal or penile irritation, you may want to try a different spermicide product. Alternatively, you could switch to condoms or see your clinician for another method of birth control.

3. Do not use spermicides to reduce risks of sexually transmitted infections. Use male or female condoms for this purpose.

Common Errors in Spermicide Use

Common errors can lead to unintended pregnancy:

- Failing to use spermicide or an alternative method such as condoms each and every time intercourse occurs, even when menstrual bleeding is present
- Failing to place spermicide high enough in the vaginal vault to be effective
- Failing to wait long enough after insertion for suppositories or film to dissolve and disperse
- Failing to use another application of spermicide if more than 1 hour has elapsed between insertion and intercourse
- Using too little spermicide or foam, or failing to shake the foam can vigorously enough
- Failing to use another applicator with every repeated act of intercourse
- Failing to recognize that the foam bottle or spermicide tube is empty
- Failing to have spermicide available

Before Intercourse

1. Check to be sure you have all the supplies you need. If you are using foam, cream, or gel, you may also need a plastic applicator. If you use foam, keep an extra container on hand. You may not be able to tell when your current container is running low.

2. Plan ahead about when to insert your method. Try to find a routine that is comfortable for you and your partner. If you are using suppositories or film, a waiting period between insertion and intercourse is essential to allow the product to melt or spread inside your vagina. The package instructions explain the exact time required. One dose of most spermicide formulations remains effective for 1 hour. If a longer time has passed, or if you have intercourse again, you must use a new dose of spermicide.

For Insertion

1. Wash your hands carefully with soap and water.

2. *Foam.* Shake the foam container vigorously then use the nozzle to fill the plastic applicator.

   Gel, Cream, or Foam. Fill the applicator by squeezing the spermicide tube. Next insert the applicator into your vagina as far as it will comfortably go; then, holding the applicator still, push the plunger to release the gel, cream, or foam. The spermicide should be deep in your vagina, close to your cervix.

Suppository. Remove the wrapping and slide the suppository into your vagina. Push it along the back wall of your vagina as far as you can so it rests on or near your cervix.

Film. Be sure your fingers are completely dry. Remove film from the package. Place one sheet of film on your fingertip and slide it along the back wall of your vagina as far as you can so the film rests on or near your cervix.

3. **Repeated intercourse.** Apply a new application of spermicide each time you have intercourse. Alternatively, you can switch to condoms for repeated intercourse if you wish.

4. **After intercourse.** Leave spermicide in place for at least 6 hours after intercourse; do not rinse your vagina. Douching is not recommended, but if you choose to douche you must wait at least 6 hours.

CARING FOR SPERMICIDE SUPPLIES

1. Store your spermicide in a convenient location that is clean, cool, and dark.

2. After each use wash your reusable applicator with plain soap and warm water. Do not use talcum powder on your applicator.

REFERENCES

1. McCormack S, Hayes R, Lacey CJ, Johnson AM. Microbicides in HIV prevention. BMJ 2001; 322(7283):410-413.
2. Microbicides 2000 conference proceedings. March 13-16, 2000, Washington, DC. AIDS 2001; 15 Suppl 1:S1-88.
3. Raymond E, Dominik R, Spermicide Trial Group. Contraceptive effectiveness of two spermicides: a randomized trial. Obstet Gynecol 1999; 93(6):896-903.
4. Raymond EG, Chen PL, Luoto J, et al. Contraceptive Effectiveness and Safety of Five Nonoxynol-9 Spermicides: A Randomized Trial. Obstet Gynecol 2004;103: 430-439.
5. Cates W Jr, Padian NS. The interrelationship of reproductive health and sexually transmitted diseases. In: Goldman MBaHMC, (eds). Women and Health. San Diego, California: Academic Press, 2000: 381-389.
6. Pauwels R, De Clercq E. Development of vaginal microbicides for the prevention of heterosexual transmission of HIV. J Acquir Immune Defic Syndr Hum Retrovirol 1996; 11(3):211-221.
7. Cates W Jr, Stewart FH, Trussell J. Commentary: the quest for women's prophylactic methods—hopes vs science [see comments]. Am J Public Health 1992; 82(11):1479-1482.
8. Roddy RE, Zekeng L, Ryan KA, Tamoufe U, Weir SS, Wong EL. A controlled trial of nonoxynol 9 film to reduce male-to-female transmission of sexually transmitted diseases. N Engl J Med 1998; 339(8):504-510.
9. Mauck C, Rosenberg Z, Van Damme L. Recommendations for the clinical development of topical microbicides: an update. AIDS 2001; 15(7):857-868.
10. Louv WC, Austin H, Alexander WJ, Stagno S, Cheeks J. A clinical trial of nonoxynol-9 for preventing gonococcal and chlamydial infections. J Infect Dis 1988; 158(3):518-523.

11. Barbone F, Austin H, Louv WC, Alexander WJ. A follow-up study of methods of contraception, sexual activity, and rates of trichomoniasis, candidiasis, and bacterial vaginosis. Am J Obstet Gynecol 1990; 163(2):510-514.
12. Van Damme L, Ramjee G, Alary M, et al. Effectiveness of COL-1492, a nonoxynol-9 vaginal gel, on HIV-1 transmission in female sex workers: a randomized controlled trial. Lancet 2002; 360:971-977.
13. Richardson BA, Lavreys L, Martin HL Jr et al. Evaluation of a low-dose nonoxynol-9 gel for the prevention of sexually transmitted diseases: a randomized clinical trial. Sex Transm Dis 2001; 28(7):394-400.
14. Roddy RE, Zekeng L, Ryan KA, Ubald T, Tweedy KG. The effect of nonoxynol-9 gel on urogenital gonorrhea and chlamydia infection. JAMA 2002; 287:1117-1122.
15. Niruthisard S, Roddy RE, Chutivongse S. Use of nonoxynol-9 and reduction in rate of gonococcal and chlamydial cervical infections. Lancet 1992; 339(8806):1371-1375.
16. Kreiss J, Ngugi E, Holmes K et al. Efficacy of nonoxynol 9 contraceptive sponge use in preventing heterosexual acquisition of HIV in Nairobi prostitutes. JAMA 1992; 268(4):477-482.
17. Roddy RE, Cordero M, Cordero C, Fortney JA. A dosing study of nonoxynol-9 and genital irritation. Int J STD AIDS 1993; 4(3):165-170.
18. Centers for Disease Control and Prevention. Male latex condoms and sexually transmitted diseases. Factsheet for public health personnel. Update December 12, 2002. www.cdcnpin.org.
19. Rockefeller Foundation. Mobilization for Microbicides: The Decisive Decade. New York, Rockefeller Foundation Microbicide Initiative, 2002.
20. Goeman J, Ndoye I, Sakho LM et al. Frequent use of menfegol spermicidal vaginal foaming tablets associated with a high incidence of genital lesions. J Infect Dis 1995; 171(6):1611-1614.
21. Hooton TM, Scholes D, Hughes JP et al. A prospective study of risk factors for symptomatic urinary tract infection in young women. N Engl J Med 1996; 335(7):468-474.
22. Strobino B, Kline J, Warburton D. Spermicide use and pregnancy outcome. Am J Public Health 1988; 78(3):260-263.
23. Simpson JL, Phillips OP. Spermicides, hormonal contraception and congenital malformations. Adv Contracept 1990; 6(3):141-167.
24. Einarson TR, Koren G, Mattice D, Schechter-Tsafriri O. Maternal spermicide use and adverse reproductive outcome: a meta- analysis. Am J Obstet Gynecol 1990; 162(3):655-660.
25. Elias C, Coggins C. Acceptability research on female-controlled barrier methods to prevent heterosexual transmission of HIV: Where have we been? Where are we going? J Womens Health Gend Based Med 2001; 10(2):163-173.
26. Steiner M, Spruyt A, Joanis C, et al. Acceptability of spermicidal film and foaming tablets among women in three countries. Int Fam Plann Perspect 1995; 21:104-107.

Vaginal Barriers

THE FEMALE CONDOM, DIAPHRAGM, CONTRACEPTIVE SPONGE, CERVICAL CAP, LEA'S SHIELD AND FEMCAP

Willard Cates Jr., MD, MPH
Felicia Stewart, MD, MPH

- Vaginal barriers are relatively simple to use and can be used intermittently with little advance planning.

- Except for the female condom, using barrier methods does not require the direct involvement of the male partner and does not interrupt lovemaking.

- Consistent and correct use is essential for vaginal barrier effectiveness; most pregnancies occur because the method is not used.

- Protection against human immunodeficiency virus (HIV) has not been documented for vaginal barriers with or without spermicide.

- Protection against some STIs by vaginal barriers has been demonstrated in observational studies.

Vaginal barriers have a rich contraceptive heritage. When Margaret Sanger and Emma Goldman visited Europe in the early 1900s, they found a wide variety of cap and diaphragm models being used. The diaphragm soon became *the* modern contraceptive method in the United States. Since then, diaphragm technology has changed little. The most recent development was the 1983 introduction of a new model, the wide-seal style, with a soft latex flange attached to the inner side of the rim.

Earlier in this century, cervical caps were made of silver, copper, or impermeable plastic. Inserted and removed by the woman's physician, they were left in place for as long as 3 to 4 weeks. These have been replaced by latex caps now manufactured in England. In 1988 the Food and Drug Administration (FDA) approved one such product, the Prentif Cavity Rim Cervical Cap, for general use in the United States. Two other cervical barrier methods, Lea's Shield and FemCap, were approved in 2002.

In 1983, the Food and Drug Administration (FDA) approved a vaginal contraceptive sponge for use in the United States. The Today Sponge, containing nonoxynol-9 (N-9) spermicide, was marketed in the U.S. until 1995 when its distribution was stopped because the manufacturer decided not to invest in needed modernization of production equipment. However, another manufacturer is currently attempting to get FDA approval to re-distribute the sponge. Vaginal contraceptive sponges containing N-9 continue to be marketed in other countries, as are similar products containing other spermicides, such as benzalkonium chloride.

The first female condom, called Reality, was approved by the FDA in 1993 for over-the-counter sale in the United States. Researchers did not include women at risk for sexually transmitted infection (STI) in the contraceptive effectiveness research required for FDA approval. Thus, available research provides only sparse evidence of its likely impact on reducing STI risk. The design of the female condom, and its physical properties, however, indicate it should protect against STI if used correctly and consistently.

MECHANISM OF ACTION

The female condom provides a physical barrier that lines the vagina entirely and partially shields the perineum. Diaphragms, caps, and sponges combine two contraceptive mechanisms: a physical barrier to shield the cervix and a chemical to kill sperm. These devices also may help to hold spermicide in place against the cervix, and in the case of the sponge, absorb and trap sperm.

VAGINAL BARRIER OPTIONS

Female condom. The Reality Female Condom is a soft, loose-fitting polyurethane sheath, 7.8 cm in diameter and 17 cm long. It contains two flexible polyurethane rings. One ring lies inside, at the closed end of the sheath, and serves as an insertion mechanism and internal anchor. The other ring forms the external, open edge of the device and remains outside the vagina after insertion (Figure 18-1). The external portion of the device provides some protection to the labia and the base of the penis during intercourse. The sheath is coated on the inside with a silicone-based lubricant; additional lubricant for the outside is provided with the device. The lubricant does not contain spermicide. Reality, approved for over-the-counter sale without prescription, is intended for one-time use. It can be inserted up to 8 hours before intercourse. Female and male condoms should not be used together; they can adhere to each other, causing slippage or displacement of one or both devices.

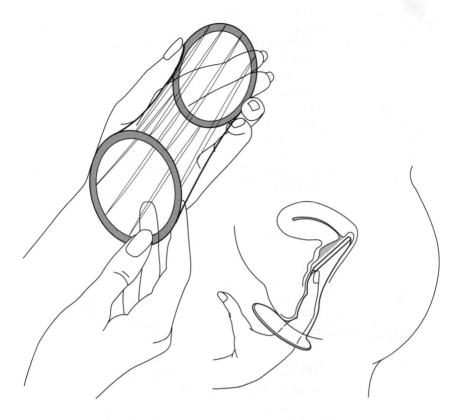

Figure 18-1 Reality Female Condom

The polyurethane used in the sheath is a thin (0.05 mm) but impermeable material with good heat-transfer characteristics. It is stronger than latex and less likely to tear or break. It does not deteriorate with exposure to oil-based products and withstands storage better than latex does.

Diaphragm. This dome-shaped rubber cup has a flexible rim; it is inserted into the vagina before intercourse so the posterior rim rests in the posterior fornix and the anterior rim fits snugly behind the pubic bone. The dome of the diaphragm covers the cervix; spermicidal cream or jelly applied to the inside of the dome before insertion is held in place near the surface of the cervix. Diaphragm purchase requires a prescription.

Once in position, the diaphragm provides effective contraceptive protection for 6 hours. If a longer interval has elapsed, insertion of additional, fresh spermicide with an applicator (without removing the diaphragm) has been previously recommended, but no evidence supports this practice. After intercourse, the diaphragm must be left in place for at least 6 hours. Wearing it for longer than 24 hours is not recommended because of the possible risk of toxic shock syndrome (TSS).

Diaphragms are available in sizes ranging from 50 millimeters (mm) to 95 mm (diameter) and in several styles (Figure 18-2). The styles differ in the inner construction of the circular rim, and in the case of the wide-seal style, the presence of a flexible flange attached to the inner edge of the rim. The thin, flat spring rim has a gentle spring strength that is comfortable for women with firm vaginal muscle tone. The sturdy coil spring rim has a firm spring strength suitable for a woman with average muscle tone and an average pubic arch depth. A plastic diaphragm introducer can be used to insert coil or flat spring styles. The sturdy and firm arcing spring folds into an arc shape that facilitates correct insertion; it can maintain a correct position despite lax muscle. Wide-seal diaphragms are available with either an arcing spring rim or a coil spring rim.

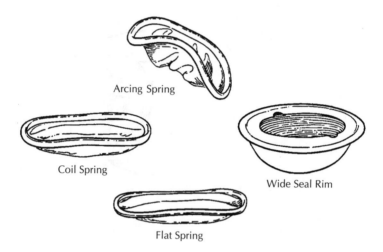

Arcing Spring

Coil Spring

Wide Seal Rim

Flat Spring

Figure 18-2 Types of diaphragms

Cervical cap. The Prentif Cavity Rim Cervical Cap is a soft, deep rubber cup with a firm round rim (Figure 18-3). A groove along the inner circumference of the rim improves the seal between the inner rim of the cap and the surface of the cervix. The Prentif cap fits with its rim snugly around the base of the cervix, close to the junction between the cervix and the vaginal fornices. Spermicide, used to fill the dome 1/3 full prior to insertion of the cap, is held in place against the cervix until the cap is removed.

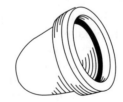

Prentif Cavity Rim Cervical Cap

Figure 18-3 Cervical cap

The cap provides continuous contraceptive protection for 48 hours, no matter how many times intercourse occurs. Additional spermicide is not necessary for repeated intercourse. Because of the possible risk of TSS, wear for longer than 48 hours is not recommended. Some women experience odor problems with more prolonged use.

Contraceptive sponge. This product is a small, pillow-shaped polyurethane sponge containing 1 gram of nonoxynol-9 spermicide. The concave dimple on one side was designed to fit over the cervix and decrease the chance of dislodgement during intercourse (Figure 18-4). The other side of the sponge incorporates a woven polyester loop to facilitate removal. The sponge is a one-size, over-the-counter product. It is moistened with tap water prior to use and inserted deep into the vagina.

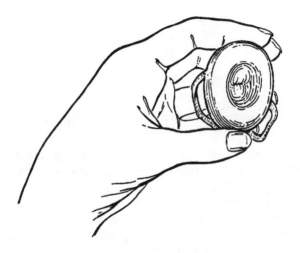

Figure 18-4 Contraceptive sponge

The sponge protects for up to 24 hours, no matter how many times intercourse occurs. After intercourse, the sponge must be left in place for at least 6 hours before it is removed and discarded. Wearing the sponge for longer than 24 to 30 hours is not recommended because of the possible risk of TSS.

Lea's Shield. This product is an oval device made of medical-grade silicone rubber, with an anterior loop that assists in removal (Figure 18-5). The device was approved by the FDA in March 2002. It is reusable and is used with spermicide much like the diaphragm. Like the cap, it blocks the cervix, but contains a central valve which allows passage of cervical secretions and air. Lea's Shield has only one size, so fitting is not required. However, in the US, the device is available by prescription only. Participants in an effectiveness study found the Lea's Shield comfortable and acceptable. The Lea's Shield's failure rate of 8.7 pregnancies per 100 women observed during this 6-month study was similar to rates observed

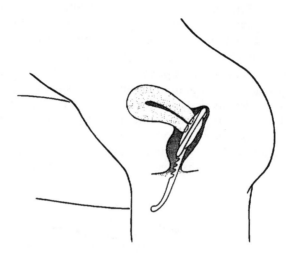

Figure 18-5 Some women prefer to use a plastic introducer for diaphragm insertion

in previous effectiveness studies for the cervical cap, diaphragm and sponge when standardized for parity in the study populations.[1]

FemCap. This product is a hat-shaped silicone rubber cap with a brim that flares outward.[2] The bowl of the FemCap covers the cervix completely, while the rim fits against the vaginal fornices. The brim is taller on one end than the other. When properly positioned, the larger brim fits into the back of the vagina. Spermicide can be placed on the inside and the outside of the cap. A strap located on the convex bowl could aid in removal. FemCap comes in 3 sizes, thus it requires clinician fitting and is available only by prescription. The FemCap can be worn for up to 48 hours.

Future barrier devices. Other products being developed include devices made of polymers that release spermicide, a custom-molded cap, and modifications of the contraceptive sponge. A sponge with a spermicide other than nonoxynol-9, or a combination of spermicide and microbicide, could have sizeable advantages, especially in STI protection.

EFFECTIVENESS

The contraceptive effectiveness of vaginal barriers is influenced by the characteristics of the individuals using them. The most important factor in determining effectiveness is correct and consistent use. About half of the women who become pregnant while using vaginal barrier methods report that contraceptive failure occurred in a context of imperfect use. The other half experience method failure despite correct use.

Table 18-1 First-year probability of pregnancy* for women using vaginal barrier methods

Method	% of Women Experiencing an Unintended Pregnancy Within the First Year of Use		% of Women Continuing Use At One Year
	Typical Use	Perfect Use	At One Year
Cap			
Parous Women	40	26	42
Nulliparous Women	20	9	56
Sponge			
Parous Women	40	20	42
Nulliparous Women	20	9	56
Female Condom	21	5	56
Diaphragm	20	6	56

* See Table 31-1 for first-year probability of pregnancy of all methods.

Emergency Contraceptive Pills: Treatment initiated within 72 hours after unprotected intercourse reduces the risk of pregnancy by at least 75%. (See Chapter 12 for more information.)

Parity also affects the efficacy of some vaginal barriers. From 5% to 9% of nulliparous users and from 5% to 26% of parous users of these methods will become pregnant during the first year of perfect use.[3-6] For parous women, the sponge and the cap are substantially less effective than the diaphragm or female condom.[7] For nulliparous women, the female condom, diaphragm, cervical cap, and sponge all provide similar contraceptive effectiveness during typical use; with perfect use, the female condom and diaphragm are somewhat more effective than the cap or sponge.

The difference between low failure rates reported in some studies and high rates reported in others is not accounted for entirely by patient diligence or parity. The wide range reflects the profound effect of differences among study populations in fertility characteristics. For example, in the diaphragm/cap comparison study, women who used the diaphragm consistently and had intercourse three times weekly or more were almost three times as likely to experience a pregnancy compared with women who had intercourse less than three times weekly.

Spermicide: essential or not essential? Many vaginal barrier users have wondered whether using spermicide with a diaphragm or cap is really necessary. Although several studies hint that spermicide may be helpful in improving contraceptive effectiveness with some of these devices, they have not been large enough to point to clear conclusions.[8] Women using the diaphragm without spermicide had a pregnancy rate of 29 pregnancies per 100 women within 12 months, while those using a diaphragm with spermicide had a rate of 21 per 100 women.[9,10] Women using the new diaphragm-like Lea's Shield device without spermicide experienced almost twice as many pregnancies as those who used spermicide (9.3 vs. 5.6 pregnancies over the 6-month study interval.[1]

COST

Reality[7] female condoms cost between $2.00 and $2.50 each. While the device is approved to be used only once, re-use after washing has been reported in a number of countries.[11] Studies have found the female condom remains structurally sound after several washings and re-use.[12,13]

Obtaining a diaphragm, cap, Lea's Shield or FemCap costs from $50 to $150, depending on the fee for the necessary medical visit and device fitting. Purchase of a cap or diaphragm alone is about $30 to $50; replacement is recommended every 2 years for the diaphragm and FemCap, and annually for the cap. The only ongoing cost for these methods is for spermicide; the amount of spermicide needed depends on intercourse frequency. Cream or jelly cost is minimal, about $0.25 per application.

Sponges, not currently marketed in the United States, cost $1.25 to $1.50 each when last sold here. A similar sponge product, called Protectaid, is available in Canada. Protectaid sponges contain benzalkonium chloride, sodium cholate, and N-9. Protectaid sponges for personal use (small quantities) can be ordered legally from Canada through the supplier's website: http://www.birthcontrol.com.

ADVANTAGES AND INDICATIONS

Vaginal barrier methods have many advantages that make them reasonable for both short-term and long-term contraception. The overall medical safety of these methods, backed up by abortion in case of failure, is comparable to consistent use of male condoms. They do not cause systemic side effects and do not alter a woman's hormone patterns. Except for the female condom, vaginal barrier methods do not require partner involvement in the decision to use them. Finally, for women who need contraception only intermittently, a vaginal barrier can be available for immediate protection whenever needed, no matter how long the interval between uses.

Sexually transmitted infection (STI) protection. Potentially, protection against spread of STIs could be the most important noncontraceptive benefit of vaginal barrier use.[14] The female condom lines the vagina completely, preventing contact between the penis and vagina. The condom traps semen and is then discarded. The polyurethane in female condoms is strong and impermeable to organisms as small as the HIV virus.[15] Unless the female condom slips out of place or is torn, or the penis gets "misrouted" between the female condom and vaginal wall, the protection against STI exposure should be equivalent to that provided by latex male condoms. Consistent, correct use of female condoms appears effective in preventing trichomonas reinfection.[16] In addition, supplementing male condoms with female condoms led to slightly lower STI rates in Thailand brothels.[17]

For women who use a diaphragm or sponge, the reduction of gonorrhea, chlamydia, and trichomoniasis differs across various observational studies.[18-20] The presence of a mechanical barrier, to reduce exposure of the fragile cervical epithelium to semen and microbes, could potentially affect infection risk.[20,21] Nonetheless, in the absence of randomized controlled trials showing effectiveness against infection, be cautious in making recommendations about using vaginal barrier methods whenever STI risk is a concern.

The role of the spermicide N-9, frequently used with vaginal barrier methods, in affecting RTI acquisition risk is discussed in Chapter 7.

Cervical neoplasia protection. Several observational studies show a lower risk of cervical dysplasia and cancer among women using the diaphragm.[22-24] Because cervical infection with certain strains of human papilloma virus (HPV) plays an etiologic part in cervical neoplasia, the protective role of diaphragm use may be similar to the reduced risk observed for other STIs. Alternatively, women who choose to use the diaphragm may be at lower risk for HPV for reasons unrelated to effects of the diaphragm itself.

DISADVANTAGES AND CAUTIONS

Few serious medical problems are associated with use of vaginal barriers. Most women are medically appropriate candidates for their use. TSS is potentially life threatening, but rare. Using vaginal barrier methods with spermicide also increases the risk for urinary tract infection (UTI), bacterial vaginosis, and vaginal candidiasis.

Common minor problems. Problems related to physical discomfort or trauma occur occasionally with use of the female condom. Among 360 women in the contraceptive efficacy study, one discontinued using the method because of vaginal discomfort and one because her partner experienced penile irritation.[25]

The most common problem associated with vaginal barriers used with spermicide is local skin irritation. Some patients are allergic or sensitive to N-9, and some women have cramps, bladder pain, or rectal pain when wearing a diaphragm or cap. Rare cases of vaginal trauma, including abrasion and laceration, have been reported with use of the Prentif cap and the diaphragm. Partners occasionally report penile pain during intercourse. For diaphragm users, refitting with an alternative size or rim type resolves the problem in some cases.

Problems with sponge removal are fairly common. Some sponge users have difficulty with vaginal dryness. Foul odor and vaginal discharge are likely to occur if a diaphragm, cap, or sponge is inadvertently left in the vagina for more than a few days. Symptoms abate promptly when the device is removed.

Latex allergy. Latex allergy is an increasingly common problem. In most cases allergy causes local cutaneous symptoms such as erythema, pruritis, and rash. For some individuals, however, latex allergy triggers serious systemic hypersensitivity with the potential for anaphylaxis that can be fatal. The incidence of latex allergy is especially high among health care workers repeatedly exposed to use of latex gloves, and among individuals who have had multiple surgeries, especially those involving latex medical equipment such as ostomy devices. Anyone who has a confirmed or suspected latex allergy should avoid exposure to latex vaginal barrier devices including latex diaphragms and caps as well as latex male condoms. Plastic female or male condoms are appropriate alternatives.

Vaginal and urinary tract infections. Using diaphragm and spermicide during sexual intercourse is associated with increased vaginal colonization with Escherichia coli.[26,27] This finding is of concern because bacterial vaginosis (BV) may be associated with increased risk for upper genital tract infection[18] and serious perinatal morbidity. It may also account for the increased risk of UTI observed among diaphragm users.[28-30]

Toxic shock syndrome. TSS is a rare but serious disorder caused by toxin(s) released by some strains of Staphylococcus aureus. Most TSS occurs in association with tampon use during menses; nonmenstrual TSS risk is increased for women who use vaginal barrier methods.[31] The absolute risk of TSS attributable to vaginal barriers, however, is very low. Three cases of TSS per year can be expected for every 100,000 women using vaginal barrier methods. These cases would result in less than 1 TSS death (0.18) annually for every 100,000 vaginal barrier users. For comparison, complications of pregnancy occurring as a result of method failure would cause almost seven times this number (1.2 deaths per 100,000 users). Nevertheless, patients using vaginal barriers need to be aware of the TSS danger signs and receive instructions consistent with recommended TSS precautions.

Systemic effects and pregnancy exposure. No serious systemic side effects have been reported in association with human use of spermicides in conjunction with vaginal barriers. Safety concerns have centered on the issue of fetal exposure related to their accidental use during early pregnancy. However, composite data show no true association exists between spermicide use and fetal defects.[32]

CAUTIONS

The following conditions may make use of one or more of the vaginal barrier methods inadvisable:

1. Allergy to spermicide, rubber, latex, or polyurethane

2. Abnormalities in vaginal anatomy that interfere with a satisfactory fit or stable placement of a female condom, diaphragm, cap or sponge

3. Inability to learn correct insertion technique

4. (For all vaginal barriers except female condom) History of TSS

5. (For all vaginal barriers except female condom) Repeated UTIs

6. (For all vaginal barriers except female condom) Need for HIV protection

7. (For the diaphragm, cap and FemCap) Lack of trained personnel to fit the device or lack of clinical time to provide instruction

8. (For the cap, Lea's Shield, FemCap and sponges) Full-term delivery within the past 6 weeks, recent spontaneous or induced abortion, or vaginal bleeding from any cause, including menstrual flow

9. (For the cap) Known or suspected cervical or uterine malignancy, an abnormal Pap smear result, or vaginal or cervical infection.

PROVIDING VAGINAL BARRIER METHODS

Help the woman choose which of the available barrier options is most likely to meet her needs. Women who plan to use female condoms or sponges do not require a pelvic exam. If you perform a routine exam, however, you can make sure the woman does not have an unusual anatomic anomaly such as a septate vagina or duplicate cervices. For a woman who wishes to use a diaphragm or cervical cap, select a device that fits well, or determine that a satisfactory fit is not possible so the patient can choose another contraceptive method.

Be sure each patient has an opportunity to practice inserting and removing her device as part of her visit. After the patient has inserted her device, verify that its position is correct and that the fit is good. Most patients find inserting a cap more difficult than inserting a diaphragm, and removal can be tricky. New cap, Lea's Shield or FemCap users should try the device initially while still using another method of birth control, such as condoms or oral contraceptives, to be sure it remains in position after intercourse.

Barrier method differences. Vaginal barriers differ in both effectiveness and in rules for their use. These differences may make one option easier or more appealing for a specific woman. For parous women, the diaphragm and female condom provide more effective contraceptive protection than do the cervical cap or contraceptive sponge. For nulliparous women, the difference in effectiveness is less striking. Because consistent use is so important, a match between the method's characteristics and the woman's personal needs and sexual patterns may improve effectiveness. For example, a woman who is sexually intimate only on weekends may find the diaphragm cumbersome because of the 24-hour limit for wear. For her, a device that can be left in place without additional spermicide may be easier to use correctly. Similarly, washing and storing a diaphragm or cap and having spermicide available may be awkward for a woman who is not at her own home.

A woman who finds spermicide irritating or does not like the messiness of other vaginal barriers may prefer the female condom. Unlike other vaginal barrier methods, the female condom prevents semen from contacting the vagina. Its use does not require the precise timing in relation to erection and intercourse that is necessary with male condoms. Thus, some couples may find the female condom easier to use since it involves less interruption in lovemaking.

Guidelines for vaginal barrier use. Guidelines for using vaginal barrier methods are based on arbitrary decisions by U.S. Food and Drug Administration (FDA) and device manufacturers. The guidelines balance concerns about possible TSS risk, spermicide effectiveness, and convenience of the method. The scientific basis for these rules is inadequate. For example, no evidence exists for specifying an unsafe duration of wear to minimize TSS risk. Similarly, the optimal spermicide dose and duration of effectiveness are unknown. Whether an extra application of spermicide for repeated intercourse improves effectiveness for diaphragm users is not known.

The guidelines also do not necessarily reflect the protocols used in studies conducted for FDA approval. Women in the cap and diaphragm study, for example, were allowed cap wear for as long as 3 days (72 hours). Most women in the study, however, reported wear of less than 40 hours, so the reviewers decided that cap efficacy with longer wear had not been documented, and a 48-hour maximum was chosen for the labeling.

Table 18-2 Vaginal barrier methods—guidelines for use

	Diaphragm	Cap	Sponge	Female Condom	Lea's Shield	FemCap
Pelvic Exam Required for Fitting	Yes	Yes	No	No	Yes	Yes
Spermicide Recommended	Yes	Yes	Yes	No	Yes	Yes
Spermicide Supplies Needed for Insertion	Yes	Yes	No	No	Yes	Yes
Equipment Needed for Storage After Use	Yes	Yes	No	No	Yes	Yes
Can be Used During Menses	Yes	No	No	Yes	Yes	Yes
Duration of Protection After Insertion	6 hours	48 hours	24 hours	8 hours	24 hours	48 hours
Longest Wear Recommended	24 hours	48 hours	30 hours	8 hours	24 hours	48 hours

CLINICIAN'S ROLE IN BARRIER SUCCESS

You play an important role in helping women make wise decisions about vaginal barrier methods and use them successfully:

1. Help the woman assess her own risk of unintended pregnancy. If her risk is low, do not discourage her confidence in vaginal barriers. If her risk is high, however, a vaginal barrier may not be a wise solo method choice. Characteristics that may be associated with higher than average risk of pregnancy using vaginal barriers include:

   - Frequent intercourse (three times or more weekly)

   - Age less than 30 years

   - Personal style or sexual patterns that make consistent use difficult

   - Previous contraceptive failure with vaginal methods

   - Known abuse of alcohol and/or other drugs

2. Help the woman assess her risk of STI exposure. If the risk is high, encourage her to use male condoms along with her female barrier. (Female condoms should not be used simultaneously with male condoms because the two condoms may stick together.)

3. If unintended pregnancy would be devastating for the woman, or if she is at high risk for vaginal barrier failure, encourage her to consider using a combination of methods such as a diaphragm, sponge, or cap plus male condoms or oral contraceptives.

4. Be sure every vaginal barrier user has an accurate understanding of ovulation timing and knows high-risk days for conception begin about 4 days before ovulation.

5. Be sure every vaginal barrier user is aware of emergency contraception (postcoital treatment) and knows how to obtain it if a contraceptive emergency arises. If possible, provide her with a kit containing an instruction sheet and a supply of oral contraceptive pills sufficient for one or more emergency treatment regimens. (See Chapter 12 on Emergency Contraception.)

PRACTICAL CAUTION: AVOID OIL-BASED LUBRICANTS AND MEDICATIONS

Lubricants such as mineral oil, baby oil, suntan oil, vegetable oil, and butter; and vaginal medications such as Femstat cream, Monistat cream, estrogen cream, and Vagisil have a rapid, deleterious effect on latex. Their effect on diaphragm or cap integrity has not been studied, but it is reasonable to warn vaginal barrier users to avoid oil products. They will not affect the silicon in Lea's Shield or the FemCap. If additional lubrication is needed, a vaginal spermicide or a product intended for use with latex condoms would be reasonable options.

FITTING A DIAPHRAGM

Choosing a style to try. The first step in fitting a diaphragm is to select an initial diaphragm style (rim type) to try. Most women find the arcing rim style easier to insert correctly than the other rim styles; it is quite difficult to insert an arcing style incorrectly. The gentle spring strength of the coil and flat spring types, however, is often more comfortable, and these styles can be inserted with a diaphragm introducer (Figure 18-5).

Diaphragm manufacturers produce sets of fitting rings (sample diaphragm rims with no dome). Whole diaphragms, however, are preferable for fitting so the patient can practice insertion and removal with the sample diaphragm. Fitting rings are not adequate for patient practice. The various products differ in rim spring strength, so prescribe precisely the same brand and rim type as was used in fitting. Although flat spring diaphragms may not be stocked in all drugstores, coil and arcing diaphragms are widely available; wide-seal diaphragms are distributed directly to physicians and clinics.

Flat spring rim. This diaphragm has a thin, delicate rim with gentle spring strength and is intended for a woman with a very firm vaginal muscle tone (nulliparous) or a shallow notch behind the pubic bone. The flat spring folds flat for insertion. Products available: Ortho-White Diaphragm, sizes 55 to 95, latex.

Coil spring rim. The coil spring has a sturdy rim with a firm spring strength intended for women with average vaginal muscle tone and an average pubic arch notch. It folds flat for insertion. Products available: Koromex Diaphragm, sizes 50 to 95, latex; Ortho Diaphragm (coil spring), sizes 50 to 100, latex; and Ramses Flexible Cushioned Diaphragm (coil spring), sizes 50 to 95, gum rubber.

Arcing spring rim. This diaphragm has a very sturdy rim with firm spring strength. Most women are able to use the arcing rim comfortably. It can often be used despite a rectocele or a cystocele or lax vaginal muscle tone. Products available: Koroflex Diaphragm, sizes 60 to 95, latex; Allflex Diaphragm (Ortho), sizes 55 to 95, latex; and Ramses Bendex Diaphragm, sizes 65 to 95, gum rubber.

The Allflex (Ortho) arcing diaphragm folds at any point along its rim and is slightly less rigid than the Koroflex (Holland Rantos) or the Ramses Bendex (Schmid) products. The Koroflex and Bendex fold at two points only (a hinge or bow-bend construction). Many women find the bow-bend rim is easier to insert because the fold compresses to a narrow leading edge and the two stiff halves of the arc can be held in the folded position close to either end of the arc, whereas the Allflex must be held in the middle.

Wide-seal rim. The wide-seal rim has a flexible flange about 1.5 cm wide attached to the inner edge of the rim. The flange is intended to hold spermicide in place inside the diaphragm and to create a better seal between the diaphragm and the vaginal wall. Wide-seal diaphragms are available in two different rim styles, arcing and coil spring. The arcing model folds at two points (bow-bend) but is similar in rigidity to the lighter Allflex arcing spring. The coil spring model folds at any point on the rim, but because of the inner flange, assumes a slight arc shape unlike other coil spring diaphragms that are flat when folded. Products available: Milex Wide-seal arcing diaphragm, sizes 60 to 95, latex; and Milex Wide-seal Omniflex coil spring diaphragm, sizes 60 to 95, latex.

Choosing a diaphragm size. Estimate the diaphragm size that will be needed:

1. Insert your index and middle fingers into the vagina until your middle finger reaches the posterior wall of the vagina.

2. Use the tip of your thumb to mark the point at which your index finger touches the pubic bone.

3. Extract your fingers.

4. Place the diaphragm rim on the tip of your middle finger. The opposite rim should lie just in front of your thumb.

Insert a sample diaphragm of the size you have selected into the patient's vagina. The device should rest snugly in the vagina, but without tension against the vaginal walls. Its rim should be in contact with the lateral walls and posterior fornix, and there should be just enough space to insert one fingertip comfortably between the inside of the pubic arch and the anterior edge of the diaphragm rim.

Choose the largest rim size that is comfortable for the patient. Try more than one rim size or type before making a final selection. Do not choose a size that is too small; vaginal depth increases during sexual arousal (3 to 5 cm in nulliparous women), and a too-small diaphragm may fail to maintain its position covering the cervix. A diaphragm that is too large, however, may cause vaginal pressure, abdominal pain or cramping, or vaginal ulceration, and may be a factor in recurrent UTI.

DISINFECTING DIAPHRAGMS AND RINGS USED FOR FITTING

Scrupulously attend to universal precautions when fitting diaphragms, as well as when cleaning and disinfecting them after fitting. Use gloves during fitting and eye splash protection and gloves during cleaning. Because they come into contact with intact mucous membrane, diaphragms and rings used for fitting are classified as semi-critical devices that require processing with a high-level disinfectant according to OSHA guidelines. After thorough scrubbing with a liquid detergent and water, three disinfection options are recommended.[33]

- Autoclave at 121 degrees Centigrade, 15 pounds per square inch (psi) for 20 minutes unwrapped or 30 minutes wrapped.

- Soak in a solution of one part Clorox to nine parts water (results in a solution of sodium hypochlorite 5,000 ppm) for 30 minutes at room temperature; rinse with tap water; then soak in 70% ethyl or isopropyl alcohol for 15 minutes. Discard all solutions.

- Immerse in Cidex (2% glutaraldehyde) for 20 minutes at room temperature; then rinse and place in boiling water for 30 minutes. Follow manufacturer's instructions concerning preparation and disposal or reuse of Cidex solution.

After disinfection, allow the diaphragms or rings to air dry, then store them in a disinfected container until later use.

FITTING A CERVICAL CAP

Prentif Cavity-Rim cervical caps are available in sizes 22 mm, 25 mm, 28 mm, and 31 mm (internal rim diameter). They are manufactured by Lamberts (Dalston) Ltd. in Luton, England, and can be purchased from the U.S. distributor: Cervical Cap Ltd., P.O. Box 38003-292, Los Gatos, California 95031.

Because of normal variations in women's cervical anatomy and the limited number of cap sizes available, it will not be possible to fit every patient properly. Factors such as average parity in each patient population affect the frequency of fitting problems; 6% to 10% of subjects could not be fitted in the large U.S. cap studies.[5]

When a Prentif cap is fitted correctly, the inner diameter of the cap rim must be almost identical to the diameter of the base of the cervix, or just a few millimeters larger. The rim forms a seal with the cervical surface to maintain the cap's position. The rim should rest at the base of the cervix so the vaginal walls surround the outer side of the rim. The cervix should be completely covered. The dome of the cap should be deep enough so that it does not rest on the cervical os.

A Prentif cap that is too tight can cause cervical trauma, and one that is too loose or fails to make a secure seal over the entire circumference of the cervix will be more likely to dislodge. Dislodgement during intercourse is also more likely if, during thrusting, the penis bumps the cap's side or rim rather than the dome. For this reason, a woman whose uterus is acutely anteflexed, so her cervical portio faces downward toward the back of her vagina, may find that her cap dislodges.

Estimating cap size. Perform a bimanual exam to determine the position and size of the uterus and cervix. Next, inspect the woman's cervix to estimate the proper cap size. The cervix must be fairly symmetrical, without extensive laceration or scarring that could interfere with uniform contact around its full diameter between the cap rim and cervix. The cervix must also be long enough to accommodate the height of the cap. A cervix that is flush or partially flush with the vaginal vault cannot be fitted with the Prentif cap. Try two or more cap sizes to determine the fit.

Inserting, checking, and removing a cap. To insert the cap, fold the rim and compress the cap dome so when it is released in place over the cervix, the unfolding dome can create suction between the rim of the cap and the cervix. After inserting the cap, check it with one finger around its entire circumference to be sure no gaps occur between the cap rim and the cervix. Next check the stability by noting its resistance to dislodgement when the cap and cervix are probed with a finger tip.

Check for evidence of suction after the cap has been in place for a minute or two. Pinch the cap dome and tug gently. The dome should remain collapsed, and the cap should resist the tug and not slide off easily. Finally, try to rotate the cap in place on the cervix. If it does not rotate at all, it is too tight; if it rotates too easily or comes off the cervix, it is too large. To be considered a good fit, the cap must cover the cervix completely, with no gaps between the rim and the cervix. It must have good suction and not dislodge easily when the dome is probed with a fingertip.

To remove the cap, probe the rim with the end of your index finger; tip the cap rim to break the seal, then gently pull the cap down and out.

DISINFECTING CAPS USED FOR FITTING

Scrupulously attend to universal precautions when fitting caps, as well as when cleaning and disinfecting them after fitting. Use gloves during fitting, and eye splash protection and gloves during cleaning. Because they come into contact with intact mucous membrane, caps used for fitting are classified as semi-critical devices that require processing with a high-level disinfectant according to OSHA guidelines. After a thorough scrubbing with a liquid detergent and water, three disinfection options are recommended.[33]

- Autoclave at 121 degrees Centigrade, 15 psi for 20 minutes unwrapped or 30 minutes wrapped.
- Soak in a solution of one part Clorox to nine parts water (results in a solution of sodium hypochlorite 5,000 ppm) for 30 minutes at room temperature; rinse with tap water; then soak in 70% ethyl or isopropyl alcohol for 15 minutes. Discard all solutions.
- Immerse in Cidex (2% glutaraldehyde) for 20 minutes at room temperature; then rinse and place in boiling water for 30 minutes. Follow manufacturer's instructions concerning preparation and disposal or reuse of Cidex solution.

After disinfection, allow the caps to air dry, then store them in a disinfected container until use.

FITTING LEA'S SHIELD

Fitting this device is quite simple. The woman inserts Lea's Shield after the clinician's instruction. The clinician then checks to see if the cervix is covered, the loop fits behind the symphysis, and the woman is comfortable. Creating a vacuum over the cervix is not necessary.

FITTING THE FEMCAP

FemCaps are available in sizes 22 mm, 26 mm, and 30 mm (internal rim diameter). When a FemCap is fitted correctly, the inner diameter of the cap rim must be almost identical to the diameter of the base of the cervix, or just a few millimeters larger. The cervix should be completely covered. The dome of the cap should be deep enough so that it does not rest on the cervical os. A FemCap that is too tight can cause cervical trauma.

Estimating cap size. Perform a bimanual exam to determine the position and size of the uterus and cervix. Next, inspect the woman's cervix to estimate the proper FemCap size. The cervix must be fairly symmetrical, without extensive laceration or scarring that could interfere with uniform contact around its full diameter between the cap rim and cervix. Try two or more cap sizes to determine the best fit.

Inserting, checking, and removing a cap. To insert the cap, fold the rim and compress the cap dome so when it is released in place over the cervix, the unfolding dome can create suction between the rim of the cap and the cervix. After inserting the cap, check it with one finger around its entire circumference to be sure it is in place.

To remove the FemCap, find the loop with the end of your index finger, then gently pull the cap down and out.

MANAGING PROBLEMS AND FOLLOW-UP

Women using vaginal barriers need no special follow-up. Labeling for the diaphragm recommends refitting annually, after a weight gain or loss of 10 pounds or more, after an abortion, or after a full-term pregnancy.[34] Weight change does not commonly require a new diaphragm size, nor does an abortion.[35] Remind women to avoid wearing vaginal barriers for the last 2 or 3 days before routine exams, if possible, to provide optimal conditions for Pap screening.

When a barrier user returns for a routine exam, ask open-ended questions about how the method is working out. If the woman finds it inconvenient or uncomfortable, offer her an opportunity to consider an alternative method. Refitting her with a different size or rim style may also be helpful.

Problems caused by vaginal barrier methods may require clinical intervention. Recurrent vaginal or introital irritation, with no evidence of vaginal infection, may indicate an allergy or sensitivity to spermicide or to latex. Recurrent UTI, recurrent yeast infection, and bacterial vaginosis may be associated with use of contraceptive sponges or a diaphragm.

If a diaphragm user experiences recurring UTIs, consider refitting her with a smaller diaphragm size, alternative rim style, or with a cervical cap. If her UTI problems persist despite these measures, changing to an alternative method of contraception that does not involve spermicide may be advisable.

A vaginal barrier user who develops signs or symptoms of TSS requires urgent and intensive evaluation and treatment. A vaginal culture can confirm the presence of Staphylococcus aureus. Treat the patient with antibiotics, and follow her carefully. If her symptoms are severe, she may need hospitalization for surveillance. Because TSS risk is increased for a woman who has had TSS in the past, the woman should avoid use of vaginal barrier methods in the future.

INSTRUCTIONS FOR USING VAGINAL BARRIERS

1. Use your method every time you have intercourse. Be sure your vaginal barrier method (female condom, diaphragm, cap, Lea's Shield or FemCap with spermicidal cream or jelly, or sponge) is in place before your partner's penis enters your vagina.

2. If you feel unsure about the proper fit or placement of your diaphragm, cap, Lea's Shield, FemCap or sponge, use male condoms until you see your clinician to be sure your insertion technique is correct.

3. If you are having problems with vaginal or penile irritation, try a different spermicide product. If you have problems with recurring bladder infections or vaginal yeast infections, discuss these with your clinician.

4. You can use male condoms along with your diaphragm, sponge, cap, Lea's Shield or FemCap if you wish. Using this combination, you will have effective protection against both pregnancy and sexually transmitted infection. Do not use a male condom along with a female condom; the two may adhere and increase the chance your female condom will dislodge or male condom will slip off.

5. No conclusive studies show just how long spermicide is fully active or exactly how long the diaphragm, cap, or sponge must be left in place after intercourse. The most important thing is consistent and correct use, protecting your cervix.

6. Douching after intercourse is not recommended. If you are using a diaphragm, sponge, or cap and choose to use a douche, wait at least 6 hours after intercourse to avoid washing away spermicide.

7. If you are using a diaphragm, cap, or sponges, learn the danger signs for toxic shock syndrome and watch for them. If you have a high fever and one or more of the danger signs, you may have early toxic shock syndrome. Remove the sponge, diaphragm, or cap and contact your clinician.

Before Intercourse

1. Check that you have all the supplies you need.

   - *Female condoms.* You need enough new, female condoms to protect each act of vaginal intercourse.

   - *Sponges.* You need clean water and a fresh, unopened sponge.

   - *Diaphragm.* You need fresh spermicidal cream or jelly, a plastic applicator for inserting additional spermicide, and a diaphragm. Check your diaphragm to be sure it has no holes, cracks, or tears.

   - *Cap.* You need fresh spermicidal cream or jelly and a cap. Check your cap to be sure it has no holes, cracks, or tears.

   - *Lea's Shield and FemCap.* You need fresh spermicidal cream or jelly and the device.

2. Plan ahead about when to insert your method. Try to find a routine that is comfortable for you.

   - *Female condoms.* You can insert the female condom for immediate protection just before intercourse or as long as 8 hours ahead of time if you prefer.

   - *Sponges.* You can insert the sponge for immediate protection just before intercourse, or ahead of time. It provides effective contraceptive protection for 24 hours, no matter how many times you have intercourse.

   - *Diaphragm.* The diaphragm may be inserted just before intercourse, or up to 6 hours beforehand.

   - *Cap, Lea's Shield and FemCap.* The device can be inserted just before intercourse, or ahead of time if you wish. It provides effective contraceptive protection for 48 hours, no matter how many times you have intercourse.

Insertion

1. Wash your hands with soap and water.

2. Insert your method carefully; it must be in the proper location in your vagina to be maximally effective.

   - *Female condom.* Remove the condom from its package and check to be sure the inner ring is at the bottom, closed end of the pouch. Follow the directions for insertion in the package; the illustrations can help you. Hold the pouch with the open end hanging down. Use the thumb and middle finger of one hand to squeeze the inner ring into a narrow oval for insertion; place your index finger between your thumb and middle finger to guide the female condom during insertion. With your other hand, spread the lips of your vagina. Insert the inner ring and the pouch of the condom into the vaginal opening and with your index finger, push the inner ring with the pouch the rest of the way up into the vagina. The outside ring lies against the outer lips when Reality[7] is in place; about 1 inch of the open end will stay outside your body. Once the penis enters, the vagina will expand and the slack will decrease.

- *Sponges.* Remove the sponge from its package, moisten it with about 2 tablespoons of clean water, and squeeze it once. Then insert the sponge into the vagina and slide it along the back wall of the vagina until it rests against your cervix. The dimple side should face your cervix, with the loop away from your cervix. Check with your finger to be sure you can feel your cervix covered by the sponge.

- *Diaphragm.* First apply spermicidal jelly or cream. Hold the diaphragm with the dome down (like a cup). Squeeze the jelly or cream from the tube into the dome (use about 1 teaspoon); spread a little bit around the rim of the diaphragm with your finger. To insert the diaphragm hold it with the dome down (spermicide in the dome) and squeeze opposite sides of the rim together so the diaphragm folds. Hold it folded in one hand between your thumb and fingers. Spread the opening of your vagina with your other hand, and insert the folded diaphragm into your vaginal canal. This can be done standing with one foot propped up (on the edge of a chair, a bathtub, or a toilet), squatting, or lying on your back.

  Push the diaphragm downward and along the back wall of your vagina as far as it will go. Then tuck the front rim up along the roof of your vagina behind your pubic bone. Once it is in place properly, you should not be able to feel the diaphragm except, of course, with your fingers. If it is uncomfortable, then most likely it is not in the correct position; take it out and reinsert it.

  After insertion, check placement. When correctly placed, the back rim of the diaphragm is below and behind the cervix, and the front edge of the rim is tucked up behind the pubic bone. Often you may not be able to feel the back rim. You should check to be sure you can feel that your cervix is covered by the soft rubber dome of the diaphragm and the front rim is snugly in place behind your pubic bone. The spermicidal cream (inside the dome of the diaphragm) should be next to your cervix.

- *Cap.* Before insertion, fill the dome of the cap 1/3 full with spermicidal cream or jelly. Next, find your cervix with your finger. It feels like a short, firm nose projecting into the vagina. This can be done standing, with one foot propped up (on the edge of a chair, a bathtub, or a toilet), squatting, or lying on your back. Separate the lips of your vagina with one hand. With the other hand, squeeze (fold) the rim of the cap between your thumb and index finger. Slide the cap into your vagina, and push it along the rear wall of the vagina as far as it will go. Using your finger to locate your cervix, press the rim of the cap around the cervix until it is completely covered. Finally, check the cap position by pressing the dome of the cap to make sure your cervix is covered. Sweep your finger around the cap rim. The cervix should not be felt outside the cap.

- *Lea's Shield and FemCap.* Before insertion, fill the bowl of the device with spermicidal cream or jelly. Separate the lips of your vagina with one hand. With the other hand, hold the device between your thumb and index finger. Slide it into your vagina, pushing it along the rear wall of the vagina as far as it will go. Using your finger to locate your cervix, press the device around the cervix until it is completely covered. Finally, check the position by sweeping your finger around the outside of the device. The cervix should not be felt outside the device.

REPEATED INTERCOURSE

- *Female condoms.* The FDA label states that a new female condom should be used for each act of intercourse.
- *Sponges.* One sponge provides continuous protection for up to 24 hours, no matter how many times you have intercourse.
- *Diaphragm.* If you have intercourse more than once within the 6 hour time your diaphragm must remain in place. Use of additional dose of spermicidal cream or jelly is optional. Do not remove your diaphragm; use the plastic applicator to insert fresh jelly or cream into your vagina in front of the diaphragm.
- *Cap.* Use of additional spermicide for repeated intercourse with the cap is optional. Do not remove your cap. If you wish to add spermicide, use the plastic introducer to insert fresh cream or jelly into your vagina in front of the cap. *Lea's Shield and FemCap.* If you have intercourse more than once within the 8 hour time your device must remain in place, and an additional dose of spermicidal cream or jelly is recommended. Do not remove your device; use a plastic applicator to insert fresh jelly or cream into your vagina in front of it.

AFTER INTERCOURSE

1. Remove your female condom immediately after intercourse, before you stand up. Squeeze and twist the outer ring to keep semen inside

the pouch. Pull the condom out gently and discard it in a trash can. Do not try to flush a used female condom down the toilet.

2. Leave the cap, diaphragm, or sponge in place for at least 6 hours after intercourse. Instructions on Lea's Shield advise leaving it in place for 8 hours. After that time, remove the device as soon as is practical. Douching is not recommended, but if you choose to douche, wait at least 6 hours.

3. Your sponge, diaphragm, or cap should not interfere with normal activities. Urination or a bowel movement should not affect its position, but you can check its placement afterward if you wish. It is fine to shower or bathe with a sponge, diaphragm, or cap in place.

4. Before removing a cap, diaphragm, Lea's Shield, FemCap or sponge, wash your hands with soap and water.

5. *Removal.* Check the position of the device. If it is dislodged, or seems not to be in correct position, you may want to contact your clinician about emergency contraception.

   • *Sponges.* Grasp the loop on the sponge with one finger and pull it gently to remove the sponge. Check to be sure the sponge is intact, then throw it away. If it is torn, remove all the pieces from the vagina.

   • *Diaphragm.* Locate the front rim of the diaphragm with your finger. Hook your finger over the rim or behind it, then pull the diaphragm down and out. Wash the diaphragm with plain soap and water, and dry it. Hold it up to the light to check for holes, tears, or cracks.

   • *Cap.* Locate the cap rim on your cervix. Press on the cap rim until the seal against your cervix is broken, then tilt the cap off the cervix. Hook your finger around the rim and pull it sideways out of the vagina. Wash the cap with plain soap and water, and dry it. Check the cap for holes, tears or cracks.

   • *Lea's Shield and FemCap.* Grasp the loop of the device with one finger and pull gently to remove it. Wash the device with soap and water, then air dry.

TAKING CARE OF YOUR VAGINAL BARRIER METHOD

1. Store your supplies in a convenient location that is clean, cool, and dark.

2. Wash your spermicide inserter, diaphragm, or cap after each use. Plain soap is best; avoid deodorant soap or perfumed soap. Do not use talcum powder on your diaphragm or cap, or in the case.

3. Contact with oil-based products can deteriorate a diaphragm or cap. Do not use oil-based vaginal medications or lubricants when you are using a diaphragm or cap. Some examples include petroleum

jelly (Vaseline), mineral oil, hand lotion, vegetable oil, cold cream, and cocoa butter as well as common vaginal yeast creams and vaginal hormone creams. If you need extra lubrication for intercourse, contraceptive jelly is a good choice, or you can try a water-soluble lubricant specifically intended for use with condoms.

Toxic Shock Syndrome Danger Signs

Caution

- Sudden high fever
- Vomiting, diarrhea
- Dizziness, faintness, weakness
- Sore throat, aching muscles and joints
- Rash (like a sunburn)

REFERENCES

1. Mauck C, Glover LH, Miller E et al. Lea's Shield: a study of the safety and efficacy of a new vaginal barrier contraceptive used with and without spermicide. Contraception 1996; 53(6):329-335.
2. Shiata AA, Trussell J. New female intravaginal barrier contraceptive device: preliminary clinical trial. Contraception 1991; 44:11-19.
3. Lane ME, Arceo R, Sobrero AJ. Successful use of the diaphragm and jelly by a young population: report of a clinical study. Fam Plann Perspect 1976; 8(2):81-86.
4. Edelman DA, McIntyre SL, Harper J. A comparative trial of the Today contraceptive sponge and diaphragm. Am J Obstet Gynecol 1984; 150(7):869-876.
5. Richwald GA, Greenland S, Gerber MM, Potik R, Kersey L, Comas MA. Effectiveness of the cavity-rim cervical cap: results of a large clinical study. Obstet Gynecol 1989; 74(2):143-148.
6. Trussell J, Strickler J, Vaughan B. Contraceptive efficacy of the diaphragm, the sponge and the cervical cap. Fam Plann Perspect 1993; 25(3):100-105, 135.
7. Trussell J, Sturgen K, Strickler J, Dominik R. Comparative contraceptive efficacy of the female condom and other barrier methods. Fam Plann Perspect 1994; 26(2):66-72.
8. Cook L, Nanda K, Grimes DA. Diaphragm versus diaphragm with spermicides for contraception (Cochrane review). In The Cochrane Library, Issue Q, 2001. Oxford: Update Software, 2001.
9. Smith C, Farr G, Feldblum PJ, Spence A. Effectiveness of the non-spermicidal fit-free diaphragm. Contraception 1995; 51(5):289-291.
10. Bounds W, Guillebaud J, Dominik R, Dalberth BT. The diaphragm with and without spermicide. A randomized, comparative efficacy trial. J Reprod Med 1995; 40(11):764-774.
11. Smith JB, Nkhama G, Sebastian P, et al. Qualitative research on female condom reuse among women in two developing countries. Research Triangle Park: Family Health International, 1999.
12. Joanis C, Latka M, Glover LH, Hamel S. Structural integrity of the female condom after a single use, washing, and disinfection. Contraception 2000; 62(2):63-72.
13. Beksinska ME, Rees HV, Dickson-Tetteh KE, Mqoqi N, Kleinschmidt I, McIntyre JA. Structural integrity of the female condom after multiple uses, washing, drying, and re-lubrication. Contraception 2001; 63(1):33-36.
14. Alexander NJ . Barriers to sexually transmitted diseases. Scientific American 1996; 3:31-41.
15. Drew WL, Blair M, Miner RC, Conant M. Evaluation of the virus permeability of a new condom for women. Sex Transm Dis 1990; 17(2):110-112.

16. Soper DE, Shoupe D, Shangold GA, Shangold MM, Gutmann J, Mercer L. Prevention of vaginal trichomoniasis by compliant use of the female condom. Sex Transm Dis 1993; 20(3):137-139.
17. Fontanet AL, Saba J, Chandelying V *et al.* Protection against sexually transmitted diseases by granting sex workers in Thailand the choice of using the male or female condom: results from a randomized controlled trial. AIDS 1998; 12(14):1851-1859.
18. Cates W Jr, Stone KM. Family planning, sexually transmitted diseases and contraceptive choice: a literature update—Part I [see comments]. Fam Plann Perspect 1992; 24(2):75-84.
19. d'Oro LC, Parazzini F, Naldi L, La Vecchia C. Barrier methods of contraception, spermicides, and sexually transmitted diseases: a review. Genitourin Med 1994; 70(6):410-417.
20. Moench TR, Chipato T, Padian NS. Preventing disease by protecting the cervix: the unexplored promise of internal vaginal barrier devices. AIDS 2001; 15(13):1595-1602.
21. Stein ZA. More on women and the prevention of HIV infection. Am J Public Health 1995; 85(11):1485-1488.
22. Celentano DD , Klassen AC, Weisman CS, Rosenshein NB. The role of contraceptive use in cervical cancer: the Maryland cervical cancer case-control study. Am J Epidemiology 1987; 70:410-417.
23. Parazzini F, Negri E, La Vecchia C, Fedele L. Barrier methods of contraception and the risk of cervical neoplasia. Contraception 1989; 40(5):519-530.
24. Peters RK, Thomas D, Hagan DG, Mack TM, Henderson BE. Risk factors for invasive cervical cancer among Latinas and non-Latinas in Los Angeles County. J Natl Cancer Inst 1986; 77(5):1063-1077.
25. Farr G, Gabelnick H, Sturgen K, Dorflinger L. Contraceptive efficacy and acceptability of the female condom. Am J Public Health 1994; 84(12):1960-1964.
26. Hooton TM, Hillier S, Johnson C, Roberts PL, Stamm WE. Escherichia coli bacteriuria and contraceptive method. JAMA 1991; 265(1):64-69.
27. Hooton TM, Roberts PL, Stamm WE. Effects of recent sexual activity and use of a diaphragm on the vaginal microflora. Clinical Infectious Diseases 1994; 19:274-278.
28. Fihn SD, Latham RH, Roberts P, Running K, Stamm WE. Association between diaphragm use and urinary tract infection. JAMA 1985; 254(2):240-245.
29. Foxman B. Recurring urinary tract infection: incidence and risk factors. Am J Public Health 1990; 80(3):331-333.
30. Vessey MP, Metcalfe MA, McPherson K, Yeates D. Urinary tract infection in relation to diaphragm use and obesity. Int J Epidemiol 1987; 16(3):441-444.
31. Schwartz B, Gaventa S, Broome CV *et al.* Nonmenstrual toxic shock syndrome associated with barrier contraceptives: report of a case-control study. Rev Infect Dis 1989; 11 Suppl 1:S43-S48; discussion S48-S49.
32. Food and Drug Administration. Data does not support association between spermicides, birth defects. FDA Drug Bulletin 1986; 11-21.
33. Bounds W, Hoffman P. Decontamination of contraceptive practice diaphragms and caps. Br J Fam Plann 1995; 21:30.
34. Ortho Diaphragm. FDA-approved product literature, 1996. In: Physician's Desk Reference, 51st Edition. Montvale, NJ: Medical Economics Co., 1997.
35. Kugel C, Verson H. Relationship between weight change and diaphragm size change. J Obstet Gynecol Neonatal Nurs 1986; 15(2):123-129.

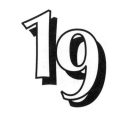

Combined Hormonal Contraceptive Methods

Robert A. Hatcher, MD, MPH
Anita Nelson, MD

- More than 100 million women throughout the world currently rely on oral contraceptives (OCs). In the United States, more than 80% of women born since 1945 have used OCs at some time in their lives, compared to 95% of French women and 4% of Japanese women. In Canada, 70% of pill users over the age of 35 have been taking OCs for more than 10 years.[1]

- OCs effectively prevent pregnancy. Of 1,000 women taking pills perfectly, only 3 will become pregnant within a year. Of 1,000 typical users initiating OC use, 80 women (8%) will become pregnant in the first year of use. However, failure rates as high as 10% to 20% have been reported.[2] Women on pills may find it reassuring to use a back-up contraceptive consistently.

- Dual protection with both condoms and any combined hormonal contraceptive will provide some protection against infection as well as excellent protection against an unintended pregnancy. A woman who misses hormonal pills, or is late starting a new cycle of pills, should consider using a back-up contraceptive until she has taken 7 consecutive pills. Emergency contraceptive pills are also an option for any woman who has missed one or more pills.

- The newer combined hormonal methods—the monthly vaginal ring and weekly patches—were developed to combine the effectiveness and non-contraceptive benefits of combined pills with longer acting delivery systems in order to reduce the demands placed by daily administration of pills.

Forty years ago, "the pill" transformed family planning by providing women with an effective method to control their own fertility for the first time in history. Over the years, the doses of the sex steroids in oral contraceptive (OC) preparations have decreased, which increased both their safety and their acceptability. In addition, numerous noncontraceptive benefits have been identified with both short- and long-term OC use.

Newer hormonal methods—the once-a-month vaginal contraceptive ring and the once-a-week transdermal contraceptive patch—are now available and combine the obvious attractiveness of OCs with longer-acting delivery systems to reduce the demands imposed by daily administration.

This chapter describes combined hormonal contraceptives: methods that contain both estrogen and progestin. Because all of these methods share the same mechanisms of action, the chapter begins with a discussion of how sex steroids influence the reproductive cycle. The effectiveness and cost sections compare OCs, the patch, and the ring. Following these reviews, each combined hormonal method is presented in detail.

MECHANISMS OF ACTION

Combined hormonal contraceptives work primarily as a contraceptive, acting before fertilization. The progestins in all combined hormonal contraceptives provide most of the birth control activity:

- Thicken cervical mucus to prevent sperm penetration into the woman's upper genital tract

- Block the luteinizing hormone (LH) surge and thus inhibit ovulation. Although there are no precise statistics concerning the occurrence of "escape ovulation" in oral contraceptive users, the incidence in earlier higher dose pills was estimated in 1980 to be around 2%.[3] Breakthrough ovulation is probably higher in current lower dose pills. In a study of 20 mcg pills, progesterone levels indicative of luteinization and ovulation were found in 2 of 24 women (8.3%).[4]

- Inhibit capacitation of the sperm, which limits the sperm's ability to fertilize the egg

- Slow tubal motility, which may delay sperm transport

Some progestin effects additionally alter the environment that would be required for embryogenesis to proceed:

- Disrupt transport of the fertilized ovum

- Induce endometrial atrophy, change underlying vascular function and structure and alter the metalloproteinase content in the endometrium

Estrogen is included in combined hormonal methods primarily to provide better cycle control (see below), but it may also boost contraceptive efficacy. Pharmacologic doses of estrogen from combined hormonal contraceptives decrease follicle-stimulating hormone (FSH) release from the pituitary, which may aid in suppressing the LH surge and thus in blocking ovulation (contraception). Estrogen at high doses may induce localized edema in the endometrial lining, which, in turn, may reduce the probability of implantation (interception); however, the clinical significance of this impact is not clear.

HORMONES IN COMBINED HORMONAL CONTRACEPTIVES

Estrogens

Only two estrogenic compounds are used in hormonal contraceptives available in the United States: ethinyl estradiol (EE) and mestranol. The patch, ring, and virtually all modern OC formulations contain EE. Mestranol, which must be metabolized into EE by the liver, is found only in a few 50 mcg pills. (Because 50 mcg of mestranol is equivalent to 35 to 40 mcg of EE, avoid using 50 mcg mestranol-containing pills when high-dose estrogen pills are needed.) The patch and vaginal ring also release EE. Only the combined injection (Lunelle), which is no longer on the market, used a different estrogen (see Chapter 24, Future Methods).

Doses of estrogen in active OCs vary from 20 to 50 mcg per day (see Figure 19-1 for a sample of pills). The transdermal contraceptive patch releases about 20 mcg EE into circulation each day. The vaginal contraceptive ring has serum levels of 15 mcg/cc of EE, or about half the circulating levels associated with that of a comparable 30 mcg OC.[5]

Progestins

In order to maintain adequate serum concentrations of progestogenic activity for daily administration, an array of progestins was developed. There are currently nine different progestins available in OCs and three other progestins in the other combined hormonal systems. The power of a particular progestin results not only from its intrinsic potency, but also from the dose that is used. Each compound has a different potency and a different balance between progesterone activity and any residual androgenicity.

In OCs, the androgen-derived compounds include norethindrone, norethindrone acetate, ethynodiol diacetate, norgestrel, levonorgestrel, norethynodrel, desogestrel, and norgestimate. OCs containing the last two are sometimes called "third-generation pills." (Other androgen-derived compounds, such as gestodene, are not available in the United States.) One new OC contains a new class of compound: drospirenone, derived from the antihypertensive compound spironolactone. Drospirenone has both anti-androgenic and anti-mineralocorticoid activity. Doses of progestins in OCs vary from 0.15 to 1 mg (see Figure 19-1).

The patch contains norelgestromin, the primary active metabolite of norgestimate, the progestin found in three OCs: Ortho-Cyclen, Ortho Tri-Cyclen, and Ortho Tri-Cyclen LO. About 150 mcg of norelgestromin is released into the circulatory system each day. The ring releases 120 mcg a day of etonogestrel, the metabolite of the progestin desogestrel found in Cyclessa and Mircette OCs. Because the bioavailability of the progestins in the patch and the vaginal ring is higher than that of OC progestins, a lower dose can produce similar serum levels. Lower doses are effective.

| Progestin (mg) | | | | | Estrogen (mcg) | | |
Greenblatt (1967) Relative Potency	Swyer (1982) Relative Potency	Dorflinger (1985) Relative Potency	Dose of Progestin (mg)	Name(s) of Pills	Dose of Estrogen (mcg)	Relative Potency	
0.35	0.35	0.35	Norethindrone 0.35	Micronor Nor-QD			1
2.2	0.15–0.22	0.375–0.75	Norgestrel 0.075	Ovrette			2
6.0	0.2–0.3	1.0–2.1	L-Norgestrel 0.1	Alesse	Ethinyl Estradiol 20		3
2.0	0.5	1.0	Norethindrone Acetate 1.0	Loestrin 1/20	Ethinyl Estradiol 20	0.7–0.8	4
1.0	1.0	1.0	Norethindrone 1.0	Norinyl 1/50 Ortho 1/50 Genora	Mestranol 50	1.0	5
3.0–7.5	0.10–0.375	0.5–2.5	L-Norgestrel 0.05/0.075/0.125	Triphasil Tri-Levlen	Ethinyl 30/40 Estradiol 30	1.0–1.2	6
9.0	0.3–0.45	1.5–3.0	L-Norgestrel 0.15	Nordette Levlen	Ethinyl Estradiol 30	1.0–1.2	7
9.0	0.6–0.9	1.5–3.0	Norgestrel 0.3	Lo/Ovral	Ethinyl Estradiol 30	1.0–1.2	8
3.0	0.75	1.5	Norethindrone Acetate 1.5	Loestrin 1.5/30	Ethinyl Estradiol 30	1.0–1.2	9
0.4	0.4	0.4	Norethindrone 0.4	Ovcon 35	Ethinyl Estradiol 35	1.2–1.4	10
0.5	0.5	0.5	Norethindrone 0.5	Brevicon Modicon	Ethinyl Estradiol 35	1.2–1.4	11
0.5–1.0	0.5–1.0	0.5–1.0	Norethindrone 0.5/1.0/0.5	Ortho 10/11	Ethinyl Estradiol 35	1.2–1.4	12
0.5–1.0	0.5–1.0	0.5–1.0	Norethindrone 0.5/1.0/0.5	Tri-Norinyl	Ethinyl Estradiol 35	1.2–1.4	13
0.5–1.0	0.5–1.0	0.5–1.0	Norethindrone 0.5/0.75/1.0	Ortho 7/7/7	Ethinyl Estradiol 35	1.2–1.4	14
1.0	1.0	1.0	Norethindrone 1.0	Norinyl 1/35 Ortho 1/35 Genora 1/35 N.E.E. 1/35	Ethinyl Estradiol 35	1.2–1.4	15
15	0.5	1.0	Ethynodiol Diacetate 1.0	Demulen 1/35	Ethinyl Estradiol 35	1.2–1.4	16
1.0	1.0	1.0	Norethindrone 1.0	Norinyl 1/80 Ortho 1/80	Mestranol 80	1.6	17
1.0	1.0	1.0	Norethindrone 1.0	Ovcon 50	Ethinyl Estradiol 50	1.7–2.0	18
2.0	0.5	1.0	Norethindrone Acetate 1.0	Norlestrin 1/50	Ethinyl Estradiol 50	1.7–2.0	19
2.0	2.0	2.0	Norethindrone 2.0	Norinyl 2 Ortho 2	Mestranol 100	2.0	20
2.7	2.5		Norethindrone 2.5	Enovid-E	Mestranol 100	2.0	21
5.0	1.25	2.5	Norethindrone Acetate 2.5	Norlestrin 2.5/50	Ethinyl Estradiol 50	1.7–2.0	22
15	1.5	2.5 -5	Norgestrel 0.5	Ovral	Ethinyl Estradiol 50	1.7–2.0	23
15	0.5	1.0	Ethyndiol Diacetate 1.0	Demulen 1/50	Ethinyl Estradiol 50	1.7–2.0	24
15	0.5	1.0	Ethynodiol Diacetate 1.0	Ovulen	Mestranol 100	2.0	25

15 10 5 0 2.0 1.5 1.0 0.5 0 5 4 3 2 1   0 1.0 2.0
Potency Units   Potency Units

Sources: Dorflinger (1985); Greenblatt (1967); Swyer (1982); Heinen (1971).

Figure 19-1 Relative potency of estrogens and progestins in selected oral contraceptives reflecting the debate about the strength of the progestins

EFFECTIVENESS

In general, combined OCs, patches, and vaginal rings belong in the second tier of contraceptive effectiveness, having higher failure rates than IUDs, implants, and injections.

Oral Contraceptives

Among women who use OCs correctly and consistently, not missing any pills and following instructions perfectly, only about 3 in 1,000 (0.3%) are expected to become pregnant within the first year. (See Table 19-1.) The first-year failure rates among typical users as observed in real world use are estimated to be 8% (see Chapter 9, The Essentials of Contraception). This means that 1 woman in 12 will become pregnant in the first year of OC use. Among these typical users, pill-taking mistakes that increase the length of the hormone-free interval are particularly likely to lead to failures. The conventional 7-day pill-free interval may also play an important role in the pill's failures. Ultrasound studies have demonstrated that by the 7th placebo pill day, 23% of women can have ovarian follicles that measure at least 10 mm in diameter.[6] If a woman misses pills early in her pack of pills, it may be much more difficult to suppress ovulation and protect against pregnancy during that cycle. Thus, OCs may be made more effective by eliminating or shortening the pill-free interval (see Starting The Pill section). Confusing this picture, however, is a recent small-scale study showing that initiation of pills early in the cycle did not reduce the risk of ovulation.[7] Larger scale studies are underway to answer this question.

Many pregnancies occur when women discontinue OCs, fail to begin another method of contraception and, therefore, have unprotected intercourse. Studies show that 11% of women discontinue their pills in the first month of use, and 19% of those who discontinue fail to adopt a new method.[8] By 6 months, 28% of pill users have stopped the pill; by one year, that percentage approaches 33% to 50%.[9] Quite disturbingly, 42% of women who discontinued OC use did so *without* consulting their clinicians. Because of these concerns, women starting the pill should also be given a second method they can implement on their own should they discontinue pill use before returning for follow-up. Instruct women in as much detail about their second method as you do their pills, and encourage them to practice using it. Also, provide new-start OC patients with a packet of or prescription for emergency contraception (Plan B) or, at a minimum, inform her about its availability.

Recently, one retrospective study has suggested that heavier women may experience higher failure rates than do lighter women.[10] The greatest difference in failure rates was seen in the use of pills with less than 35 mcg EE, with which heavier women were noted to have 4.5 (1.4 - 14.4) times higher pregnancy rates (6.8% vs. 1.8%) than did lighter women. These results have not yet been substantiated by any other studies. Consensus is that it is not prudent to prescribe higher dose pills based on these preliminary data because of the increased risk of thrombosis with high doses of estrogen.[11] Heavier women who used extended cycles of OCs had no increase in pregnancy risk.[12]

Transdermal Patch and Contraceptive Ring

The patch and the vaginal ring have not been in use long enough to permit precise measurements of typical-use failure rates. In comparative trials, the failure rates for patches, vaginal rings, and OCs were low[13,14] and roughly equivalent. Successful utilization rates were statistically higher with the longer acting agents than with the pills that were taken daily. Overall, women who used the patch or vaginal ring were more likely to use their methods correctly and consistently for 13 cycles than were OC users.[15,16] These observations suggest that, in routine practice, the newer long-acting delivery systems may be associated with lower typical-use pregnancy rates than are the pills. However, since this tantalizing possibility has not yet been demonstrated, the authors have decided to quote the same typical failure rates for the pill, the patch, and the vaginal ring (see Chapter 9, The Essentials of Contraception).

One group of potential patch users deserves special counseling. Heavier women, weighing >198 lbs, comprised 3% of the study population but experienced 30% of all the pregnancies in the clinical trial.[17] This decrease in efficacy does not preclude use of the patch by heavier women but does suggest that these women may benefit from additional counseling,[18] including recommending back-up contraception.

Table 19-1 First-year probability of pregnancy* for women using combined hormonal contraceptives compared with other hormonal contraceptives

Method	% of Women Experiencing an Unintended Pregnancy Within the First Year of Use		% of Women Continuing Use at One Year
	Typical Use	Perfect Use	
Combined pill and minipill	8	0.3	68
Evra Patch and Nuva Ring	8**	0.3	68
Depo-Provera	3	0.3	56
IUD			
Paragard (Copper T)	0.8	0.6	78
Mirena (LNG-IUS)	0.1	0.1	81

* See Table 9-2 for pregnancy year failure rates of all methods.
** No data available; assumed to be same as combined oral contraceptives.

Emergency Contraceptive Pills: Treatment initiated within 72 hours after unprotected intercourse reduces the risk of pregnancy by at least 75%. (See Chapter 12 for more information.)

COST

Health department family planning programs in Washington State have paid much less for OCs than for other hormonal contraceptives. In 2001, they reported paying $1.35 per cycle of combined pills, just over one third of the cost of Depo-Provera. In Washington, the discounted cost of OCs to health departments is about 1/20th of the price charged to a private pharmacy chain.[19] The cost of the pills to women paying full price at pharmacies varies somewhat but is becoming higher all the time, ranging from $15 to $50 or even higher per cycle. Generic brands are typically less expensive. Usually, pills cost from $30 to $35 per cycle, one ring costs $40, and a pack of 3 patches (one cycle) costs $42. This means women paying full price pay $390 to $455 per year out of pocket for OCs, just over $500 for the ring and about $550 for the patch. Women whose contraceptives are covered by insurance have to pay a co-pay each month. Purchase of OCs from the Internet, when 3 cycles are bought at a time, can reduce the price to under $20 per cycle with delivery charges extra. Some women travel to Mexico to purchase pills over-the-counter for as little as $3 to $5 per cycle.

ORAL CONTRACEPTIVES

OCs are safe and effective for the vast majority of reproductive-aged women. They are the most extensively studied medications in the history of medicine. Over 80% of U.S. women born after 1945 have used the pill at some time.[1] In the United States, OCs are available only by prescription; in some other countries, they are available over the counter. The keys to successful and safe OC use are selection of appropriate OC candidates, patient motivation, and effective counseling.

Oral Contraceptive Formulations

OCs are available in either monophasic or multiphasic packaging:

- **Monophasic formulations.** Each active pill contains the same doses of the estrogen and progestin.
- **Multiphasic formulations.** The amounts of hormones in the active pills can vary throughout the cycle.
  - Biphasic pills have 2 different combinations of estrogen and progestin in the pills.
  - Triphasic formulations have 3 different combinations. Sometimes the progestin content increases in stepwise progression during the cycle, but some other formulations may also alter the amounts of estrogen given during the cycle. One formulation (Estrostep) holds the progestin dose constant and increases the estrogen content in tablets late in the cycle.

Most pill packs contain 21 active (hormone containing) pills with or without 7 placebo pills (21-pill packs versus 28-pill packs). However, one brand (Mircette) includes 21 active pills, 2 placebo pills and 5 pills with 10 mcg EE each. Another preparation (Seasonale) has 84 active pills followed by 7 placebo pills, which reduces the number of withdrawal bleeds to 4 episodes a year. Under development are preparations containing 24 active pills and 4 placebo pills per pack.

A DVANTAGES AND INDICATIONS

Many women harbor profound misinformation about the safety and utility of OCs. A 2000 survey revealed that 41% of those interviewed believed the pill was associated with significant health hazards.[20] However, OCs have numerous attractive features:

General Advantages

1. **Effectiveness.** When taken correctly and consistently, OCs are very effective contraceptives that give women control over their own fertility.

2. **Safety.** Through prudent selection of users (see below), OCs are safer for a woman's health than are pregnancy and delivery. Recent large-scale studies show that OC use does not increase the risk of death among non-smokers.[21]

3. **An option throughout the reproductive years.** Healthy women can safely use OCs throughout their reproductive lives. Age itself is not a reason to avoid OCs. The noncontraceptive benefits of the pill meet the varying needs of women of all ages. Young women may benefit from reduction in severe dysmenorrhea and acne, while at the other end reproductive life, perimenopausal women may benefit from cycle control and hot flash reduction provided by OCs.

4. **Rapid reversibility.** On average, women who stop taking OCs have only a 2-week delay in return of ovulation. Some women (<3%) have a slower return to fertility—the so-called "post-pill amenorrhea"—that is diagnosed 6 months after stopping the pills. Women need to understand that OC use neither hastens nor delays the onset of menopause.

Contraceptive health benefits

1. **Reduction of maternal deaths.** The CDC calculated that there were 11.8 pregnancy-related deaths per 100,000 live births in the last decade of the 20th century, but that there was significant under-reporting.[22] Embolism, hemorrhage, and pregnancy-induced hypertension were the 3 leading causes of death. Considering that nearly half the pregnancies in this country are unintended, prevention of those pregnancies could significantly decrease maternal deaths.

2. **Reduction of ectopic pregnancies.** OCs reduce the risk of ectopic pregnancy by over 90%.[23-25] At least one in 80 pregnancies in the United States is an ectopic pregnancy, the leading cause of maternal death in the first trimester. The CDC reports that 25 women died of ectopic pregnancy in 1992.

Menstrually-related health benefits

1. **Decreased dysmenorrhea.** OCs significantly decrease menstrual cramps and pain. Although the original studies used high-dose formulations, even low-dose formulations help when given in the conventional cyclic fashion.[26] OC use reduces the incidence of all degrees of dysmenorrhea by 60%.[27] Severe dysmenorrhea was reduced by almost 90%.[28] In a randomized clinical trial, low-dose OC users reported fewer absences from school and work and used less pain relief medicine than placebo users. More significant relief of symptoms can be achieved by continuous or extended use, which eliminates withdrawal periods for prolonged periods of time.

2. **Decreased menstrual blood loss.** OCs decrease the number of days of bleeding and the amount of blood women lose each cycle. In women with menorrhagia, high-dose OC use reduced blood loss by 53%.[29] In more recent studies with low dose OCs (30 mcg EE), menstrual blood loss and duration of flow were also decreased.[30] Overall, a 38% to 49% reduction in menstrual blood loss was seen in another study with a 30 mcg EE preparation.[31,32] In addition, nearly 50% of women experience a reduction in duration of menstrual bleeding with OC use.[33] Decreased menstrual blood loss reduces a woman's risk for iron deficiency anemia. If women use any of the extended cycle options, the number of withdrawal bleeds decreases, enhancing these benefits even more.

3. **Reduction in menstrually-related PMS symptoms.** OCs can reduce menstrually-related PMS symptoms such as mastalgia, bloating, cramping, and pain. Drospirenone-containing pills have also been shown to improve symptoms of water retention, negative affect, and increased appetite associated with menses.[34,35]

4. **Decreased anovulatory bleeding.** Low-dose OC use was associated with a more than 80% improvement in dysfunctional uterine bleeding in a randomized, double blind, placebo-controlled study.[36]

5. **Mittelschmerz relief.** By preventing ovulation, OCs can eliminate the midcycle pain some women experience with ovarian follicle swelling and oocyte extrusion.

6. **Fewer ovarian cyst problems.** Because OCs suppress ovulation, they reduce the risk of hemorrhagic corpora luteal cysts, a condition which can require surgery. Because OCs decrease stimulation of the ovaries by FSH and LH, the incidence of other functional ovarian cysts among women using high-dose OCs was also reduced. Low-dose and multiphasic formulations may help reduce postovulatory cysts;[37,38] however, they do not protect against follicular cyst formation.[39,40]

7. **Improvement in menstrual migraines.** Menstrual migraines are caused by estrogen withdrawal. Cyclic OC use may worsen the intensity of a woman's migraine during her menses; on the other hand, menstrual migraine symptoms may be prevented if she takes active pills every day continuously. (See the section on Headaches, in Managing Side Effects.)

General health benefits

1. **Endometrial and ovarian cancer risk reductions.** When compared with women who have never used OCs, OC users are 40% less likely to develop epithelial ovarian cancer.[41] Ten years or more of use of all monophasic formulations reduces a woman's risk of developing such cancers by 80%.[42] This protection lasts for up to two decades beyond the time the woman takes her last OC.[42,43] Studies that focus on the newer lower dose formulations (<35 mcg EE) have found similar protection levels[43] even in women genetically at higher risk for developing ovarian cancer (BRCA1 mutation cancers).[43,44] Formulations with high doses of progestins protected more than twice as well as OCs with a lower dose of progestins.[45] Women with a family history of ovarian cancer enjoy a greater benefit of ovarian cancer risk reduction than women with no family history.[46] Women with first-degree relatives with ovarian cancer who use OCs for 4 years had a 90% reduction in ovarian cancer risk.[47] One study found that increased duration of OC use did not reduce further the risk of ovarian cancer in BRCA1 or BRCA2 mutation carriers and cautioned against routine use of OCs for chemoprevention.[48] On the other hand, current information has led some to suggest that OCs should be offered to women at high risk for ovarian cancer even if contraceptive benefit is not required.[49]

   OC use for at least 12 months reduces a woman's risk of developing endometrial cancer by about 40%.[50] That risk reduction is increased to 80% in women who use OCs for at least a decade.[41] This protection also endures for up to 20 years after OC discontinuation.[51]

2. **Decreased risk of benign breast conditions.** OC users are less likely to develop fibrocystic breast changes, cysts, or fibroadenoma and are less likely to experience progression of those breast

conditions.[52] In one case-controlled study with over 500 women, the risk of benign breast conditions was lower in the OC users, and significantly less in women who started OC use before their first full-term pregnancy.[53] Women who have hyperplasia with atypia are a notable exception; OC use does not confer any protection to these women.[54]

3. **Improvement of androgen sensitivity or androgen-excess conditions** (e.g., polycystic ovary syndrome). In prospective, randomized, placebo-controlled, double-blind trials, women who use OCs have been shown to have a reduction in the numbers and size of acne lesions.[55,56] Dutch surveys reported that OC use reduced the prevalence of acne by over two-thirds.[57] Only 2 formulations have received FDA approval for treatment of mild to moderate acne (OrthoTri-Cyclen and Estrostep), but other formulations with little or no androgenicity and relatively high estrogenicity increase sex hormone binding globulin (SHBG), which is understood to be the main mechanism for OC use in acne treatment. Women with excessive facial or body hair (hirsutism) have reduction in the hair shaft diameter with OC use.[58,59]

4. **Reduced risk of hospitalization for gonorrheal PID.** The risk of cervical gonorrhea infection spreading into the uterus (endometritis), fallopian tubes (salpingitis) or other pelvic organs (PID) is reduced. In studies conducted in the 1980s, when fewer women with PID were treated on an outpatient basis, the risk of hospitalization for PID was reduced by 50% to 60% in current users after 12 months of use.[61] The exact mechanism of this protection is not known. It may be due to thickened cervical mucus blocking sperm penetration, atrophy of the endometrium (fewer days of bleeding), and/or reduction of movement of pathogens into the tube. Similar reductions are not seen in the risk of chlamydial PID.[60]

5. **Suppression of endometriosis.** Current or recent OC use is associated with a lower incidence of symptomatic endometriosis, especially among parous women (see Chapter 6, Menstrual Problems and Common Gynecologic Concerns).[62] The risk of endometrioma was found to be significantly reduced in current OC users over age 25.[63] OCs reduce menstrual flow and presumably decrease retrograde menses, which is generally believed to contribute to endometriosis. Women who have endometriosis can be treated with extended or continuous use of strong progestogenic OCs to induce pseudo-decidualization of the endometriotic implants and to reduce symptoms during use.[64] Such treatment is not curative, however; the implants undergo atrophy during treatment but remain ready for reactivation when OCs are stopped.[65]

6. **Decrease risk of iron deficiency anemia.** By reducing menstrual blood loss, women increase their hemoglobin and ferritin

levels.[66] This benefit is especially important for women with sickle cell anemia or Von Willebrand's disease, women using anticoagulants or anticonvulsants, and women with fibroids or other causes of primary or secondary menorrhagia (see Chapter 6, Menstrual Problems and Common Gynecologic Concerns).

7. **Treatment of hot flashes and other hormonal fluctuation symptoms** in perimenopausal women.[67,68] (See Chapter 5 on Menopause for more discussion.)

Other potential health benefits

1. **Reduced risk of developing rheumatoid arthritis** (RA). Although early studies suggested that OC use was associated with a reduced risk of RA, there is still controversy about this benefit. One meta-analysis suggested that instead of protecting against the condition, OC use slowed progression of RA,[69] and a later metaanalysis found no protective effect.[70]

2. **Reduced risk of uterine fibroids.** OC users have fewer fibroids, especially with long-term use,[71] but use early in life may increase risk.[72] OCs may control menorrhagia due to uterine myoma. In fact, in many settings, women with moderate-sized fibroids must fail to respond to medical management for menorrhagia (usually with OCs) before they can be considered for surgery.

3. **Reduced risk of fractures.** The impact OC use has on the risk for fracture is still under question. Studies have shown a lower risk for postmenopausal hip fractures,[73] increased bone mineral density (BMD) especially in the lumbar spine,[74] and a slight reduction in osteoporosis.[75] However, one prospective study reported an increased risk of osteoporosis.[76] A comprehensive review of 13 studies of low-dose OCs use found 9 studies showed favorable impact on BMD, and 4 were neutral.[77] If there is a benefit, it may only be in at-risk women with low estrogen levels. OC use increases BMD in young women with hypothalamic amenorrhea.[78] OC use in women with osteopenia due to anorexia nervosa is not sufficient to protect bone, but when added to anabolic agents such as insulin growth factor (IGF), OC use significantly improves that agent's effectiveness.[79] OC use modulates the negative impact of smoking in young women and improves BMD in young women with irregular menses.[80]

4. **Favorable impact on lipids.** EE increases HDL cholesterol and reduces LDL cholesterol. Progestins diminish the magnitude of this favorable impact; the more androgenic formulations have a more pronounced negative effect. Although triglyceride levels increase somewhat with estrogen-containing contraception, there is little concern because those remnants are not atherogenic. However, estrogen-containing contraceptives should be avoided

if their use will be anticipated to raise triglyceride levels to 500 mg/dl and place the woman at risk for pancreatitis.

5. **Improved lung mechanics.**[81]

6. **Possible reduced risk for colorectal cancer.**[82]

7. **Influence on sexual enjoyment.** OC use may increase sexual pleasuring, either by increasing libido (less concern about pregnancy) or increasing lubrication. On the other hand, some OC users report decreased libido and more vaginal dryness.

8. **Fewer episodes of seizures, porphyria, and asthma.** These conditions may worsen during a woman's menses. Continuous use of OCs can prevent these problems for months at a time.

9. **Vitamin fortification.** Iron has been added to some placebo pills at the end of the cycle. Work is underway to add 400 mcg of folic acid to both active and placebo pills. Iron deficiency is associated with anemia, and maternal folic acid deficiency contributes to neural tube defects in offspring.

INDICATIONS

Considering the wide range of benefits OCs offer, their use can be particularly attractive for women who desire reversible contraception and have hormone-related problems. It should be noted that OCs might be beneficial in treatment of some of the following conditions (after underlying pathology has been ruled out), even if the woman is not at risk for pregnancy:

- Heavy, painful, irregular menstrual bleeding, or menorrhagia (dysmenorrhea, oligomenorrhea)
- Dysfunctional uterine bleeding
- Recurrent luteal phase ovarian cysts
- Family history of ovarian cancer
- Personal risk for endometrial cancer
- Acne or hirsutism
- Polycystic ovary syndrome (PCOS)

In addition, extended use OC may be particularly helpful for women with

- Premenstrual symptoms (PMS)
- Endometriosis
- Mentally challenged women whose monthly menstruations terrify them and provide a hygiene challenge to their caregivers.
- Anemia due to menorrhagia
- Dysmenorrhea

Finally, OCs with levonorgestrel or norgestrel may be used for emergency contraception. New studies suggest that OCs with norethindrone may be used for emergency contraception if the more effective formulations are not available (see Chapter 12 on Emergency Contraception).[83]

D ISADVANTAGES AND HEALTH COMPLICATIONS

Inform women that OC use may be associated with some disadvantages, many of which can be overcome or managed. Consult the section on Managing Side Effects. Some disadvantages are also discussed in the section on Special Issues.

General Disadvantages

1. **Daily administration.** Inconsistent or incorrect use of OCs reduces protection from the risk of pregnancy and increases the incidence of side effects, such as breakthrough bleeding.

2. **Expense and access.** In many states, insurance plans are not required to cover contraception, so women must pay for their OCs. Often, women are required to return to pharmacies each month to purchase another package. The mismatch between calendar months with 30 to 31 days and pill packs with only 28 pills can present challenges in use.

3. **Need for storage and ready access.** Adolescent women or women whose partners do not want them to use contraception may not have a place to hide their pills. Practitioners need to confirm that the patient's plans for storage are realistic (school lockers are not an answer) and guide them to more private contraceptive methods, if needed. Homeless women and women who travel extensively may have difficulty storing their pill packs.

4. **No protection against STIs.** Women at risk for STIs may use OCs, but they should be advised to reduce their risk for infection by confining their activity to mutually monogamous, uninfected partners, or by using condoms with every act of coitus.

Health Complications

1. **Myocardial infarction (MI).** A pivotal U.S. study showed that low-dose OCs (<50mcg EE) do not significantly increase the risk of MI or stroke in healthy, non-smoking women.[84] Compared to never-users, current users as a group had a relative risk of 1.3 for MI; most of the increased risk was seen in women with known risk factors. A second study supported those findings.[85] Recent metaanalysis of the literature demonstrated that overall current use of OCs increased the risk of MI by 2.48 times. Pills with 20 mcg EE did not increase the risk of MI.[86] Large increases, by

factors of 7 to more than 100, have been observed in the relative risk (RR) of MI and ischemic stroke among OC users who also smoke or have hypertension.[87] The attributable risk of death from cardiovascular disease from low-dose OC use is 0.06 per 100,000 nonsmokers age 15 to 34 and 3.0 per 100,000 nonsmokers aged 35 to 44. However, the risk of death attributable to OC use by low-risk women of any age is less than their risk of mortality from pregnancy.[88]

In an interesting analysis of those data, it was observed that nearly 75% of cases of MI could be attributed to smoking.[89] The third-generation OCs showed no increase in the risk of MIs, but the second-generation formulations apparently doubled the risk.[86] The increase in heart attacks seen with use of combined hormonal contraceptives is due to arterial thrombosis caused by estrogen. This is why women with underlying atherosclerotic coronary vessel damage from smoking, hypertension, and hyperlipidemia are more vulnerable. The effect is reversible. After women stop taking the pill, their risks for MI return to baseline. Once women over age 40 have stopped smoking for 3 to 12 months, they may be candidates for OC use if they have no other contraindications. Women with risk factors for MI may still be candidates for progestin-only methods.

2. **Stroke in high-risk women.** In 2002, a World Health Organization (WHO) panel found no significant increased risk of ischemic or hemorrhagic stroke among nonsmoking women with no history of migraine headaches who use low-dose (<35 mcg EE) OCs,[90] as did a subsequent study.[91] However, OC users who smoke or are hypertensive have a three-fold risk of hemorrhagic stroke compared to those who do not have those risk factors. WHO studies found a significant increase in the risk of ischemic stroke, but not hemorrhagic stroke, among OC users who experienced migraine with aura (odds ratio 3.0, CI 1.3–11.3) and a nonsignificant increase in OC users who reported migraine without aura (OR 3.0, CI 0.7–148) (see Headache section in Managing Side Effects, below).[92] The WHO panel stated that migraineurs with aura have a higher risk of stroke than those without aura, but no study had sufficient proof to examine risk of stroke by type of migraine.[93] There is no difference between second- and third-generation formulations.[94] OC patient package inserts state that the relative risk of hemorrhagic stroke associated with OC use is reported to be 1.2 for non-smokers, 7.6 for smokers, and 25.7 for severe hypertensives. The risk is also greater in older women.[95]

3. **Venous thromboembolism** (VTE). VTE can develop in different organ systems and present with different symptoms as listed on Table 19-2. The rate of thrombosis is 4 to 5 for every 100,000 reproductive-age women, 12 to 20 for low-dose OC users, and 48

Table 19-2 Circulatory diseases attributable to pills

Diagnosis	Location of Pathology	Symptoms
Thrombophlebitis	Lower leg	Calf pains, swelling, heat or tenderness
Thrombophlebitis	Thigh	Pain, heat, or redness
Pulmonary embolism	Lung	Cough, including coughing up blood, chest pain; shortness of breath
Myocardial infarction	Heart	Chest pain, left arm and shoulder pain, shortness of breath, weakness
Thrombotic stroke	Brain	Headache, weakness or numbness, visual problem, sudden intellectual impairment
Hemorrhagic stroke, including subarachnoid hemorrhage	Brain	Headache, weakness or numbness, visual problem, sudden intellectual impairment
Retinal vein thrombosis	Eye	Headache, complete or partial loss of vision
Mesenteric vein thrombosis	Intestines	Abdominal pain, vomiting, weakness
Pelvic vein thrombosis	Pelvis	Lower abdominal pain, cramps

Source: Stewart F, et al. (1987).

to 60 for pregnant women.[96,97] Pills with 35 mcg EE are associated with a lower risk of VTE than are 50 mg formulations.[98–100] The risk for VTE is highest in the first 1 to 2 years of OC use and then decreases over time. The effects are reversible. Past use of OCs is not associated with increased risk. Smoking does not add to the risk.

Estrogen increases liver production of a variety of clot promoting factors (such as factor VII, factor VIII, factor X and fibrinogen), decreases the production of clot lysing factors (such as antithrombin III and protein S), and increases platelet activity. Progestins alone have no impact on the clotting system, but when combined with estrogen they generally temper estrogen's actions or maintain neutrality. In the mid 1990s, international studies indicated that pills containing the progestins desogestrel and gestodene (not available in the United States) may be associated with higher rates of thrombosis than the formulations containing levonorgestrel and norgestrel.[98–100] U.S. labeling reflects these findings. Since then, it has been shown that there were confounding factors such as duration of use, selection bias (healthy user effect), and detection biases that may have influenced those study outcomes. Norgestimate was not included in the early international studies but was implicated in a subsequent transnational study.[101] Because the new compound, drospirenone, has antiandrogenic effects, it may also allow fuller expression of estrogen's thrombotic impact.[102,103]

In most healthy women, estrogen and progestin together have no clinically significant impact on the coagulation system. Risk factors that place a woman at increased risk for venous thrombosis include obesity, previous venous compromise, and immobilization. However, the increase in VTE risk seen with OC use is most frequently due to inherited disorders such as factor V Leiden mutation or Protein S and C synthesis disorders. The factor V Leiden mutation explains 30% of all deep venous thromboses. In the United States, it is estimated that 5.3% of Caucasians, 2.2% of Hispanics, 1.2% of Blacks and Native Americans, and 0.5% of Asians carry Leiden mutations. Caucasians have a common genetic mutation in prothrombin, which affects 0.7% to 4% of that population.[104] Heterozygous factor V Leiden mutation carriers have thrombotic risk 6 to 8 times higher (24 to 40/100,000), and homozygous carriers have risk about 10 times greater than in the general population. When a carrier uses OCs, her VTE risk rises to 120 to 150/100,000 a year.[105] (For further discussion, see section on Patient Selection.)

4. **Hypertension.** OCs increase circulating levels of angiotensin II. Some women are very sensitive to angiotensin II levels, which can increase both their diastolic and systolic blood pressure readings. Both estrogen and progestin enhance aldosterone activity, which results in fluid retention, which, in turn, also contributes to an increase in blood pressure. The vast majority of women who use OCs will have no significant increase in either diastolic or systolic blood pressure measurements, although a 3 to 5 mm rise is not uncommon. However, 1% to 3% of women who use modern, low-dose OCs will, over time, experience increases in their blood pressure readings, which, if attributable to OC use, will normalize within 3 months of stopping estrogen-containing contraceptives. The women whose readings do not return to normal should undergo a standard work-up, although most will be found to have essential hypertension. Some women may need to begin antihypertensive agents as well as discontinuing OCs.

5. **Glucose tolerance and diabetes.** OCs currently available in the United States do not adversely affect carbohydrate metabolism.[106] Older OC formulations with high doses of sex steroids had a more profound impact on glucose tolerance and in some instances resulted in hyperglycemia with hyperinsulinemia. In the CARDIA study, current use of OCs was associated with lower glucose levels and perhaps with a lower odds ratio of diabetes.[107] Concerns have been raised about OC use in women at risk for developing diabetes because progesterone is a competitive inhibitor of the insulin

receptor and estrogen influences the release of insulin from the pancreatic islet cells and decreases insulin sensitivity.[108] High-risk women, such as those with a history of gestational diabetes who used OCs with low progestin content (Ovcon-35), had no higher risk of developing glucose intolerance or overt diabetes than the controls who used non-hormonal methods when both groups were studied for up to 7 years.[109]

6. **Gallbladder disease.** Recent studies of low-dose OCs do not show the increased risk of cholelithiasis and cholecystitis associated earlier with high-dose OCs. However, it may still be possible that low-dose OCs accelerate the development of symptomatic gallbladder disease in women with preexisting stones or sludge. OCs do not increase the risk of gallbladder cancer.[110]

7. **Cholestatic jaundice.** The active transport of bile can be impaired by high-dose combined hormonal contraceptives, resulting in cholestatic jaundice with pruritus. This condition reverses with discontinuation of hormones. The incidence in the general population using low-dose formulations is not known but is assumed to be very rare.

8. **Hepatic neoplasms.** Benign liver tumors have been associated with the use of high-dose OCs, especially long-term use. Focal nodular hyperplasia may be increased nearly 3-fold in OC users.[111] Adenomas are the most significant, since they can cause rupture of the liver capsule, extensive intraperitoneal hemorrhage, and even death. Women may or may not have abdominal pain with adenomas; their liver function tests are usually normal. Palpate the liver edge as part of the annual physical exam. If the liver is enlarged or tender, discontinue hormonal contraception and evaluate with MRI or CT tests; ultrasound is not reliable. Tumor regression is expected after stopping OCs.

   Hepatocellular carcinoma risk is not increased with OC use.[112] Use of hormonal contraception by high-risk women (with chronic hepatitis B virus) did not appear to increase the risk of hepatitis cellular carcinoma beyond their baseline elevated risk.

9. **Chlamydia/HIV.** Women who use OCs are at increased risk for acquiring chlamydia cervicitis.[113,114] In a study of Kenyan professional sex workers, users of OCs had an increased risk (hazard ratio 1.8, C1.1–2.9) of becoming infected with chlamydia when compared with women using no contraceptives.[115]

   OCs influence transcription of natural antimicrobials in the human endometrium, which might increase a woman's vulnerability to upper-tract chlamydia or HIV infection.[116] Although a recent study shows that OCs thicken the vaginal epithelium,[117] hormonal contraception might increase a woman's vulnerability to HIV infection by reducing its barrier protection, by increasing the number or permissiveness of susceptible cells, or by directly affecting viral expression.[118] Clearly, all women at risk for STIs should limit their sexual activity to one uninfected, monogamous partner or, at a minimum, use latex or polyurethane condoms with every sexual act.

10. **Melanoma.** A pooled analysis of 10 case-controlled studies involving nearly 2,400 cases of melanoma revealed no correlation between OC use and the development of melanoma. No effect of duration of use or current use was observed.[119] However, it is recommended that women with a history of melanoma refrain from getting pregnant or using hormonal contraception for at least 3 years after their original therapy, since the risk of recurrence is highest at this time.

11. **Leiomyoma** (uterine fibroids) contain both estrogen and progesterone receptors. Since fibroids often shrink after menopause, when estrogen levels decrease, it has been suggested that estrogen-containing contraceptives might increase the growth of these benign uterine tumors. However, clinical studies with low-dose OCs have found no impact on the risk of developing new fibroids or increasing the size of pre-existing fibroids.[120–122] In fact, OCs are often used to control excessive menstrual bleeding caused by fibroids.

12. **Cervical dysplasia and cervical carcinoma.** OC users have a statistically significant higher risk of developing cervical dysplasia compared to women who use no method of contraception or who rely on tubal ligation. Cervical dysplasia and cervical carcinoma are caused by the human papillomavirus (HPV), especially HPV 16 and 18. OC users may have more unprotected intercourse with multiple partners. However, combined hormonal methods cause eversion of the cervical os, which not only increases metaplasia in nulliparous women but exposes those vulnerable metaplastic cells to HPV. OC use may be associated with artifacts that mimic ASC-US (glycogen vacuoles create perinuclear halos in OC users) on liquid-based cytology tests. Reflex HPV testing will demonstrate that two-thirds of those women have no virus.[123]

OC users do not need to have cervical cytology testing more frequently than required by their other risk factors. Similarly, they do not need to be tested with more sensitive cytologic modalities because they use OCs.

Women who use OCs for more than 5 years and who are infected with HPV have a 3- to 4-fold increased risk for in situ and invasive squamous cell cervical carcinoma.[124] However, a similarly large increase in the risk of cervical cancer was seen in another study in women with HPV infection who had 7 or more pregnancies (RR 8.29). Pregnancy before 18 years of age increases the relative risk (RR) for cervical cancer to 10.71.[125] A large meta-analysis of 28 studies including 12,531 women with cervical cancer found a 1.1 relative risk after 5 years of OC use, RR 1.6 after 5 to 10 years, and RR 2.2 more than 10 years.[126] Studies demonstrate that OC use may increase the risk of adenocarcinoma (cancer of the "glandular" cells of the cervix).[127]

13. **Breast cancer.** A recent study shows that among women aged 35 to 64 years, current or former use of OCs is not associated with an increased risk for developing breast cancer.[128] An older meta-analysis of 90% of the women's literature found that current users had a 25% increased risk of being diagnosed with breast cancer, although all the excess risk disappeared 10 years after stopping the pills. The cancers diagnosed in those studies were more localized.[129] The remaining question is the effect OCs may have on the development of breast cancer in women under age 35, when the disease is very rare. (See Most Frequently Asked Questions, below).

14. **Special issues for drospirenone-containing OCs.** Drospirenone has antimineralocorticoid activity, which introduces the potential for hyperkalemia in high-risk patients; the 3 mg of drospirenone found in Yasmin has the same impact on electrolytes as a 25 mg dose of spironolactone. Women receiving daily, long-term treatment for chronic conditions or diseases with medications that may increase serum potassium should have their serum potassium levels checked during the first treatment cycle. Drugs that may increase serum potassium include ACE inhibitors, angiotensin-II receptor antagonists, potassium-sparing diuretics, heparin, aldosterone antagonists, and NSAIDS. Note that *intermittent* use of NSAIDS does not pose any problems.

PATIENT SELECTION

Patient selection is the key to safe OC use. The benefits of OCs generally far outweigh any significant adverse events. However, some women have medical conditions or personal habits that increase their risk of developing serious complications with use of combined hormonal contraception.

Cigarette smokers over age 40 face a greater mortality risk with ongoing OC use than they would experience with pregnancy and, therefore, should not use OCs or other estrogen-containing contraceptives. Similarly, heavy smokers (>15 cigarettes/day) over age 35 should avoid estrogen-containing methods, according to product labeling. Many clinicians will not provide combined pills for women over the age of 35 if they smoke at all. (See discussion on Smokers in section on Special Populations.)

Combined hormonal contraceptives should not be used by women with an increased propensity to form blood clots, polycythemia vera, or a personal history of thrombosis, stroke or heart attack, advanced diabetes, labile hypertension, estrogen sensitive malignancies (such as breast cancer), active liver problems, and migraines with focal neurologic symptoms. Although the relative risk of thrombosis is greatly increased in women who have factor V Leiden mutations, routine screening for these rare mutations is not recommended prior to prescribing estrogen-containing contraceptives. However, it may be very appropriate to test (not screen) women who have a strong family history of multiple, unexplained clots in many family members, especially at a young age. Table 19-3 lists conditions from pill package labeling that are listed as contraindications.

PRECAUTIONS

To guide family planning programs, WHO has developed a more comprehensive list of precautions in providing combined hormonal contraceptives, which are summarized in Table 19-4.[130] Use of hormonal contraception by women who have medical conditions are ranked into four different categories. Category 4 conditions preclude the use of combined hormonal contraceptives. Conditions in Category 3 may be adversely impacted by combined hormonal contraceptives, and the risks generally outweigh the benefits. Providers should exercise caution if these agents are used and carefully monitor these OC users for adverse effects. The WHO recognized in its Category 2 that some conditions may trigger potential concerns with hormonal contraceptives, but the benefits of contraceptive use with these conditions usually outweigh the risks. Category 1 conditions raise no concerns about OC use, and OC use should not be restricted.

PROVIDING ORAL CONTRACEPTIVES

Explore the patient's medical and reproductive health history and her family history to ensure that she has no reason to avoid using combined hormonal contraception (see Tables 19-3 and 19-4 on WHO Medical Eligibility Criteria). Discuss the potential noncontraceptive benefits and examine all her lifestyle issues to ensure that she has a secure plan for where to keep her pill pack and can realistically expect to take a pill a day. Anticipatory counseling about safety concerns can reduce later discontinuation. Determine if she wants to have monthly withdrawal bleeding or if she would prefer less frequent bleeding episodes. Ask if she has any other complaints that need to be addressed at this visit. In particular, find out if she needs any STI testing or if she needs emergency contraception now or may need it in the future. Advise her to follow safer sex practices.

Measure the woman's blood pressure. It may be prudent to do a breast examination, but a pelvic examination is *not* needed for an asymptomatic woman prior to initiating OCs,[131,132] even if the woman has not had a recent Pap smear. STI screening, if needed, can be urine-based. No other screening tests are routinely needed unless her history or blood pressure indicate a need for further assessment.[133]

Table 19-3 Medical conditions precluding OC use, as listed in pill package inserts (PPI)

There are specific medical conditions that indicate a woman should not use OCs. The FDA-approved pill package inserts (PPI) list a somewhat different set of medical conditions that preclude OC use than do the WHO medical eligibility criteria. Below is the FDA-approved package insert list of medical conditions that indicate OCs "should not be used." The category assigned in the WHO medical eligibility criteria (Table 19-4) is included in the adjacent column.

Medical Conditions Precluding OC Use (PPI)	WHO Category
• Thrombophlebitis or thromboembolic disorder	4
• Past history of deep vein thrombosis or thromboembolic disorders	4
• Cerebrovascular or coronary artery disease	4
• Valvular heart disease with thrombogenic complications	4
• Uncontrolled hypertension	4
• Diabetes with vascular involvement	3/4
• Headaches with focal aura	4
• Major surgery with prolonged immobilization	4
• Breast cancer	4
• Carcinoma of the endometrium	1
• Other known or suspected estrogen-dependent neoplasia	Not discussed
• Undiagnosed abnormal genital bleeding	2
• Cholestatic jaundice of pregnancy	2
— Jaundice with prior pill use	3
• Acute or chronic hepatocellular disease with abnormal liver function, hepatic adenomas, or hepatic carcinomas	4
• Known or suspected pregnancy	"Not applicable"
• Hypersensitivity to any component of the product	Not discussed

Table 19-4 WHO Medical eligibility criteria for low-dose combined oral contraceptives (COCs), patches and rings, 2004

LOW-DOSE COMBINED ORAL CONTRACEPTIVES (COCs) <35 mcg of ethinylestradiol	COCs do not protect against STI/HIV. If there is risk of STI/HIV (including during pregnancy or postpartum), the correct and consistent use of condoms is recommended, either alone or with another contraceptive method. Male latex condoms are proven to reduce the risk of STI/HIV.
CONDITION	CATEGORY I = Initiation C = Continuation

PERSONAL CHARACTERISTICS AND REPRODUCTIVE HISTORY

PREGNANCY	NA
AGE	
a) Menarche to <40 years	1
b) ≥ 40 years	2
PARITY	
a) Nulliparous	1
b) Parous	1
BREASTFEEDING	
a) < 6 weeks postpartum	4
b) ≥ 6 weeks to <6 months postpartum (primarily breastfeeding)	3
c) ≥ 6 months postpartum	2
POSTPARTUM (in non-breastfeeding women)	
a) <21 days	3
b) ≥ 21 days	1
POST-ABORTION	
a) First trimester	1*
b) Second trimester	1
c) Immediate post-septic abortion	1
PAST ECTOPIC PREGNANCY	1
HISTORY OF PELVIC SURGERY (including Caesarean section)	1
SMOKING	
a) Age <35 years	2*
b) Age ≥ 35 years	
(i) < 15 cigarettes/day	3*
(ii) ≥ 15 cigarettes/day	4*

(continued)

* For more detailed clarifications, consult the WHO website.

Table 19-4 WHO Medical eligibility criteria for low-dose combined oral contraceptives (COCs), patches and rings, 2004—*(cont'd)*

CONDITION	CATEGORY I = Initiation C = Continuation
OBESITY	
≥ 30 kg/m^2 body mass index (BMI)	2
CARDIOVASCULAR DISEASE	
MULTIPLE RISK FACTORS FOR ARTERIAL CARDIOVASCULAR DISEASE (such as older age, smoking, diabetes and hypertension)	3/4*
HYPERTENSION	
a) History of hypertension, where blood pressure CANNOT be evaluated (including hypertension during pregnancy)	3*
b) Adequately controlled hypertension, where blood pressure CAN be evaluated	3*
c) Elevated blood pressure levels (properly taken measurements)	
(i) systolic 140–159 or diastolic 90–99	3
(ii) systolic ≥160 or diastolic ≥100	4
d) Vascular disease	4
HISTORY OF HIGH BLOOD PRESSURE DURING PREGNANCY (where current blood pressure is measurable and normal)	2
DEEP VENOUS THROMBOSIS (DVT)/ PULMONARY EMBOLISM (PE)	
a) History of DVT/PE	4
b) Current DVT/PE	4
c) Family history of DVT/PE (first-degree relatives)	2
d) Major surgery	
(i) with prolonged immobilization	4
(ii) without prolonged immobilization	2
e) Minor surgery without immobilization	1
KNOWN THROMBOGENIC MUTATIONS (e.g., Factor V Leiden, prothrombin, protein S, protein C, and antithrombin deficiency)	4*

(continued)

* For more detailed clarifications, consult the WHO website.

Table 19-4 WHO Medical eligibility criteria for low-dose combined oral contraceptives (COCs), patches and rings, 2004—*(cont'd)*

CONDITION	CATEGORY I = Initiation C = Continuation	
SUPERFICIAL VENOUS THROMBOSIS		
a) Varicose veins	1	
b) Superficial thrombophlebitis	2	
CURRENT AND HISTORY OF ISCHAEMIC HEART DISEASE	4	
STROKE (history of cerebrovascular accident)	4	
KNOWN HYPERLIPIDAEMIAS (screening is *not* necessary for safe use of contraceptive)	2/3*	
VALVULAR HEART DISEASE		
a) Uncomplicated	2	
b) Complicated (pulmonary hypertension, atrial fibrillation, history of subacute bacterial endocarditis)	4	

NEUROLOGIC CONDITIONS

	I	C
HEADACHES		
a) Non migrainous (mild or severe)	1*	2*
b) Migraine		
(i) *without aura*		
Age < 35	2*	3*
Age ≥ 35	3*	4*
(ii) *with aura (at any age)*	4*	4*
EPILEPSY	1*	
DEPRESSIVE DISORDERS	1*	

(continued)

* For more detailed clarifications, consult the WHO website.

Table 19-4 WHO Medical eligibility criteria for low-dose combined oral contraceptives (COCs), patches and rings, 2004—*(cont'd)*

CONDITION	CATEGORY I = Initiation C = Continuation
REPRODUCTIVE TRACT INFECTIONS AND DISORDERS	

VAGINAL BLEEDING PATTERNS

a)	Irregular pattern *without* heavy bleeding	1
b)	Heavy or prolonged bleeding (includes regular and irregular patterns)	1*

UNEXPLAINED VAGINAL BLEEDING (suspicious for serious condition)

Before evaluation	2*

ENDOMETRIOSIS	1
BENIGN OVARIAN TUMOURS (including cysts)	1
SEVERE DYSMENORRHOEA	1

TROPHOBLAST DISEASE

a)	Benign gestational trophoblastic disease	1
b)	Malignant gestational trophoblastic disease	1

CERVICAL ECTROPION	1
CERVICAL INTRAEPITHELIAL NEOPLASIA (CIN)	2
CERVICAL CANCER (awaiting treatment)	2

BREAST DISEASE

a)	Undiagnosed mass	2*
b)	Benign breast disease	1
c)	Family history of cancer	1
d)	Cancer	
	(i) current	4
	(ii) past and no evidence of current disease for 5 years	3

ENDOMETRIAL CANCER	1
OVARIAN CANCER	1

(continued)

* For more detailed clarifications, consult the WHO website.

Table 19-4 WHO Medical eligibility criteria for low-dose combined oral contraceptives (COCs), patches and rings, 2004—*(cont'd)*

CONDITION	CATEGORY I = Initiation C = Continuation
UTERINE FIBROIDS	
a) Without distortion of the uterine cavity	1
b) With distortion of the uterine cavity	1
PELVIC INFLAMMATORY DISEASE (PID)	
a) Past PID (assuming no current risk factors for STIs)	
(i) with subsequent pregnancy	1
(ii) without subsequent pregnancy	1
b) PID-current or within the last 3 months	1
STIs	
a) Current purulent cervicitis or chlamydial infection or gonorrhea	1
b) Other STIs (excluding HIV and hepatitis)	1
c) Vaginitis without purulent cervicitis	1
d) Increased risk of STIs (e.g., multiple partners or partner who has multiple partners)	1
HIV/AIDS	
HIGH RISK OF HIV	1
HIV-INFECTED	1
AIDS	1*
OTHER INFECTIONS	
SCHISTOSOMIASIS	
a) Uncomplicated	1
b) Fibrosis of liver	1
TUBERCULOSIS	
a) Non-pelvic	1*
b) Known pelvic	1*
MALARIA	1

(continued)

* For more detailed clarifications, consult the WHO website.

Table 19-4 WHO Medical eligibility criteria for low-dose combined oral contraceptives (COCs), patches and rings, 2004—*(cont'd)*

CONDITION	CATEGORY I = Initiation C = Continuation
ENDOCRINE CONDITIONS	
DIABETES	
a) History of gestational disease	1
b) Non-vascular disease	
(i) non-insulin dependent	2
(ii) insulin dependent	2
c) Nephropathy/retinopathy/neuropathy	3/4*
d) Other vascular disease or diabetes of >20 years' duration	3/4*
THYROID	
a) Simple goiter	1
b) Hyperthyroid	1
c) Hypothyroid	1
GASTROINTESTINAL CONDITIONS	
GALL-BLADDER DISEASE	
a) Symptomatic	
(i) treated by cholecystectomy	2
(ii) medically treated	3
(iii) current	3
b) Asymptomatic	2
HISTORY OF CHOLESTASIS	
a) Pregnancy-related	2
b) Past COC-related	3
VIRAL HEPATITIS	
a) Active	4
b) Carrier	1
CIRRHOSIS	
a) Mild (compensated)	3
b) Severe (decompensated)	4

(continued)

* For more detailed clarifications, consult the WHO website.

Table 19-4 WHO Medical eligibility criteria for low-dose combined oral contraceptives (COCs), patches and rings, 2004—*(cont'd)*

CONDITION	CATEGORY I = Initiation C = Continuation
LIVER TUMORS	
a) Benign (adenoma)	4
b) Malignant (hepatoma)	4
ANAEMIAS	
THALASSAEMIA	1
SICKLE CELL DISEASE	2
IRON DEFICIENCY ANEMIA	1
DRUG INTERACTIONS	
COMMONLY USED DRUGS WHICH AFFECT LIVER ENZYMES	
a) Certain antibiotics (rifampicin)	3*
b) Certain anticonvulsants (phenytoin, carbamezapine, barbiturates, primidone, topiramate, oxcarbazepine)	3*
OTHER ANTIBIOTICS (excluding rifampicin)	1
a) Griseofulvin	2
b) Other antibiotics	1
ANTIRETROVIRAL THERAPY	2*

* For more detailed clarifications, consult the WHO website.

Source: WHO (2004),[131] with permission.
For references and update, please consult
http://www.who.int/reproductive-health/publications/MEC_3

FOLLOW-UP

Because side effects can appear in the first few months of OC use, a follow-up visit at 3 or 6 months is quite commonly recommended. A woman who has used the pill for 3 to 6 months, has no problems, and wants to continue the pill, may be given 7 to 13 packets (a 6-month to 1-year supply). One author of this chapter strongly recommends providing only 3 cycles of pills at the first visit with a 9-month refill, followed by a 12-month supply every subsequent year. Recent suggestions that it may be appropriate to provide OCs over-the-counter also suggest that new OC users may not need such frequent reassessment.[134,135] An alternative approach is to prescribe or give a woman a full year's supply of pills the very first visit and then encourage a revisit or two in the first year for a blood pressure and headache check. After a woman has used OCs for 1 year, you could consider prescribing a full year's supply of pills (or even 18 cycles) in an effort to increase OC continuation rates.

Women who are planning major surgery requiring prolonged immobilization should discontinue use of estrogen-containing OCs 1 month prior to surgery. Similarly, women being treated with anticoagulants should stop their OCs 1 month prior to finishing their anticoagulant.

CHOICES FOR PILL INITIATION

Quick start. For the Quick Start method, the patient takes the *first* pill in the pill pack on the day of her office visit, as long as she is not pregnant and not in need of emergency contraception. If she needs emergency contraception, she should take both tablets of Plan-B or its equivalent at once on the visit day, and start her pills no later than the next day. Tell her to use a back-up method with her pills for at least 7 days. Her next menses will be delayed until she completes the active pills in her pack and starts the placebo pills. If she has concern about an undetectable early pregnancy, she can start her pills and be instructed to return for a urine pregnancy test in 2 to 3 weeks, or do one at home. Alternatively, she can use a first-day start. The hormones in the pills will not adversely affect an early pregnancy and the prompt repeat pregnancy testing will detect the pregnancy early enough to begin the pregnancy care she chooses.

The Quick Start approach was more successful getting women started on the pill than are the two methods discussed below; more women were using the pill in the third cycles, especially if they had menstrually-related problems.[136] However, it is an off-label practice. The reason Quick Start is preferred is because other approaches leave a time gap between the time the patient is prescribed her pills and the time she is intended to start taking them. As many as 25% of young women starting by one of the conventional start methods (see below) failed to begin taking the pills as instructed because they had conceived in the interim, forgot the pill-taking instructions, failed to fill the prescription, or were worried about taking the pill after their visit.[137,138] Quick Start does not increase irregular spotting or bleeding.[139]

First-day start. The first-day start was introduced to gain early control of ovarian follicles during the first cycle. In this approach, a woman takes her first pill on the first day of her next period. It is important to have the woman determine that her period is normal—that it occurs at the predicted time and is preceded by symptoms that are usual for her. If there is any question that the menses is not normal, have her rule out pregnancy before she starts her pills.

Sunday start. The Sunday start was the most common method for starting pills for decades. Women were told to start their first active pill on the first Sunday of their menses. For example, if a woman were to start bleeding on Friday, she should take her first pill two days later on Sunday. If her period were to start on Sunday, she should start on that day. Make sure the patient understands that she should not wait to start the first pill on the Sunday after her menses ends. Today, the Sunday start is not generally recommended because it is often difficult for women to get refills when they need them on weekends. In addition, many women are working outside the home and prefer not to menstruate during their work week. A Sunday start often requires that a back-up method be used for 7 days.

SWITCHING FROM OTHER METHODS

Women who switch from other methods can start OCs immediately, using the guidelines for the pill Quick Start initiation. For example, women who have implants or IUDs removed can start their OCs that same day and be told to use a back-up contraceptive method for the next week. Women who have had recent unprotected intercourse can be given Plan B emergency contraception (EC) immediately and start their OCs no later than the next day coupled with a back-up method for at least 7 days. A urine pregnancy test in 2 to 3 weeks may be offered to detect any EC failures. Women using injectable methods generally start their OCs at the end of the effective period of the injection. However, if a woman is amenorrheic as a result of the injection and is late for reinjection, she can start the OCs the same day with a 7-day course of a back-up method. For any woman with a recent history of unprotected intercourse, provide EC, OCs, and back-up methods followed by a repeat pregnancy test in 2 to 3 weeks.

CHOOSING A PATTERN OF PILL USE

1. **Monthly cycling 21/7.** Conventional pill packaging contains 3 weeks of active pills followed by 7 placebo pills to provide a predictable, coordinated withdrawal bleed that women will interpret to be a normal menses. Pioneers in the development of the birth control pill touted this feature as a distinct benefit for women,[140] which it was at the time.

2. **Shortened pill-free interval.** It is possible that the 7-day pill-free interval allows too much time for follicular development and increases to the failure rate with low-dose OCs. Shortening the pill-free interval with 20 mcg EE pills from 7 to 5 days suppressed ovarian activity more effectively.[141] One way to implement this approach is to have the patient use the "first-day start" for every cycle, in which she begins a new pill pack each month on the first day of her withdrawal bleeding. If she has no menses by the 5th placebo pill day, she should start her new pack that day. A pregnancy test is not necessary, but may provide comfort to the woman. In a trial comparing a 23-day regimen to the traditional 21-day regimen of 20 mcg EE pills, the withdrawal bleeding was shorter in the group using more active pills.[142] Mircette has 21 active pills, 2 placebos, and 5 pills with 10 mcg EE.

3. **Extended use.** Recent studies have found that many of the "pill side effects" (such as headache, cramping, breast tenderness, bloating

and/or swelling) occur during the week women take their placebo pills.[143] Because recent surveys have shown that many women would prefer to bleed less frequently than once a month,[144] it is time to re-evaluate the need for monthly withdrawal bleeding.[145] The purpose of menstruation in spontaneously cycling women is to resolve the prior unsuccessful cycle (no pregnancy) and to prepare for the next cycle (which may result in pregnancy). With OC use, however, conception is not desired; there is no biological need to provoke artificial withdrawal bleeding on a monthly basis. Unless the patient wants to use bleeding as a reassurance that she is not pregnant, monthly cycling is *not* necessary and may be replaced by extended OC use.[146] In clinical studies, women with prolonged flow had fewer menstrually related problems, and the majority of those women continued to use the extended cycle.[147] The regimen using extra packs of pills is cost-effective for women with menorrhagia.[148] Other women for whom extended use would be particularly attractive are those with dysmenorrhea or menstrual migraines, and those on active military duty or who have similarly demanding jobs.

Options for extended use include the following:

- *Brief manipulation of a cycle for convenience* such as for a honeymoon, trip, athletic event, camping experience, business meetings, exams or presentations.

- *Bicycling*, which is the back-to-back of 2 packs of active pills by taking the first pack of 21 active pills, throwing away the 7 placebo pills in that first pack and immediately starting the second pack of 21 active pills followed by the 7 placebo pills at the end of the second package. Recent studies of extended cycles ("bicycling") found that the longer cycles had significant reduction in the days of bleeding and in annual expenditures for female hygiene.

- *Tricycling*, meaning taking the 21 active pills from 3 packages followed by the 7 placebo pills from the third package.

- *Taking Seasonale*, which contains 84 active pills followed by 7 placebo pills. A woman using this regimen has four periods a year, hence the name, Seasonale.

- *No-cycling*, meaning taking active pills indefinitely (for many months or years) with no placebo pills as long as the woman has no troublesome spotting. Seasonale or any strong progestin monophasic pills may be used in this off-label manner.

CHOOSING A FORMULATION

Clinicians in the United States have numerous OCs from which to choose. (See the color insert for photographs and formulations of pills available in the United States). Select an OC based on the hormonal dose and on the woman's clinical picture. Figure 19-2 gives an algorithm to help clinicians.

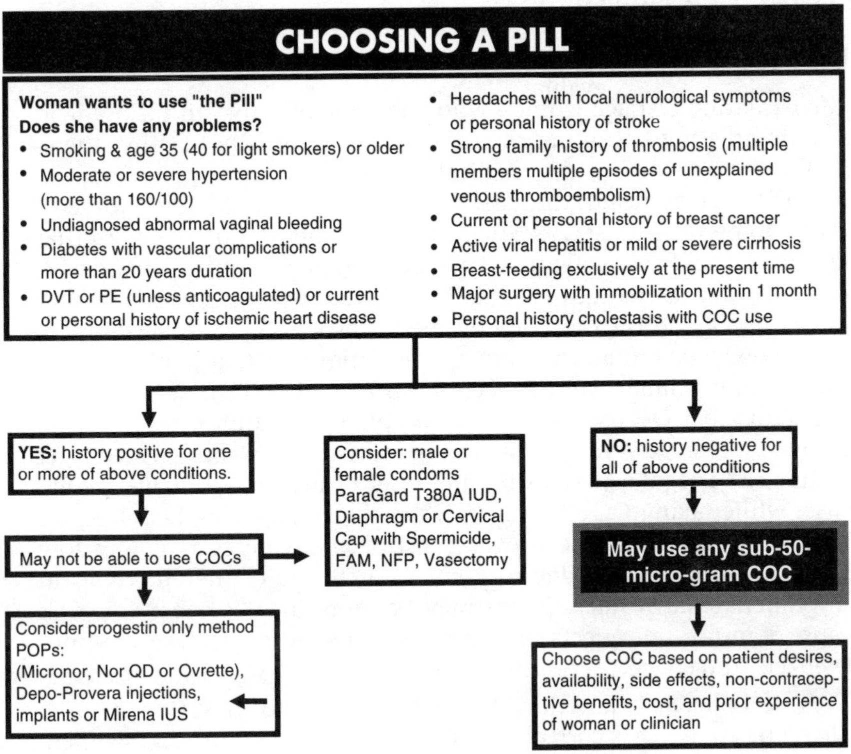

CHOOSING A PILL

Woman wants to use "the Pill"
Does she have any problems?
- Smoking & age 35 (40 for light smokers) or older
- Moderate or severe hypertension (more than 160/100)
- Undiagnosed abnormal vaginal bleeding
- Diabetes with vascular complications or more than 20 years duration
- DVT or PE (unless anticoagulated) or current or personal history of ischemic heart disease

- Headaches with focal neurological symptoms or personal history of stroke
- Strong family history of thrombosis (multiple members multiple episodes of unexplained venous thromboembolism)
- Current or personal history of breast cancer
- Active viral hepatitis or mild or severe cirrhosis
- Breast-feeding exclusively at the present time
- Major surgery with immobilization within 1 month
- Personal history cholestasis with COC use

YES: history positive for one or more of above conditions.

↓

May not be able to use COCs →

↓

Consider progestin only method
POPs:
(Micronor, Nor QD or Ovrette),
Depo-Provera injections,
implants or Mirena IUS ←

Consider: male or female condoms ParaGard T380A IUD, Diaphragm or Cervical Cap with Spermicide, FAM, NFP, Vasectomy

NO: history negative for all of above conditions

↓

May use any sub-50-micro-gram COC

↓

Choose COC based on patient desires, availability, side effects, non-contraceptive benefits, cost, and prior experience of woman or clinician

---

- The World Health Organization and the Food and Drug Administration both recommend using the **lowest dose pill** that is effective. All combined pills with less than 50 pg of estrogen are effective and safe.

- There are no studies demonstrating a decreased risk of deep vein thrombosis (DVT) in women on 20 mcg pills. Data on higher dose pills (50 mcg EE vs. 30 mcg) have demonstrated that the less the etrogen dose, the lower the risk for DVT.

- All COCs lower free testosterone. In the US, only Ortho Tri-Cyclen and Estrostep have FDA labeling indicating it as a treatment of moderate acne vulgaris, based on results of randomized, placebo controlled trials. Other formulations are under study. Class labeling in Canada for all combined pills states that use of pills may improve acne. In Canada, only Tri-Cyclen has "treatment of moderate acne vulgaris" as an indication for use.

- To minimize discontinuation due to spotting and breakthrough bleeding, warn women in advance, reassure that spotting and breakthrough bleeding become better over time.

- To attain the most favorable lipid profile, consider norgestimate, desogestrel pill or low dose norethindrone acetate, or norethindrone (Ovcon-35) or ethnodiol diacetate (Demulen 1/35 or Zovia 35). No clinical benefits have been demonstrated to be attributable to difference in lipids caused by these pills. Estrogen has a beneficial effect on the walls of blood vessels. All currently available COCs raise triglycerides.

Source: Modified from Hatcher RA, et al. (2003),[149] with permission.

Figure 19-2 Choosing a pill

SPECIAL POPULATIONS

ADOLESCENT WOMEN

Menstruating teenage women who are sexually active and those who are contemplating becoming sexually active are usually healthy; therefore, for young women, the medical and social risks of pregnancy far outweigh the small health risks associated with OC use. Explore the teen's decision to become (or stay) sexually active. Is she comfortable with that decision or would she prefer to delay sexual intercourse? (See Chapter 13, Abstinence and the Range of Sexual Experience.) Many teens can benefit from taking OCs to treat primary dysmenorrhea, anovulatory cycling, or acne. A pelvic examination is not needed prior to OC initiation for an asymptomatic woman (see the section on Pill Initiation). Reassure anxious parents that OC use for noncontraceptive indications has not been shown to encourage young women to become sexually active. A teenager who has had irregular periods or late onset of menses will have regular menses while taking OCs; however, when she stops taking her OCs, her periods may again become irregular. Estrogen in the current low-dose OCs do not limit height due to premature closure of the epiphyses in young, menarchal women. Teens may be more likely to abandon OCs because of minor side effects such as nausea or spotting, so take all minor side effects in teenagers seriously.

Provide concrete counseling to adolescents, who may find it more challenging to use OCs correctly and consistently than do older women. Instruct each teen who wants to use OCs about condom use, both for reducing the risk of acquiring STIs and for back-up in case she discontinues taking the pill. Provide emergency contraception and instructions on how to use it if she needs it. Studies have shown that women of all ages are more able to successfully use the once-a-week or once-a-month methods than they are able to remember to take a pill once a day. However, in the patch study, 18- and 19-year-olds showed the greatest improvement in successful utilization rates. For this reason, offer the vaginal ring and patch to teens considering OCs.

PERIMENOPAUSAL WOMEN

Healthy, nonsmoking women in their 40s are candidates for combined hormonal contraception. OCs can help regulate menstrual bleeding and reduce the risks of irregular bleeding and endometrial hyperplasia associated with anovulatory cycling during the perimenopausal years. Women in their 40s are at highest risk for menorrhagia due to leiomyoma and adenomyosis; OCs can provide medical alternatives to hysterectomy. OCs also help reduce the risk of ovarian and endometrial cancers. Another significant advantage OCs offer many women who are experiencing hormonal fluctuations is reduction of vasomotor symptoms, especially if OCs are used on an extended cycle basis. (See the Menopause Chapter.)

No special testing is required prior to prescribing OCs for women in their 40s, except for blood pressure measurement. Screening measures such as clinical breast exams, mammograms, serum lipids, and pelvic exam with Pap smears are important elements of well-woman care, but need not be performed in apparently healthy women of any age prior to OC initiation.

OC users in their late 40s or early 50s may not experience traditional symptoms of menopause while taking OCs. They will not experience menstrual irregularities or hot flashes, especially if the OCs are used on an extended basis. In this context, it may be difficult to detect when menopause occurs. Do not rely on blood tests to diagnose menopause in perimenopausal women. (See Chapter 5 on Menopause.)

SMOKERS

Heavy smoking by women older than 35 precludes the use of estrogen-containing hormonal methods. *Any* smoking by women older than 40 precludes use of estrogen-contining contraceptive on an ongoing basis. Light smoking by women age 35 to 40 merits caution (WHO category 3). For example, smoking increases an OC user's risk of heart attack nearly 13- to 14-fold.[150] Indeed, women who smoke as few as 1 to 4 cigarettes a day have a 2.5 fold increased risk of coronary heart disease.[151] The older the smoker, the more cigarettes she smokes, and the more concomitant cardiovascular problems she faces, the less likely she is to be a candidate for OCs, especially if she can use more effective methods such as progestin-only injections or IUDs. In otherwise healthy young women, the absolute risk of cardiovascular disease is low, so that estrogen-containing contraceptives in women who smoke are still safer than the risks of pregnancy. The first priority in caring for a woman who smokes is to encourage and aid her to stop smoking, or to significantly reduce the number of cigarettes she smokes each day. Three to 12 months after stopping smoking, past smokers have the same OC-related cardiovascular risks as nonsmokers.

In selecting a pill for smokers, the clinician is conflicted. On the one hand, the ideal pill would have the lowest estrogen content (to reduce arterial thrombosis) and the lowest androgenicity (to minimize any adverse impacts on lipids). Smokers tend to metabolize estrogen more rapidly and to increase SHBG levels more than nonsmokers do, so that the 20-mcg EE dose pill may not provide as much contraceptive efficacy for a smoker. However, there are no clinical trials to provide guidance. It may be prudent to start smokers and nicotine patch/gum/etc. users on 20 mcg EE formulation with a strong (low androgenic) progestin, advise them to use a back-up method during the first 2 to 3 months, and monitor breakthrough bleeding as a marker of adequate serum levels. If she has persistent breakthrough bleeding on a 20-mcg EE pill, use of a 25 to 30 mcg EE formulation or delivery system may be advisable. Shortening the pill-free interval may be helpful.

POSTPARTUM WOMEN

Pregnancy is a hypercoagulable state. Estrogen increases the risk of venous thrombosis and embolism (VTE). As a result, it is generally recommended that postpartum women delay use of estrogen-containing contraception until 3 to 4 weeks postpartum, when those pregnancy-induced changes in the coagulation system have waned.

BREASTFEEDING WOMEN

Although many progestin-only methods may be used immediately postpartum, estrogen may decrease the quantity and quality of breast milk (see Chapter 23 on Postpartum Contraception and Lactation). Therefore, the American Academy of Pediatrics advises against use of estrogen as long as the woman is exclusively breast-feeding. Estrogen can be used as soon as supplemental sources of nutrition are introduced into the infant's diet (if the mother is at least 3 to 4 weeks postpartum).

WOMEN WITH MEDICAL PROBLEMS

Diabetes. As the WHO guidelines state, only women with uncomplicated diabetes can be considered for OC use. Women with advanced diabetes complicated by nephropathy (proteinuria), retinopathy, neuropathy, or diabetes of more than 20-years duration are not candidates for estrogen-containing methods (WHO:4). If uncomplicated diabetes is combined with hypertension, smoking, or other major risk factors for cardiovascular disease, estrogen-containing contraceptives may not be used.

For diabetic women who are candidates for OCs, consider each of the components of the pill. Progesterone is a competitive inhibitor of insulin at the insulin receptor; therefore, a pill with low progesterone activity is important. Estrogen can decrease insulin release by the islet cells of the pancreas, so a relatively low-dose estrogen formulation may be favored. Androgens can have an adverse impact on lipids and increase the woman's risk for cardiovascular disease. However, any low-dose pill with similar properties is quite reasonable.

Sickle cell anemia. Women with sickle cell disease are predisposed to occlusion of the microvasculature. However, OC users and non-users appear to have no differences with regard to coagulation studies, blood viscosity measurements, or incidence or severity of painful sickle cell crises. In addition, women with sickle cell anemia can ill afford to lose menstrual blood. Sickle cell disease (WHO:1) and thallasemia (WHO:2) are not reasons to avoid OCs.[130]

Gallbladder disease. WHO recommends that women with symptoms of gallbladder disease and those who are being treated medically for gallbladder disease not use estrogen-containing contraception if more appropriate methods are acceptable (WHO:3). Similarly, women who have experienced cholestatic jaundice in pregnancy may use OCs with caution (WHO:2), although those who experienced jaundice with past OC use fall into category 3.

Cervical dysplasia. Women who have cervical dysplasia or who have a history of previously treated cervical dysplasia may still use combined hormonal contraception (WHO:2).

Special issues for drospirenone-containing OCs. Do not prescribe Yasmin or such formulations to patients with conditions that predispose to hyperkalemia (i.e., renal insufficiency, hepatic dysfunction, and adrenal insufficiency).

MANAGING SIDE EFFECTS

A double-blind trial showed no difference in the incidence of any of the traditionally "hormonally-related" side effects during the 6-month comparison of OC users and placebo pills users. Similar percentages of women in each group developed headaches, nausea, vomiting, mastalgia, weight gain, etc.[152] This finding differs from the impression given by the pill package labeling, because the side effect numbers in labeling come from clinical trials and reflect the events that women had *while* they use pills that could possibly be related to pill use, not events that occur *because* of the pill. Similarly, when women with "pill side effects" such as nausea, headache, irritability, fatigue, weight gain, breast tenderness, and breakthrough bleeding were treated in another study with either Vitamin B6 or sugar pill, both groups improved in all symptoms.[153]

However, 59% to 81% of women who discontinued OC use in one study reported that they stopped due to side effects. Therefore, management of side effects on OCs is crucial to successful use of hormonal contraceptives. Counsel all potential hormonal contraceptive users that side effects are possible (Table 19-5), but not necessarily to be expected. Advise women that side effects are usually transient and often respond to changes in pill formulation.

Absence of withdrawal bleeding

Advise women that the amount of withdrawal bleeding may be significantly lower with hormonal methods. Even scant bleeding or spotting on the placebo pills counts as withdrawal bleeding. The incidence of complete lack of withdrawal bleeding varies with different formulations and increases with duration of use. Some women deliberately extend the numbers of active pills they use (bicycling, tricycling, or extended use) to achieve amenorrhea. For women using cyclic regimens of hormonal contraceptives who fail to have withdrawal bleeding, obvious causes of amenorrhea (such as pregnancy) must be excluded. Other specific conditions, such as cervical stenosis, need to be evaluated, particularly if the patient has recently had cervical surgery (e.g., D&C, cone biopsy, LEEP,etc). When women use hormonal contraceptives, it is far less likely that other common causes of amenorrhea are present. For example, thyroid problems, prolactinoma, and hypothalamic amenorrhea due to stress or excessive exercise or anovulatory states such as PCOS or obesity are important considerations when a woman not using hormonal contraceptives develops amenorrhea. However, combined hormonal contraceptives restore predictable menstrual cycling in women with these problems.

Women who enjoy the lack of withdrawal bleeding but just want to reassure themselves periodically that they are not pregnant may use home pregnancy tests or may want to monitor their basal body temperature (BBT) during 3 sequential days of placebo pills. If that BBT is <98°F, the likelihood of pregnancy is very low. If women desire to have cyclic withdrawal bleeding, switching to a more estrogenic formulation or to a triphasic formulation may decrease the likelihood of amenorrhea.

Table 19-5 Estrogenic, progestogenic, and combined effects of oral contraceptive pills

Estrogenic effects	Estrogen + progestin effects	Progestin effects
• Nausea • Increased breast size (ductal and fatty tissue) • Leukorrhea • Cervical eversion or ectopy • Hypertension • Rise in cholesterol concentration in gallbladder bile • Telangiectasia • Hepatocellular adenomas • Cerebrovascular accidents (rare) • Thromboembolic complications including DVT or pulmonary emboli (rare) • Decreased libido and/or enjoyment of intercourse • Pruritus (Most pills with less than 50 mcg of ethinyl estradiol are less likely to produce troublesome estrogen-mediated side effects or complications.	Both the estrogenic and the progestational components of oral contraceptives may contribute to the development of the following adverse effects: • Breast tenderness • Headaches • Hypertension • Myocardial infarction (rare) • Cyclic weight gain due to fluid retention • Growth of leiomyomata • Stimulation of breast neoplasia (exceedingly rare)	All low-dose combined pills suppress a woman's production of testosterone, which has a beneficial effect on acne, oily skin and hirsutism. The progestin component may have androgenic as well as progestational effects: • Increased appetite and weight gain • Depression, fatigue, tiredness • Acne, oily skin • Increased LDL cholesterol levels • Decreased HDL cholesterol levels • Decreased carbohydrate tolerance; increased insulin resistance • Bloating • Constipation

Acne, oily skin, hirsutism

Two formulations have FDA approval for the treatment of acne (Ortho TriCyclen and Estrostep). Progestin inhibits LH release, which decreases ovarian androgen production. Estrogen increases hepatic production of sex hormone-binding globulin, which binds testosterone and other androgens in the woman's circulation. Occasionally (<10%) women will report worsening or new onset of acne, oily skin, or hair growth. Consider other causes of androgen exposure (other medications, ovarian tumors, etc.). If it appears her OC may be contributing to her problem, switch to a less androgenic formulation (e.g., Yasmin, Ortho Tri-Cyclen, Desogen, Ovcon-35).

Gastrointestinal complaints

Working at the level of the central nervous system, estrogen can cause nausea or vomiting. Sex steroid hormones do not directly affect the gastric lining, although new research has demonstrated a hormonal impact on the intrinsic firing rate of the gastric pacemaker cells. Progesterone slows peristalsis and can induce constipation and sensations of bloating and distention. Most affected women acclimate to the hormones, and nausea resolves within 1 to 3 months of use. If a woman complains of nausea, she can try taking her pills with food or at night. Avoid double dosing. Counsel the patient to "catch up" any pills she forgets by taking pills at 12-hour intervals, rather than 2 pills at one time, which increases the likelihood of nausea. In addition, advise more fluids and fresh fruits and vegetables. Women with recent onset of severe gastrointestinal symptoms should be evaluated promptly to rule out problems, such as cholecystitis, appendicitis and diverticulitis.

If vomiting or diarrhea is related to taking the pill, try the following approaches:

- Decrease hormone dose. A 20 mcg OC dramatically decreases nausea for many women, although it may also lead to more spotting and breakthrough bleeding.
- Bloating and constipation may be helped with a reduction in the progestin component in the pill. Bloating associated with menses can be diminished by extended cycle or continuous active pill use.
- Try progestin-only formulations to control nausea and other symptoms.
- Consult the Instructions for Using Oral Contraceptives for guidance on how to manage missed pills due to vomiting or poor absorption due to diarrhea.

Headaches

Headaches occur commonly. Controlled trials found that women using placebo pills experienced as many headaches as did OC users.[152] Nonetheless, headaches in an OC user deserve evaluation, because they are the major warning sign that precedes stroke. (See Figure 19-3.) If a woman begins having headaches or her headaches worsen after she starts OCs, consider all differential diagnoses. Measure the patient's blood pressure to rule out hypertension.

- Determine the type of headache. Ask about the severity of the headache, aura, duration, character (throbbing or constant), cyclicity, and location (including asymmetry). Ask about associated symptoms, such as photophobia, nausea, vomiting, dizziness, scotomata, blurred vision, watering of the eyes, loss of vision or speech, weakness or numbness. Can the patient function when the headaches are most severe? What medication provides relief?

- Rule out other causes, such as transient ischemic attacks, migraine headaches, vascular headaches, or cerebrovascular accident; hypertension; cyclic fluid retention induced by OCs; sinusitis, viremia, sepsis, or allergy; temporomandibular joint (TMJ) disorders or dental problems; drug use, alcohol or caffeine withdrawal, or central nervous system tumor.

Tension headache. The most common headache is the tension headache, which usually starts as a neck pain late in the day and radiates through the occipital area over the scalp to involve the forehead. There are no associated neurologic sensations, but women with tension headaches may experience nausea or vomiting from the intensity of the pain. These headaches usually respond to over-the-counter analgesics and/or rest. Rarely is it necessary to change pill formulations.

Migraine headache. The headache that causes most medical concern is the migraine headache, which tends to occur in the temporal region and is more frequently unilateral. Although the word "migraine" has become almost synonymous with severe headaches, it is important to identify the true migraines. If a woman develops new-onset migraine or a worsening in the severity or frequency of her headache, promptly reassess if she is still a candidate for using estrogen-containing contraceptives. If she has any associated neurological auras (flashing lights, tingling sensation, paraesthesias, etc), stop the OCs and provide contraception without estrogen. On the other hand, if her symptoms develop or worsen on the days she takes placebo pills (when the estrogen levels drop), it maybe possible to offer her extended-use, low-dose OCs to reduce her menstrual migraines.

Stroke. Strokes are often preceded for weeks or months by either visual symptoms or headaches or both. If a patient has experienced transient, total, or partial loss of vision; elevated blood pressure; or other neurologic symptoms, discontinue estrogen-containing hormonal contraceptives immediately and refer her to a neurologist. If visual impairment accompanies migraine headaches that have become worse, discontinue OCs immediately.

If the headaches are not serious and are related to OC use, consider the following approaches:

- Discontinue the OCs.
- Lower the dose of estrogen.
- Lower the dose of progestin.
- Tricycle. Eliminate the pill-free interval for 2 to 3 consecutive cycles of pills. This recommendation is helpful only if a woman's headaches occur during the pill-free interval.

NEW ONSET OR WORSENING HEADACHES IN COC USERS

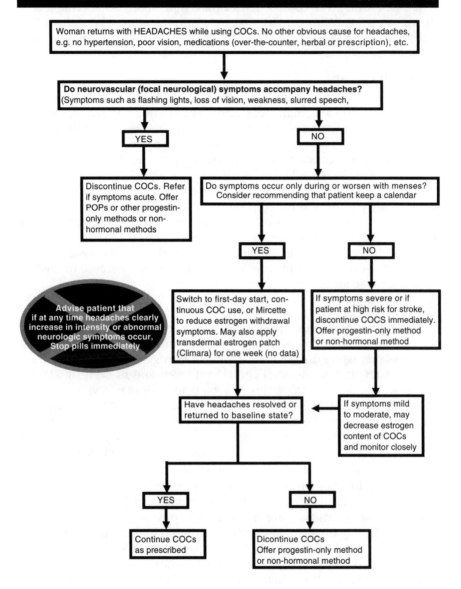

Woman returns with HEADACHES while using COCs. No other obvious cause for headaches, e.g. no hypertension, poor vision, medications (over-the-counter, herbal or prescription), etc.

Do neurovascular (focal neurological) symptoms accompany headaches? (Symptoms such as flashing lights, loss of vision, weakness, slurred speech,

YES

NO

Discontinue COCs. Refer if symptoms acute. Offer POPs or other progestin-only methods or non-hormonal methods

Do symptoms occur only during or worsen with menses? Consider recommending that patient keep a calendar

YES

NO

Advise patient that if at any time headaches clearly increase in intensity or abnormal neurologic symptoms occur, Stop pills immediately

Switch to first-day start, continuous COC use, or Mircette to reduce estrogen withdrawal symptoms. May also apply transdermal estrogen patch (Climara) for one week (no data)

If symptoms severe or if patient at high risk for stroke, discontinue COCS immediately. Offer progestin-only method or non-hormonal method

Have headaches resolved or returned to baseline state?

If symptoms mild to moderate, may decrease estrogen content of COCs and monitor closely

YES

NO

Continue COCs as prescribed

Dicontinue COCs Offer progestin-only method or non-hormonal method

Source: Hatcher RA, et al. (2003),[149] with permission.

Figure 19-3 New onset or worsening headaches in OC users

Lens effects

Women who wear contact lenses may note some visual changes or change in lens tolerance with OC use. Normal saline eye drops often provide adequate treatment, but consultation with an ophthalmologist may be helpful.

Libido decrease

Though infrequent, decreased libido is occasionally a problem and may be the reason a woman seeks a different pill or a different contraceptive. When a patient notes a decrease in libido, also ask about depression as both symptoms may occur in the same patient. In some women, the pill alters vaginal secretions and decreases levels of free testosterone, both of which may decrease libido.[154] An estrogen deficiency may decrease vaginal lubrication and make sexual intercourse less comfortable and occasionally painful. Consider using the vaginal ring to increase lubrication. Even if the initiation of OCs is accompanied by a clear loss of interest in sex or an inability to have orgasms, evaluate other potential causes of the decreased libido or anorgasmia, including depression. Many women, however, may find more enjoyment from sex because the risk of pregnancy is reduced.

Hyperlipidemia

Routine screening for lipids is not necessary before prescribing OCs unless a patient has pre-existing hyperlipidemia or a very strong family history of premature cardiovascular disease. Estrogen is known to increase HDL-C, triglycerides, and total cholesterol levels and to decrease LDL-C. The androgen-derived progestins may be neutral or may reverse some of estrogen's effects on HDL-C and triglycerides and increase LDL-C. The net effect depends upon the dose, potency, and estrogen/androgen balance of each formulation. If LDL levels rise or HDL levels drop significantly with OC use, change to a more estrogenic, less androgenic formulation.

Hypertriglyceridemia is an independent risk factor for early cardiovascular disease in women. Although most modern formulations increase triglycerides by about 30%, these estrogen-induced triglycerides are differently sized fragments than are endogenously produced triglycerides, and they do not increase a woman's risk for atherosclerosis. However, excessively high serum triglycerides (>500 mg/dl) can cause pancreatitis. Therefore, women with triglycerides of >350 mg/dl should use estrogen-containing hormonal contraceptives only with caution. Lower dose pills (20–25 mcg EE) would clearly be preferred to higher dose ones; progestin-only formulations may be necessary.

Mastalgia

Both estrogen and progestin affect the breast. The average woman experiences up to a 20% increase in breast volume in the luteal phase due to venous and lymphatic engorgement. Estrogen causes hypertrophy of the adipose cells in the breast and can cause increase in breast size. In addition, both hormones stimulate the terminal ductal lobular tuft growth especially in nulliparous women. Nearly 30% of women experience mastalgia or breast tenderness after they start taking OCs. A proper fitting bra is the first recommendation. Reduction of the doses of both steroids may be necessary if symptoms do not resolve rapidly enough to satisfy the patient. Lower dose pills (20 mcg) produced less mastalgia than higher dose (35 mcg) pills in one comparative trial.[155] If the symptoms develop just before menses, extended cycle length can help.

Melasma and chloasma

Estrogen stimulates the production of melanocytes and can cause darkening of pigmented areas (linea nigra). Darkening of patches on the face, often called the "mask of pregnancy," chloasma, or melasma can also develop. Women with darker skin pigment are more susceptible. The melasma fades slowly and incompletely after discontinuation of estrogen. Progestin-only methods may be preferable for at-risk women. Recommend consistent use of sunscreen and hats.

Mood swings, depression

Multiple studies have demonstrated no increase in the risk of clinical depression in women using OCs. Both estrogen and progestin in high-dose pills interact with tryptophans and serotonin; however, low-dose pills have not been implicated in any of these complaints.[55,155] Women on OCs remain solidly within normal ranges for all vitamins and do not require vitamin B supplementation.[156] Some women do report an increase in depressive symptoms, moodiness, and other emotional states when on OCs. This may represent an idiosyncratic response to hormones, which may warrant a decrease in hormone doses or pill cessation. However, it is important to identify when in a woman's cycle these symptoms develop. If the symptoms appear just before the menses, then extended or continuous use of active pills may dampen the hormonal swings.[147] If the patient desires withdrawal bleeding, restart her active pills each month on the first day of her menses. If there is any concern about an underlying depressive or anxiety disorder, these conditions deserve an explicit evaluation and treatment; cessation of hormonal contraceptives is not adequate therapy. Suicidal women need emergency treatment by specialists. Less acutely ill women may be managed locally with close follow-up.

Pregnancy

There is no evidence that OC users have higher rates of spontaneous abortion, preterm delivery, birth defects,[157–161] or compromise of fertility of offspring.[162] The risk of significant congenital anomalies is no higher than in the general population; no extra testing during prenatal care is needed because of early pregnancy exposure to steroidal hormones. Women should consider all their pregnancy options (keeping the baby, adoption, foster care, and abortion) based on their own personal situations; combined hormonal use should not influence that decision process.

Women who want to become pregnant should seek preconceptional care. They should start folic acid supplementation at least 1 to 3 months before they stop taking their pills. A routine dose of 0.4 mg folic acid supplement as found in prenatal vitamins is usually adequate. However, adolescent women who have had poor diets and prolonged OC use may benefit from 1 mg doses of folic acid preconceptionally and in the first trimester of pregnancy.

Once a woman discontinues the OCs, patches, or rings, her fertility returns rather rapidly to baseline rates. On average, there is a 2-week delay in the resumption of ovulation, but the normal time to ovulation ranges from 0 to 26 weeks. Barrier methods used to be suggested until a woman had her first spontaneous withdrawal bleed after stopping the pills. This was recommended to permit dating the pregnancy from the last menses. However, if a woman conceives the first month after stopping the pills, a dating ultrasound can be used to confirm the accuracy of her expected due date.

Vaginal discharge

Some women notice an increase in vaginal secretions with estrogen-containing contraceptives. These secretions generally are not an indication of infection. Women who use low OCs are not at any increased risk for developing uncomplicated candidal infections or bacterial vaginosis (BV). Reassurance is generally the only intervention needed once infection has been ruled out. Point out to the woman that these secretions are healthy and serve as lubricant during coitus.

Vaginal spotting and bleeding

Breakthrough spotting and bleeding are common (30% to 50%) in the first few months of OC use and generally resolve by the third to fourth month of use. Progestins administered early in the cycle reduce estrogen's proliferative influence and induce atrophy (thinning) of the uterine lining. When women first start to use OCs, their endometria must adjust to the exogenous hormones, so irregular spotting and bleeding is understandable. However, by the third pack of pills, 70% to 90% of women (depending upon the formulation) have no further breakthrough bleeding or spotting.

Before changing OC type, rule out more likely and more serious causes: pregnancy, infection (such as vaginitis and cervicitis), medications that block hormone aborption (olestin) or increase their metabolism by the liver (anticonvulsants, cigarette smoking, St. John's Wort, rifampin, griseofulvin), and gastrointestinal problems such as vomiting and diarrhea that may prevent adequate hormone absorption to sustain the uterine lining. *One of the most common causes of pill-associated spotting and bleeding is missed pills.*

For women with persistent irregular bleeding after 2 to 3 months of use, consider changing to other formulations, although no research indicates that any specific OC is best at eliminating spotting or bleeding.

- Women who report spotting or bleeding before they complete their active pills probably need more endometrial support. Increase the progestin content of their pills, either by changing to a different monophasic formulation or by switching to a triphasic formulation that increases progestin levels in the last active pills.
- Women with continued spotting after the withdrawal bleed need more estrogen support. Increase the estrogen in each tablet or decrease the progestin in the early pills (especially with a triphasic formulation). The cause of mid-cycle spotting/bleeding is not clear. One approach to this relatively uncommon bleeding pattern is to increase both estrogen/progestin mid-cycle with agents such as Triphasil and Tri-Levlen.

Seasonale. Some women experience spotting and breakthrough bleeding while using an extended-use pill such as Seasonale. Here are two suggestions to reduce these problems:

- Inform users that, as with all other pills, they will have more spotting initially when they begin taking pills. This spotting will decrease rapidly over time.
- One approach for Seasonale users is to take one pill every day for the first 21 days whether or not spotting occurs. Thereafter, on the first day of significant spotting, they can stop taking pills for 2-3 days to allow a withdrawal bleed to start, and then they should restart the active pills, taking at least 1 full pack each time before they stop again. As they take pills in this pattern, the length of time between spotting will increase and they will be able to eventually take pills for the full 84 days.

Weight change

A placebo-controlled, randomized clinical trial has demonstrated that there is no difference in weight gain due to low-dose OC use.[163] Similarly, a prospective trial of women using triphasic OCs with daily weight measurements for 4 months showed no change in mean weight at the end of the trial compared to baseline, although some weight fluctuations were noted during the cycle.[164] Oral contraceptive use by adolescent women has been shown not to be associated with either weight gain or increased body fat in a 9-year study.[165] In clinical trials, women who use OCs do not typically gain any more weight than women living in the United States typically gain in the same time interval.

However, some women may respond robustly to any of the pill's hormones. Increased measurements in the breasts, hips, and thighs reflect estrogen's impact on adipose cells (hypertrophy). Decreasing estrogen in the pill can reduce this impact. Weight gain similar to premenstrual fluid retention is due to increased aldosterone release and results from estrogen activity augmented by progesterone. In this situation, switch to a pill with both lower estrogen and progestin levels. Drospirenone-containing OCs, which have an antimineralocorticoid activity (mild diuretic effect), may also be an appropriate choice in this condition. Steadily increasing weight may be attributed to the nitrogen retention and increase in muscle mass stimulated by androgens. Although it is unlikely that the pill would be responsible for this type of weight gain, switching to a low androgenic pill (Ortho Tri-Cyclen, Ovcon-35, Modicon, Yasmin, etc.) may address that patient's concerns. Every woman should be encouraged to adopt a healthy diet and to exercise routinely to achieve and maintain a healthy weight.

PILLS AND DRUG INTERACTIONS

Some drugs may negatively influence the effectiveness of combined hormonal contraceptives:

Anti-tuberculosis. Rifampicin (Rifampin) and rifabutin increase hepatic clearance of EE and progestins.[166] Although rifampicin did not permit break-through ovulation in one small study,[167] product labeling and several published reports recommend women using these agents avoid taking OCs.

Antifungal (systemic). Griseofulvin increases microsomal enzyme activity and theoretically may decrease OC efficacy.

Anticonvulsants. Many of the anticonvulsants, such as barbituates, carbamazepine (Tegretol), oxcarbazepine, (Trileptal), phenobarbital, phenytoin (Dilantin), primidone (Mysoline), topiramate (Topamax) and felbamate (Felbatol) induce various cytochrome p450 activities and reduce circulating levels of contraceptive hormones. In some women, low doses can induce profound changes in circulating estrogen levels; in others, high doses of anticonvulsants produce minimal effect. Do not offer low-dose (<35 mg EE) formulations to a woman using these anticonvulsants unless she uses a back-up contraceptive method. If she has no breakthrough bleeding while using a 35-mcg EE pill with a back-up barrier method for 3 months, she may rely on the pills exclusively. However, many women using these anticonvulsants do require 50 mcg EE (not mestranol) pills to control breakthrough bleeding and possibly prevent escape ovulation. These drugs also affect the circulating levels of estrogen and progestin from the patches and vaginal rings. No data are available yet about efficacy of these methods in women using anticonvulsants. Therefore, exercise caution and recommend barriers. Progestin-only injections and IUDs are generally better choices. It should be noted that neither valproic acid nor gabapentin affects serum levels of estrogen or progestin.

Anti-HIV protease inhibitors. Several of the anti-HIV protease inhibitors can change (either increase or decrease) serum levels of estrogen and progestins. Consult the labeling for specific anti-HIV protease inhibitors to see if OC use requires additional back-up methods or if different methods may need to be considered.

Broad-spectrum antibiotics. Broad-spectrum antibiotics such as amoxicillin and tetracycline, which alter the intestinal flora thought to be instrumental in promoting absorption of the sex steroids, do *not* reduce the efficacy of OCs. Women using the antibiotics do have statistically significant but *not* clinically significant lower serum levels of estrogen and progestins. However, virtually every woman taking these antibiotics has remained well within the therapeutic range for the sex steroids.[168-170] As a result, back-up methods should not be necessary unless the patient has problems taking her pills, e.g., if her underlying medical condition interferes with pill taking or absorption. Long-term use of broad-spectrum antibiotics (such as erythromycin or tetracycline for acne) is compatible with OC use; back-up methods are not routinely needed for pregnancy prevention.[171]

Over-the-counter drugs. St. John's Wort is taken by many women to treat mild depression. Since this botanical agent does not require a prescription, women sometimes neglect to tell their health care providers that they are using it. St. John's Wort greatly increases hepatic metabolism of exogenous estrogen and progestin. Although little published data are available about the impact of this agent on pregnancy rates with OC use, some experts have recommended increasing the dose of emergency contraceptives by 50% in women using this over-the-counter antidepressant. The FDA has alerted providers that St. John's Wort may decrease the therapeutic effect of OCs.[172]

Another unanswered concern is that women who use Orlistat to block fat absorption may also reduce intestinal absorption of OC hormones. This concern is magnified if the woman experiences diarrhea from Orlistat use.

On a lighter note, the German National Chemists Association has advised women who use OCs to avoid eating too much licorice. Eating more than 10 to 50 gm a day of black licorice may trigger edema or elevate blood pressure, and OCs may do likewise.

OC effects on drug metabolism

The estrogen in combined hormonal contraceptives may alter hepatic clearance of other medications. Serum levels of fluoroquinolones, such as moxifloxacin and trovafloxacin, are significantly lower in OC users.[173] Similarly, estrogen promotes more marked metabolic clearance of some anticonvulsants, which would reduce circulating levels. Women starting these methods should have their anticonvulsant levels checked 1 month after OC initiation to insure that their medications are still in the therapeutic range. Conversely, estrogen-containing hormonal contraceptives may increase the effect of theophylline (used to treat asthma), the antipsychotic drugs diazepam (Valium) and chlordiazepoxide (Librium), and cyclic antidepressants. Doses of these drugs may need to be lowered with combined hormonal contraceptive use.

Drospirenone acts as an antimineralocorticoid and can interact with other potassium-sparing drugs to cause hyperkalemia. Women using ACE inhibitors, angiotensin-II receptor antagonists, potassium-sparing diuretics, heparin, aldosterone antagonists, and NSAIDS on a daily basis to treat chronic conditions or diseases should have their serum potassium checked during the first cycle of drospirenone use.

INSTRUCTIONS FOR USING COMBINED PILLS

Pills work primarily by stopping ovulation (release of an egg), and they thicken a woman's mucus in her cervix to keep sperm out of the upper genital track. Pills have less than a 1% rate of failure if taken every day on schedule. In addition to preventing pregnancy, pills lower your risk of ovarian cancer, cancer of the lining of the uterus (endometrium), benign breast masses, and some kinds of ovarian cysts. Pills decrease menstrual blood loss, cramps, and pain. Pills tend to make acne and oily skin better. Pills also decrease your chance of having a dangerous ectopic pregnancy—a pregnancy outside of the uterus.

Remember: pills do not protect you from AIDS (acquired immunodeficiency syndrome) or other sexually transmitted infections. Use a latex or polyurethane male condom or a female condom every time you have sexual intercourse that could expose you or your partner to infection.

Be sure you know your clinician's telephone number in case of questions or problems.

Getting started

Your clinician will suggest one of three ways to begin taking pills:

- *Quick Start.* Take your first pill while you are in your clinician's office. This is the preferred method. Use a back-up contraceptive method for 7 days. You will not get your period until you finish taking the active pills.

- *First-day start.* Take your first pill on the first day of your next period.

- *Sunday start.* Take your first pill on the first Sunday, during your period. Use a backup method for 7 days.

Daily pill routine

1. Take 1 pill a day until you finish the pack. Then:

   - If you are using a 28-day pack, begin a new pack immediately. Skip no days between packages.

   - If you are using a 21-day pack, stop taking pills for 1 week and then start your new pack.

   - An alternative is to begin each new pack the day withdrawal bleeding begins.

2. Associate taking your pill with something else that you do at about the same time every day, like going to bed, eating a meal, or brushing your teeth.

3. Mark your calendar to remind yourself of the days you will begin a new pack of pills. Some women mark their calendar each day as they take their pills.

4. Check your pack of pills each morning to make sure you took your pill the day before.

5. Use a back-up contraceptive method if any of the following occur to make your pills less effective: you missed taking pills, were late starting your new pill pack, had severe vomiting or diarrhea, or are taking medications that lower the ability of the body to absorb contraceptive hormones (see the instructions on these specific problems). If you think you may have had sexual intercourse that was not adequately protected, consider emergency contraception. Call 1-888-NOT-2-LATE for more information.

6. Use condoms if you suspect, even a little, that you or your partner may be exposed to a sexually transmitted infection.

7. If you see a clinician for any reason or are hospitalized, be sure to mention that you are taking birth control pills.

8. You do *not* need to take a "rest" from taking pills. If you stop taking your pills, you risk becoming pregnant.

Missed pills

OC pills should be taken every day at about the same time. Missing a pill means taking it after an interval of more than 24 hours or not at all (completely missing a pill). The impact of a missed pill depends upon when in the pill packet you miss a pill (which week), how many pills you may have missed earlier in the pack, and whether you need to use emergency contraception. If you had only one episode of missed pills in packet, follow these directions:

# Pills Missed	Week Pills Missed	OC Recommendation	Finish this pack	Emergency contraception	7-day Back-up
1	1	Take 2 pills ASAP	Yes	Yes*	Yes
1	2-3	Take 2 pills ASAP	Yes	No	No
1	4	Skip placebo pills	Yes	No	No
2-4	1	Take 2 pills ASAP	Yes	Yes*	Yes
2-4	2	Take 2 pills ASAP	Yes	No	No
2-4	3	Start new pack	N/A	No	No
2-4	4	Skip placebo	Yes	No	No
5	Any	Take 2 pills – start new pack	N/A	Yes*	Yes

* Start emergency contraception as soon as possible. No need to double up on pills. Take the the next pill on the next day.

While these instructions are very complete, they are also very complicated. The odds are that if you miss a pill late in the pack, you probably missed a pill or took it late sometime earlier in the pill pack. For this reason, it has been suggested that if you miss active pills, think about whether you had intercourse in the last 120 hours:

- If you had no intercourse in the last 5 days, take 2 active OCs all at once, use a back-up method for 7 days, and finish the pill pack by taking 1 pill daily. You can skip the placebo pills in this pack and start a new pack immediately if you missed more than 4 pills.

- If you had intercourse in the last 5 days, use emergency contraception today (call your clinician to get some if you do not have any on hand). Restart daily OCs the next day to finish the pack. Use a back-up method for 7 days. You can skip the placebo pills of this pack and start a new pack immediately if you missed more than 4 pills.

Vomiting or diarrhea

Repeated vomiting or severe diarrhea can decrease the absorption of the hormones in pills. The longer you have vomiting or diarrhea, the greater the concern and the more important it would be to avoid intercourse, use condoms as a back-up contraceptive, and/or use emergency contraceptive pills.

Pills and your periods

1. *Short and scanty.* A drop of blood, or a brown stain on your panty liner, pad or on your underwear during the week you are taking no hormonal pills is counted as a period when you are on the pills.

2. *Spotting.* You may have very light bleeding between periods for the first few months you are on pills. If you have bleeding between periods, try to take your pills at the same time every day. Spotting is generally not a sign of any serious problem. If after the first few months you suddenly begin to have bleeding between periods (especially after intercourse) and have not missed pills or taken pills late, have your clinician check you for an infection or other problems. Spotting between periods may also signal decreased pill effectiveness. *Start each new package of pills on time.* Some clinicians recommend a back-up contraceptive when you have spotting, especially if you are taking a medication that may make the pill less effective.

3. *Missed period.* If you have not missed any pills and you miss one period without any other signs of pregnancy, pregnancy is very unlikely, but you may wish to get a pregnancy test if you are worried. Many women miss one period now and then. Call your clinician if you are worried. You are fairly safe and can start a new pack of pills on your regular day.

Pills and pregnancy

1. If you decide you want to become pregnant, stop taking pills. Use prenatal vitamins for 1 to 3 months before you try to get pregnant. It is safe to become pregnant immediately after you stop the pill. The pill does not decrease your fertility; however, after you stop taking pills, you may have a 1- to 2-month delay before your periods become regular. You may wish to use another contraceptive method until you have at least 1 normal menstrual period off the pill. That way, when you become pregnant, your date of delivery can be calculated more easily.

2. If you become pregnant while taking pills, do not worry about the pills' impact on your pregnancy. It does not seem to increase the risk of having a baby with birth defects or of having a spontaneous abortion.

ACHES—PILL WARNING SIGNALS

Call your clinician if you have any of the Pill Warning Signs (next page) or if you develop depression, yellow jaundice, a breast lump, a bad fainting attack or collapse, a seizure (epilepsy), difficulty speaking, a blood pressure above 160/95 mm Hg, a severe allergic skin rash, or if you are immobilized (in a wheelchair or bedridden) after an accident or major surgery. If major surgery is planned, switch from an estrogen containing contraceptive method 4 weeks before the operation. The risk of a blood clot in a vein is greatest if any of the following conditions are present: if you are overweight, immobile, have severe varicose veins, or if several members of your family have had a blood clot in a vein before age 45. Usually these warning signs have an explanation other than pills; get checked to be sure. *Do not ignore these problems or wait to see if they disappear.*

Pills and future fertility

1. Pills are a good option for women who want to become pregnant in the future.

2. By reducing the risk of causes of infertility such as pelvic infections, uterine fibroids, ectopic pregnancies, ovarian cysts, ovarian cancer, endometrial cancer, and endometriosis, OCs may improve your future ability to become pregnant.

PILL WARNING SIGNALS

Pills have been studied extensively and are very safe. However, very rarely pills lead to serious problems. Here are the warning signals to watch out for while using pills. These warning signals spell out the word **ACHES**. If you have one of these symptoms, it may or may not be related to pill use. You need to check with your clinician as soon as possible. The problems that could possibly be related to using pills are as follows:

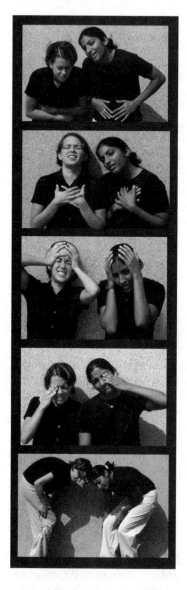

ABDOMINAL PAIN
- Blood clot in the pelvis or liver
- Benign liver tumor or gall bladder disease

CHEST PAIN
- Blood clot in the lungs
- Heart attack
- Angina (heart pain)
- Breast lump

HEADACHES
- Stroke
- Migraine headache with neurological problems (blurred vision, spots, zigzag lines, weakness, difficulty speaking)
- Other heaches caused by pills
- High blood pressure

EYE PROBLEMS
- Stroke
- Blurred vision, double vision, or loss of vision
- Migraine headache with neurological problems (blurred vision, spots, zigzag lines)
- Blood clots in the eyes
- Change in shape of cornea (contacts don't fit)

SEVERE LEG PAIN
- Inflammation and blood clots of a vein in the leg

You should also return to the office if you develop severe mood swings or depression become jaundiced (yellow-color skin), miss 2 periods or have signs of pregnancy.

Source: Hatcher RA, et al. (2003),[149] with permission.

3. If your periods are irregular prior to taking pills, they may again become irregular after you stop taking pills.

4. Return of fertility is not improved by taking a break from pills.

5. You may experience some delay (an average of 2 to 3 months) in becoming pregnant compared with the amount of time it would have taken if you had not taken the pills. Do *not* count on this; if you do not want to become pregnant now, start using another contraceptive method right after you stop taking pills.

6. Between 1% and 2% of women will not menstruate for 6 months or more after stopping pills. However, it is not certain that OCs are responsible for this lack of periods.

Pills and smoking

If you smoke, stop. This is the single most important thing you can do for your health. If you cannot stop, try to cut back on the number of cigarettes you smoke. It is all the more important that you watch for the pill warning signals. If you smoke, you should probably *stop* taking pills at age 35, and definitely by age 40.

Pills and mood changes

If you notice mood changes—depression, irritability, or a change in sex drive—see your clinician. Switching pill brands may help if your mood changes are related to the pill. Depression, premenstrual symptoms (PMS), and sexual pleasure can improve on pills, but in some women they become worse.

Pills and Drug Interactions

A few drugs you may need to take for medical conditions may decrease the effectiveness of your pills. Be sure to tell all your clinicians that you are using OCs. If you are using drugs such as rifampin, griseofulvin, Dilantin (phenytoin), phenobarbital, topirimate, Tegretol (carbamazepine), or St. John's Wort, tell your clinician, because you may need to use stronger pills or a back-up method of contraception. Women using antiretroviral drugs may need lower or higher dose OCs.

DO BIRTH CONTROL PILLS CAUSE BREAST CANCER?

After more than 50 studies, most experts believe that *pills have little, if any, effect on the risk of developing breast cancer.* The Woman's Care Study found no increased risk for breast cancer among women currently using pills and a decreased risk of breast cancer for those women who had previously used pills. Use of pills by women with a family history of breast cancer was not associated with an increased risk for breast cancer, nor was the initiation of pill use at a young age.[174]

A recent summary of studies suggested that current users of pills are slightly more likely to be *diagnosed* with breast cancer.[175] Two factors may explain the increased risk of breast cancer being diagnosed in women currently taking pills: 1) a *detection bias,* meaning that pill users are simply more likely to have existing breast cancer identified because they have more breast exams or more mammography, or 2) *promotion* of an existing lesion that is nearly cancer into one that is cancer, usually an early cancer. Most authorities think the first explanation is most likely because the duration of pill use has no effect on risk and the excess risk seen in current users is restricted to breast cancers that are localized. Breast cancers diagnosed in women currently on pills or women who have taken pills in the past are more likely to be localized.[175] *By the age of 55,* the risk of having had breast cancer diagnosed is the *same* for women who have used pills and those who have not.

The conclusion of several studies of the risk for breast cancer in women on pills is that women with a strong family history of breast cancer do not further increase their risk for breast cancer risk by taking pills.[174–179]

While there are still unanswered questions about pills and breast cancer, today, four decades after their arrival on the contraceptive scene, the overall conclusion is that pills have little or no effect on breast cancer. *"Many years after stopping oral contraceptive use, the main effect may be protection against metastatic disease."* [175,180]

TRANSDERMAL CONTRACEPTIVE PATCH

The Ortho Evra transdermal contraceptive patch is a lightweight, wafer-thin, flexible, beige-colored, 20 cm^2 matrix patch. The patch consists of three layers: an outer protective layer of polyester; a medicated, adhesive layer; and a clear, polyester release liner, which protects the adhesive layer and is removed prior to application. Once the hormones are in circulation, they act the same way as orally administered hormones do to prevent pregnancy.

Each patch lasts 7 days. Women replace the patch each week for 3 weeks each cycle, then have a 7 day patch-free week, during which time they will start their withdrawal bleeding.

ADVANTAGES AND INDICATIONS

The transdermal patch system is safe, effective, and rapidly reversible and can be used by healthy, nonsmoking women throughout the reproductive years. Because the hormonal mechanisms of action are similar, it is expected that the patch may provide many of the same advantages and non-contraceptive health benefits that OCs do, although data about long-term health benefits may not be documented for decades.

The patch offers the clear advantage of once-a-week dosing, which makes it easier to use successfully. In addition, the user can easily verify the presence of the patch, which can reassure her of continued protection. This reduces the anxiety many women report with OCs—questioning if they remembered to take today's pill and worrying that they might forget to take it. Given that by the third cycle of OCs, studies show that 54% of women missed more than 2 pills,[181] this concern seems justified. In a comparison of the clinical 3 trials, perfect use with the patch ranged from 92.9% to 93.6% whereas OCs were taken correctly by only 77.2% to 88.77% of women.

D ISADVANTAGES AND CAUTIONS

Although the patch avoids the challenges of daily administration, it still needs to be changed every week. It is difficult to conceal, so privacy is sub-optimal. Costs, storage and access issues are still present. The patch, as with all hormonal contraceptive methods, provides no protection against sexually transmitted infections. At-risk women should be counseled about safer sex practice and offered male condoms to reduce their vulnerability.

In addition to the health complications associated with combined hormonal contraceptives (myocardial infarction, stroke, VTE, hypertension, diabetes, gallbladder disease, cholestatic jaundice, hepatic neoplasms, etc.), the transdermal delivery system is associated with an increased risk of local skin irritation, redness or rash. The residual adhesive clinging to the skin after the patch is removed may need to be lifted off with baby oil.

Side effects

In the comparative clinical trials done in the United States, side effects reported by patch users were similar to those reported by pill users except that 20% of the patch users had unique complaints related to reactions at the application site. In addition, women using the patch were more likely than OC users to experience breast tenderness, vaginal spotting, and dysmenorrhea in the first 2 cycles. Within 3 months of use, the occurrence of these hormone-related side effects was similar between patch and pill users. The numbers of women who withdrew from the trial due to serious adverse effects were relatively small. However, overall more patch users than OC users withdrew from the study due to adverse effects (8.6% vs. 1.8%) or for specific complaints such as skin reactions (2.6% vs. 0%), nausea (1.5% vs. 0.3%), and dysmenorrhea (1.5% vs. 0.3%). Hyperpigmentation may develop under the patch application site. It is reversible but may take some time.

PRECAUTIONS

None of the women with medical contraindications to pill use is a candidate for the patch, unless the problem with pills relates to intestinal absorption of hormones. Additionally, women with conditions that affect the skin beneath the patch should not use the patch. The patch should not be placed over skin that is red, irritated, or cut. Women with psoriasis, eczema or sunburn may not be able to use the patch. Women should periodically confirm that the patch is firmly adherent and avoid using any creams, lotion, or oils near the patch since those agents may cause the patch to detach. The effectiveness of the patch is reduced in women who weigh more than 198 pounds.

PROVIDING THE TRANSDERMAL PATCH

Talk to the patient about how and where to store her patches. Remind her that when she removes a patch, she should fold it closed to reduce release of the hormones. She should not flush the used patch into the water system, but should dispose of it in the garbage as solid waste.

The patient can start her patch on the Sunday following the first day of her menses or on the first day of her flow. If she starts on Sunday, she should use a back-up method for 7 days; if she starts on the first day of her flow, she needs no back-up method. The calendar reminders that accompany the patches can accommodate either approach. The Quick Start for the patch may be reported soon.

Switching from other methods. Contraceptive sex hormone levels reach reliably therapeutic levels about 48 hours after patch placement; therefore, women switching from OCs should apply their first patch as soon as their pill withdrawal period starts, but no later than 4 to 5 days after their last active pill. If they use the Sunday start method, they will need 7 days of back-up contraception. They should *not* wait until they complete their last pack of pills to start the patch. Women switching from injectable contraceptives (DMPA) should apply their patches when they are due for their next injection.

MANAGING PROBLEMS AND FOLLOW UP

Dislodged or detached patches. During clinical trials involving over 70,000 patches, fewer than 3% required replacement for partial detachment and fewer than 2% were replaced because they became fully detached. Patches adhered well in humid conditions (saunas), in exercise conditions, and during swimming. In freezing weather, the patch should be worn beneath clothing.

- If the patch is partially detached, it should be firmly pressed in place for 10 seconds. Reconfirm that the edges are sticking well. If it sticks well, the woman can continue to use it for the full 7 days. If it does not stick well, tell her to remove it and apply a replacement patch.

- If the patch is completely detached, she should try to reapply the same patch if it is clean and usable. If it cannot be used, tell her to apply a new patch immediately.

If the patch has been partially or completely detached for more than 24 hours or if the woman does not know how long it has been loose, instruct her to use a back-up method for 7 days. Consider the need for emergency contraception.

Missed patches and late patches. Management of missed patches depends upon which patch is forgotten and how long it is missed:

When patched missed	Management
1st week patch.	• If a patch is forgotten or late the first week, give emergency contraception if the woman has had unprotected intercourse.
	• Tell her to place the patch immediately.
	• She should use a back-up method for 7 days.
	• The woman will change her patch each week on the day of the week she started this new patch from now on.
2nd—3rd week patch	• *1-2 days late*: the woman must remove the old patch and place a new one immediately. No back-up method or emergency contraception is needed.
	• *More than 2 days late*: Have her remove the old patch and place a new one on immediately. Provide emergency contraception if she has had unprotected intercourse (especially if she is 4 days or more late applying her patch). She should use back-up method for 7 days. Tell her to change the patch each week on the day of the week that she placed this new patch.
4th week patch	• Tell her to remove the patch.
	• She should place a new one on the usual day.
	• No back-up method or emergency contraception is needed.

USING THE TRANSDERMAL SYSTEM

One patch is used for 7 days. Apply a new patch once a week on the same day for 3 weeks in a row. During the 4th week, do not wear a patch. At the end of the week, start another cycle of patches.

Applying the patch

1. Each patch is packaged in an individual foil packet. To place the patch, open the pouch by tearing along the top edge and one side edge. Peel the foil pouch apart and open it. Lift the patch and its clear plastic cover out of the foil pouch together by using a fingernail to peel the unit off the foil pouch.

2. Fold the patch open. Hold onto one half and peel the plastic off the other half. Apply the sticky side of the opened patch to the skin. Press it in place. The patch can be placed on the buttock, abdomen, upper torso (excluding the breasts), or on the outside

of the upper arm. Avoid placing patches in areas of friction such as under bra straps or thongs. The patch should be applied only to clean, dry skin. Do not put it over skin that is irritated, sunburned, red or infected. Make sure there are no creams, oils, sunscreen, or sweat on the skin or the patch will not adhere.

3. Fold the patch in half, remove the clear plastic cover, open it and apply the rest of the sticky side of the patch to the skin. Press firmly on the patch for 10 seconds. Run your finger around the edges of the patch to make sure that all parts of the patch are sticking properly.

Wearing the patch

1. Keep the patch in the same place for 7 days; then remove it. Check the patch every day to make sure it is fully adherent.

2. Apply a new patch in a different spot on your body. Wear it for 7 days. Repeat the procedure for a third week.

3. During the fourth week, do not wear a patch. You will begin your menstrual period.

4. After a week without wearing a patch, apply a new "first-week" patch on the same day of the week you applied your other patches.

5. Store the patches in their protective pouches at room temperature.

Removing the patch

1. To remove the patch, grasp it by an edge and pull it off. Fold it closed on itself on the adhesive side to seal in the medication.

2. Discard the patch in the solid waste garbage; do not flush it into the waste water system.

3. If any stickiness or adhesive remains on your skin, remove it by using baby oil; do not use harsh chemicals such as nail polish remover, alcohol, etc.

VAGINAL CONTRACEPTIVE RING

The vaginal contraceptive ring (NuvaRing) is a flexible, soft, transparent ring made of the plastic ethylene vinyl acetate. The ring has an outer diameter (side to side) of 54 mm and a cross-sectional diameter of 4 mm. The ring releases ethinyl estradiol and etonorgestrel in steady, low doses so that serum levels are lower than the patch or pills.

The woman places one ring high in the vaginal once every 28 days. The ring is kept in place for 21 days and removed for a 7-day ring-free period to permit withdrawal bleeding. Hormonal levels needed to suppress ovulation are achieved within the first day of vaginal ring use, so there is no delay in onset of contraceptive protection, as seen with the transdermal patch. The ring has a steady release rate, so serum hormone levels do not fluctuate during the day the way they do with OCs.

The eight color pages of pills are organized as follows:

Color photos of pills from lowest to highest estrogen dose

- Progestin-only pills with **no estrogen**: Micronor, NOR-QD, and Ovrette
- Lowest estrogen pills with **20 micrograms** of the estrogen, ethinyl estradiol: Alesse, Levlite, LoEstrin 1/20, and Mircette
- All of the **30- and 35-microgram** pills (all ethinyl estradiol)
- All of the **phasic** pills
- Highest estrogen pills, with **50 micrograms** of estrogen (ethinyl estradiol OR mestranol). Mestranol is converted in the body to ethinyl estradiol; 50 mcg of mestranol is equivalent to 35 mcg of ethinyl estradiol

* There are prominent horizontal or vertical parallel lines ("equal signs") between pills which are pharmacologically exactly the same. The color and packaging of pills dispensed in clinics may differ from pills in pharmacies.

Pills you can prescribe as emergency contraceptive pills

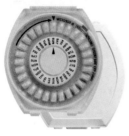 =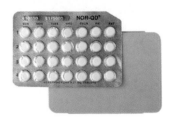

**MICRONOR® TABLETS
28-DAY REGIMEN**
(0.35 mg norethindrone) (lime green)
Ortho-McNeil

NOR-QD® TABLETS
(0.35 mg norethindrone) (yellow)
Watson

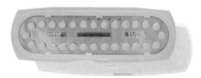

OVRETTE® TABLETS
(0.075 mg norgestrel) (yellow)
Wyeth

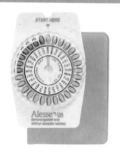 = 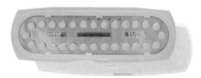 = **AVIANE**
(0.1 mg
levonorgestrel/
20 mcg ethinyl
estradiol)
(active pills
orange)
Barr
Laboratories

LEVLITE™ - 28 TABLETS
(0.1 mg levonorgestrel/20 mcg ethinyl estradiol)
(active pills pink)
Berlex

ALESSE - 28 TABLETS
(0.1 mg levonorgestrel/20 mcg ethinyl estradiol)
(active pills pink)
Wyeth

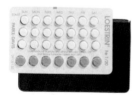 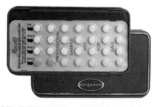

LOESTRIN® FE 1/20
(1 mg norethindrone acetate/20 mcg ethinyl
estradiol/75 mg ferrous fumarate [7d])
(active pills white)
Pfizer

MIRCETTE - 28 TABLETS
(0.15 mg desogestrel/ 20 mcg ethinyl estradiol X 21 (white)/
placebo X 2 (green)/10 mcg ethinyl estradiol X 5 (yellow)
Organon

(B)

COMBINED PILLS - 30 microgram PILLS

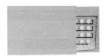 =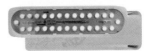

LEVLEN® 28 TABLETS
(0.15 mg levonorgestrel/30 mcg ethinyl estradiol)
(active pills light orange)
Berlex

LO/OVRAL®-28 TABLETS
(0.3 mg norgestrel/30 mcg ethinyl estradiol)
(active pills white)
Wyeth

=

=

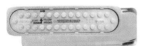

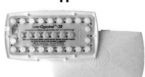

NORDETTE®-28 TABLETS
(0.15 mg levonorgestrel/30 mcg ethinyl estradiol)
(active pills light orange)
Monarch

LOW-OGESTREL - 28
(0.3 mg norgestrel/30 mcg ethinyl estradiol)
(active pills white)
Watson

=

=

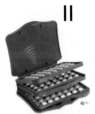

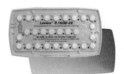

=

SEASONALE
(0.15 mg levonorgestrel/30 mcg ethinyl estradiol)
84 active pills followed by 7 placebo pills
Barr Laboratories

LEVORA TABLETS
(0.15 mg levonorgestrel/30 mcg ethinyl estradiol)
(active pills white)
Watson

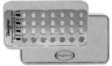

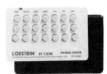

DESOGEN® 28 TABLETS
(0.15 mg desogestrel/30 mcg ethinyl estradiol)
(active pills white)
Organon

LOESTRIN® 21 1.5/30
(1.5 mg norethindrone acetate/ 30 mcg ethinyl estradiol)
(active pills green)
Pfizer

=

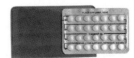

ORTHO-CEPT® TABLETS
28-DAY REGIMEN
(0.15 mg desogestrel/30 mcg ethinyl estradiol)
(active pills orange)
Ortho-McNeil

YASMIN 28 TABLETS
(3.0 mg drospirenone/30 mcg ethinyl estradiol)
(active pills yellow)
Berlex

(C)

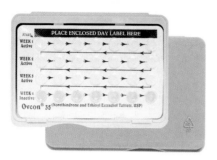

OVCON® 35 28-DAY
(0.4 mg norethindrone/35 mcg ethinyl estradiol)
(active pills peach)
Warner-Chilcott
Now there is a chewable Ovcon-35 pill! ◄——

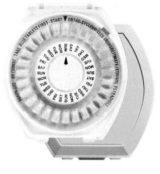

ORTHO-CYCLEN®
28 TABLETS
(0.25 mg norgestimate/35 mcg ethinyl estradiol)
(active pills blue)
Ortho-McNeil

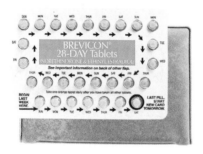

BREVICON®
28-DAY TABLETS
(0.5 mg norethindrone/35 mcg ethinyl estradiol)
(active pills blue)
Watson

=

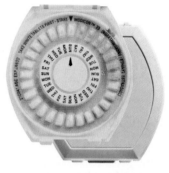

MODICON® TABLETS
28-DAY REGIMEN
(0.5 mg norethindrone/35 mcg ethinyl estradiol)
(active pills white)
Ortho-McNeil

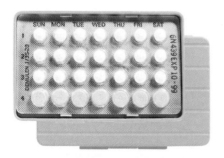

DEMULEN® 1/35-28
(1 mg ethynodiol diacetate/35 mcg ethinyl estradiol)
(active pills white)
Pharmacia
A Division of Pfizer

=

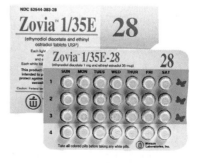

ZOVIA® 1/35E–28
(1 mg ethynodiol diacetate/35 mcg ethinyl estradiol)
(active pills light pink)
Watson

(D)

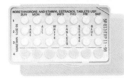

NORETHIN 1/35E–28
(1 mg norethindrone/35 mcg ethinyl estradiol)
(active pills white)
Shire

=

ORTHO-NOVUM® 1/35 28 TABLETS
(1 mg norethindrone/35 mcg ethinyl estradiol)
(active pills peach)
Ortho-McNeil

||

||

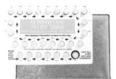
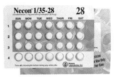

NORINYL® 1+35 28-DAY TABLETS
(1 mg norethindrone/35 mcg ethinyl estradiol)
(active pills yellow-green)
Watson

=

NECON 1/35-28
(1 mg norethindrone/35 mcg ethinyl estradiol)
(active pills dark yellow)
Watson

COMBINED PILLS – PHASIC PILLS

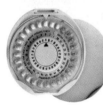

ORTHO TRI-CYCLEN® LO - 28 TABLETS
(norgestimate/ethinyl estradiol)
0.18 mg/25 mcg (7d) (white),
0.215 mg/25 mcg (7d) (light blue),
0.25 mg/25 mcg (7d) (dark blue)
remaining 7 placebo pills are green
Ortho-McNeil

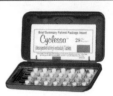

CYCLESSA
(desogestrel/ethinyl estradiol–triphasic regimen)
0.1 mg/25 mcg (7d) (light yellow)
0.125 mg/25 mcg (7d) (orange)
0.150 mg/25 mcg (7d) (red)
Organon

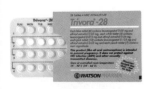

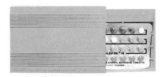

TRIVORA®
(levonorgestrel/ethinyl estradiol–triphasic regimen)
0.050 mg/30 mcg (6d), 0.075 mg/40 mcg (5d),
0.125 mg/30 mcg (10d) (pink)
Watson

=

TRIPHASIL®- 28 TABLETS
(levonorgestrel/ethinyl estradiol–triphasic regimen)
0.050 mg/30 mcg (6d) (brown),
0.075 mg/40 mcg (5d) (white),
0.125 mg/30 mcg (10d)
(light yellow)
Wyeth

=

TRI-LEVLEN® 28 TABLETS
(levonorgestrel/ethinyl estradiol– triphasic regimen)
0.050 mg/30 mcg (6d) (brown),
0.075 mg/40 mcg (5d) (white),
0.125 mg/30 mcg (10d)
(light yellow)
Berlex

(E)

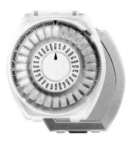

ORTHO-NOVUM® 10/11
28 TABLETS
(norethindrone/ethinyl estradiol)
0.5 mg/35 mcg (10d) (white),
1 mg/35 mcg (11d) (peach)
Ortho-McNeil

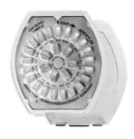

JENEST 28 TABLETS
(norethindrone/ethinyl estradiol)
0.5 mg/35 mcg (7d) (white),
1 mg/35 mcg (14d) (peach)
Organon

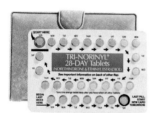

TRI-NORINYL®
28-DAY TABLETS
(norethindrone/ethinyl estradiol)
0.5 mg/35 mcg (7d) (blue),
1 mg/35 mcg (9d) (yellow-green),
0.5 mg/35 mcg (5d) (blue)
Watson

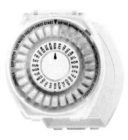

ORTHO-NOVUM® 7/7/7
28 TABLETS
(norethindrone/ethinyl estradiol)
0.5 mg/35 mcg (7d) (white),
0.75 mg/35 mcg (7d) (light peach),
1 mg/35 mcg (7d) (peach)
Ortho-McNeil

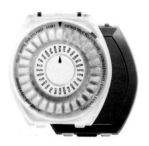

ORTHO TRI-CYCLEN®
28 TABLETS
(norgestimate/ethinyl estradiol)
0.18 mg/35 mcg (7d) (white),
0.215 mg/35 mcg (7d) (light blue),
0.25 mg/35 mcg (7d) (blue)
Ortho-McNeil

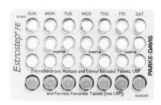

ESTROSTEP® FE
28 TABLETS
(norethindrone acetate/ethinyl estradiol)
1 mg/20 mcg (5d) (white triangular),
1 mg/30 mcg (7d) (white square),
1 mg/35 mcg (9d), 75 mg ferrous
fumarate (7d) (white round)
Pfizer

COMBINED PILLS – 50 microgram PILLS

Pills with 50 micrograms of mestranol are not as strong as pills with 50 micrograms of ethinyl estradiol

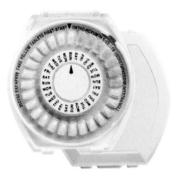

ORTHO-NOVUM® 1/50
28 TABLETS
(1 mg norethindrone/50 mcg mestranol)
(active pills yellow)
Ortho-McNeil

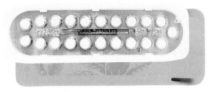

OVRAL - 21 TABLETS
(0.5 mg norgestrel/50 mcg ethinyl estradiol)
(active pills white)
Wyeth

=

OGESTREL
Watson

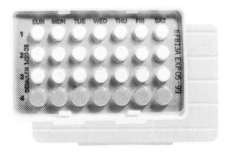

DEMULEN® 1/50-28
(1 mg ethynodiol diacetate/50 mcg ethinyl estradiol)
(active pills white)
Pharmacia
A Division of Pfizer

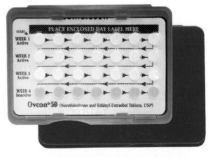

OVCON® 50 28-DAY
(1 mg norethindrone/50 mcg ethinyl estradiol)
(active pills yellow)
Warner-Chilcott

PILLS AS EMERGENCY CONTRACEPTIVES:
2 Different Approaches: Progestin-Only Pills OR Combined Pills

PROGESTIN-ONLY PILLS

Plan B

1 + 1 pill 12 hours apart OR
2 Plan B pills ASAP
after unprotected sex

20 + 20 pills 12 hours apart

Ovrette *(yellow pills)*

(Plan B and Ovrette are NOT carried
in all pharmacies. Check in advance.
Ask your pharmacy to carry Plan B

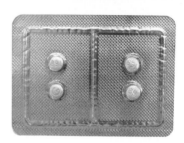

plan B˜
(LEVONORGESTREL)
[2 tablets, 0.75 mg]

PLAN B

Antinausea meds <u>not</u> necessary ←

COMBINED ORAL CONTRACEPTIVES

2 + 2 pills 12 hours apart

Preven* *(blue pills)* OR
Ogestrel *(white pills)*
Ovral *(white pills)*

(Preven Ogestrel and Ovral are NOT carried
in all pharmacies. Check in advance.)*

4 + 4 pills 12 hours apart
Low-Ogestrel *(white pills)*
Lo-Ovral *(white pills)*,
Levora *(white pills)* OR
Levlen *(light orange pills)* OR
Nordette *(light orange pills)* OR
Triphasil *(yellow pills)*,
Tri-Levlen *(yellow pills)* OR
Trivora *(pink pills)*

PREVEN*

> Have your patient take
> antinausea medication an
> hour before the first dose if
> using any of the combined
> oral contraceptives as
> emergency contraception.
> This is <u>not</u> necessary if
> using Plan B.

5 + 5 pills 12 hours apart
Alesse *(pink pills)* OR
Levlite *(pink pills)* OR
Aviane *(orange pills)*

• NOTE: Preven Discontinued in 2004

ADVANTAGES

The once-a-month self-administered use permits convenience, privacy, and ease of use. It is relatively easy for a woman to confirm that the device is in place. The NuvaRing releases low, steady amounts of ethinyl estradiol and etonorgestrel. Cycle control is another advantage; in every cycle, fewer than 10% of women experienced any untimely spotting or bleeding. In a comparative trial of vaginal ring versus a 30 mcgEE/0.15 levonorgestrel OC, the NuvaRing provided significantly better cycle control.[182] Overall satisfaction with the method was relatively high (85%); 96% to 98% of users reported that the ring was easy to insert and remove; and 83% said they rarely or never felt the ring during intercourse. Nine out of 10 study participants said they would recommend the vaginal ring to a friend.[183]

DISADVANTAGES AND CAUTIONS

Some women may be hesitant to touch their genitalia to place and remove the rings. Although the rings may be stored at room temperature for up to 4 months, it is generally preferred that rings be kept refrigerated to prolong their active life. This may pose challenges for women who need private methods.

Health complications. In addition to the health complications associated with combined hormonal contraceptives (myocardial infarction, stroke, VTE, hypertension, diabetes, cholestatic jaundice, hepatic neoplasms, etc.), the vaginal delivery system may be associated with localized conditions such as vaginal discomfort and vaginal discharge.

Side effects. Overall, relatively few users reported hormone-related side effects: headaches (5.8%), nausea (3.2%), and breast tenderness (2.0%). Local side effects specific to the ring were also reported at the following rates: vaginitis (5.6%), leukorrhea (4.6%), other device-related problems (4.4%), and vaginal discomfort (2.4%).

In the combined (North American and European) clinical trial, 15.1% of women withdrew because of adverse events such as the sensation of a foreign body, coital problems and expulsion; headaches (1.3%); emotional lability (1.2%); and weight increase (1%). Fewer than 1% of women stopped because of bleeding irregularity, vaginitis, or leukorrhea.

Precautions

Women who have medical contraindications to OC use (except for those contraindications related to intestinal absorption problems) are not candidates for the vaginal ring, nor are women who have significant pelvic relaxation, are unable to touch their genitalia, or who have vaginal obstruction. The NuvaRing may not be suitable for women with conditions that make the vagina more susceptible to infection or ulceration. The NuvaRing should not be used in conjunction with a diaphragm, since it may prevent correct placement of that barrier.

PROVIDING THE VAGINAL RING

The NuvaRing should be inserted no later than cycle day 5, even if the patient has not finished her menstrual bleeding. If a woman has not used a hormonal method of contraception the cycle before she starts NuvaRing, she should use a back-up method of contraception (male or female condom or spermicide) for the first 7 days of continuous ring use.

Switching from other methods. If a woman switches from OCs, she should place the NuvaRing on the day she would start a new pack of pills. If she is switching from progestin-only pills, she should place the first ring on the same day she takes the last pill. Similarly, she should place the first ring on the day the implants or IUDs are removed. If she is switching from a copper IUD, she may also need emergency contraception if she has had recent intercourse, and she may need to use a back-up method for 7 days if she is not having her menses. If she is switching from injections, she should start the ring the day she is due for her next injection. The ring may be started within 5 days of completion of a first-trimester elective abortion or pregnancy loss. Postpartum women who are not breastfeeding or women who have second trimester losses may start begin the patch 4 weeks after delivery.

MANAGING PROBLEMS AND FOLLOW UP

If the NuvaRing is removed or expelled during the 21 days it should be in place, it should be rinsed with cool to lukewarm (not hot) water and reinserted as soon as possible, but at the latest within 3 hours from the time it was lost. If the NuvaRing is lost, a new vaginal ring should be inserted for a new 21-day period.

If a NuvaRing is out of the vagina for more than 3 hours, a back-up method must be used for the next 7 days. If the NuvaRing is inserted late and the woman has had unprotected intercourse prior to placement, administer emergency contraception.

USING THE VAGINAL RING

1. Insert one ring into your vagina. Use any position you find most comfortable: standing with one leg up, squatting, or lying down. Compress the rim of the ring and place the leading edge into the opening of the vagina.

2. Place the ring high in the vault of your vagina, against the wall. The exact position of the NuvaRing is not critical for its function.

3. Leave the ring in place for 3 weeks. Do not remove the ring for intercourse.

4. After 3 weeks, remove the vaginal ring for 7 days. During this break, you will experience withdrawal bleeding. Remove the

NuvaRing by hooking your index finger under the forward rim or by grasping the rim between your index and middle finger and pulling it out. Place the used ring in the sachet (foil pouch) and discard it in a waste receptacle out of the reach of children and pets (do not flush it down the toilet).

5. After the 7-day break, insert a new vaginal ring to begin the cycle again. Insert the new NuvaRing on the same day of the week you inserted the previous ring, even if you have not finished your period.

6. If the NuvaRing is out of your vagina for more than 3 hours during the 21-day period, re-insert it and use back-up contraception for the next 7 days. If you have had unprotected intercourse, use emergency contraception.

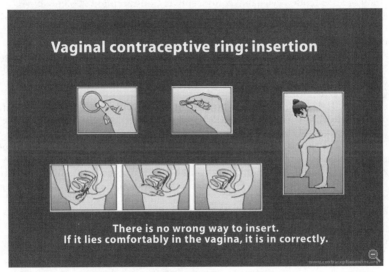

Figure 19-4 Vaginal contraceptive ring: insertion

Source: Ballagh SA (2002),[184] with permission courtesy of Organon USA.

REFERENCES

1. Blackburn RD, Cunkelman A, Zlidar VM. Oral contraceptives—an update. Popul Rep A 2000;28(1):1-16, 25-32.
2. Speroff L, Darney P. A clinical guide for contraception. Third Edition. Baltimore MD: Williams & Wilkins, 2001.
3. Bronson RA. Oral contraception: mechanism of action. Clin Obstet Gynecol 1981;24(3):869-877.
4. Killick SR, Fitzgerald C, Davis A. Ovarian activity in women taking an oral contraceptive containing 20 micrograms ethinyl estradiol and 150 microg desogestrel: effects of low estrogen doses during the hormone-free interval. Am J Obstet Gynecol 1998;179(1):S18-24.
5. Timmer CJ, Mulders TM. Pharmacokinetics of etonogestrel and ethinylestradiol released from a combined contraceptive vaginal ring. Clin Pharmacokinet 2000;39(3):233-242.

6. Tayob Y, Robinson G, Adams J, Nye M, Whitelaw N, Shaw RW et al. Ultrasound appearance of the ovaries during the pill-free interval. Br J Family Planning 1990;16:94-96.

7. Schwartz JL, Creinin MD, Pymar HC, Reid L. Predicting risk of ovulation in new start oral contraceptive users. Obstet Gynecol 2002;99(2):177-182.

8. Rosenberg MJ, Waugh MS. Oral contraceptive discontinuation: a prospective evaluation of frequency and reasons. Am J Obstet Gynecol 1998;179(3 Pt 1):577-582.

9. Potter LS, Oral contraceptive compliance and its role in the effectiveness of the method. In Cramer JA, Spilker B eds, Patient Compliance In Medical Practice And Clinical Trials. New York: Raven Press, 1991 pp 195-207.

10. Holt VL, Cushing-Haugen KL, Daling JR. Body weight and risk of oral contraceptive failure. Obstet Gynecol 2002;99(5 Pt 1):820-827.

11. Zieman M, Nelson AL. Contraceptive efficacy and body weight. Female Patient 2002;27(10):36-38.

12. Anderson FD, Hait H; The Seasonale-301 Study Group. A multicenter, randomized study of an extended cycle oral contraceptive. Contraception 2003;68:89-96.

13. Smallwood GH, Meador ML, Lenihan JP, Shangold GA, Fisher AC, Creasy GW; ORTHO EVRA/EVRA 002 Study Group. Efficacy and safety of a transdermal contraceptive system. Obstet Gynecol 2001;98(5 Pt 1):799-805.

14. Audet MC, Moreau M, Koltun WD, Waldbaum AS, et al.; ORTHO EVRA/EVRA 004 Study Group. Evaluation of contraceptive efficacy and cycle control of a transdermal contraceptive patch vs an oral contraceptive: a randomized controlled trial. JAMA 2001;285(18):2347-2354.

15. Creasy G, Hall N, Shangold G. Patient adherence with the contraceptive patch dosing schedule versus oral contraceptives [abstract]. Obstet Gynecol 2000;95 (suppl):60S.

16. Dieben TO, Roumen FJ, Apter D. Efficacy, cycle control, and user acceptability of a novel combined contraceptive vaginal ring. Obstet Gynecol 2002;100(3):585-593.

17. Zacur HA, Hedon B, Mansour D, Shangold GA, et al. Integrated summary of Ortho Evra/Evra contraceptive patch adhesion in varied climates and conditions. Fertil Steril 2002;77(2 Suppl 2):S32-35.

18. Zieman M, Guillebaud J, Weisberg E, Shangold GA, et al. Contraceptive efficacy and cycle control with the Ortho Evra/Evra transdermal system: the analysis of pooled data. Fertil Steril 2002;77(2 Suppl 2):S13-18.

19. Margulies R, Miller L. Increased depot medroxyprogesterone acetate use increases family planning program pharmaceutical supply costs. Contraception 2001;63(3): 147-149.

20. American College of Obstetricians and Gynecologists. The pill at 40: Women say it's safer, has extra benefits, but not covered by insurance. Press release. Washington DC: ACOG, May 2, 2001.

21. Vessey M, Painter R, Yeates D. Mortality in relation to oral contraceptive use and cigarette smoking. Lancet 2003;362(9379):185-191.

22. Chang J, Elam-Evans LD, Berg CJ, Herndon J, et al. Pregnancy-related mortality surveillance—United States, 1991–1999. MMWR Surveill Summ. 2003;52(2):1-8.

23. Franks AL, Beral V, Cates W Jr, Hogue CJ. Contraception and ectopic pregnancy risk. Am J Obstet Gynecol 1990;163(4 Pt 1):1120-1123.

24. Sivin I. Dose- and age-dependent ectopic pregnancy risks with intrauterine contraception. Obstet Gynecol 1991;78(2):291-298.

25. Marchbanks PA, Annegers JF, Coulam CB, Strathy JH, Kurland LT. Risk factors for ectopic pregnancy. A population-based study. JAMA 1988;259(12):1823-1827.

26. Milsom I, Sundell G, Andersch B. The influence of different combined oral contraceptives on the prevalence and severity of dysmenorrhea. Contraception 1990;42(5):497-506.

27. Mishell DR Jr. Noncontraceptive health benefits of oral steroidal contraceptives. Am J Obstet Gynecol 1982;142(6 Pt 2):809-816.

28. Robinson JC, Plichta S, Weisman CS, Nathanson CA, Ensminger M. Dysmenorrhea and use of oral contraceptives in adolescent women attending a family planning clinic. Am J Obstet Gynecol 1992;166(2):578-583.

29. Nilsson L, Rybo G. Treatment of menorrhagia. Am J Obstet Gynecol 1971;110(5):713-720.

30. Larsson G, Milsom I, Lindstedt G, Rybo G. The influence of a low-dose combined oral contraceptive on menstrual blood loss and iron status. Contraception 1992;46(4):327-334.

31. Fraser IS, McCarron G. Randomized trial of 2 hormonal and 2 prostaglandin-inhibiting agents in women with a complaint of menorrhagia. Aust N Z J Obstet Gynaecol 1991;31(1):66-70.

32. Iyer V, Farquhar C, Jepson R. Oral contraceptive pills for heavy menstrual bleeding. Cochrane Database Syst Rev 2000;(2):CD000154.

33. Runnebaum B, Grunwald K, Rabe T. The efficacy and tolerability of norgestimate/ethinyl estradiol (250 micrograms of norgestimate/35 micrograms of ethinyl estradiol): results of an open, multicenter study of 59,701 women. Am J Obstet Gynecol 1992;166(6 Pt 2):1963-1968.

34. Parsey KS, Pong A. An open-label, multicenter study to evaluate Yasmin, a low-dose combination oral contraceptive containing drospirenone, a new progestogen. Contraception 2000;61(2):105-111.

35. Borenstein J, Yu HT, Wade S, Chiou CF, Rapkin A. Effect of an oral contraceptive containing ethinyl estradiol and drospirenone on premenstrual symptomatology and health-related quality of life. J Reprod Med 2003;48(2):79-85.

36. Davis A, Godwin A, Lippman J, Olson W, Kafrissen M. Triphasic norgestimate-ethinyl estradiol for treating dysfunctional uterine bleeding. Obstet Gynecol 2000;96(6):913-920.

37. Lanes SF, Birmann B, Walker AM, Singer S. Oral contraceptive type and functional ovarian cysts. Am J Obstet Gynecol 1992;166(3):956-961.

38. Vessey M, Metcalfe A, Wells C, McPherson K, et al. Ovarian neoplasms, functional ovarian cysts, and oral contraceptives. Br Med J (Clin Res Ed). 1987;294(6586):1518-1520.

39. Young RL, Snabes MC, Frank ML, Reilly M. A randomized, double-blind, placebo-controlled comparison of the impact of low-dose and triphasic oral contraceptives on follicular development. Am J Obstet Gynecol 1992;167(3):678-682.

40. Chiaffarino F, Parazzini F, La Vecchia C, Ricci E, Crosignani PG. Oral contraceptive use and benign gynecologic conditions. A review. Contraception 1998;57(1):11-18.

41. Vessey MP, Painter R. Endometrial and ovarian cancer and oral contraceptives--findings in a large cohort study. Br J Cancer 1995;71(6):1340-1342.

42. Rosenberg L, Palmer JR, Zauber AG, Warshauer ME, et al. A case-control study of oral contraceptive use and invasive epithelial ovarian cancer. Am J Epidemiol 1994;139(7):654-661.

43. Ness RB, Grisso JA, Klapper J, Schlesselman JJ, et al. Risk of ovarian cancer in relation to estrogen and progestin dose and use characteristics of oral contraceptives. SHARE Study Group. Steroid Hormones and Reproductions. Am J Epidemiol 2000;152(3):233-241.

44. Narod SA, Risch H, Moslehi R, Dorum A, et al. Oral contraceptives and the risk of hereditary ovarian cancer. Hereditary Ovarian Cancer Clinical Study Group. N Engl J Med 1998;339(7):424-428.

45. Schildkraut JM, Calingaert B, Marchbanks PA, Moorman PG, Rodriguez GC. Impact of progestin and estrogen potency in oral contraceptives on ovarian cancer risk. J Natl Cancer Inst 2002;94(1):32-38.

46. Gross TP, Schlesselman JJ. The estimated effect of oral contraceptive use on the cumulative risk of epithelial ovarian cancer. Obstet Gynecol 1994;83(3):419-424.

47. Walker GR, Schlesselman JJ, Ness RB. Family history of cancer, oral contraceptive use, and ovarian cancer risk. Am J Obstet Gynecol 2002;186(1):8-14.

48. Modan B, Hartge P, Hirsh-Yechezkel G, Chetrit A, et al; National Israel Ovarian Cancer Study Group. Parity, oral contraceptives, and the risk of ovarian cancer among carriers and noncarriers of a BRCA1 or BRCA2 mutation. N Engl J Med 2001;345(4):235-240.
49. Jensen JT, Speroff L. Health benefits of oral contraceptives. Obstet Gynecol Clin North Am 2000;27(4):705-721.
50. Combination oral contraceptive use and the risk of endometrial cancer. The Cancer and Steroid Hormone Study of the Centers for Disease Control and the National Institute of Child Health and Human Development. JAMA 1987;257(6): 796-800.
51. Schlesselman JJ. Risk of endometrial cancer in relation to use of combined oral contraceptives. A practitioner's guide to meta-analysis. Hum Reprod 1997;12(9): 1851-1863.
52. Brinton LA, Vessey MP, Flavel R, Yeates D. Risk factors for benign breast disease. Am J Epidemiol 1981;113(3):203-214.
53. Charreau I, Plu-Bureau G, Bachelot A, Contesso G, et al. Oral contraceptive use and risk of benign breast disease in a French case-control study of young women. Eur J Cancer Prev 1993;2(2):147-154.
54. Rohan TE, Miller AB. A cohort study of oral contraceptive use and risk of benign breast disease. Int J Cancer 1999;82(2):191-196.
55. Redmond GP, Olson WH, Lippman JS, Kafrissen ME, et al. Norgestimate and ethinyl estradiol in the treatment of acne vulgaris: a randomized, placebo-controlled trial. Obstet Gynecol 1997;89(4):615-622.
56. Lucky AW, Henderson TA, Olson WH, Robisch DM, et al. Effectiveness of norgestimate and ethinyl estradiol in treating moderate acne vulgaris. J Am Acad Dermatol 1997;37(5 Pt 1):746-754.
57. Jemec GB, Linneberg A, Nielsen NH, Frolund L, et al. Have oral contraceptives reduced the prevalence of acne? A population-based study of acne vulgaris, tobacco smoking and oral contraceptives. Dermatology 2002;204(3):179-184.
58. Dewis P, Petsos P, Newman M, Anderson DC. The treatment of hirsutism with a combination of desogestrel and ethinyl oestradiol. Clin Endocrinol (Oxf) 1985;22(1):29-36.
59. Lobo RA. The androgenicity of progestational agents. Int J Fertil 1988;33 Suppl:6-12.
60. Washington AE, Gove S, Schachter J, Sweet RL. Oral contraceptives, Chlamydia trachomatis infection, and pelvic inflammatory disease. A word of caution about protection. JAMA 1985;253(15):2246-2250.
61. Panser LA, Phipps WR. Type of oral contraceptive in relation to acute, initial episodes of pelvic inflammatory disease. Contraception 1991;43(1):91-99.
62. Sangi-Haghpeykar H, Poindexter AN 3rd. Epidemiology of endometriosis among parous women. Obstet Gynecol 1995;85(6):983-992.
63. Westhoff C, Britton JA, Gammon MD, Wright T, Kelsey JL. Oral contraceptive and benign ovarian tumors. Am J Epidemiol 2000;152(3):242-246.
64. Parazzini F, Ferraroni M, Bocciolone L, Tozzi L, Rubessa S, La Vecchia C. Contraceptive methods and risk of pelvic endometriosis. Contraception 1994;49(1):47-55.
65. Nisolle-Pochet M, Casanas-Roux F, Donnez J. Histologic study of ovarian endometriosis after hormonal therapy. Fertil Steril 1988;49(3):423-426. Erratum in: Fertil Steril 1988 Jul;50(1):184.
66. Task Force for Epidemiological Research on Reproductive Health, United Nations Development Programme/United Nations Population Fund/World Health Organization/World Bank Special Programme of Research, Development and Research Training in Human Reproduction, World Health Organization, Geneva, Switzerland. Effects of contraceptives on hemoglobin and ferritin. Contraception 1998;58(5):262-273.
67. Shargil AA. Hormone replacement therapy in perimenopausal women with a triphasic contraceptive compound: a three-year prospective study. Int J Fertil 1985;30(1):15, 18-28.

68. Casper RF, Dodin S, Reid RL, Study Investigators. The effect of 20 μg ethinyl estradiol/1 mg norethindrone acetate (Minestrin™), a low-dose oral contraceptive, on vaginal bleeding patterns, hot flashes, and quality of life in symptomatic perimenopausal women. Menopause 1997;4(3):139-147.

69. Spector TD, Hochberg MC. The protective effect of the oral contraceptive pill on rheumatoid arthritis: an overview of the analytic epidemiological studies using meta-analysis. J Clin Epidemiol 1990;43(11):1221-1230.

70. Pladevall-Vila M, Delclos GL, Varas C, Guyer H, Brugues-Tarradellas J, Anglada-Arisa A. Controversy of oral contraceptives and risk of rheumatoid arthritis: meta-analysis of conflicting studies and review of conflicting meta-analyses with special emphasis on analysis of heterogeneity. Am J Epidemiol 1996;144(1):1-14.

71. Chiaffarino F, Parazzini F, La Vecchia C, Marsico S, Surace M, Ricci E. Use of oral contraceptives and uterine fibroids: results from a case-control study. Br J Obstet Gynaecol 1999;106(8):857-860.

72. Marshall LM, Spiegelman D, Goldman MB, Manson JE, Colditz GA, Barbieri R, et al. A prospective study of reproductive factors and oral contraceptive use in relation to the risk of uterine leiomyomata. Fertil Steril 1998;70(3):432-439.

73. Seeman E, Szmukler GI, Formica C, Tsalamandris C, Mestrovic R. Osteoporosis in anorexia nervosa: the influence of peak bone density, bone loss, oral contraceptive use, and exercise. J Bone Miner Res 1992;7(12):1467-1474.

74. Pasco JA, Kotowicz MA, Henry MJ, Panahi S, Seeman E, Nicholson GC. Oral contraceptives and bone mineral density: A population-based study. Am J Obstet Gynecol 2000;182(2):265-269.

75. Mallmin H, Ljunghall S, Persson I, Bergstrom R. Risk factors for fractures of the distal forearm: a population-based case-control study. Osteoporos Int 1994;4(6):298-304.

76. Cooper C, Hannaford P, Croft P, Kay CR. Oral contraceptive pill use and fractures in women: a prospective study. Bone 1993;14(1):41-45.

77. Kuohung W, Borgatta L, Stubblefield P. Low-dose oral contraceptives and bone mineral density: an evidence-based analysis. Contraception 2000;61(2):77-82.

78. Hergenroeder AC, Smith EO, Shypailo R, Jones LA, Klish WJ, Ellis K. Bone mineral changes in young women with hypothalamic amenorrhea treated with oral contraceptives, medroxyprogesterone, or placebo over 12 months. Am J Obstet Gynecol 1997;176(5):1017-1025.

79. Grinspoon S, Thomas L, Miller K, Herzog D, Klibanski A. Effects of recombinant human IGF-I and oral contraceptive administration on bone density in anorexia nervosa. J Clin Endocrinol Metab 2002;87(6):2883-2891.

80. Elgan C, Samsioe G, Dykes AK. Influence of smoking and oral contraceptives on bone mineral density and bone remodeling in young women: a 2-year study. Contraception 2003;67(6):439-447.

81. Strinic T, Eterovic D. Oral contraceptives improve lung mechanics. Fertil Steril 2003;79(5):1070-1073.

82. Fernandez E, La Vecchia C, Balducci A, Chatenoud L, Franceschi S, Negri E. Oral contraceptives and colorectal cancer risk: a meta-analysis. Br J Cancer 2001;84(5):722-727.

83. Ellertson C, Webb A, Blanchard K, Bigrigg A, Haskell S, Shochet T, Trussell J. Modifying the Yuzpe regimen of emergency contraception: a multicenter randomized controlled trial. Obstet Gynecol 2003;101(6):1160-1167.

84. Tanis BC, van den Bosch MA, Kemmeren JM, Cats VM, Helmerhorst FM, Algra A, et al. Oral contraceptives and the risk of myocardial infarction. N Engl J Med 2001;345(25):1787-1793.

85. Rosenberg L, Palmer JR, Rao RS, Shapiro S. Low-dose oral contraceptive use and the risk of myocardial infarction. Arch Intern Med 2001;161:1065-1070.

86. Khader YS, Rice J, John L, Abueita O. Oral contraceptives use and the risk of myocardial infarction: a meta-analysis. Contraception 2003;68(1):11-17.

87. Petitti DB. Combination estrogen-progestin oral contraceptives. N Engl J Med 2003;349:1443-1450.

88. Schwingl PJ, Ory HW, Visness CM. Estimates of the risk of cardiovascular death attributable to low-dose oral contraceptives in the United States. Am J Obstet Gynecol 1999;180(1 Pt 1):241-249.

89. Chasan-Taber L, Stampfer M. Oral contraceptives and myocardial infarction--the search for the smoking gun. N Engl J Med. 2001;345(25):1841-1842.

90. Lidegaard O, Kreiner S. Contraceptives and cerebral thrombosis: a five-year national case-control study. Contraception 2002;65(3):197-205.

91. Siritho S, Thrift AG, McNeil JJ, You RX, Davis SM, Donnan GA; Melbourne Risk Factor Study (MERFS) Group. Risk of ischemic stroke among users of the oral contraceptive pill: The Melbourne Risk Factor Study (MERFS) Group. Stroke 2003;34(7):1575-1580.

92. Chang CL, Donaghy M, Poulter N. Migraine and stroke in young women: case-control study. The World Health Organisation Collaborative Study of Cardiovascular Disease and Steroid Hormone Contraception. BMJ 1999;318(7175):13-18.

93. Curtis KM, Chrisman CE, Peterson HB, WHO Programme for Mapping Best Practices in Reproductive Health. Contraception for women in selected circumstances. Obstet Gynecol 2002;99(6):1100-1112.

94. Kemmeren JM, Tanis BC, van den Bosch MA, Bollen EL, Helmerhorst FM, van der Graaf Y, et al. Risk of Arterial Thrombosis in Relation to Oral Contraceptives (RATIO) study: oral contraceptives and the risk of ischemic stroke. Stroke 2002;33(5):1202-1208.

95. Patient package inserts for Ortho Tricyclen, Ortho Cyclen, Ortho-Cept, Ortho Novum and Yasmin. August 2003.

96. Schlesselman JJ. Net effect of oral contraceptive use on the risk of cancer in women in the United States. Obstet Gynecol 1995;85(5 Pt 1):793-801.

97. Schwingl PJ, Shelton J. Modeled estimates of myocardial infarction and venous thromboembolic disease in users of second and third generation oral contraceptives. Contraception 1997;55(3):125-129.

98. World Health Organization Collaborative Study of Cardiovascular Disease and Steroid Hormone Contraception. Effect of different progestagens in low oestrogen oral contraceptives on venous thromboembolic disease. Lancet 1995;346(8990):1582-1588.

99. Spitzer WO, Lewis MA, Heinemann LA, Thorogood M, MacRae KD. Third generation oral contraceptives and risk of venous thromboembolic disorders: an international case-control study. Transnational Research Group on Oral Contraceptives and the Health of Young Women. BMJ 1996;312(7023):83-88.

100. Jick H, Jick SS, Gurewich V, Myers MW, Vasilakis C. Risk of idiopathic cardiovascular death and nonfatal venous thromboembolism in women using oral contraceptives with differing progestagen components. Lancet 1995;346(8990):1589-1593.

101. Lewis MA, Heinemann LA, MacRae KD, Bruppacher R, Spitzer WO. The increased risk of venous thromboembolism and the use of third generation progestagens: role of bias in observational research. The Transnational Research Group on Oral Contraceptives and the Health of Young Women. Contraception. 1996 Jul;54(1):5-13. Erratum in: Contraception 1996 Aug;54(2):121.

102. Sheldon T. Dutch GPs warned against new contraceptive pill. BMJ 2002;324(7342):869.

103. CBG website , March 28, 2002.

104. Ridker PM, Miletich JP, Hennekens CH, Buring JE. Ethnic distribution of factor V Leiden in 4047 men and women. Implications for venous thromboembolism screening. JAMA 1997;277(16):1305-1307.

105. Vandenbroucke JP, van der Meer FJ, Helmerhorst FM, Rosendaal FR. Factor V Leiden: should we screen oral contraceptive users and pregnant women? BMJ 1996;313(7065):1127-1130.

106. Troisi RJ, Cowie CC, Harris MI. Oral contraceptive use and glucose metabolism in a national sample of women in the United States. Am J Obstet Gynecol 2000;183(2):389-395.

107. Kim C, Siscovick DS, Sidney S, Lewis CE, Kiefe CI, Koepsell TD; CARDIA Study. Oral contraceptive use and association with glucose, insulin, and diabetes in young adult women: the CARDIA Study. Coronary Artery Risk Development in Young Adults. Diabetes Care 2002;25(6):1027-1032.

108. Kojima T, Lindheim SR, Duffy DM, Vijod MA, Stanczyk FZ, Lobo RA. Insulin sensitivity is decreased in normal women by doses of ethinyl estradiol used in oral contraceptives. Am J Obstet Gynecol 1993;169(6):1540-1544.

109. Kjos SL, Peters RK, Xiang A, Thomas D, Schaefer U, Buchanan TA. Contraception and the risk of type 2 diabetes mellitus in Latina women with prior gestational diabetes mellitus. JAMA 1998;280(6):533-538.

110. Milne R, Vessey M. The association of oral contraception with kidney cancer, colon cancer, gallbladder cancer (including extrahepatic bile duct cancer) and pituitary tumours. Contraception 1991;43(6):667-693.

111. Scalori A, Tavani A, Gallus S, La Vecchia C, Colombo M. Oral contraceptives and the risk of focal nodular hyperplasia of the liver: a case-control study. Am J Obstet Gynecol 2002;186(2):195-197.

112. The WHO Collaborative Study of Neoplasia and Steroid Contraceptives. Combined oral contraceptives and liver cancer. Int J Cancer 1989;43(2):254-259.

113. Bontis J, Vavilis D, Panidis D, et al. Detection of Chlamydia trachomatis in asymptomatic women: relationship to history, contraception, and cervicitis. Adv Contracept 1994;10(4):309-315.

114. Kinghorn GR, Waugh MA. Oral contraceptive use and prevalence of infection with Chlamydia trachomatis in women. Br J Vener Dis 1981;57(3):187-190.

115. Baeten JM, Nyange PM, Richardson BA, Lavreys L, Chohan B, Martin HL Jr, et al. Hormonal contraception and risk of sexually transmitted disease acquisition: results from a prospective study. Am J Obstet Gynecol 2001;185(2):380-385.

116. Fleming DC, King AE, Williams AR, Critchley HO, Kelly RW. Hormonal contraception can suppress natural antimicrobial gene transcription in human endometrium. Fertil Steril 2003;79(4):856-863.

117. Ildgruben AK, Sjoberg IM, Hammarstrom ML. Influence of hormonal contraceptives on the immune cells and thickness of human vaginal epithelium. Obstet Gynecol 2003;102(3):571-582.

118. Baeten JM Hormonal contraception increases HIV risk and disease progression. 10th Conference on Retroviruses and Opportunistic Infections, Abstract 116. Boston: presented February 12, 2003.

119. Karagas MR, Stukel TA, Dykes J, Miglionico J, Greene MA, Carey M, et al. A pooled analysis of 10 case-control studies of melanoma and oral contraceptive use. Br J Cancer 2002;86(7):1085-1092.

120. Ross RK, Pike MC, Vessey MP, Bull D, Yeates D, Casagrande JT. Risk factors for uterine fibroids: reduced risk associated with oral contraceptives. Br Med J (Clin Res Ed). 1986;293(6543):359-362. Erratum in: Br Med J (Clin Res Ed) 1986; 293(6553):1027.

121. Parazzini F, Negri E, La Vecchia C, Fedele L, Rabaiotti M, Luchini L. Oral contraceptive use and risk of uterine fibroids. Obstet Gynecol 1992;79(3):430-433.

122. Marshall LM, Spiegelman D, Goldman MB, et al. A prospective study of reproductive factors and oral contraceptive use in relation to the risk of uterine leiomyomata. Fertil Steril 1998;70(3):432-439.

123. Morrison C, Prokorym P, Piquero C, Wakely PE Jr, Nuovo GJ. Oral contraceptive pills are associated with artifacts in ThinPrep Pap smears that mimic low-grade squamous intraepithelial lesions. Cancer 2003;99(2):75-82.

124. Moreno V, Bosch FX, Munoz N, Meijer CJ, Shah KV, et al.; International Agency for Research on Cancer. Multicentric Cervical Cancer Study Group. Effect of oral contraceptives on risk of cervical cancer in women with human papillomavirus infection: the IARC multicentric case-control study. Lancet 2002;359(9312):1085-1092.

125. Munoz N, Franceschi S, Bosetti C, Moreno V, et al.; International Agency for Research on Cancer. Multicentric Cervical Cancer Study Group. Role of parity and human papillomavirus in cervical cancer: the IARC multicentric case-control study. Lancet 2002;359(9312):1093-1101.

126. Smith JS, Green J, Berrington de Gonzalez A, Appleby P, Peto J, Plummer M, et al. Cervical cancer and use of hormonal contraceptives: a systematic review. Lancet 2003;361(9364):1159-1167.
127. Ursin G, Peters RK, Henderson BE, d'Ablaing G 3rd, et al. Oral contraceptive use and adenocarcinoma of cervix. Lancet 1994;344(8934):1390-1394.
128. Marchbanks PA, McDonald JA, Wilson HG, Folger SG, et al. Oral contraceptives and the risk of breast cancer. N Engl J Med 2002;346(26):2025-2032.
129. Collaborative Group on Hormonal Factors in Breast Cancer. Breast cancer and hormonal contraceptives: collaborative reanalysis of individual data on 53,297 women with breast cancer and 100,239 women without breast cancer from 54 epidemiological studies. Lancet 1996;347(9017):1713-1727.
130. World Health Organization. Medical eligibility criteria. http://www.who.int/ reproductive-health/publications/MEC_3/index.htm. Accessed 7/3/2004.
131. Stewart FH, Harper CC, Ellertson CE, Grimes DA, Sawaya GF, Trussell J. Clinical breast and pelvic examination requirements for hormonal contraception: Current practice vs evidence. JAMA 2001;285(17):2232-2239.
132. Harper C, Balistreri E, Boggess J, Leon K, Darney P. Provision of hormonal contraceptives without a mandatory pelvic examination: the first stop demonstration project. Fam Plann Perspect 2001;33(1):13-18.
133. Hannaford PC, Webb AM. Evidence-guided prescribing of combined oral contraceptives: consensus statement. An International Workshop at Mottram Hall, Wilmslow, U.K., March, 1996. Contraception 1996;54(3):125-129.
134. Adesanya O, Colie CF. Evaluating oral contraceptive use at 6 and 12 months. J Reprod Med 1996;41:431-434.
135. Grimes. DA. Editorial: Over the counter oral contraceptives—an immodest proposal? Amer J Public Health 1993;83:1092-1103.
136. Lara-Torre E, Schroeder B. Adolescent compliance and side effects with Quick Start initiation of oral contraceptive pills. Contraception 2002;66(2):81-85.
137. Oakley D, Sereika S, Bogue EL. Oral contraceptive pill use after an initial visit to a family planning clinic. Fam Plann Perspect 1991;23(4):150-154.
138. Polaneczky M, Slap G, Forke C, Rappaport A, Sondheimer S. The use of levonorgestrel implants (Norplant) for contraception in adolescent mothers. N Engl J Med 1994;331(18):1201-1206.
139. Westhoff C, Morroni C, Kerns J, Murphy PA. Bleeding patterns after immediate vs. conventional oral contraceptive initiation: a randomized, controlled trial. Fertil Steril 2003;79(2):322-329.
140. Gladwell M. John Rock's Error: What the co-inventor of the Pill didn't know about menstruation can endanger women's health. New Yorker Magazine 2000 Mar 10:52-63.
141. Spona J, Elstein M, Feichtinger W, Sullivan H, et al. Shorter pill-free interval in combined oral contraceptives decreases follicular development. Contraception 1996;54(2):71-77.
142. Endrikat J, Cronin M, Gerlinger C, Ruebig A, et al. Open, multicenter comparison of efficacy, cycle control, and tolerability of a 23-day oral contraceptive regimen with 20 microg ethinyl estradiol and 75 microg gestodene and a 21-day regimen with 20 microg ethinyl estradiol and 150 microg desogestrel. Contraception 2001;64(3):201-207.
143. Sulak PJ, Scow RD, Preece C, Riggs MW, Kuehl TJ. Hormone withdrawal symptoms in oral contraceptive users. Obstet Gynecol 2000;95(2):261-266.
144. Extended Regimen Contraception Clinical Proceedings. ARHP Clinical Proceedings. 2003 May 2. Available at: http://www.arhp.org/healthcareproviders/cme/onlinecme/ extendedregimencp/index.cfm?ID=328.
145. Coutinho E, Segal S. Is menstruation obsolete? New York: Oxford University Press; 1999.
146. Miller L, Notter KM. Menstrual reduction with extended use of combination oral contraceptive pills: randomized controlled trial. Obstet Gynecol 2001;98(5 Pt 1):771-778.

147. Sulak PJ, Kuehl TJ, Ortiz M, Shull BL. Acceptance of altering the standard 21-day/7-day oral contraceptive regimen to delay menses and reduce hormone withdrawal symptoms. Am J Obstet Gynecol 2002;186(6):1142-1149.
148. Schwartz JL, Creinin MD, Pymar HC. The trimonthly combination oral contraceptive regimen: is it cost effective? Contraception 1999;60(5):263-267.
149. Hatcher RA, Nelson AL, Zieman M, et al. Managing contraception. Tiger, GA: Bridging the Gap Foundation, 2003.
150. Chasan-Taber L, Stampfer M. Oral contraceptives and myocardial infarction--the search for the smoking gun. N Engl J Med 2001;345(25):1841-1842.
151. Willett WC, Green A, Stampfer MJ, Speizer FE, Colditz GA, Rosner B, et al. Relative and absolute excess risks of coronary heart disease among women who smoke cigarettes. N Engl J Med 1987;317(21):1303-1309.
152. Redmond G, Godwin AJ, Olson W, Lippman JS. Use of placebo controls in an oral contraceptive trial: methodological issues and adverse event incidence. Contraception 1999;60(2):81-85.
153. Villegas-Salas E, Ponce de Leon R, Juarez-Perez MA, Grubb GS. Effect of vitamin B6 on the side effects of a low-dose combined oral contraceptive. Contraception 1997;55(4):245-248.
154. Graham CA, Ramos R, Bancroft J, Maglaya C, Farley TMM. The effects of steroidal contraceptives on the well-being and sexuality of women: A double-blind, placebo-controlled, two-centre study of combined and progestogen-only methods. Contraception 1995;52:363-369.
155. Rosenberg MJ, Meyers A, Roy V. Efficacy, cycle control, and side effects of low- and lower-dose oral contraceptives: a randomized trial of 20 micrograms and 35 micrograms estrogen preparations. Contraception 1999;60(6):321-329.
156. Mooij PN, Thomas CM, Doesburg WH, Eskes TK. Multivitamin supplementation in oral contraceptive users. Contraception 1991;44(3):277-288.
157. Raman-Wilms L, Tseng AL, Wighardt S, Einarson TR, Koren G. Fetal genital effects of first-trimester sex hormone exposure: a meta-analysis. Obstet Gynecol 1995; 85(1):141-149.
158. Lammer EJ, Cordero JF. Exogenous sex hormone exposure and the risk for major malformations. JAMA 1986;255(22):3128-3132.
159. Contraceptives and congenital anomalies. ACOG Committee Opinion: Committee on Gynecologic Practice. Number 124-July 1993. Int J Gynaecol Obstet 1993;42(3):316-317.
160. Bracken MB. Oral contraception and congenital malformations in offspring: a review and meta-analysis of the prospective studies. Obstet Gynecol 1990;76(3 Pt 2):552-557.
161. Cardy GC. Outcome of pregnancies after failed hormonal postcoital contraception—an interim report. Br J Fam Plann 1995;21(3):112-115.
162. Hemminki E, Gissler M, Merilainen J. Reproductive effects of in utero exposure to estrogen and progestin drugs. Fertil Steril 1999;71(6):1092-1098.
163. Redmond G, Godwin AJ, Olson W. Lippman JS. Use of placebo controls in an oral contraceptive trial: methodological issues and adverse event incidence. Contraception 1999;60:81-85.
164. Rosenberg M. Weight change with oral contraceptive use and during the menstrual cycle. Results of daily measurements. Contraception 1998;58(6):345-349.
165. Lloyd T, Lin HM, Matthews AE, Bentley CM, Legro RS. Oral contraceptive use by teenage women does not affect body composition. Obstet Gynecol 2002;100(2): 235-239.
166. Back DJ, Breckenridge AM, Crawford FE, Hall JM, et al. The effect of rifampicin on the pharmacokinetics of ethynylestradiol in women. Contraception 1980;21(2): 135-143.
167. Barditch-Crovo P, Trapnell CB, Ette E, Zacur HA, et al. The effects of rifampin and rifabutin on the pharmacokinetics and pharmacodynamics of a combination oral contraceptive. Clin Pharmacol Ther 1999;65(4):428-438.
168. Murphy AA, Zacur HA, Charache P, Burkman RT. The effect of tetracycline on levels of oral contraceptives. Am J Obstet Gynecol 1991;164(1 Pt 1):28-33.

169. Neely JL, Abate M, Swinker M, D'Angio R. The effect of doxycycline on serum levels of ethinyl estradiol, norethindrone, and endogenous progesterone. Obstet Gynecol 1991;77(3):416-420.
170. Friedman CI, Huneke AL, Kim MH, Powell J. The effect of ampicillin on oral contraceptive effectiveness. Obstet Gynecol 1980;55(1):33-37.
171. Helms SE, Bredle DL, Zajic J, Jarjoura D, et al. Oral contraceptive failure rates and oral antibiotics. J Am Acad Dermatol 1997;36(5 Pt 1):705-710.
172. Henney JE. From the Food and Drug Administration. Risk of drug interactions with St. John's wort. JAMA. 2000;283(13):1679. (Also available at http://www.fda.gov/cder/drug/advisory/stjwort.htm)
173. Amsden GW, Mohamed MA, Menhinick AM. Effect of hormonal contraceptives on the pharmacokinetics of trovafloxacin in women. Clin Drug Invest. 2001;21(4):281-6. (Available at http://www.medscape.com/viewarticle/406222)
174. Marchbanks PA, McDonald JA, Wilson HG, Folger SG, et al. Oral contraceptives and the risk of breast cancer. N Engl J Med 2002; 346: 2025-2032.
175. Collaborative Group on Hormonal Factors in Breast Cancer. Breast cancer and hormonal contraceptives: collaborative reanalysis of individual data on 53,297 women with breast cancer and 100,239 women without breast cancer from 54 epidemiological studies. Lancet 1996; 347:1713-1727.
176. Lipnick RJ, Buring JE, Hennekens CH, et al. Oral contraceptives and breast cancer: a prospective cohort study. JAMA 1986;255:58-61.
177. Colditz GA, Rosner BA, et al. Risk factors for breast cancer according to family history of breast cancer. J Natl Cancer Inst 1996;88:365-371.
178. Murray PP, Stadel BV, Schlesselman JJ. Oral contraceptive use in women with a family history of breast cancer. Obstet Gynecol 1989;73:977-983.
179. The Centers for Disease Control Cancer and Steroid Hormone Study. Long-term oral contraceptive use and the risk of breast cancer. JAMA 1983;249:1591-1595.
180. Speroff L, Darney PD. A Clinical Guide for Contraception, 3rd edition 2001. Lippincott Williams and Wilkins, Philadelphia, PA.
181. Potter L, Oakley D, de Leon-Wong E, Canamar R. Measuring compliance among oral contraceptive users. Fam Plann Perspec. 1996;28(4):154-158.
182. Bjarnadottir RI, Tuppurainen M, Killick SR. Comparison of cycle control with a combined contraceptive vaginal ring and oral levonorgestrel/ethinyl estradiol. Am J Obstet Gynecol 2002;186(3):389-395.
183. Szarewski A. High acceptability and satisfaction with NuvaRing use. Eur J Contracept Reprod Health Care 2002;7 Suppl 2:31-6; discussion 37-39.
184. Ballagh SA. NuvaRing vaginal contraceptive ring: insertion. Contraception online slide series. Posted December 31, 2002. Accessed at http://www.contraceptiononline.org/slides/slide01.cfm?tk=7&dpg =

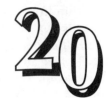

Depo-Provera
Injections, Implants,
and Progestin-Only Pills
(Minipills)

Robert A. Hatcher, MD, MPH

- Progestin-only contraceptives are particularly important for women who cannot use a contraceptive that contains estrogen.

- Counsel clients at initial and at each follow-up visit about menstrual cycle changes associated with progestin-only methods; counseling can contribute substantially to lower discontinuation rates.[1] Ask each woman considering a progestin-only method, "Will it be acceptable to you if your periods change dramatically?"

- Lactating women may use progestin-only contraceptives. Just how soon after delivery they should start remains controversial.

- Progestin-only methods provide no protection against sexually transmitted infections (STIs). Condoms should be used consistently and correctly if intercourse poses any risk of transmitting STIs, including infection with the human immunodeficiency virus (HIV).

- Norplant implants are no longer available in the United States, and there are no plans to reintroduce them. Implanon, the single implant elaborating etonogestrel is now available in 9 European countries and may be available soon in the United States.

Depo-Provera (DMPA). The most commonly used injectable contraceptive is depot medroxyprogesterone acetate (DMPA), marketed as Depo-Provera, given in a deep intramuscular injection of 150 milligrams (mg) every 12 weeks (or 3 months). Depo-Provera is extremely effective, in part because it is forgiving for some women who return late for an injection.[2,3]

Implanon. With a single decision a woman can elect to have 3 years of effective contraception. Implanon is a single 4 cm long implant that releases the progestin etonogestrel at a rate of 60 micrograms (mcg) daily. The method can be reversed any time by removing this one implant.

Progestin-only pills (minipills). Minipills consisting of 0.35 mg of norethindrone (Micronor and NOR QD) or 0.075 mg of norgestrel (Ovrette) are taken every day with no hormone-free days.

Intrauterine contraception. The levonorgestrel intrauterine system (LNG IUS) elaborates 20 micrograms a day of levonorgestrel. The LNG IUS (Mirena) and the copper T 380A (Paragard) are discussed in Chapter 21 on Intrauterine Devices.

MECHANISM OF ACTION

The mechanisms of action of progestin-only contraceptives, which may be administered by mouth, injection, implants, intrauterine devices, and vaginal rings, is summarized in Table 20-1. Progestins may prevent pregnancy by causing the following conditions:

- Ovulation inhibited by decreased GnRH pulse frequency and inhibition of positive feedback of estradiol on luteinizing hormone (LH) and follicle stimulating hormone (FSH)
- Midcycle peaks of LH and FSH suppressed[4]
- Cervical mucus thickened and decreased (an anti-estrogen effect that prevents sperm penetration[4]
- Endometrial changes, including development of an atrophic endometrium[4]

Depo-Provera. Depo-Provera inhibits ovulation by suppressing levels of FSH and LH and by eliminating the LH surge. The pituitary gland remains responsive to gonadotropin-releasing hormone, which suggests that the site of action of Depo-Provera is the hypothalamus.[5]

Implanon. The etonogestrel in Implanon suppresses ovulation (greater suppression than the anovulatory effect provided by Norplant implants), thickens cervical mucus within 24 hours of insertion and leads to an atrophic endometrium.

Minipills. The effectiveness of minipills is greatest when ovulation is inhibited consistently, causing amenorrhea or prolonged periods of time between menstrual bleeding episodes. When ovulation is not suppressed, menstrual bleeding occurs as it had before the woman initiated minipills.

EFFECTIVENESS
DEPO-PROVERA

Depo-Provera is an extremely effective contraceptive option (see Table 9-2 and 20-2). Among perfect users, the probability of pregnancy is only 0.3%. Among typical users the failure rate is 3%. These estimates apply to a 12-week regimen, with each injection providing 150 mg of DMPA per 1 cc.

Table 20-1 Delivery systems for progestin-only contraceptives and combined pills

	Injectable	Implant	Oral	
	Depo-Provera	Implanon	Progestin-only Pill	Combined OC
Administration				
Frequency	Every 3 months	Every 3 years	Daily	Daily
Progestin dose	High	Ultra-low	Ultra-low	Low
Blood levels	Initial peak then decline	Constant	Rapidly fluctuating	
1st pass through liver	No	No	Yes	Yes
Major Mechanisms of Action				
Ovary: ↓ ovulation	+++	+++	+	+++
Cervical mucus: ↓ sperm penetrability	Yes	Yes	Yes	Yes
Endometrium: ↓ receptivity to blastocyst	Yes	Yes	Yes	Yes
First-year failure rate (perfect use)	0.3	0.0	0.5	0.1
Menstrual pattern	Very irregular	Very Irregular	Often irregular	Regular
Amenorrhea during use	Very common	Common	Occasional	Rare
Reversibility				
Immediate termination possible	No	Yes	Yes	Yes
By woman herself at any time	No	No	Yes	Yes
Median time to conception from first omitted dose, removal	6 months	c.1 month	< 3 months	3 months

Adapted from Guilleband (1985).[6]

* By several mechanisms—LH and FSH surges suppressed; preovulatory follicles suppressed

Questions have been raised about the effectiveness of less expensive, more concentrated solutions that provide 400 mg DMPA per 1 cc. This concentrated solution, which is not approved as a contraceptive, does not appear to offer suitable contraceptive efficacy,[7] and administration is more painful. Moreover, it is difficult to provide the exact volume (0.37 cc) required to deliver 150 mg DMPA.

In the largest U.S. study of Depo-Provera use, reported in 1973, continuation rates were 59.4% at 1 year, 41.5% at 2 years, 30.2% at 3 years, and 24.1% at 4 years.[8] More recent studies report lower continuation rates: from 26% to 53% at 1 year.[9-11] Counseling may improve DMPA continuation rates. In rural Mexico, 175 women received detailed, structured counseling at both pre-treatment and each injection visit about the hormonal effects of Depo-Provera, while 175 received routine counseling and information. Over 12 months, only 8% of women receiving structured counseling discontinued use due to amenorrhea or irregular or heavy bleeding, compared to 32% of women receiving routine counseling. The total termination rate was 17% among women receiving structured counseling vs. 43% among women receiving routine counseling.[1]

IMPLANON

An extremely effective contraceptive, Implanon has no scope for user error, so the typical-use and perfect-use estimates are the same. No pregnancies occurred in the first 70,000 cycles studied.

NORPLANT

Although no longer currently available, Norplant is an extremely effective contraceptive, with a perfect-use probability of pregnancy of 0.05%. Because there is no scope for user error, the typical-use and perfect-use estimates are the same. Norplant has a higher rate of pregnancy among heavy women: 2.4% after 5 years among women weighing more than 154 pounds and 1.5% among women weighing 131 to 153 pounds.[12] In Colorado, almost one-third (30%) of teens covered by Medicaid in 1992 chose the implant as their contraceptive. The repeat birth rate was 2.5% after 24 months compared with 22.1% for teens not using the implant.[13] Approximately 84% of women continue to use Norplant implants at 1 year.

MINIPILL

Progestin-only pills are slightly less effective than combined oral contraceptives (OCs). In the first year of use, the probability of pregnancy among typical users is 8%. With perfect use, only 0.3% of women would become pregnant in the first year. A multicenter, double-blind study compared progestin-only pills (containing levonorgestrel [0.03 mg] or norethindrone [0.35 mg]) with two combined OCs (containing 50 mcg mestranol and 1 mg norethindrone or 30 mcg ethinyl estradiol and 0.15 mg levonorgestrel). The pregnancy rates for the progestin-only pills were only slightly higher than the rates for combined OCs; at 670 days, the pregnancy rate for progestin-only pills containing levonorgestrel was lower than the rate for OCs containing mestranol and norethindrone (9.5% vs. 12.9%).[14] A study of 358 nonlactating women who used progestin-only pills for up to 150 months and for a total of 18,125 woman-months of use found a Pearl-index pregnancy rate of 0.2 per 100 woman-years.[15] In lactating women, the progestin-only pill is nearly 100% effective because of the added contraceptive effect of breastfeeding.[16] Drugs that induce liver enzymes, and therefore increase hepatic clearance of progestins, are likely to reduce the efficacy of progestin-only pills. It is not known if increasing the dose of hormone alleviates this concern.[17]

Table 20-2 First-year probability of pregnancy* for women using hormonal contraceptives

Method	% of Women Experiencing an Unintended Pregnancy Within the First Year of Use		% of Women Continuing Use at One Year
	Typical Use	Perfect Use	
Pill (Combined and Progestin only)	8	0.3	68
Evra Patches	8	0.3	68
IUD Copper T 380A (Paragard)	0.8	0.6	78
LNG 20 (Mirena)	0.1	0.1	81
Depo-Provera Injections	3.0	0.3	56
Norplant and Norplant-2	0.05	0.05	84

*See Table 9-2 for first-year pregnancy rates of all methods.

COST

Depo-Provera. In the state of Washington, health departments pay $14.25 for Depo-Provera for one injection. The per-month cost of Depo-Provera is therefore four times greater than the cost of one pack (one month) of pills for the same clinics.[18] If a woman buys Depo-Provera from a pharmacy, she will pay $55 to $65 per vial. In some pharmacies the cost of the co-pay for a woman whose Depo-Provera is covered by insurance is three times the co-pay for a cycle of pills. She will also pay her clinician's office a fee to perform the injection. These expenses do not include routine laboratory tests, the cost of her annual examination, transportation, loss of work necessitated by repeat visits, or pregnancy tests performed by a clinic.

Implanon. The cost of Implanon has not been determined.

Norplant. The Contraception Foundation (1-800-760-9030) provides funds to pay for simple or complicated removals for some uninsured women. *If a woman wants her implants removed, removal must be done regardless of her ability to pay.*

Minipills. Minipills cost more than combined pills, both in pharmacies and in sales to public family planning programs.

A DVANTAGES AND INDICATIONS

Progestin-only contraceptives offer several advantages:

Advantages of All Progestin-Only Methods

1. **No estrogen.** Because progestin-only contraceptives contain no estrogen, they do not appear to cause the rare but serious complications attributable to estrogenic agents (including thrombophlebitis and pulmonary embolism). Studies thus far have not shown that serious cardiovascular effects are associated with use of progestin-only contraceptives.[5,19,20]

2. **Noncontraceptive benefits.** Implanon, Norplant, Depo-Provera, and minipills may lead to several noncontraceptive benefits, including the following:
   - Scanty menses or no menses; less anemia
   - Decreased cyclic menstrual cramps, pain, mood changes, headaches, breast tenderness, and/or nausea
   - Suppression of pain associated with ovulation (mittelschmerz)
   - Decreased risk of endometrial cancer, ovarian cancer, and pelvic inflammatory disease (PID)
   - Management of pain associated with endometriosis

3. **Reversibility.** The contraceptive effects of minipills are immediately reversible. The contraceptive effect of Norplant implants ends immediately when the implants are removed. Depo-Provera is reversible once the effect of the last shot wears off. Depo-Provera does not cause long-term loss of fertility; however, ovulation may not return until 9 to 10 months after the last shot.[3]

4. **Long-term effective contraception.** Implanon and Norplant implants are extremely effective long-term contraceptives. Depo-Provera provides 3 months of highly effective contraception per injection. Minipills provide contraception only for 1 day at a time as long as they are taken.

5. **Low risk of ectopic pregnancy.** Norplant and Depo-Provera reduce a woman's risk for having an ectopic pregnancy compared with women using no contraceptive at all. While the overall risk of ectopic pregnancy is lowered by most progestin-only methods, any pregnancy that does occur is more likely to be ectopic. As many

as 10% of pregnancies among women taking minipills are ectopic.[19] The risk of ectopic pregnancy may be greater in heavier women or in long-term Norplant users (which reinforces the importance of removal or use of a back-up contraceptive in heavier women after 5 years of use).[21] The overall incidence of ectopic pregnancy in women taking minipills is similar to that of women using no contraceptive.[19]

6. **Absence of menstrual bleeding.** Progestin-only contraceptives cause women to have very light periods or to miss periods entirely. This pattern of bleeding is considered by many women to be an advantage, if they have an opportunity to discuss it at counseling sessions. Depo-Provera is especially likely to cause amenorrhea. During the first year of Depo-Provera use, for example, 30% to 50% of women are amenorrheic; by the end of the second year, 70%; and by the end of the fifth year, 80% are amenorrheic.[22] Although clinicians and some women consider the absence of menstrual bleeding an advantage of using Depo-Provera, others do not. In a study of teenagers, nearly two-thirds of Depo-Provera users and one-third of Norplant users reported amenorrhea at 6 months.[23] Over time, Norplant users are less likely to miss periods. Amenorrhea is least common among minipill users.[19]

Advantages of Depo-Provera

1. **Culturally acceptable.** In some cultures, a woman may consider medication by injection desirable. Some women wish to use a contraceptive without the knowledge of their partner. Many couples find Depo-Provera use attractive because it is not coitally dependent. A subcutaneous formulation of Depo-Provera that women could self-inject is being evaluated.

2. **Minimal drug interactions.** There has been no demonstrated interaction between Depo-Provera and antibiotics or enzyme-inducing drugs.[24] The only drug that decreases the effectiveness of Depo-Provera is aminoglutethimide (Cytadren), which is usually used to suppress adrenal function in selected cases of Cushing's disease.

3. **Fewer seizures.** Depo-Provera has been found to decrease the frequency of grand mal seizures.[25,26] Improvement in seizure control is probably due to the sedative properties of progestins. Taking anti-seizure medicine has no impact on the efficacy of Depo-Provera.

4. **Fewer sickle cell crises.**[27]

Advantages of Norplant

1. **Continuation rates.** Norplant has higher continuation rates than do other hormonal contraceptives.[28]

2. **Not coitus-dependent.** Implants are an excellent contraceptive option for women who have difficulty using a contraceptive at the time of intercourse or on a daily basis, including adolescents or for women who are injection drug users.[28-30]

Advantages of Minipills

1. **Not confusing.** Users take the same type of pill every day (same color and hormone content) and do not have a pill-free week or hormone-free week.

2. **Health benefits.** Most of the health benefits of progestin-only pills are similar to combined OCs: decreased menstrual cramps or pain, less heavy bleeding, decreased premenstrual syndrome symptoms, and decreased breast tenderness. In theory, the thick, less penetrable cervical mucus in women on progestin-only pills should decrease the risk of PID.

INDICATIONS

Breastfeeding women. Although non-hormonal methods are generally preferable during breastfeeding, progestin-only hormonal methods may be quite appropriate if care is taken in the timing of initiation so as to avoid fetal effects or a diminution in the production of breast milk. (See the discussion in the section on Special Issues.) If breast milk production decreases, consider switching to a nonhormonal method.

Older women. The decreased risk of thrombotic complications makes Depo-Provera, Norplant and Implanon, and progestin-only pills an advantageous choice for older women. For a woman who may choose sterilization in the next 3 to 12 months, Depo-Provera may be a better option than an implant. Progestin-only pills may also be an excellent option for women who are late in their reproductive years.[31]

Women who cannot take estrogen. Progesterone-only methods may be options for women who want to use a hormonal contraceptive but who have to reasons to avoid estrogen. Women who have developed nausea, breast tenderness, severe headaches, or hypertension while taking combined OCs may be candidates for progestin-only pills. Advise lactating women who desire a hormonal contraceptive that progestin-only contraceptives can be a better choice than combined pills.

Women who need excellent temporary contraception. Depo-Provera provides excellent short-term contraception for women who require maximum protection after rubella immunization, while using Accutane, while awaiting sterilization, for the 3 months following female sterilization using the Essure technique, or at the time the partner is undergoing vasectomy. The 3% failure rate in typical users and high rates of discontinuation strongly suggest that Depo-Provera *not* be the sole contraceptive for women taking Accutane.

DISADVANTAGES AND PRECAUTIONS

1. **Lack of protection against sexually transmitted infections (STIs)**, including infection with the human immunodeficiency virus (HIV). Progestin-only contraceptives provide no known protection against STIs, including HIV. It is possible that vaginal thinning caused by progestin-only contraceptives may increase a woman's risk of acquiring HIV and may increase viral shedding if a woman has HIV disease.[32-34]

2. **Menstrual cycle disturbances.** Menstrual irregularity is the most common reason for discontinuation. Many women experience either an increased number of days of light bleeding or amenorrhea. While amenorrhea becomes less common over time among women using Norplant, it becomes more common over time among Depo-Provera users (Table 20-3).[35] Amenorrhea is more common in women who take minipills punctually. Rarely do women using Norplant or Depo-Provera experience an increased number of days of heavy bleeding. In a very large (18,125 woman-months) study of progestin-only pills, only 40% of cycles were regular[15] (structure counseling helps improve continuation rates).

Table 20-3 Bleeding patterns over a 5-year period among women using Depo-Provera injections and Norplant implants

	DMPA Injections		Norplant Implants	
	1 Yr.	5 Yr.	1 Yr.	5 Yr.
Regular cycles*	30%	17%	27%	67%
Amenorrhea	25%	80%	5%	9%

Sources: Shoup et al. (1993).[36]
Depo-Provera NDA 20-246

* Regular cycle Norplant: 21-35 days
Regular cycle DMPA: 25-34 days

3. **Weight gain.** Some women using progestin-only methods, particularly women receiving Depo-Provera injections, gain weight or complain of feeling bloated. The weight gain is probably due to increased appetite rather than fluid retention.[24] Weight gain is predictable in women using DMPA: 5.4 pounds (average) in the first year, 8.1 pounds after 2 years of use, and 13.8 pounds after 4 years of use (according to the Depo-Provera package insert). Over 5 years, the weight gain among Norplant users averages just less than 5 pounds, close to the average weight gain for women in their early to mid-reproductive years. Weight gain is not an important problem in women taking minipills.

4. **Breast tenderness.** Some women using Norplant, Depo-Provera, and minipills experience breast tenderness.

5. **Depression.** Individual women may experience an increase in depression when they use progestin-only contraceptives although overall levels of depression are not increased. This is because some women become less depressed using a given hormonal contraceptive while others using the same method become more depressed. Depression becomes a particular concern when it occurs in a woman following a Depo-Provera injection because it is not possible to discontinue Depo-Provera immediately.[37] Use caution in providing DMPA for a woman with a history of severe postpartum depression, and consider waiting until 6 weeks postpartum for the first injection. If depression is a concern, try 2.5 or 5 mg tablets of medroxyprogesterone acetate (Provera) orally for 10 days prior to the first Depo-Provera injection.

Disadvantages of Depo-Provera

1. **Not possible to discontinue immediately.** Weight gain, depression, breast tenderness, allergic reactions, and menstrual irregularities may continue until Depo-Provera is cleared from a woman's body, about 6 to 8 months after her last injection. After discontinuing Depo-Provera, women also have a 6- to 12-month delay in return of fertility.[3,8,24] To prevent severe allergic reactions to DMPA, ask women if they have experienced significant itching or redness at site of previous Depo-Provera injections.

2. **Return visits are required every 11 to 13 weeks.** For some women, visits for repeated injections of Depo-Provera are unacceptable. Only from 24% to 70% of women continue to use Depo-Provera at 1 year.[7,9-11] Home visits for injections have been scheduled for some wheelchair-bound patients.

3. **Lipid changes.** Decreases in high density lipoprotein (HDL), and increases in total and LDL cholesterol levels have been found in some studies of women using Depo-Provera.[5,38] These adverse changes in lipids do not occur in women using Norplant.

4. **Allergic reactions.** Although rare, severe allergic reactions may occur. Some programs encourage women to remain in the vicinity of the clinic for 20 minutes after an injection. Ask patients to report itching at injection sites.

5. **Bone density decrease.** Long-term Depo-Provera users may develop decreased bone density.[39] Smoking may be a risk factor. (See section on bone density in Special Issues.)

Disadvantages of Norplant (unavailable at the present time)

1. **Difficult removal.** Both insertion and removal require a minor surgical procedure. Removal is particularly likely to be difficult if an implant was inserted too deeply. Norplant removal requires a clinic visit and occasionally more than one visit.

2. **Drug interactions.** The average release rate of 35 mcg per day is less than 25% of the dose provided by a low-dose combination OC containing levonorgestrel. Because of its low dose, Norplant's effectiveness is more significantly lowered by antiseizure medicines (except for valproic acid) and by rifampin than are other hormonal contraceptives. Norplant failure rates increase to unacceptable levels when a user takes drugs such as carbamazepine, primidone, griseofulvin, phenytoin (Dilantin), phenylbutazone, St. John's Wort, phenobarbital, rifampin, and aminoglutetethemide.[40,41]

3. **Local inflammation or infection.** A pooled analysis of 2,674 first-year users in seven countries found that 0.8% experienced infection, 0.4% experienced expulsion of a capsule, and 4.7% had skin irritation at the insertion site. Complications did not always occur immediately after insertion. Some 35% of infections and 64% of expulsions occurred after the first 2 months of use.[42] Slightly increased pigmentation of the skin occasionally appears over the site of the implants.

4. **Ovarian cysts.** Norplant causes less suppression of the hypothalamic pituitary axis, particularity FSH, than do combined OCs. Most ovarian cysts regress spontaneously and do not need to be evaluated sonographically or laparoscopically unless they become large and painful or fail to regress.[38]

Disadvantages of Minipills

1. **Vulnerable efficacy.** The primary disadvantage of minipills is the need for obsessive regularity in pill-taking.

2. **Extremely low-dose contraceptive.** Certain medications decrease the effectiveness of low-dose contraceptives such as minipills (see Disadvantage 12 above).

3. **Less availability.** Minipills are less likely to be stocked by pharmacies and public family planning clinics. Clinicians are less likely to have had experience prescribing minipills.

PRECAUTIONS

The 2004 World Health Organization (WHO) Medical Eligibility Criteria (Table 20-4) guide health care providers in determining who can safely use various progestin-only methods. In the WHO guidelines, category 1 means no restrictions, category 2 implies a condition where the benefits of using the method generally outweigh the theoretical or proven risks, category 3 means the risks usually outweigh the benefits, and category 4 indicates an unacceptable health risk.[17] As is the case with combined oral contraceptive pills, FDA precautions for progestin-only methods differ from those in the WHO criteria; consult product package labeling for FDA precautions.

Table 20-4 WHO medical eligibility criteria for progestogen-only contraceptives

P   = Progestogen-only pill (POP)

D/NE   = Depot medroxyprogesterone acetate (DMPA)/norethisterone enantate (NET-EN)

PROGESTOGEN-ONLY CONTRACEPTIVES (POCs)	POCs do not protect against STI/HIV. If there is risk of STI/HIV (including during pregnancy or postpartum), the correct and consistent use of condoms is recommended, either alone or with another contraceptive method. Male latex condoms are proven to protect against STI/HIV.	
CONDITION	**CATEGORY** I = Initiation C = Continuation	
	P	**D/NE**

PERSONAL CHARACTERISTICS AND REPRODUCTIVE HISTORY		
PREGNANCY	NA	
AGE		
a) Menarche to <18 years	1	2
b) 18 to 45 years	1	1
c) > 45 years	1	2
PARITY		
a) Nulliparous	1	1
b) Parous	1	1
BREASTFEEDING		
a) < 6 weeks postpartum	3	3
b) 6 weeks to <6 months postpartum (primarily breastfeeding)	1	1
c) ≥ 6 months postpartum	1	1
POSTPARTUM (in non-breastfeeding women)		
a) < 21 days	1	1
b) ≥ 21 days	1	1
POST-ABORTION		
a) First trimester	1	1
b) Second trimester	1	1
c) Immediate post-septic abortion	1	1
PAST ECTOPIC PREGNANCY	2	1
HISTORY OF PELVIC SURGERY	1	1
SMOKING		
a) Age <35 years	1	1
b) Age ≥ 35 years		
(i) < 15 cigarettes/day	1	1
(ii) ≥ 15 cigarettes/day	1	1

(continued)

Table 20-4 Progestogen-only contraceptives—*(cont'd)*

CONDITION	CATEGORY I = Initiation C = Continuation	
	P	**D/NE**
OBESITY		
≥ 30 kg/m² body mass index (BMI)	1	1
BLOOD PRESSURE MEASUREMENT UNAVAILABLE	NA	NA
CARDIOVASCULAR DISEASE		
MULTIPLE RISK FACTORS FOR ARTERIAL CARDIOVASCULAR DISEASE (such as older age, smoking, diabetes and hypertension)	2	3
HYPERTENSION		
a) History of hypertension, where blood pressure CANNOT be evaluated (including hypertension during pregnancy)	2	2
b) Adequately controlled hypertension where blood pressure CAN be evaluated	1	2
c) Elevated blood pressure levels (properly taken measurements)		
(i) systolic 140–159 or diastolic 90–99	1	2
(ii) systolic ≥ 160 or diastolic ≥ 100	2	3
d) Vascular disease	2	3
HISTORY OF HIGH BLOOD PRESSURE DURING PREGNANCY (where current blood pressure is measurable and normal)	1	1
DEEP VENOUS THROMBOSIS (DVT)/ PULMONARY EMBOLISM (PE)		
a) History of DVT/PE	2	2
b) Current DVT/PE	3	3
c) Family history of DVT/PE (first-degree relatives)	1	1
d) Major surgery		
(i) with prolonged immobilization	2	2
(ii) without prolonged immobilization	1	1
e) Minor surgery without immobilization	1	1
KNOWN THROMBOGENIC MUTATIONS (e.g., Factor V Leiden, prothrombin, protein S, protein C, and antithrombin deficiency)	2	2

(continued)

Table 20-4 Progestogen-only contraceptives—*(cont'd)*

CONDITION	CATEGORY I = Initiation C = Continuation			
	P		**D/NE**	
SUPERFICIAL VENOUS THROMBOSIS				
a) Varicose veins	1		1	
b) Superficial thrombophlebitis	1		1	
CURRENT AND HISTORY OF ISCHAEMIC HEART DISEASE	I 2	C 3	3	
STROKE (history of cerebrovascular accident)	I 2	C 3	3	
KNOWN HYPERLIPIDAEMIAS	2		2	
VALVULAR HEART DISEASE				
a) Uncomplicated	1		1	
b) Complicated (pulmonary hypertension, risk of atrial fibrillation, history of subacute bacterial endocarditis)	1		1	
NEUROLOGIC CONDITIONS				
HEADACHES	I	C	I	C
a) Non migrainous (mild or severe)	1	1	1	1
b) Migraine				
(i) without focal neurologic symptoms				
Age < 35	1	2	2	2
Age ≥ 35	1	2	2	2
(ii) with focal neurologic symptoms (at any age)	2	3	2	3
EPILEPSY	1		1	
DEPRESSIVE DISORDERS	1		1	
REPRODUCTIVE TRACT INFECTIONS AND DISORDERS				
VAGINAL BLEEDING PATTERNS				
a) Irregular pattern *without* heavy bleeding	2		2	
b) Heavy or prolonged bleeding (includes regular and irregular patterns)	2		2	

(continued)

Table 20-4 Progestogen-only contraceptives—*(cont'd)*

CONDITION	CATEGORY I = Initiation C = Continuation	
	P	D/NE
UNEXPLAINED VAGINAL BLEEDING (suspicious or serious underlying condition)		
Before evaluation	2	3
ENDOMETRIOSIS	1	1
BENIGN OVARIAN TUMOURS (including cysts)	1	1
SEVERE DYSMENORRHOEA	1	1
TROPHOBLAST DISEASE		
a) Benign gestational trophoblastic disease	1	1
b) Malignant gestational trophoblastic disease	1	1
CERVICAL ECTROPION	1	1
CERVICAL INTRAEPITHELIAL NEOPLASIA (CIN)	1	2
CERVICAL CANCER (awaiting treatment)	1	2
BREAST DISEASE		
a) Undiagnosed mass	2	2
b) Benign breast disease	1	1
c) Family history of cancer	1	1
d) Cancer		
(i) current	4	4
(ii) past and no evidence of current disease for 5 years	3	3
ENDOMETRIAL CANCER	1	1
OVARIAN CANCER	1	1
UTERINE FIBROIDS		
a) Without distortion of the uterine cavity	1	1
b) With distortion of the uterine cavity	1	1
PELVIC INFLAMMATORY DISEASE (PID)		
a) Past PID (assuming no current risk factors of STIs)		
(i) with subsequent pregnancy	1	1
(ii) without subsequent pregnancy	1	1
b) PID—current or within the last 3 months	1	1

(continued)

Table 20-4 Progestogen-only contraceptives—*(cont'd)*

CONDITION	CATEGORY	
	I = Initiation	
	C = Continuation	
	P	D/NE
STIs		
a) Current or within 3 months (including purulent cervicitis)	1	1
b) Vaginitis without purulent cervicitis	1	1
c) Increased risk of STIs (e.g., multiple partners or partner who has multiple partners)	1	1
HIV/AIDS		
HIGH RISK OF HIV	1	1
HIV-POSITIVE	1	1
AIDS (clinically well on ARV therapy)	1	1
OTHER INFECTIONS		
SCHISTOSOMIASIS		
a) Uncomplicated	1	1
b) Fibrosis of liver (if severe, see cirrhosis)	1	1
TUBERCULOSIS		
a) Non-pelvic	1	1
b) Known pelvic	1	1
MALARIA	1	1
ENDOCRINE CONDITIONS		
DIABETES		
a) History of gestational disease	1	1
b) Non-vascular disease		
(i) non-insulin dependent	2	2
(ii) insulin dependent	2	2
c) Nephropathy/retinopathy/neuropathy	2	3
d) Other vascular disease or diabetes of >20 years' duration	2	3
THYROID		
a) Simple goiter	1	1
b) Hyperthyroid	1	1
c) Hypothyroid	1	1

(continued)

Table 20-4   Progestogen-only contraceptives—*(cont'd)*

CONDITION	CATEGORY I = Initiation C = Continuation	
	P	D/NE
GASTROINTESTINAL CONDITIONS		
GALL-BLADDER DISEASE		
a) Symptomatic		
(i) treated by cholecystectomy	2	2
(ii) medically treated	2	2
(iii) current	2	2
b) Asymptomatic	2	2
HISTORY OF CHOLESTASIS		
a) Pregnancy-related	1	1
b) Past COC-related	2	2
VIRAL HEPATITIS		
a) Active	3	3
b) Carrier	1	1
CIRRHOSIS		
a) Mild (compensated)	2	2
b) Severe (decompensated)	3	3
LIVER TUMORS		
a) Benign (adenoma)	3	3
b) Malignant (hepatoma)	3	3
ANAEMIAS		
THALASSAEMIA	1	1
SICKLE CELL DISEASE	1	1
IRON DEFICIENCY ANAEMIA	1	1
DRUG INTERACTIONS		
DRUGS WHICH AFFECT LIVER ENZYMES		
a) Rifampicin	3	2
b) Certain anticonvulsants (phenytoin, carbamezapine, barbiturates, primidone, topiramate, oxcarbazepine)	3	2
ANTIBIOTICS (excluding rifampicin)		
a) Griseofulvin	2	1
b) Other antibiotics	1	1
ANTIRETROVIRAL THERAPY	2	2

Source: WHO (2004),[131] with permission.

For references and update, please consult http://www.who.int/reproductivehealth/
publications/RHR_00_2_medical_eligibility_criteria_third_edition/index.htm

S PECIAL ISSUES
BREASTFEEDING WOMEN

In theory, progestin-only methods may thwart lactogenesis if they are initiated before the post-delivery decline in natural progesterone, which functions as the trigger for milk synthesis.[43] A prudent approach may be to wait until breastfeeding is well established. Unlike the use of combined OCs, use of progestin-only contraceptives once breastfeeding has been established has not been shown to have an adverse effect on breast milk volume; in some studies, milk production has been enhanced. The quality of breast milk is not affected. Because of theoretical concerns over early neonatal exposure to exogenous steroids, several international organizations have urged that progestin-only methods not be initiated until at least 6 weeks postpartum.[17,44,45] It is unlikely that a lactating woman will conceive during this time. (See Chapter 23 on Postpartum Contraception and Lactation.)

Depo-Provera. Studies of Depo-Provera initiated within 7 days postpartum[46] or within 6 weeks postpartum[47] have found no adverse effects.

Minipills. When initiated in the first week postpartum but after withdrawal of natural progesterone, minipills have demonstrated no adverse effects on lactation, infant growth,[16,19,48] or duration of breastfeeding.[49] In one study, 83% of minipill users breastfed for 4 months or longer compared with 40% of combined pill users.[50] Breasfeeding women from 6 weeks on and women with a history of gestational diabetes both received a Category 1 rating in the World Health Organization medical eligibility criteria.[51] However, in one study progestin-only pills have been associated with an increased risk of diabetes in breastfeeding Latinas with recent gestational diabetes.[52]

BREAST CANCERS AND DEPO-PROVERA

Toxicologic studies of beagle dogs given DMPA that showed an increase in mammary gland tumors, some of which became malignant, raised the concern that humans may also be at risk.[53] Several international studies found no effect in humans (Table 20-5). In a New Zealand study, the overall relative risk associated with the use of DMPA was 1.0; however, among women aged 25 to 34 years, the relative risk was 2.0.[54] The risk was greatest among women who used the drug for 6 years or longer. This study suggests that Depo-Provera may accelerate the presentation of breast cancer in young women, perhaps acting as a promoter in the late stages of carcinogenesis. The WHO Collaborative Study failed to demonstrate a significantly increased risk for either breast cancer or cervical cancer among women using Depo-Provera.[55,56] (See Table 20-5.)

BONE DENSITY AND DEPO-PROVERA

In one study, Depo-Provera use was associated with a 3.1% decrease in lumbar bone mineral density (compared to a 9.5% increase among control subjects) after 2 years among women with an average age of 14.2.[57] A large cross-sectional study of women aged 18 to 54 that found a 7.2% decrease in lower spinal bone density suggested the deficit was greater for women who had initiated DMPA use before the age of 21 and for women who had used DMPA for more than 15 years.[58] Since the effects of contraceptives on bone mass may be particularly important for adolescents who have not yet reached peak bone mass, it is important to know if teenagers who have used Depo-Provera regain bone mass after discontinuing DMPA.[59] At this time the World Health Organization medical eligibility criteria suggest that for women from menarche to under 18, the advantages of Depo-Provera generally outweigh the theoretical or proven risk (category 2).[51]

A 12-month study of women in their mid-twenties demonstrated a lumbar bone mineral density loss of 2.74% in users of Depo-Provera compared to a gain of 2.33% in combined pill users on a norethindrone pill, an increase of 0.33% in pill-users on a desogestrel pill, and a loss of 0.37% in controls on no hormonal contraception.[60] *Calcium intake and exercise need to be addressed with each woman receiving Depo-Provera.*

Table 20-5 Risks of 5 types of cancers in DMPA users

Site of Cancer	No. of Cases Who Used DMPA/ All Cases (%)	No. of Controls Who Used DMPA/ All Controls (%)	Relative Risk for Women Who Have Ever Used DMPA*
Breast	39/427 (9)	557/5,951 (9)	1.0
Cervix	126/920 (14)	545/5,833 (9)	1.2
Ovary	7/105 (7)	74/637 (12)	0.7
Endometrium	1/52 (2)	30/316 (9)	0.3
Liver	7/57 (12)	34/920 (12)	1.0

Source: Liskin (1987).[61]

DEPO-PROVERA

PROVIDING DEPO-PROVERA

Before Depo-Provera was approved by the Food and Drug Administration, it was used to minimize menstrual bleeding for adolescents who were mentally retarded or who had emotional or behavioral problems.[29] Take special care in making certain that a woman's use of Depo-Provera is completely voluntary.

Depo-Provera is usually provided from vials of 150 mg in each 1 cc. The label states a 2-year shelf-life (in Belgium, the label states a 5-year shelf-life). Using a sterile needle and syringe, inject the Depo-Provera deeply into the deltoid or the gluteus maximus muscle. Injections into the deltoid are less embarrassing but may be slightly more painful. The 21- to 23-gauge needle should be 2.5 to 4 cm long.[24] Do not massage the area over the injection, because it could lower the effectiveness of Depo-Provera and also cause pain. A subcutaneous formulation of Depo-Provera that women can self-inject is being evaluated.

Schedule injections every 11 or 12 weeks (3 months), although the contraceptive effect usually lasts longer. Some programs provide injections to women who are as many as 4 weeks late. These women are informed that they could have become pregnant during the time they were late. Because ovulation does not occur for at least 14 weeks after a 150-mg injection of DMPA, there is a 2-week grace period for women receiving injections every 3 months. Although the 2-week grace period is supported by published literature, the manufacturer recommends excluding pregnancy before proceeding with re-injection in women who return more than 13 weeks after the previous injection.[62] Some women are late for injections because of fear of cancer, changes in the pattern of menstrual bleeding or other side effects, cost of injections, time lost coming to the clinic, or partner or family disapproval of the method. At Grady Memorial Hospital in Atlanta, clinicians schedule injections at 11-week intervals so that a woman can be as late as 2 weeks for her appointment and still receive her next shot without having to take a pregnancy test or recount her sexual activity during that time.

At each and every 11- to 13-week follow-up visit, ask about weight gain, any problems or concerns, the date of the last menstrual period, and any risk of HIV infection and other STIs. Record the patient's weight and blood pressure. At the time of the annual exam, perform a pelvic examination, take a Papanicolaou (Pap) smear, and, at appropriate intervals, order a mammogram. If the client is not gaining weight excessively or having any unacceptable symptoms or problems, she may continue getting Depo-Provera injections.

MANAGING DEPO-PROVERA PROBLEMS AND FOLLOW-UP

In one of the largest studies of Depo-Provera users, 17% of the 3,875 women complained of headaches, 11% of nervousness, 5% of decreased libido, 3% of breast discomfort, and 2% of depression.[8]

Menstrual changes. Inform women in advance that changes will occur in their menstrual cycles. Do not dismiss the impact of bleeding changes: they are the major reason that women discontinue this method. Spotting or breakthrough bleeding may be managed most easily in a family planning clinic by offering women one or more cycles of combined OCs. Other options include exogenous estrogen or a prostaglandin inhibitor. Five days of pills may be enough. Counseling definitely helps continuation rates (see section on Effectiveness.) Inform women that the irregular bleeding may return. At each return visit inform all women on Depo-Provera that amenorrhea will increase over time, but that it is not harmful.

Allergic reactions. *The Physicians' Desk Reference (PDR) notes that ana-phylactic and anaphylactoid reactions may occur immediately following Depo-Provera injection.* Fortunately, severe anaphylactic reactions are rare. However, because Depo-Provera is irretrievable once injected, have on hand emergency supportive measures such as epinephrine, steroids, and diphenhydramine. One possibility is to encourage patients to stay in the clinic/office area for 20 minutes following an injection.

Common Questions About Depo-Provera

1. *Can a woman who is breastfeeding her baby receive Depo-Provera injections?*

   Yes. Depo-Provera is a reasonable option for breastfeeding mothers. Fully breastfeeding is an effective contraceptive, so as long as the woman will return for her postpartum exam, a fully breastfeeding woman can delay her injection until her 4 to 6 week postpartum exam. Many clinicians in the United States initiate DMPA for postpartum women prior to discharge from the hospital.

2. *Does Depo-Provera cause weight gain, and what can be done about it if it does?*

   Yes, it does appear that some women on Depo-Provera gain weight. All women on Depo-Provera should be encouraged to be careful about food intake and to exercise regularly.

INSTRUCTIONS FOR USING DEPO-PROVERA

Depo-Provera injections are very effective if you return every 12 weeks (3 months) for a repeat injection. Of 1,000 women who consistently get repeat injections on time, only 3 will become pregnant over a year's time. Depo-Provera injections confer a number of noncontraceptive benefits by decreasing the following:

- Menstrual blood flow
- Menstrual cramping
- Risk of anemia
- Risk of endometrial cancer
- Risk of pelvic infection
- Risk of ectopic pregnancy (a pregnancy outside of your uterus)
- Risk of a sickle cell crisis
- Frequency of grand mal seizures

On the other hand, you must be willing to accept unpredictable, frequent, or absent bleeding to use Depo-Provera. About 50% of women using Depo-Provera will stop having any bleeding after a year of injections. This is to be expected and is not harmful. Depo-Provera injections do not protect you from sexually transmitted infections, including infection with the virus that causes AIDS (acquired immune deficiency syndrome). Use a latex or plastic male or female condom every time that sexual intercourse may expose you or your partner to infection.

1. **Have on hand a back-up contraceptive method** such as foam, spermicidal tablets or suppositories, condoms, or a diaphragm. You will need to use your back-up method for 1 week after your first injection. (This precaution may not be necessary if the first shot is given during the first 5 days after the beginning of a normal menstrual period.) Ask your clinician to give you a package of the emergency contraceptive pill, Plan B, or a prescription for Plan B.

2. Because of the rare possibility of an allergic reaction, some programs ask that women remain in the vicinity of the clinic for 20 minutes after having their Depo-Provera injections.

3. **Return to the clinic every 11 to 12 weeks** (3 months) for another injection. Mark your calendar for your next Depo-Provera shot to be sure you will be on time. You may want to get your partner to mark his calendar too. Some programs are beginning to offer women (who have been using Depo-Provera successfully) the opportunity to take home enough Depo-Provera and syringes to last for a full year. If you would like to learn to give yourself your injections of Depo-Provera, ask your clinician.

4. Have a latex or plastic condom ready if you:
   - Are late for your injection
   - May be at risk for a sexually transmitted infection, including infection with the virus that causes AIDS
   - Are using Accutane. *Be sure you have a package of the emergency contraceptive pill Plan B so that you may take it immediately should you ever need it.*

5. See your clinician regularly for routine checkups. Be sure to have a blood pressure check, Pap smear, breast exam, and pelvic exam.

6. Depression and premenstrual symptoms may improve or become worse. If you become severely depressed, see your clinician immediately.

7. There are still some unanswered questions about the long-term effects of Depo-Provera injections on women's estrogen levels and on their bones. This is very important because estrogen is important in preventing heart disease and osteoporosis. Exercise regularly and vigorously and take in adequate amounts of calcium from foods like milk, cheese, yogurt, or ice cream or from several tablets of Tums or calcium citrate a day.

8. Depo-Provera users may gain weight due to an increased appetite. Pay close attention to what you eat and exercise regularly.

Late for Injection

1. **If you realize after intercourse that you have missed your injection or are late for it,** use emergency contraception right away and another contraceptive (or do not have intercourse). You can also call 1-888-NOT- 2-LATE to find the phone numbers of 5 providers of emergency contraception nearest to you. Return as soon as possible for your shot.

2. Schedule your next appointment for 11 weeks so that you have 2 extra weeks of protection should you be late for your appointment.

Depo-Provera and Your Periods

1. Depo-Provera makes a woman's periods less regular, and spotting between periods is fairly common. Eventually most women stop having periods completely. This is not harmful. Do *not* choose Depo-Provera unless it will be acceptable to you to have your periods change.

2. If your pattern of bleeding concerns you, return to the clinic to get a blood test for anemia and to rule out the possibility of pregnancy or infection.

3. If the pattern of bleeding you experience is annoying, contact your clinician. There are medications you can take to make you have a more acceptable pattern of bleeding.

4. When you discontinue taking Depo-Provera, it may be a number of months before your periods return to normal after your last Depo-Provera injection.

Discontinuing Depo-Provera

1. If you are more than 1 week late for your injection, use a back-up method of contraception as soon as you realize that you are going to be late. Visit your clinician as soon as possible for your injection. You will need to continue using a back-up method until you get your injection and for a week after your next injection. Many

clinicians will give you a pregnancy test to make sure you are not pregnant. If you have any questions about whether intercourse may have been unprotected, see emergency contraception.

2. If you discontinue Depo-Provera and do not want to become pregnant, start using a new contraceptive 13 weeks after your last shot. You may start pills or another contraceptive *before* 13 weeks from your last injection.

3. If you are discontinuing Depo-Provera because you want to become pregnant, remember that the contraceptive effect may take a number of months to go away. Be patient.

Depo-Provera and Pregnancy

1. Depo-Provera injections may keep you from getting pregnant for more than 12 weeks (3 months) after your last shot. The average delay in return of fertility is about 10 months from the last injection. Depo-Provera does not decrease your fertility in the long run.

2. If you are 35 to 45 years old and want to become pregnant in the future, you may want to use a contraceptive that has minimal or no delay in return of fertility after you stop using that other method.

Depo-Provera Warning Signals

1. See your clinician if you develop any of the warning signals or any other symptoms that concern you.

Depo-Provera® (The Shot) Warning Signals

Caution

■ Repeated, very painful headaches

■ Heavy bleeding

■ Depression

■ Severe, lower abdominal pain (may be a sign of pregnancy)

■ Pus, prolonged pain, or bleeding at injection site

NORPLANT IMPLANTS

Norplant is no longer available on the U.S. market. However, because the implants are effective for 5 years of use, some women still have the implants in place and continue to rely on them for contraceptive protection. Users have noted a number of side effects that may occur (including headache, ovarian enlargement, dizziness, breast tenderness, nervousness, nausea, acne, dermatitis, etc.), especially during the first year of

Norplant use.[19,21] Occasionally, Norplant implants must be removed to eliminate these complications. This section details the methods for removing implanted Norplant implants. For more information about Norplant in general and about insertion, please consult the 17th edition of *Contraceptive Technology*, published in 1998.

Norplant Removal: 20 Helpful Hints

Most of these suggestions for removal also apply to removal of the Implanon implant.

1. Use the arm model to practice removal.

2. When you perform your first Norplant removal, try to have someone at your side who has experience. Initially, it may take you 45 to 60 minutes to remove the implants.

3. Remind the client that removal may be more difficult than insertion and could require a second visit.

4. Raise the head of the examining table. The patient will be more comfortable.

5. Be sure you are comfortable. You may be more at ease sitting rather than standing.

6. An assistant may be helpful during the removal procedure.

7. Mark both the proximal and distal ends of each of the six implants.

8. Add sodium bicarbonate to the local anesthetic to decrease stinging.

9. Inject the local anesthetic slowly under the proximal 1/3 of the implants. Package instructions recommend that you initially inject approximately 3 cc of 1% xylocaine. Have an additional 3 to 5 cc of xylocaine available in case you need it later.

10. Rather than making your incision at exactly the same site as the location of the incision used to insert implants, you may want to make the incision as close as possible to the tips of all 6 implants. Some clinicians use the same incision so as to avoid a second scar.

11. Make an incision 4 to 10 mm long (see Hint #17, below, for more discussion).

12. Make a second incision if one implant is far from the others.

13. Throughout the procedure, ask the client if she feels any pain and provide additional local anesthetic as needed.

14. With your finger, apply pressure to the distal end of each implant as you remove it. Push the implant toward the incision (Figure 20-1).

15. With a sharp blade, a gauze pad, or Adson's forceps remove the scar tissue covering the implants.

16. Do not pull an implant too hard. It may break.

17. The Emory method of Norplant removal can speed up the procedure. Some clinicians average less than 15 minutes per removal.[63]
    - Use 6 to 8 cc of local anesthesia rather than 3 cc.
    - Make a 8 mm to 1 cm incision rather than a 4 mm incision.
    - Before attempting to remove the implants, gently disrupt adhesions for 30 seconds by repeatedly opening and closing a small curved hemostat in the tissue near the end of the implants.[63]

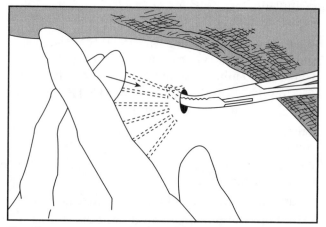

Use of hemostat to remove implant while clinician's finger pushes implant toward incision

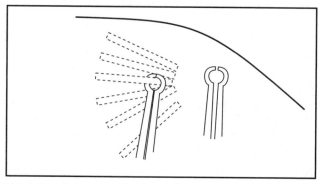

U-technique for removing Norplant implants (similar to use of forceps during a vasectomy)

Figure 20-1 Norplant removal techniques

18. The "U" Technique can also facilitate Norplant removal.[64,65] The instrument is available through Wyeth Laboratories at no cost (see Figure 20-1).

19. Warn your client that she may develop a bruise after removal, but that it will go away completely. Prostaglandin inhibitors may ease any pain in her arm following removal.

20. Remind your client that she may become pregnant immediately following Norplant removal. If she does not want to become pregnant, discuss contraception.

Common Question About Norplant Implants

Is Norplant going to be reintroduced as an option in the United States?

Probably not. This is unfortunate, but perhaps we will soon have the single etonogestrel implant, Implanon.

INSTRUCTIONS FOR USING NORPLANT

See the last edition (17th) of *Contraceptive Technology.*

PROGESTIN-ONLY PILLS (MINIPILLS)
PROVIDING MINIPILLS

Because of the small number of women who use minipills, large-scale studies that document benefits and side effects are unavailable. In general, progestin-only pills have slightly lower effectiveness than combined OCs, more breakthrough bleeding, fewer noncontraceptive benefits, and fewer serious complications.[19] Consult the color insert for photographs and formulations of the minipills available in the United States.

Minipills must be taken on time. Figure 20-2 illustrates how more sperm penetrate cervical mucus if the interval between progestin-only pills is longer than 24 hours. Because minipills must be taken at close to the same hour each day, they may not be the best choice for women who are disorganized. However, an advantage of minipills is that each day, whether or not she is bleeding, the woman takes exactly the same type of pill, with no pill-free interval.

MANAGING MINIPILL PROBLEMS AND FOLLOW-UP

The approaches for managing increased days of light or heavy bleeding, spotting, or amenorrhea are the same as would be considered for the woman using implants or injectable contraceptives: switch to a combined OC, use supplemental estrogen, or use prostaglandin inhibitors. Rule out pregnancy and provide counseling.

As in the case with Norplant and IUD users, when a pregnancy occurs in a woman using minipills, it is more likely to be ectopic because of the contraceptive effect of minipills on the endometrial lining.

INSTRUCTIONS FOR USING MINIPILLS

Minipills are theoretically safer than combined OCs because they have not been shown to increase the risk of either cardiovascular complications or malignant disease and are less likely to cause headaches, blood pressure elevation, depression, and other side effects.[19,66]

Common Questions About Minipills

1. *What effect do minipills have on ovulation?*
   - Users may ovulate every month. Women who have regular periods may be more likely to become pregnant using minipills.
   - Users may never ovulate. A woman may go months without any bleeding.
   - Users may ovulate some months and not others, in which case their periods are irregular.
2. *When are back-up methods of contraception a good idea?*
   - Women with regular periods ovulate regularly and are more likely to become pregnant, so a back-up method would enhance the efficacy of minipills.
   - During the first cycle of taking minipills, a woman may forget pills or take them late.
   - When a woman is several hours late taking a minipill, she should use a back-up contraceptive for 48 hours until she is back on schedule. If in doubt, she should consider emergency contraceptive pills.
   - If the woman becomes anxious every time a period is late, a back-up method will allow her to feel more secure.
   - Anyone at risk for HIV infection or other STIs should use condoms consistently.

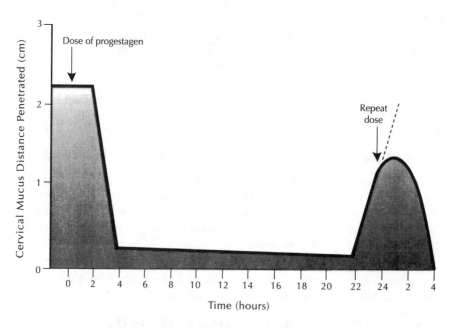

Note: Minimum reduction in sperm penetration between 4 hours and 22 hours after a single dose of megestrol acetate

Figure 20-2 Sperm penetration test following progestin-only pill

INSTRUCTIONS FOR USING MINIPILLS

Minipills are contraceptive pills that do not contain estrogen. When they are taken about the same time every day, only 1 out of 200 women will become pregnant over a year's time.

Minipills have a number of noncontraceptive benefits by decreasing the following:

- Menstrual blood flow
- Menstrual cramping
- Risk of anemia
- Risk of endometrial cancer
- Risk of pelvic infection

On the other hand, you must be willing to accept unpredictable, frequent, or absent bleeding to use minipills. Minipills do not protect you from sexually transmitted infections, including infection with the virus that causes AIDS (acquired immune deficiency syndrome). Use a latex or plastic male or female condom every time that sexual intercourse may expose you or your partner to infection.

1. **Have on hand a back-up contraceptive method** such as condoms, foam, spermicidal tablets or suppositories, or a diaphragm. You will need to use your back-up method:
   - While you are waiting to start your first pack of minipills
   - During your first 7 to 28 days on minipills
   - If you miss a minipill (See the instructions for Late or Missed Pill, below.)

2. You may be able to take your first pill today or on the first day of your next period. Be sure you know when your clinician wants you to take your first pill.

3. Swallow one pill each day until you finish your pill pack. Then start your new pack the next day. Never miss a day and try to take pills at about the same time each day. The evening meal may be the best time to take minipills.

4. Minipills are very low-dose contraceptives. You have a very narrow margin of error, so do not rely on minipills for contraception unless you will be able to take pills *every single day*. Some women use a back-up method at all times to increase the effectiveness of minipills.

5. Have a latex or plastic condom ready if you:
   - Have missed pills
   - May be at risk for a sexually transmitted infection, including infection with the virus that causes AIDS
   - Ask your clinician to provide you with a package of the emergency contraceptive pill, Plan B, or a prescription for Plan B.

6. Depression and premenstrual symptoms may improve or become worse. If you become severely depressed, see your clinician immediately.

7. See your clinician regularly for routine checkups. Be sure to have a blood pressure check, Pap smear, breast exam, and pelvic exam.

Late or Missed Minipills

1. Start taking your minipills as soon as possible.

2. If you miss 1 minipill, take it (yesterday's minipill) as soon as you remember. Also take today's minipill at the regular time, even if that means taking two pills in 1 day. If you are more than 3 hours late taking a minipill, use your back-up birth control method for the next 48 hours (2 days).

3. If you miss 2 or more minipills in a row, there is an increased chance you could become pregnant. Immediately start using your back-up method. Restart your minipills right away and take 2 pills a day for 2 days. If your menstrual period does not begin within 4 to 6 weeks, see your clinician for an exam and a pregnancy test.

4. If you have already had intercourse without adequate protection because you missed pills, call your clinician immediately. You may be able to use an emergency contraceptive. Call 1-888-NOT-2-LATE to find the phone numbers of 5 providers of emergency contraception nearest to you.

Minipills and Your Periods

1. Minipills tend to make a woman's periods less regular, and spotting between periods is fairly common. Some women stop having periods completely. This is not harmful.

2. If your pattern of bleeding concerns you, return to the clinic to get a blood test for anemia and to rule out the possibility of pregnancy or infection.

3. If the pattern of bleeding you experience is annoying, contact your clinician. There are medications you can take to make you have a more acceptable pattern of bleeding.

4. Your periods will return to normal (and you will be able to get pregnant) very quickly after your minipills are discontinued.

Discontinuing Minipills

1. If you discontinue minipills and do not want to become pregnant, start using another contraceptive immediately. Your ability to become pregnant returns right away after stopping minipills.

Minipill Warning Signals

1. See your clinician right away if you have severe lower abdominal pain while using minipills.

2. Return to see your clinician if you develop any of the following warning signals:

Progestin-Only Pills (Minipills) Warning Signs

Caution

- Abdominal pain-May be due to an ovarian cyst or an ectopic pregnancy (Don't stop pills but contact us right away.)
- Delayed period after several months of regular cycles may be a sign of pregnancy
- Repeated, very severe headaches
- Pill taken too late-Even if only 3 hours late, use a back-up contraceptive for the next 2 days. Be careful to use minipill *on time.*

REFERENCES

1. Canto De Cetina TE, Canto P, Luna MO. Effect of counseling to improve compliance in Mexican women receiving depot medroxyprogesterone acetate. Contraception 63; 2001:143-146.
2. Hatcher RA, Rinehart W, Blackburn R, Geller JS. The Essentials of Contraceptive Technology. Baltimore, Johns Hopkins School of Public Health, Population Information Program, 1997.
3. Mishell DR. Pharmacokinetics of depot medroxyprogesterone acetate contraception. J. Reprod Med [suppl] 1996;41:381-390.
4. Croxatto HB. Mechanisms that explain the contraceptive action of progestin implants for women. Contraception 2002;65:21-27.
5. Mishell DR. Long-acting contraceptive steroids. Postcoital contraceptives and antiprogestins. In: Mishell DR, Davajan V, Lobo RA (eds). Infertility, contraception, and reproductive endocrinology. Cambridge: Blackwell Scientific Publications, 1991.
6. Guillebaud J. Contraception: your questions answered. New York NY: Pitman, 1985.
7. Antal EG. Personal communication from Drug Information Clinical Pharmacist at the Upjohn Company to Robert A. Hatcher; March 18, 1993.
8. Schwallie PC, Assenzo JR. Contraceptive use-efficacy study utilizing medroxyprogesterone acetate administered as an intramuscular injection once every 90 days. Fertil Steril 1973;24(5):331-339.
9. Koo HP, Griffith JD, Nennstiel M. Adolescents' use of Norplant and Depo-Provera: how do they do? Poster session at the 1996 APHA meeting.
10. Polaneczky M, Guarnaccia M, Alon J, Wiley J. Early experience with the contraceptive use of depo-medroxyprogesterone acetate in an inner-city population. Family Planning Perspectives 1996;28:174-178.
11. Potter L, Dalberth B, Canamar R, Betts M. DMPA acceptors: a retrospective study at a North Carolina health department (forthcoming).
12. Sivin I, Lahteenmaki P, Ranta S, Darney P, et al. Levonorgestrel concentrations during use of levonorgestrel rod (LNG ROD) implants. Contraception 1997;55:81-85.
13. Sivin I, Viegas O, Campodonico I, Diaz S, et al. Clinical performance of a new two-rod levonorgestrel contraceptive implant: a three-year randomized study with Norplant implants as controls. Contraception 1997;55:73-80.
14. Sheth A, Jain U, Sharma S, Adatia A, et al. A randomized, double-blind study of two combined and two progestogen-only oral contraceptives. Contraception 1982; 25(3):243-252.
15. Broome M, Fotherby K. Clinical experience with the progestogen-only pill. Contraception 1990;42:489-495.

16. Moggia AV, Harris GS, Dunson TR, Diaz R, et al. A comparative study of a progestin-only oral contraceptive versus non-hormonal methods in lactating women in Buenos Aires, Argentina. Contraception 1991;44(1):31-43.
17. World Health Organization. Improving access to quality care in family planning: medical eligibility criteria for contraceptive use. Geneva: WHO 2000 [www.who. int/ reproductive-health/publications/RHR_00_2_medical_eligibility_crieteria_second _edition/index.htm]. Accessed October 14, 2003.
18. Margulies R, Miller L. Increased depot medroxy-progesterone acetate use increases family planning program pharmaceutical supply costs. Contraception 2001(63): 147-149.
19. McCann MF, Potter LS. Progestin-only oral contraception: a comprehensive review. Contraception 1994;Suppl 50:S1-S195.
20. Speroff L, Darney PD. A clinical guide for contraception. Third edition. Philadelphia: Lippincott Williams & Wilkins, 2001.
21. McCauley AP, Geller JS. Decisions for Norplant programs. Popul Rep 1992;Series K(4).
22. Mishell DR, Kletzky OA, Brenner PF, Roy S, Nicoloff J. The effect of contraceptive steroids on hypothalamic-pituitary function. Am J Obstet Gynecol 1977:128(1):60-74.
23. Cromer VE, Smith RD, Blair JM, Dwyer J, Brown RT. A prospective study of adolescents who choose among levonorgestrel implants (Norplant), medroxy-progesterone acetate (Depo-Provera), or the combined oral contraceptive pill as contraception. Pediatrics 1994;94:687-694.
24. World Health Organization. Injectable contraceptives: their role in family planning. Monograph. Geneva, 1990.
25. Mattson RH, Cramer JA, Darney PD, Naftolin F. Use of oral contraceptives by women with epilepsy. JAMA 1986;256(2):238-240.
26. Mattson RH, Rebar RN. Contraceptive methods for women with neurologic disorders. Am J Obstet Gynecol 1993; 168: 2027-2032.
27. de Abood M, de Castillo Z, Guerrero F, Espinoso M, Austin KL. Effect of Depo-Provera or Microgynon on the painful crises of sickle cell anemia patients. Contraception 1997;56:313.
28. Darney PD, Atkinson E, Tanner ST, MacPherson S, Hellerstein S, Alvarado AM. Acceptance and perceptions of Norplant among users in San Francisco, USA. Stud Fam Plann 1990;21(3):152-160.
29. Isart F, Weber FT, Merrick CL, Rowe S. Use of injectable progestin (medroxy-progesterone acetate) in adolescent health care. Contraception 1992;46(1):41-48.
30. Ricketts, SA. Repeat fertility and contraceptive implant use among Medicaid recipients in Colorado. Family Planning Perspectives 1996;28(6):278-280, 284.
31. Bertrabet SS, Shikary ZK, Toddywalla VS, et al. Transfer of norethisterone (NET) and levonorgestrel (LNG) from a single tablet into the infant's circulation through the mother's milk. Contraception 1987;35(6):517-522.
32. Anonymous. More research needed in link between progesterone and HIV infection: clinical recommendations unchanged by monkey study. Contraceptive Technology Update 1996;178:89-92 and Counseling Supplement.
33. Duerr A, Warren D, Smith D, Nagachinta T, Marx PA. Contraceptives and HIV transmission [letter]. Nature Medicine 1997;3:124.
34. Marx PA, Spira AI, Gettie A, Dailey PJ, et al. Progesterone implants enhance SIV vaginal transmission and early virus load. Nature Medicine 1996;2:1084-1089.
35. Sivin I. Internation experience with Norplant and Norplant II. Contraception 1988;19(2):81-94.
36. Shoup D, Mishell DR, Bopp B, Fielding M. The significance of bleeding patterns in Norplant implant users. Obstet Gynecol 1993;77:256-265.
37. Archer B, Irwin D, Jensen K, Johnson ME, Rorie JA. Depo medroxyprogesterone: management of side-effects commonly associated with its contraceptive use. J Nurse Midwifery 1997;42;2:104-111.
38. Speroff L, Darney P. A clinical guide for contraception. Third Edition. Baltimore MD: Williams & Wilkins, 2001.

39. Cundy T, Evans M, Roberts H et al. Bone density in women receiving depo medroxyprogesterone acetate for contraception. BMJ 1991;303:13-16.
40. Haukkamaa M. Contraception by Norplant subdermal capsules is not reliable in epileptic patients on anticonvulsant treatment. Contraception 1986;33(6):559-565.
41. Norplant Consensus Background Paper. July 3, 1997.
42. Klavon SL, Grubb G. Insertion site complications during the first year of Norplant use. Contraception 1990;41(1):27-37.
43. Kennedy KL, Short RV, Tully MR. Premature introduction of progestin-only contraceptive methods during lactation. Contraception 1997;55:347-350.
44. International Planned Parenthood Federation. IMAP statement on breast feeding, fertility and postpartum contraception. IPPF Medical Bulletin 1996; 30(3)1-3.
45. Technical Guidance/Competence Working Group and the World Health Organization/Family Planning and Population Unit. Family planning methods: New guidance. Population Reports, Series J, No. 44. Baltimore, Johns Hopkins School of Public Health, Population Information Program, October 1996.
46. McCann MF, Liskin LS, Piotrow PT, Rinehart W, Fox G. Breastfeeding, fertility and family planning. Popul Reports 1984;12(2),Series J(24):525-575.
47. Koetsawang S, Boonyaprakob V, Suvanichati S, Paipeekul S. Long term study of growth and development of children breast-fed by mothers receiving Depo-Provera (medroxyprogesterone acetate) during lactation. In: Zatuchni GI, Goldsmith A, Shelton JD, Sciarra JJ (eds). Long-acting contraceptive delivery systems: proceedings from an international workshop on long-acting contraceptive delivery systems, May 31-June 3, 1983, New Orleans LA. Philadelphia PA: Harper & Row, 1983: 378-387.
48. McCann MF, Moggia AV, Higgins JE, Potts M, Becker C. The effects of a progestin-only oral contraceptive (levonorgestrel 0.03 mg) on breast-feeding. Contraception 1989;40(6):635-648.
49. Blackburn RD, Cunkelman JA, Zlidar VM. Oral contraceptives—an update. Population Reports Series A, Number 9;28:1, Spring, 2000.
50. Coy JF,Mair H, and Ratkowsky, DA. Breastfeeding and oral contraceptives: Tasmanian survey. Australian Paediatric journal 19(3): 168-171. Sep. 1983.
51. World Health Organization. Improving access to quality care in family planning. Medical eligibility criteria for contraceptive use. Second edition. World Health Organization, Geneva. 2000.
52. Kjos SL, Peters RK, Xiang A, Thomas D, Schaefer U, Buchanan TA. Contraception and the risk of type 2 diabetes mellitus in Latina women with prior gestational diabetes mellitus. JAMA. 1998;280(6):533-538.
53. Finkel MJ, Berliner VR. The extrapolation of experimental findings (animal to man): the dilemma of the systemically administered contraceptives. Bulletin of the Society of Pharmacological and Environmental Pathologists, December 1973.
54. Paul C, Skegg DCG, Spears GFS. Depot medroxyprogesterone (Depo-Provera) and risk of breast cancer. Br Med J 1989;299(6702):759-762.
55. World Health Organization Collaborative Study of Neoplasia and Steroid Contraceptives. Breast cancer and depo-medroxyprogesterone acetate: a multinational study. Lancet 1991;338(8771):833-838.
56. World Health Organization Collaborative Study of Neoplasia and Steroid Contraceptives. Depo-medroxyprogesterone acetate (DMPA) and risk of invasive squamous cell cervical cancer. Contraception 1992;45(4):299-312.
57. Cromer B, Blair JM, Mahan JD, Zibners L, Naumovski Z. A prospective comparison of bone density in adolescent girls receiving depo medroxyprogesterone acetate (Depo-Provera), levonorgestrel (Norplant), or oral contraceptives. J Pediatr 1996;129:671-676.
58. Cundy T, Cornish J, Roberts H, Elder H, Reid I. Spinal bone density in women using depo medroxyprogesterone acetate contraception. Obstet Gynecol 1998;92:569-73.
59. Curtis KM, Chrisman CE, Peterson HB, for the WHO Programme for Mapping Best Practices in Reproductive Health. Obstet Gynecol 2002;99:1100-1112.

60. Berenson AB, Radecki CM, Grady JJ, Rickert VI, Thomas A. A prospective, controlled study of the effects of hormonal contraception on bone mineral density. Obstet Gynecol 2001;98:576-582.
61. Liskin L, Blackburn R. Hormonal contraception: new long-acting methods. Popul Rep 1987;Series K(3).
62. Fotherby K, Koetsawang S, Mathrubutham M. Pharmacokinetic study of different doses of Depo Provera. Contraception 1980;22:527-536.
63. Sarma SP, Hatcher RA. The Emory method for rapid removal of Norplant implants. Contraception 1994;49:J 551-556.
64. Blumenthal PD, Gafikin L, Affandi B, Bongiovanni A, et al. Training for Norplant removal: assessment of learning curves and competancy. Obstet Gynecol 1997; 89:174-178.
65. Praptohardjo U, Wibowo S. The "U"technique: a new method for Norplant implants removal. Contraception 1993;48(6):526-536.
66. Vessey MP, Lawless M, Yeates D, McPherson K. Progestin-only oral contraception: findings in a large prospective study with special reference to effectiveness. Br J Fam Plann 1985;10:117-121.

Intrauterine Devices (IUDs)

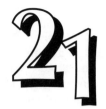

David A. Grimes, MD

- The Cu T 380A and levonorgestrel-releasing intrauterine system rival surgical sterilization in efficacy.
- Intrauterine contraception is highly convenient.
- Intrauterine contraception provides long-term protection against pregnancy yet is promptly reversible.
- In properly selected IUD users, the risk of upper-genital-tract infection is negligible.

Intrauterine contraception is poised for a major renaissance in the United States, due in part to the growing good news about safety, efficacy, and possible non-contraceptive therapeutic benefits. The recent introduction of the levonorgestrel intrauterine system (LNG-IUS) has boosted interest in intrauterine contraception as well.

Opinions about IUDs in the United States are paradoxical. Surveys among women reveal that only a minority of women view IUDs favorably . . . except among those women using IUDs. Among women using an IUD for contraception, 99% reported being "very" or "somewhat satisfied" with the method compared with 92% of implant users and 91% of oral contraceptive users who held these views.[1] An important responsibility for health care providers—and the media—is to provide correct information to consumers and professionals and thus increase the availability and use of this excellent method. In Turkey the media had a large impact, with an information campaign leading to a 30% increase in IUD use.[2]

Options in the United States

Two highly effective intrauterine contraceptives are available in the United States: the Copper T 380A (ParaGard, FEI Women's Health LLC,

New York, NY), and the LNG-IUS (Mirena, Berlex Laboratories, Montville, New Jersey). The progesterone T (Progestasert, ALZA Pharmaceuticals, Mountain View, California), first introduced in 1976, was discontinued in July 2001.

More than 25 million Copper T 380A IUDs (TCu380A) have been distributed in 70 countries. Introduced in the United States in 1988, the TCu 380A is made of polyethylene with barium sulfate added to create x-ray visibility. Fine copper wire is wound around the vertical stem of the T. Each of the two horizontal arms has a sleeve of copper as well. The combined copper surface area of the wire and sleeves is 380 +/- 23 mm^2. The device measures 36 mm tall and 32 mm wide. The bottom of the vertical stem has a 3 mm bulb into which a monofilament polyethylene string is tied; these two strands enable easy removal of the device. The approved duration of use of the device is 10 years, although data indicate high effectiveness as long as 12 years.[3]

The LNG-IUS was approved for use in the United States in 2000. This system has been available in Europe for a decade, and an estimated 3 million women have used it to date. The system releases levonorgestrel directly into the endometrial cavity at an initial rate of 20 mcg per day. This release rate provides high contraceptive effectiveness while minimizing side effects. The rate declines to about 14 mcg per day after 5 years, which is still in the therapeutic range.

The approved life span of the levonorgestrel system is 5 years, although the protection with the system in place may last at least 7 years.[4] The product is based on a NOVA T model polyethylene frame, with a cylinder of a polydimethylsiloxane-levonorgestrel mixture molded around its vertical arm. The cylinder is coated with a membrane that regulates the release of the hormone. Measuring 32 mm in both height and width, the T-shaped frame contains barium sulfate for visibility on X-ray. The base of the vertical stem has dark monofilament polyethylene threads to assist with removal.

Because small amounts of levonorgestrel are systemically absorbed, some systemic side effects can occur. However, the daily dose of levonorgestrel is about 10% that of an oral contraceptive containing 150 mcg levonorgestrel, and the mean plasma concentration is only 5%. Moreover, the plasma concentrations of levonorgestrel are lower than those achieved with either the subdermal levonorgestrel implants or the progestin-only pill.

MECHANISM OF ACTION

IUDs work primarily by preventing sperm from fertilizing ova.[5] Stated alternatively, IUDs are not abortifacients.[6] The TCu 380A causes an increase in uterine and tubal fluids containing copper ions, enzymes, prostaglandins, and white blood cells (macrophages) that impair sperm function and prevent fertilization. The levonorgestrel intrauterine system may have an array of contraceptive actions, including thickening the cervical mucus, inhibiting sperm capacitation and survival, and suppressing the endometrium. The system has a local effect in the endometrium, causing release of foreign-body mediators. In addition, some women do not ovulate as a result of systemic absorption of levonorgestrel.[7]

Two lines of evidence indicate that IUDs work earlier in the reproductive process than previously thought.[6] First, sensitive assays for early pregnancy do not reveal "chemical pregnancies."[8,9] Second, and more compelling, are tubal flushing studies. Investigators have studied women undergoing tubal sterilization at mid-cycle. The fallopian tubes were then flushed and the fluid examined with a microscope to look for sperm and fertilized eggs. In women not using contraception, eggs were recovered from about half. In women using IUDs, no fertilized, normally-dividing eggs were recovered.[10] In addition, IUD users have a marked decrease in the risk of ectopic pregnancies, which implies that IUDs inhibit fertilization.

EFFECTIVENESS

Both of the intrauterine contraceptives available in the United States rank in the top tier of contraceptive methods in effectiveness (including surgical sterilization, implants, and injectable contraceptives). In combined trials by the World Health Organization (WHO) and the Population Council, the rates of accidental pregnancy in the first-year of TCu 380A use was only 0.7 per 100 women, and even lower rates occurred in years 2 through 10.[11] In the WHO trials, the cumulative 12-year failure rate with the TCu 380A was 2.2 pregnancies per 100 women.[3] In three trials conducted by Leiras, the Finnish manufacturer of the LNG-IUS, the first-year cumulative failure rate was 0.14 per 100 women, and the cumulative 5-year failure rate was only 0.71 per 100 women. In the Population Council's randomized trial of the LNG-IUS vs. the TCu 380A, the seven-year cumulative failure rates were 1.1 and 1.4 per 100 women, respectively.[4] In contrast, the overall 10-year failure rate with all methods of tubal sterilization in the United States is 1.9 per 100 women.[12] Thus, contemporary intrauterine contraceptives rival the effectiveness of tubal sterilization.

COST

The initial cost of intrauterine contraception can be expensive. In addition to the expense of the device, the insertion process carries a fee as well. However, when the initial costs are amortized over the life of the device, intrauterine contraception becomes inexpensive—even when compared with condoms. A landmark analysis of the direct medical costs of contraception found the TCu 380A to be the most cost-effective method of contraception over 5 years of use.[13] The costs considered included method use, side effects, and unintended pregnancies. Compared with use of no contraception, the TCu 380A saved more than $14,000. Thus, the acquisition costs of contraception do not accurately predict the real costs of various methods of contraception.

ADVANTAGES OF INTRAUTERINE CONTRACEPTION

- Highly effective
- Protective against ectopic pregnancy
- Long-lasting
- Convenient
- Well-liked by users
- Low risk of side effects
- Cost-effective

Intrauterine contraception is "first-line" family planning. One office visit can provide a decade or more of superb contraception, at a low daily cost. Few methods are as convenient: no need for taking a pill daily or using a barrier method with each coitus. Fertility rebounds promptly upon discontinuation. Modern intrauterine contraceptives have an enviable safety record.

Not only are contemporary intrauterine contraceptives effective against intrauterine pregnancies, they also prevent extrauterine pregnancies as well. The notion that intrauterine contraceptives increase the risk of ectopic pregnancy was debunked long ago.[14] Both the copper and levonorgestrel-releasing contraceptives dramatically reduce a woman's risk of an ectopic pregnancy, compared with use of no contraception.[4,15] For example, in the World Health Organization trials of the TCu 380A, the 12-year cumulative discontinuation rate for ectopic pregnancy was only 0.4 per 100 women.[3]

In addition, intrauterine contraception is often an excellent choice for women who cannot use oral contraceptives because of medical disorders.[16] Women who are poor surgical candidates for sterilization (e.g., because of obesity or severe asthma) are often ideal candidates for this method.

Cancer Protection. One of the most exciting aspects of contemporary intrauterine contraception is the evolving story of cancer prophylaxis. Six case-control studies around the world have examined the potential association between IUD use and development of endometrial cancer.[17–22]

Five of the six found protection against endometrial cancer from devices, and the effect was statistically significant in two (including the Cancer and Steroid Hormone Study of the Centers for Disease Control and Prevention). While the mechanism of action is unknown, it may relate to the altered endometrium associated with intrauterine contraception. Similarly, progestin-releasing intrauterine contraceptives should also protect against this cancer,[23] as is true of contraceptives that deliver a progestin systemically.[24] Two studies examining the risk of cervical cancer among IUD users[25,26] found a 40% reduction in risk, which was not statistically significant.

Medical Benefits of the LNG-IUS. Topical delivery of progestin to the uterine cavity has therapeutic benefits aside from contraception. Some therapeutic indications are well-established and approved overseas, while others are still being explored.

While average menstrual blood loss increases among users of the TCu 380A, the opposite occurs among users of the LNG-IUS. Overall blood loss drops about 90%, and about 20% of women stop bleeding altogether. This translates into clinically important increases in hemoglobin and iron stores. Some evidence supports a benefit in treating heavy bleeding associated with adenomyosis[27] and leiomyomas.[28]

Indeed, the LNG-IUS can be used to treat heavy menses, not just prevent them. Trials have compared this approach to medical treatments with an oral progestin, a nonsteroidal anti-inflammatory drug, or tranexamic acid (not available in the United States). The LNG-IUS proved superior to the other alternatives. In addition, this system has been found an acceptable (and inexpensive) alternative to endometrial ablation or hysterectomy.[29,30]

Another logical use of the LNG-IUS is as part of hormone replacement therapy in menopause. Many women suffer from unpleasant side effects of oral progestins given along with estrogen. In addition, nuisance bleeding is the primary reason women abandon hormone replacement therapy. Use of the LNG-IUS leads to profound suppression of the endometrium, which then ceases to bleed.[29] Lack of uterine bleeding during hormone replacement therapy is desirable for the woman and her clinician.

DISADVANTAGES OF INTRAUTERINE CONTRACEPTION

Menstrual problems. Bleeding problems constitute some of the more common IUD complications. Altered bleeding patterns may be a normal side effect of intrauterine contraception or may signal pregnancy, infection, or partial expulsion. Irregular bleeding is common in the early months of intrauterine contraception. Women using the TCu 380A usually have heavier menses, and irregular bleeding can occur during early use. Irregular but light bleeding or spotting is the norm in the early months of using the LNG-IUS because endometrial suppression takes several months to achieve. Thereafter, bleeding decreases markedly. Counsel women thoroughly about these effects, which tend to be self-limiting.

Cramping and pain. At the time of IUD insertion, the woman may feel discomfort followed by cramping pain over the next 10 to 15 minutes.

Expulsion. Between 2% to 10% of IUD users spontaneously expel their IUD within the first year. An IUD expulsion can occur without the woman detecting it. Nulliparity, abnormal amount of menstrual flow, and severe dysmenorrhea are risk factors for Cu T 380A expulsion.[31] A woman who has expelled one IUD has a 30% chance of subsequent expulsions.[32]

Perforation. Perforation of the uterus can occur at the time of IUD insertion; no evidence supports that notion that IUDs "migrate" outside the uterus thereafter. The most important determinant of the risk of perforation is skill of the person doing the insertion. In experienced hands, this risk is 1 per 1,000 insertions or less. [6]

S PECIAL ISSUES
UPPER-GENITAL-TRACT INFECTION

Flaws in early IUD research exaggerated the risk of upper-genital-tract infection. Rigorous randomized controlled trials[33,34] and reviews of the literature[35] have established that the risk of infection and infertility among IUD users is very low.

Both epidemiological[36] and bacteriological evidence[37] indicate that the insertion process, and not the modern devices or their strings, poses the transient risk of infection. Adherence to "strict asepsis" (widely recommended for the insertion process) is unrealistic. Although sterile technique should be used, endocervical bacteria are routinely introduced to the endometrial cavity, regardless of technique,[37] because no procedure traversing the cervical canal can be devoid of all pathogenic organisms.

Antibiotic prophylaxis should not be used routinely before insertion.[38] Strong evidence supports the benefit of prophylactic antibiotics around the time of induced abortion;[39] by analogy, the same might hold for endometrial contamination at IUD insertion.[40] A large randomized controlled trial in Los Angeles County evaluated the potential benefit of prophylactic azithromycin given before IUD insertion.[33] Overall, no benefit was evident. The more important finding, however, was that salpingitis was rare with or without prophylaxis: only one women out of about a thousand in each group developed salpingitis in the early months of IUD use.

International experience with IUDs has similarly been favorable. In large, WHO-sponsored trials of IUDs, the risk of upper-genital-tract infection was limited to the first 20 days after insertion.[34] Afterwards, the risk returned to a low level and remained there for years. Both randomized controlled trial and cohort studies have revealed that the monofilament string does not increase the risk of upper-genital-tract infection.[35]

Three persistent biases led to the wrong conclusion about the risk of IUD-related infection.[35] First, many studies used an inappropriate comparison group for IUD users: women using other contraceptives. Many of these contraceptives, such as the pill or condom, decrease the risk of salpingitis,[41] thus biasing the comparison against the IUD. Second, systematic over-diagnosis of salpingitis among IUD users is probable. When objective diagnostic procedures are used for diagnosis, the apparent risk of salpingitis associated with IUD use is greatly reduced. This indicates that diagnostic bias accounted for much of the apparent risk. Third, salpingitis is a sexually transmitted infection (STI) in most cases, but many early studies failed to take sexual behavior into account.

The powerful effect of these biases is evident in the Oxford-Family Planning Association cohort study. An early report documented more than a ten-fold increase in the risk of salpingitis among IUD users.[42] After taking into account these biases and after updating their data, the same investigators reported no significant increase in the risk of salpingitis among copper IUD users.[43]

Early assessments of the risk of tubal infertility among IUD users appear exaggerated as well.[44,45] Recent follow-up studies of IUD users discontinuing their contraception have found no significant differences in return to fertility, whether the IUD was removed because of a desire for pregnancy or because of problems with the IUD. This was true in both New Zealand[46] and Norway.[47] Indeed, the common problem among former IUD users was *excess* fertility, leading to induced abortions and unplanned births.

A landmark case-control study from Mexico City[48] was the first to perform *Chlamydia* serology on all cases and controls. The investigators found that prior copper IUD use was not significantly related to documented tubal pathology, even in nulliparous users, whereas the presence of *Chlamydia* antibodies was. Again, this underscores the point that STIs, not IUDs, cause salpingitis.

Little is known about the potential effect of an IUD on acquiring a cervical or vaginal STI. Fair evidence refutes an increased risk of chlamydial infection, but no evidence is available concerning gonorrhea.[35] Women who harbor pathogens in their cervices have an increased risk of upper-genital-tract infection, regardless of their IUD status. However, whether the IUD contributes in any way to that risk is unknown, because no study to date has used the appropriate groups for comparison. Studies to date have compared the risk of salpingitis among IUD users who have an STI vs. IUD users who do not have an STI. The correct comparison would be the risk of salpingitis among IUD users who have an STI vs. women who have an STI but do *not* use the IUD. Few would argue that women harboring an STI have higher rates of upper genital tract infection than do uninfected women; what remains unknown is whether the presence of an IUD influences that risk of salpingitis.

ACTINOMYCES-LIKE ORGANISMS SEEN ON PAPANICOLAOU SMEAR

Several decades ago, a pseudo-epidemic of genital actinomycosis occurred among IUD users. Cytologists and cytopathologists[49] began reporting *Actinomyces* organisms on routine cytology smears, creating alarm and confusion. Current evidence supports the following points[50]:

- The Papanicolaou smear is an invalid test for *Actinomyces*.

- The presence of *Actinomyces*-like organisms on Papanicolaou smear does not predict clinical illness.

- Actinomyces species are normal inhabitants of the female genital tract.

- Vaginal culture is not helpful in diagnosing actinomycosis.

- Pelvic actinomycosis is a very rare, serious, and poorly understood infection.

An asymptomatic IUD user who has "*Actinomyces*-like organisms" reported on Papanicolaou smear should be notified and informed about the significance of the finding. If she is asymptomatic, nothing more need be done. If she has evidence of infection, remove the device and prescribe a course of oral antibiotics. The reason for removal is that, unlike usual gynecological pathogens, this genus of bacterium preferentially grows on foreign bodies. *Actinomyces* species are sensitive to a variety of antibiotics, including penicillin.

PROVIDING THE IUD

WHO GUIDELINES FOR INTRAUTERINE DEVICES[51]

The World Health Organization (WHO) Medical Eligibility Criteria guides health care providers in determining who can safely use an IUD. In the WHO guidelines, category 1 means no restrictions, category 2 implies a condition where the benefits of using the method generally outweigh the theoretical or proven risks, category 3 means the risks usually outweigh the benefits, and category 4 indicates an unacceptable health risk.

SPECIAL POPULATIONS

Women who have not been pregnant. Although "nulliparity" is often cited as a relative contraindication to IUD use, the real issue appears to be "nulligravidity," i.e., never having been pregnant before. Uterine enlargement by pregnancy, even one lost through miscarriage or induced abortion, seems to promote successful IUD use. Sexual lifestyle, e.g., number of sex partners, appears to be a more important risk factor for upper-genital-tract infection than age or parity per se.[52] After its review of the evidence, the WHO[51] listed nulliparity (not having given birth) as category 2, meaning that, in general, the benefits of IUD use outweigh the potential or known risks. However, the WHO noted that nulliparous women have an increased risk of expulsion.

Because of the small diameter of their cervical canals or size of their endometrial cavities, women who have not been pregnant may have a higher rate of mechanical problems with IUDs than do other women. Several steps can facilitate IUD insertion in nulliparous women and thus minimize the risk of a vasovagal reaction. Cervical priming with misoprostol 400 mcg either a few hours or the night before insertion can open the canal. Similarly, one or more osmotic dilators, such as laminaria, left in overnight will gently dilate the canal to a small diameter. Prophylaxis with an oral nonsteroidal anti-inflammatory drug and paracervical anesthesia[53] can help as well.

Women infected with human immunodeficiency virus. IUD use appears safe and effective for selected HIV-infected women who have access to medical care. Because of theoretical increases in the risk of pelvic inflammatory disease among users or female-to-male transmission of HIV to an uninfected partner, several major international medical organizations have discouraged IUD use among HIV-infected women. In contrast, a cohort study in Nairobi showed that these women had no significant increase in the risk of complications, including infection, in the early months of IUD use, as compared with uninfected IUD users.[54] This group of women used the IUD safely for 2 years.[55] Moreover, viral shedding of HIV did not increase in these IUD users.[56] Thus, published evidence does not support the category 3 rating given HIV infection by the WHO.[51]

Women with heart valve abnormalities or shunts. The risk of infectious complications, such as bacterial endocarditis, following IUD insertion or removal is unknown but presumably negligible among women with heart valve abnormalities or shunts. No bacteremia has been found after manipulation of an IUD in the absence of obvious infection.[57] Hence, no evidence suggests that antibiotic prophylaxis is warranted. The question of whether bacteremia can develop after removal of an "infected IUD" is controversial, and prophylaxis may be reasonable.[58] Should prophylaxis be desired, patients deemed at high risk (e.g., prosthetic heart valve) should receive parenteral ampicillin and gentamicin. For those at moderate risk (e.g., rheumatic heart disease), a single dose of amoxicillin 2 g can be given by mouth 1 hour before insertion or removal.[58]

Women with diabetes. Good evidence supports the use of copper-bearing IUDs for women with Type 1 and 2 diabetes.[59–62] Earlier concerns about possible decreased contraceptive effectiveness and increased risk of infection have now been allayed. Data are limited on use of the LNG-IUS in such women, although the low plasma levels of levonorgestrel should not adversely affect carbohydrate metabolism.

Women who have new sexual partners. Women who are at risk of acquiring STIs from a new partner or partners should be advised to use condoms. This is sound advice for any woman, independent of the contraceptive she uses.

Women who acquire chlamydial infection or gonorrhea. No evidence suggests that an IUD should be removed from a woman infected with chlamydia or gonorrhea. Standard treatment and counseling of the woman and her partner(s) are indicated.[63]

COUNSELING ABOUT THE IUD

- Make all presentations, counseling, and educational materials (handouts, flipcharts, and posters) compatible with the language, culture, and education of the patient. Manufacturers provide Patient Package Inserts in Spanish and several other foreign languages.

- During the initial visit, a woman needs counseling to help her select a method, then additional counseling after the IUD insertion to learn about ongoing IUD use.

- Let women handle and examine sample IUDs. Many are surprised at how small IUDs are.

- Be aware of the local myths and misconceptions about IUDs (e.g., that the IUD can "float off" and lodge in distant parts of the body, such as the heart and the brain). Address these sensitively but directly. (See Myths and Misconceptions About the IUD).

- Use a standard checklist to remember important information to tell the user.

- Ask the woman to repeat important information.

- Give each woman an identification card with the name and picture of her IUD, date of insertion, and date recommended for removal.

MYTHS AND MISCONCEPTIONS ABOUT THE IUD

Myth	Fact
IUDs are abortifacients.	IUDs prevent fertilization and thus are true contraceptives.
IUDs increase the risk of ectopic pregnancy.	IUDs significantly reduce a woman's risk of an ectopic pregnancy, because the IUD prevents all types of pregnancies. Should a pregnancy occur with an IUD in place, the ratio of ectopic to intrauterine pregnancies may be increased.
IUDs expose the provider to medicolegal risk.	In past decades, product liability suits against manufacturers alleged inherently unsafe products and/or failure to warn of risks. Today, IUDs have been judged safe by the Food and Drug Administration. Package inserts and patient brochures provide extensive information about risks and benefits. Hence, litigation related to IUDs has virtually disappeared.
IUDs increase the risk of PID.	The IUD itself appears to have no effect on the risk of upper-genital-tract infection. Rather, the insertion process carries a small, transient risk in some women. The risk of PID in appropriately selected IUD candidates is so small that prophylactic antibiotics are not warranted.

PROVIDER TRAINING

With appropriate training, a broad range of trained personnel including nurses, nurse-midwives, physician assistants, and paramedical personnel can safely insert the IUD. Practice IUD insertions first on a model, then counsel women and insert an adequate number of IUDs under supervision to demonstrate your proficiency. Rather than an absolute number requirement, a level of proficiency in varying insertion situations (different uterine positions) should be the criterion for certification. Because the levonorgestrel system has a different insertion device and process than the TCu 380A, clinicians should be trained before beginning to insert the devices.

INSERTION TIMING

No scientific reason supports the common practice of inserting the IUD only during menstrual bleeding.[6,64] The inconvenience and cost to the woman caused by such a policy can be substantial. Allowing insertion at any time during the entire menstrual cycle gives the woman and her provider more flexible appointment times. An IUD can be inserted provided reasonable assurance (e.g., negative results on a sensitive pregnancy test) exists that the woman is not pregnant.

Extensive experience overseas has shown that IUD insertion immediately after abortion or delivery is both feasible and safe. A recent systematic review[65] of randomized controlled trials of immediate post-abortal insertion showed low rates of perforation and pelvic inflammatory disease (PID), however, IUD insertion after second-trimester abortions was associated with high expulsion rates. Only one trial directly compared the success of IUD insertion immediately after abortion vs. having the woman return at a later date (delayed insertion). The performance of the Copper 7 inserted immediately was inferior to that of delayed insertion, although the difference was not statistically significant. Of note, however, 42% of women scheduled to return for delayed insertion did not return. Evidence is insufficient to compare immediate post-abortal vs. delayed interval insertion of IUDs.

Insertion of IUDs immediately after delivery is popular in many countries, including China, Mexico, and Egypt. Another systematic review[66] of randomized controlled trials found no direct comparisons of immediate vs. delayed vs. interval insertion. Nevertheless, immediate insertions appeared both safe and practical. Advantages of this practice include convenience, high motivation, and assurance that the woman is not pregnant. On the other hand, expulsions appear to be higher than with interval insertions. Modifications to existing IUDs did not improve performance. Whether insertion was done by hand or by instrument made little difference in subsequent outcomes.

A case-control study from the United States suggested a dramatic increase in the risk of IUD perforation if the woman was breastfeeding.[67] However, other large cohort studies have not confirmed this conclusion.[68] Thus, breastfeeding is not a contraindication to IUD insertion.[69]

INSERTION TECHNIQUE

Review the IUD insertion procedure with the woman. Consider administering a non-steroidal anti-inflammatory drug (NSAID) an hour before procedure.

Before inserting the IUD, perform a careful pelvic examination to judge the direction of the uterus and its axial length. In general, a length of 6-9 cm leads to successful use; a shorter length may increase the risk of expulsion and other mechanical problems. Anatomic abnormalities that distort the uterine cavity, such as a bicornuate uterus or submucous leiomyomas, are considered contraindications. More detailed information is available in the World Health Organization guidelines (Table 21-1).

Table 21-1 WHO medical eligibility criteria

Intrauterine Devices (IUDs)

Cu	= Copper-bearing IUD
LNG	= Levonorgestrel-releasing IUD (20 µg/24hours)
COC	= Combined oral contraceptives
POC	= Progestin-only contraceptives

INTRAUTERINE DEVICES (IUDs)	IUDs do not protect against STI/HIV. If there is risk of STI/HIV (including the postpartum period), the correct and consistent use of condoms is recommended, either alone or with another contraceptive method. Male latex condoms are proven to protect against STI/HIV.	
CONDITION	**CATEGORY** I=Initiation, C=Continuation **Cu LNG**	**NEW EVIDENCE /COMMENTS**

PERSONAL CHARACTERISTICS AND REPRODUCTIVE HISTORY			
PREGNANCY	4	4	The IUD is not indicated during pregnancy and should not be used because of the risk of serious pelvic infection and septic spontaneous abortion.
AGE			
a) Menarche to < 20 years	2	2	There is concern both about the risk of expulsion due to nulliparity and risk of STIs due to sexual behaviour in younger age-groups.
b) ≥ 20 years	1	1	
PARITY			
a) Nulliparous	2	2	Nulliparity is related to an increased risk of expulsion.
b) Parous	1	1	
POSTPARTUM (breastfeeding or non-breastfeeding, including post-caesarean section)			
a) < 48 hours	2	3	There is an increased risk of expulsion for IUD insertion done within the first 48 hours postpartum.
b) 48 hours to < 4 weeks	3	3	

(continued)

Table 21-1 WHO medical eligibility criteria — (cont'd)

INTRAUTERINE DEVICES (IUDs)	IUDs do not protect against STI/HIV. If there is risk of STI/HIV (including the postpartum period), the correct and consistent use of condoms is recommended, either alone or with another contraceptive method. Male latex condoms are proven to protect against STI/HIV.		
CONDITION	**CATEGORY** I=Initiation, C=Continuation		**NEW EVIDENCE /COMMENTS**
	Cu	**LNG**	

POSTPARTUM—*(cont'd)*

c) ≥ 4 weeks	1	1	There is a lack of data on the local effects of LNG-IUDs on uterine involution. Concern that the neonate may be at risk due to exposure to steroid hormones during the first 6 weeks postpartum is the same as for other POCs.
			There is an increased risk of perforation for IUD insertions done after 48 hours and up to 4 weeks postpartum.
			If breastfeeding, LNG-IUD is a category 3 until 6 weeks postpartum.
d) Puerperal sepsis	4	4	Insertion of an IUD may substantially worsen the condition.

POST-ABORTION

a) First trimester	1	1	IUDs can be inserted immediately after first trimester spontaneous or induced abortion.
b) Second trimester	2	2	There is some concern about the risk of expulsion after second trimester abortion. There is a lack of data on the local effects of LNG-IUD on uterine involution.
c) Immediate post-septic abortion	4	4	Insertion of an IUD may substantially worsen the condition.
PAST ECTOPIC PREGNANCY	1	1	The absolute risk of ectopic pregnancy is extremely low due to the high effectiveness of IUDs. However, when a woman becomes pregnant during IUD use the relative likelihood of ectopic pregnancy is increased.

(continued)

Table 21-1 WHO medical eligibility criteria — *(cont'd)*

INTRAUTERINE DEVICES (IUDs)	IUDs do not protect against STI/HIV. If there is risk of STI/HIV (including the postpartum period), the correct and consistent use of condoms is recommended, either alone or with another contraceptive method. Male latex condoms are proven to protect against STI/HIV.		
CONDITION	**CATEGORY** I=Initiation, C=Continuation		**NEW EVIDENCE/COMMENTS**
	Cu	**LNG**	
HISTORY OF PELVIC SURGERY (see postpartum, including caesarean section)	1	1	
SMOKING			
a) Age < 35 years	1	1	
b) Age ≥ 35 years			
(i) < 15 cigarettes/day	1	1	
(ii) ≥ 15 cigarettes/day	1	1	
OBESITY ≥ 30 kg/m2 body mass index (BMI)	1	2	
ANATOMICAL ABNORMALITIES			
a) Distorted uterine cavity (any congenital or acquired uterine abnormality distorting the uterine cavity in a manner that is incompatible with IUD insertion)	4	4	In the presence of an anatomic abnormality that distorts the uterine cavity, proper IUD placement may not be possible.
b) Other abnormalities (including cervical stenosis or cervical lacerations) not distorting the uterine cavity or interfering with IUD insertion	2	2	
BLOOD PRESSURE MEASUREMENT UNAVAILABLE	NA	NA	While a blood pressure measurement may be appropriate for good preventative health care, it is not materially related to safe and effective IUD use. Women should not be denied use of IUDs simply because their blood pressure cannot be measured.

(continued)

Table 21-1 WHO medical eligibility criteria — *(cont'd)*

INTRAUTERINE DEVICES (IUDs)	IUDs do not protect against STI/HIV. If there is risk of STI/HIV (including the postpartum period), the correct and consistent use of condoms is recommended, either alone or with another contraceptive method. Male latex condoms are proven to protect against STI/HIV.		
CONDITION	CATEGORY I=Initiation, C=Continuation		NEW EVIDENCE /COMMENTS
	Cu	LNG	

CARDIOVASCULAR DISEASE

	Cu	LNG	
MULTIPLE RISK FACTORS FOR ARTERIAL CARDIOVASCULAR DISEASE (such as older age, smoking, diabetes and hypertension)	1	2	When multiple major risk factors exist, risk of cardiovascular disease may increase substantially. Some progestogens may increase the risk of thrombosis, although this increase is substantially less than for COCs.
HYPERTENSION			
a) History of hypertension where blood pressure CANNOT be evaluated (Including hypertension in pregnancy)	1	2	There is theoretical concern about the effect of LNG on lipids. There is no restriction for copper IUDs. LNG use may decrease HDL levels.
b) Adequately controlled hypertension where blood pressure CAN be evaluated	1	1	
c) Elevated blood pressure levels (properly taken measurements)			
(i) systolic 140-159 or diastolic 90-99	1	1	
(ii) systolic ≥ 160 or diastolic ≥ 100	1	2	
d) Vascular disease	1	2	
HISTORY OF HIGH BLOOD PRESSURE DURING PREGNANCY (where current blood pressure is measurable and normal)	1	1	

(continued)

Table 21-1 WHO medical eligibility criteria — *(cont'd)*

INTRAUTERINE DEVICES (IUDs)	IUDs do not protect against STI/HIV. If there is risk of STI/HIV (including the postpartum period), the correct and consistent use of condoms is recommended, either alone or with another contraceptive method. Male latex condoms are proven to protect against STI/HIV.		
CONDITION	**CATEGORY** I=Initiation, C=Continuation		**NEW EVIDENCE/COMMENTS**
	Cu	**LNG**	

CONDITION	Cu	LNG	NEW EVIDENCE/COMMENTS
DEEP VENOUS THROMBOEMBOLISM (DVT)/ PULMONARY EMBOLISM (PE)			
a) History of DVT/PE	1	2	Some progestogens may increase the risk of venous thrombosis, although this increase is substantially less than for COCs.
b) Current DVT/PE	1	3	
c) Family history of DVT/PE (first-degree relatives)	1	1	
d) Major surgery			
(i) *with prolonged immobilization*	1	2	
(ii) *without prolonged immobilization*	1	1	
e) Minor surgery without immobilization	1	1	
SUPERFICIAL VENOUS THROMBOSIS			
a) Varicose veins	1	1	
b) Superficial thrombophlebitis	1	1	

CONDITION	Cu	LNG I	LNG C	NEW EVIDENCE/COMMENTS
CURRENT AND HISTORY OF ISCHAEMIC HEART DISEASE	1	2	3	LNG may reduce HDL levels.
STROKE (history of cerebrovascular accident)	1	2		LNG may reduce HDL levels. Some progestogens may increase the risk of thrombosis, although this increase is substantially less than for COCs.
KNOWN HYPERLIPIDAEMIAS	1	2		Routine screening is not appropriate because of the rarity of the condition. Some types of hyperlipidaemias are a risk factor for vascular disease, which may be affected by LNG.

(continued)

Table 21-1 WHO medical eligibility criteria — (cont'd)

INTRAUTERINE DEVICES (IUDs)	IUDs do not protect against STI/HIV. If there is risk of STI/HIV (including the postpartum period), the correct and consistent use of condoms is recommended, either alone or with another contraceptive method. Male latex condoms are proven to protect against STI/HIV.		

CONDITION	CATEGORY I=Initiation, C=Continuation		NEW EVIDENCE/COMMENTS
	Cu	LNG	
VALVULAR HEART DISEASE			
a) Uncomplicated	1	1	
b) Complicated (pulmonary hypertension, risk of arterial fibrillation, history of subacute bacterial endocarditis, on anti-coagulant treatment)	2	2	Prophylactic antibiotics to prevent endocarditis are advised for insertion.

NEUROLOGIC CONDITIONS

HEADACHES		I	C	
a) Non migrainous (mild or severe)	1	1	1	
b) Migraine				There is concern that migraine headaches may increase with use of LNG-IUDs, although there is less concern than with POCs. Some POCs may increase the risk of thrombosis, although this increase is substantially less than with COCs. Any new headaches or marked changes in headaches should be evaluated.
(i) without focal neurologic symptoms				
Age < 35	1	2	2	
Age ≥ 35	1	2	2	
(ii) with focal neurologic symptoms (at any age)	1	2	3	
EPILEPSY	1	1		

REPRODUCTIVE TRACT INFECTIONS AND DISORDERS

VAGINAL BLEEDING PATTERNS		I	C	
a) Irregular pattern *without* heavy bleeding	1	1	1	

(continued)

Table 21-1 WHO medical eligibility criteria — *(cont'd)*

INTRAUTERINE DEVICES (IUDs)	IUDs do not protect against STI/HIV. If there is risk of STI/HIV (including the postpartum period), the correct and consistent use of condoms is recommended, either alone or with another contraceptive method. Male latex condoms are proven to protect against STI/HIV.			
CONDITION	**CATEGORY** I=Initiation, C=Continuation			**NEW EVIDENCE/COMMENTS**
	Cu		**LNG**	
b) Heavy or prolonged bleeding (includes regular and irregular patterns)	2		1 2	Unusually heavy bleeding should cause suspicion of a serious underlying pathology. LNG-IUD use may actually be indicated to correct heavy bleeding. LNG-IUD use may induce irregular bleeding patterns, especially during the first 3–6 months, but these patterns may persist longer. The amount of blood loss is always reduced, which may be a desirable effect in many women.
UNEXPLAINED VAGINAL BLEEDING (suspicion for serious condition)				If pregnancy or an underlying pathological condition (such as pelvic malignancy) is suspected, it must be evaluated and the category adjusted after evaluation. There is no need to remove the IUD before evaluation.
	I	**C**	**I** **C**	
Before evaluation	4	2	4 2	
ENDOMETRIOSIS	2		1	Copper IUD use may worsen dysmenorrhoea associated with the condition.
BENIGN OVARIAN TUMOURS (including cysts)	1		1	
SEVERE DYSMENORRHOEA	2		1	Dysmenorrhoea may intensify with copper IUD use. LNG-IUD use has been associated with reduction of dysmenorrhoea.
TROPHOBLAST DISEASE				
a) Benign gestational trophoblastic disease	3		3	
b) Malignant gestational trophoblastic disease	4		4	There is an increased risk of perforation since the treatment for the condition may require multiple uterine curettages.
CERVICAL ECTROPION	1		1	

(continued)

Table 21-1 WHO medical eligibility criteria — *(cont'd)*

INTRAUTERINE DEVICES (IUDs)	IUDs do not protect against STI/HIV. If there is risk of STI/HIV (including the postpartum period), the correct and consistent use of condoms is recommended, either alone or with another contraceptive method. Male latex condoms are proven to protect against STI/HIV.				
CONDITION	**CATEGORY** I=Initiation, C=Continuation				**NEW EVIDENCE/COMMENTS**
	Cu		**LNG**		

CONDITION	Cu		LNG		NEW EVIDENCE/COMMENTS
CERVICAL INTRAEPITHELIAL NEOPLASIA (CIN)	1		2		There is some theoretical concern that LNG-IUDs may enhance progression of CIN.
CERVICAL CANCER (awaiting treatment)	**I**	**C**	**I**	**C**	There is concern about the increased risk of infection and bleeding at insertion, which may make the condition worse. The IUD will likely need to be removed at the time of treatment but, until then, the woman is at risk of pregnancy.
	4	2	4	2	
BREAST DISEASE					
a) Undiagnosed mass	1		2		
b) Benign breast disease	1		1		
c) Family history of cancer	1		1		
d) Cancer:					Breast cancer is a hormonally sensitive tumour. Concerns about progression of the disease may be less with LNG-IUDs than with COCs or higher-dose POCs.
(i) current	1		4		
(ii) past and no evidence of current disease for 5 years	1		3		
ENDOMETRIAL CANCER	**I**	**C**	**I**	**C**	
	4	2	4	2	There is concern about the increased risk of infection, perforation and bleeding at insertion, that may make the condition worse. The IUD will likely need to be removed at the time of treatment but, until then, the woman is at risk of pregnancy.
OVARIAN CANCER	3	2	3	2	The IUD will likely need to be removed at the time of treatment but, until then, the woman is at risk of pregnancy.
UTERINE FIBROIDS					
a) Without distortion of the uterine cavity	2		2		
b) With distortion of the uterine cavity	4		4		Pre-existing uterine fibroids that distort the uterine cavity may be incompatible with IUD insertion.

(continued)

Table 21-1 WHO medical eligibility criteria — (cont'd)

INTRAUTERINE DEVICES (IUDs)	IUDs do not protect against STI/HIV. If there is risk of STI/HIV (including the postpartum period), the correct and consistent use of condoms is recommended, either alone or with another contraceptive method. Male latex condoms are proven to protect against STI/HIV.				
CONDITION	**CATEGORY** I=Initiation, C=Continuation				**NEW EVIDENCE/COMMENTS**
	Cu		**LNG**		
	I	C	I	C	
PELVIC INFLAMMATORY DISEASE (PID)					
a) Past PID (assuming no known current risk factors for STIs)					Barrier methods, especially condoms, are always recommended for prevention of STI/HIV/PID.
(i) with subsequent pregnancy	1	1	1	1	
(ii) without subsequent pregnancy	2	2	2	2	In women at low risk of STIs, IUD insertion poses little risk of PID. Current risk of STIs and desire for future pregnancy are relevant considerations.
b) PID—current or within the last 3 months	4	3	4	3	There is serious concern that IUD use may worsen current PID. Recent PID is a strong risk factor for subsequent PID. Continued use of an IUD depends on the client's current risk factors for STIs and PID and her informed choice.
STIs					
a) Current or within 3 months (including purulent cervicitis)	4		4		There is serious concern that IUD use increases risk of PID in women with current STIs, or who are at high risk of acquiring these infections.
b) Vaginitis without purulent cervicitis	2		2		Where background incidence of STIs is high, vaginitis may indicate an STI.
c) Increased risk of STIs (e.g., multiple partners or partner who has multiple partners)	3		3		
HIV/AIDS					
HIGH RISK OF HIV	3		3		Women at high risk of HIV are also at high risk of other STIs.

(continued)

Table 21-1 WHO medical eligibility criteria — *(cont'd)*

INTRAUTERINE DEVICES (IUDs)	IUDs do not protect against STI/HIV. If there is risk of STI/HIV (including the postpartum period), the correct and consistent use of condoms is recommended, either alone or with another contraceptive method. Male latex condoms are proven to protect against STI/HIV.				
CONDITION	CATEGORY I=Initiation, C=Continuation				NEW EVIDENCE/COMMENTS
	Cu		LNG		
HIV-POSITIVE	3		3		There are theoretical concerns about increased risks of STIs and PID and increased risks of transmission to uninfected partners, particularly for immunosuppressed women.
AIDS	3		3		

OTHER INFECTIONS

SCHISTOSOMIASIS

	Cu		LNG		
a) Uncomplicated	1		1		
b) Fibrosis of the liver (if severe, see cirrhosis)	1		1		

TUBERCULOSIS	I	C	I	C	
a) Non-pelvic	1	1	1	1	
b) Known pelvic	4	3	4	3	Insertion of an IUD may substantially worsen the condition.

	Cu		LNG		
MALARIA	1		1		

ENDOCRINE CONDITIONS

DIABETES

	Cu		LNG		
a) History of gestational disease	1		1		LNG use may slightly influence carbohydrate and lipid metabolism. Whether the amount of LNG released by the IUD causes such change is unclear.
b) Non-vascular disease					
(i) non-insulin dependent	1		2		
(ii) insulin dependent	1		2		
c) Nephropathy / retinopathy / neuropathy	1		2		Some progestogens may increase the risk of thrombosis, although this increase is substantially less than for COCs.
d) Other vascular disease or diabetes of > 20 years' duration	1		2		

(continued)

Table 21-1 WHO medical eligibility criteria — *(cont'd)*

INTRAUTERINE DEVICES (IUDs)	IUDs do not protect against STI/HIV. If there is risk of STI/HIV (including the postpartum period), the correct and consistent use of condoms is recommended, either alone or with another contraceptive method. Male latex condoms are proven to protect against STI/HIV.		
CONDITION	CATEGORY I=Initiation, C=Continuation		NEW EVIDENCE/COMMENTS
	Cu	LNG	

CONDITION	Cu	LNG	NEW EVIDENCE/COMMENTS
THYROID			
a) Simple goitre	1	1	
b) Hyperthyroid	1	1	
c) Hypothyroid	1	1	
GASTROINTESTINAL CONDITIONS			
GALL-BLADDER DISEASE			
a) Symptomatic			**New evidence:** Some progestogens may cause a small increase in risk of gall bladder disease. There is also concern that progestogens may worsen existing gall-bladder disease.
(i) *treated by cholecystectomy*	1	2	
(ii) *medically treated*	1	2	
(iii) *current*	1	2	
b) Asymptomatic	1	2	
HISTORY OF CHOLESTASIS			
a) Pregnancy-related	1	1	
b) Past COC-related	1	2	There is concern that history of COC-related cholestasis may predict subsequent cholestasis with LNG use. Whether there is any risk with use of LNG-IUD is unclear.
VIRAL HEPATITIS			
a) Active	1	3	There is concern about hormonal load associated with LNG-IUD use in active liver disease, but it is less than for COCs.
b) Carrier	1	1	
CIRRHOSIS			
a) Mild (compensated)	1	2	There is concern about hormonal load associated with LNG-IUD use in active liver disease, but it is less than for COCs.
b) Severe (decompensated)	1	3	

(continued)

Table 21-1 WHO medical eligibility criteria — (cont'd)

INTRAUTERINE DEVICES (IUDs)	IUDs do not protect against STI/HIV. If there is risk of STI/HIV (including the postpartum period), the correct and consistent use of condoms is recommended, either alone or with another contraceptive method. Male latex condoms are proven to protect against STI/HIV.		
CONDITION	**CATEGORY** I=Initiation, C=Continuation		**NEW EVIDENCE/COMMENTS,**
	Cu	**LNG**	

LIVER TUMOURS

	Cu	LNG	
a) Benign (adenoma)	1	3	Progestogens are metabolized by the liver, and their use may adversely affect women whose liver function is compromised. In addition, progestogen use may enhance the growth of tumours. This concern is similar to, but less than, that for COCs.
b) Malignant (hepatoma)	1	3	

ANAEMIAS

	Cu	LNG	
THALASSAEMIA	2	1	There is concern about an increased risk of blood loss with copper IUDs.
SICKLE CELL DISEASE	2	1	There is concern about an increased risk of blood loss with copper IUDs.
IRON DEFICIENCY ANAEMIA	2	1	There is concern about an increased risk of blood loss with copper IUDs.

DRUG INTERACTIONS

COMMONLY USED DRUGS WHICH AFFECT LIVER ENZYMES

	Cu	LNG	
a) Certain antibiotics (rifampicin and griseofulvin)	1	1	LNG-IUDs function chiefly by local levonorgestrel effect; systemic progestogen metabolism will not affect local efficacy.
b) Anticonvulsants (phenytoin, carbamazepine, barbiturates, primidone)	1	1	
OTHER ANTIBIOTICS (excluding rifampicin and griseofulvin)	1	1	

Always insert an IUD slowly and gently. Insertion methods differ depending on the size and shape of the IUD, inserter barrel, plunger, packaging, and strings. Read and follow the manufacturer's instructions on insertion. Detailed handbooks and videos from manufacturers are available on insertion, withdrawal, and management techniques.

General Preparation

1. Perform a careful bimanual examination to exclude pelvic infection and to identify the position of the uterus. An unrecognized retroflexed uterus may increase the possibility of uterine perforation at the time of the IUD insertion.

2. After you have inserted a warm speculum and viewed the cervix, apply a topical antiseptic solution to the cervix and vagina. Some providers recommend also cleansing the internal cervical os by inserting a cotton-tipped swab dipped in antiseptic, although no evidence supports this practice.

3. If appropriate, inject a paracervical block. If using lidocaine, the upper limit should be 2 mg per pound or 4.5 mg per kg, not to exceed 300 mg of lidocaine plain. If using bupivacaine, a common dose is 20 cc of 0.25% bupivacaine.

4. Anesthetize the cervix at the 12:00 position. Grasp the lip of the cervix with a tenaculum about 1.5 to 2.0 cm from the os. Close the single-tooth tenaculum slowly. Before sounding the uterus, straighten the axis of the uterus by applying traction to the tenaculum.

TCu 380A Insertion Instructions

The following instructions for the TCu 380A are reproduced with permission from the package insert for the ParaGard T:

Step 1

To minimize chance of introducing contamination, do not remove the ParaGard T 380A from the inserter tube prior to placement in the uterus. Do not bend the arms of the ParaGard T 380A earlier than 5 minutes before it is to be introduced into the uterus.

In the absence of sterile gloves, the device can be loaded without destroying sterility by folding the arms in the partially opened package. Place the partially opened package on a flat surface and pull the solid rod partially from the package so it will not interfere with assembly. Place thumb and index finger on top of package on ends of the horizontal arms. Push insertion tube against arms of ParaGard T 380A as indicated by arrow in Figure 21-1 to start arms folding.

Complete the bending by bringing the thumb and index finger together using the other hand to maneuver the insertion tube to pick up the arms of the ParaGard T 380A (Figure 21-2). Insert no further than necessary to insure retention of the arms. Introduce the solid rod into the insertion tube from the bottom alongside the threads until it touches the bottom of the ParaGard T 380A.

Step 2

Adjust the movable flange so that it indicates the depth to which the ParaGard T 380A should be inserted and the direction in which the arms of the ParaGard T 380A will open. At this point, make certain that the horizontal arms of the ParaGard T 380A and the long axis of the flange lie in the same horizontal plane. Introduce the loaded insertion tube through the cervical canal and upwards until the ParaGard T 380A lies in contact with the fundus. The movable flange should be at the cervix (Figure 21-3). *Do not force the insertion.*

Step 3

To release the arms of the ParaGard T 380A, withdraw the insertion tube not more than ½ inch while the solid rod is not permitted to move. This releases the arms of the ParaGard T 380A (Figure 21-4).

Step 4

After the arms are released, the insertion tube should be moved upward gently until the resistance of the fundus is felt. This will assure placement of the T at the highest possible position within the endometrial cavity (Figure 21-5).

Step 5

Withdraw the solid rod while holding the insertion tube stationary (Figure 21-6).

Step 6

Withdraw the insertion tube from the cervix. Be sure sufficient length of the threads are (sic) visible (approximately 1 in. or 2.5 cm.) to facilitate checking for the presence of the ParaGard T 380A (Figure 21-7). Notation of length of the threads should be made in patient record.

Copper T 380A Insertion

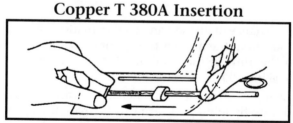

Figure 21-1 *Step 1*

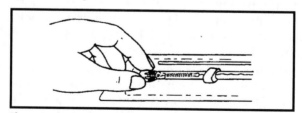

Figure 21-2 *Step 1, continued*

Copper T 380A Insertion—*continued*

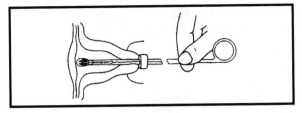

Figure 21-3 *Step 2*

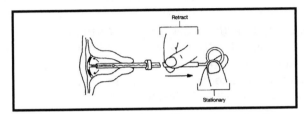

Figure 21-4 *Step 3*

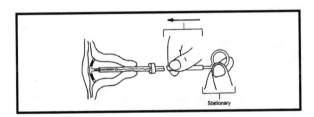

Figure 21-5 *Step 4*

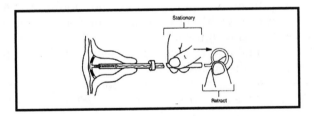

Figure 21-6 *Step 5*

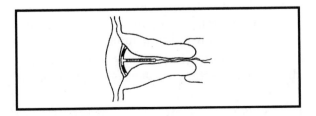

Figure 21-7 *Step 6*

LNG-IUS Insertion Instructions

The following insertion instructions for the LNG-IUS are reproduced with permission from the package insert for the Mirena system:

Insertion procedure

- Open the sterile package.
- Place sterile gloves on your hands.
- Pick up the inserter containing Mirena.
- Carefully release the threads from behind the slider, so that they hang freely.
- Make sure that the slider is in the furthest position away from you (positioned at the top of the handle nearest the IUS).
- While looking at the insertion tube, check that the arms of the system are horizontal. If not, align them on a sterile surface (Figure 21-8) or with sterile gloved fingers.

Checking that the arms of the system are horizontal

- Pull on both threads to draw the Mirena system into the insertion tube (Figure 21-9).
- Note that the knobs at the ends of the arms now cover the open end of the inserter (Figure 21-10).
- Fix the threads tightly in the cleft at the end of the handle (Figure 21-11).

Set the flange to the depth measured by the sound, as indicated in (Figure 21-12).

Mirena is now ready to be inserted.

Hold the slider firmly in the furthermost position (at the top of the handle). Grasp the cervix with the tenaculum and apply gentle traction to align the cervical canal with the uterine cavity. Gently insert the inserter into the cervical canal and advance the insertion tube into the uterus until the flange is situated at a distance of about 1.5–2 cm from the external cervical os to give sufficient space for the arms to open (Figure 21-13). **NOTE!** *Do not force the inserter.*

While holding the inserter steady release the arms of Mirena (Figure 21-14) by pulling the slider back until the top of the slider reaches the mark (raised horizontal line on the handle) (Figure 21-15).

Push the inserter gently into the uterine cavity until the flange touches the cervix. Mirena should now be in the fundal position (Figure 21-16).

Holding the inserter firmly in position release Mirena by pulling the slider down all the way. The threads will be released automatically (Figure 21-17).

Remove the inserter from the uterus. Cut the threads to leave about 2 to 3 cm visible outside the cervix (Figure 21-18).

Post-insertion Instructions

Plan for a follow-up visit after the woman's next menses. Check that the IUD is still in place and that no signs of infection are evident. Further routine visits are not required;[70,71] however, encourage women to return at any time if they have problems, questions, or concerns. In particular, tell women to return for a check-up if they cannot feel the IUD strings, the strings seem too long, or the plastic IUD is palpable in the cervix.

The one-month visit can be strategically important in identifying women at increased risk of discontinuing IUD use because of side effects. Women with excessive menstrual flow or intermenstrual bleeding or spotting are significantly more likely to discontinue than are other women.[72] Counseling and use of non-steroidal anti-inflammatory drugs may help promote continued use.

IUD Removal

When removing an IUD, grasp the IUD strings with a sponge forceps, apply gentle, steady traction, and remove the IUD slowly. If you cannot remove the IUD with gentle traction, a paracervical block may make the removal easier and less painful. After placing the block, use a tenaculum to steady the cervix and straighten the anteversion or retroversion of the uterus and try again. If this technique does not work, dilate the cervix to a small amount with misoprostol, osmotic dilators, rigid dilators, or other appropriate instrument (dilators should always be available in a family planning clinic using IUDs).

Levonorgestrel-Releasing Intrauterine System (LNG-IUS) Insertion

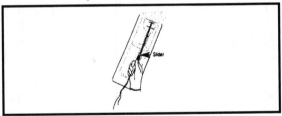

Figure 21-8

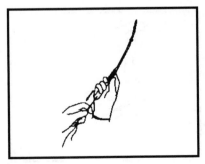

Figure 21-9

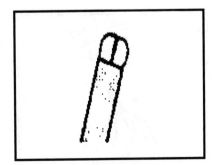

Figure 21-10

Levonorgestrel-Releasing
Intrauterine System (LNG-IUS) Insertion—*continued*

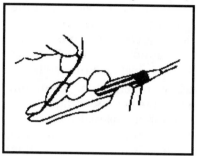

Figure 21-11

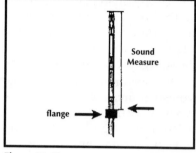

Figure 21-12

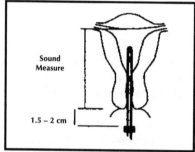

Figure 21-13

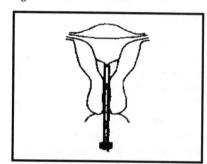

Figure 21-14

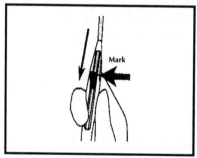

Figure 21-15

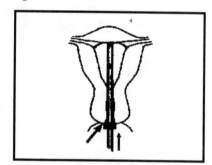

Figure 21-16

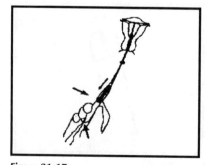

Figure 21-17

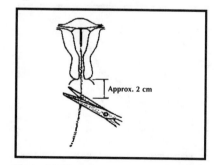

Figure 21-18

MANAGING PROBLEMS AND FOLLOW UP

Excessive bleeding. Excessive bleeding with the TCu 380A can be treated with non-steroidal anti-inflammatory drugs;[73] trials have not demonstrated the superiority of one product over another. Because local prostaglandin production is involved with excessive bleeding, any prostaglandin synthetase inhibitor should help. If the woman's hemoglobin levels drop, she can take oral iron supplementation.

Not all nuisance bleeding can be attributed to the IUD. Other gynecologic disorders, such as endometrial polyps, accidental pregnancy (including an ectopic pregnancy), or endometritis, may be responsible. Of note, endometrial biopsy performed with small catheters can be done without removal of the device. Persistent abnormal bleeding requires clinical evaluation.

Cramping and pain. One approach is preventive therapy with oral non-steroidal anti-inflammatory drugs, local anesthesia, or both. While the literature is divided on the usefulness of topical application of local anesthesia to the endometrial cavity,[74,75] more evidence supports the use of paracervical anesthesia for intrauterine manipulation.[76] Use of a long-acting local anesthetic, such as bupivacaine, may be preferable to shorter-acting drugs, such as lidocaine. Should a woman have pain or vasovagal symptoms immediately after insertion, a paracervical block can be placed at that time. Rarely, the IUD needs to be removed at the insertion visit. Pain that develops later may reflect threatened or partial expulsion, dislodgment, infection, or a complicated pregnancy.

Expulsion. The symptoms of an IUD expulsion include unusual vaginal discharge, cramping or pain, intermenstrual spotting, postcoital spotting, dyspareunia (for the man or the woman), absence or lengthening of the IUD string, and presence of the hard plastic of the IUD at the cervical os or in the vagina.[77] If the menstrual period is delayed, check for IUD strings. A missed period may be the first indication of a "silent" expulsion. If the woman is not pregnant, another IUD can be inserted immediately.

Perforation. Copper-bearing IUDs found to be outside the endometrial cavity should be removed promptly. Copper in the peritoneal cavity induces adhesion formation, which may involve the adnexa, omentum, and bowel. Laparoscopy is the preferred approach for removal. In contrast, non-medicated and progestin-bearing devices do not evoke similar intraperitoneal adhesions. No clear medical indication exists for removal of extra-uterine T-shaped IUDs not containing copper,[78] although this is commonly done.

String problems. Missing strings may signal an unsuspected perforation or spontaneous expulsion; alternatively, some strings ascend into the endometrial cavity, or descend, without known explanation. Ultrasound examination can quickly confirm the presence of an IUD within the endometrial cavity. If the IUD is in place, nothing need be done. Should the woman request removal of an IUD whose strings have ascended into the uterine cavity, a cotton swab or endometrial biopsy instrument can sometimes tease the strings from the endometrium to the endocervix.

Removal of a T-shaped device without visible strings has two prerequisites: the patient's comfort and cervical dilation. A paracervical block, supplemented by an oral analgesic, decreases the pain associated with the procedure. Osmotic dilators left in the os overnight or misoprostol 400 mcg (vaginally or orally) will dilate the cervix. Gentle exploration with an alligator forceps usually yields the device quickly; if not, ultrasound guidance may be helpful. Rarely are the expense and inconvenience of hysteroscopy required for IUD removal.

Several mechanical problems relate to string length. If the male partner complains of penile discomfort from the string being cut too short, one option is to cut the strings off even shorter within the endocervical canal. This may eliminate the barb-like sensation and obviate the need to replace the IUD; however, the lack of string will make it difficult for the woman to monitor the ongoing presence of her device. If the strings initially are too long, simply trim them. If the strings become longer at a later time, check for partial expulsion of the IUD.

Pregnancy complications. If a woman becomes pregnant with an IUD in place, confirm that the pregnancy is intrauterine and not ectopic. Remove the IUD promptly if the woman is in the early stages of pregnancy, regardless of her plans for the pregnancy. Early removal reduces the risk of spontaneous miscarriage or preterm delivery should the woman plan to continue the pregnancy.[6,79] If the woman plans to continue the pregnancy, tell her to look for symptoms of an influenza-like syndrome, which may suggest that she is having a septic spontaneous abortion. A copper IUD in place during pregnancy carries no risk of teratogenesis. If the woman plans to have an induced abortion, remove the IUD promptly rather than delay the removal until the time of abortion.

Upper genital-tract infection. Upper-genital-tract infection needs prompt treatment and follow-up. Accurate diagnosis is often difficult, and widely used diagnostic criteria for salpingitis[80] have been found invalid.[81] Hence, when in doubt, treat. The Centers for Disease Control and Prevention has published recommendations for both inpatient and outpatient therapy.[63] All involve two antibiotics in order to provide an adequate spectrum of coverage. Male partners of women thought to have salpingitis should be contacted, examined, and treated presumptively according to guidelines. Although many clinicians remove the IUD along with giving antibiotics, no evidence supports this practice. Indeed, one small randomized controlled trial showed no benefit of IUD removal as an adjunct to antibiotic therapy.[82]

REFERENCES

1. Forrest JD. U.S. women's perceptions of and attitudes about the IUD. Obstet Gynecol Surv 1996;51:S30-34.
2. Trieman K, Liskin L, Kols A, et al. IUDs—an update. Popul Rep 1995;Series B, No. 5.
3. World Health Organization. Long-term reversible contraception. Twelve years of experience with the TCu380A and TCu220C. Contraception 1997;56:341-352.
4. Sivin I, Stern J, Coutinho E, Mattos CE, el Mahgoub S, Diaz S, et al. Prolonged intrauterine contraception: a seven-year randomized study of the levonorgestrel 20 mcg/day (LNG 20) and the Copper T380 Ag IUDS. Contraception 1991;44:473-480.
5. Rivera R, Yacobson I, Grimes D. The mechanism of action of hormonal contraceptives and intrauterine contraceptive devices. Am J Obstet Gynecol 1999;181:1263-1269.
6. World Health Organization. Mechanism of action, safety and efficacy of intrauterine devices: technical report series 753. Geneva: World Health Organization, 1987.
7. Barbosa I, Olsson SE, Odlind V, Goncalves T, Coutinho E. Ovarian function after seven years' use of a levonorgestrel IUD. Adv Contracept 1995;11:85-95.
8. Segal SJ, Alvarez-Sanchez F, Adejuwon CA, Brache de Mejia V, Leon P, Faundes A. Absence of chorionic gonadotropin in sera of women who use intrauterine devices. Fertil Steril 1985;44:214-218.
9. Wilcox AJ, Weinberg CR, Armstrong EG, Canfield RE. Urinary human chorionic gonadotropin among intrauterine device users: detection with a highly specific and sensitive assay. Fertil Steril 1987;47:265-269.
10. Alvarez F, Brache V, Fernandez E, Guerrero B, Guiloff E, Hess R, et al. New insights on the mode of action of intrauterine contraceptive devices in women. Fertil Steril 1988;49:768-773.
11. Sivin I, Schmidt F. Effectiveness of IUDs: a review. Contraception 1987;36:55-84.
12. Peterson HB, Xia Z, Hughes JM, Wilcox LS, Tylor LR, Trussell J. The risk of pregnancy after tubal sterilization: findings from the U.S. Collaborative Review of Sterilization. Am J Obstet Gynecol 1996;174:1161-1168; discussion 1168-1170.
13. Trussell J, Leveque JA, Koenig JD, London R, Borden S, Henneberry J, et al. The economic value of contraception: a comparison of 15 methods. Am J Public Health 1995;85:494-503.
14. Ory HW. Ectopic pregnancy and intrauterine contraceptive devices: new perspectives. The Women's Health Study. Obstet Gynecol 1981;57:137-144.
15. Franks AL, Beral V, Cates W Jr, Hogue CJ. Contraception and ectopic pregnancy risk. Am J Obstet Gynecol 1990;163:1120-1123.
16. Nelson AL. Intrauterine device practice guidelines: medical conditions. Contraception 1998;58:59S-63S; quiz 72S.
17. Shu XO, Brinton LA, Zheng W, Gao YT, Fan J, Fraumeni JF Jr. A population-based case-control study of endometrial cancer in Shanghai, China. Int J Cancer 1991; 49:38-43.
18. Castellsague X, Thompson WD, Dubrow R. Intra-uterine contraception and the risk of endometrial cancer. Int J Cancer 1993;54:911-916.
19. Parazzini F, La Vecchia C, Moroni S. Intrauterine device use and risk of endometrial cancer. Br J Cancer 1994;70:672-673.
20. Rosenblatt KA, Thomas DB. Intrauterine devices and endometrial cancer. The WHO Collaborative Study of Neoplasia and Steroid Contraceptives. Contraception 1996;54:329-332.
21. Sturgeon SR, Brinton LA, Berman ML, Mortel R, Twiggs LB, Barrett RJ, et al. Intrauterine device use and endometrial cancer risk. Int J Epidemiol 1997;26:496-500.
22. Hill DA, Weiss NS, Voigt LF, Beresford SA. Endometrial cancer in relation to intra-uterine device use. Int J Cancer 1997;70:278-281.
23. Gardner FJ, Konje JC, Abrams KR, Brown LJ, Khanna S, Al-Azzawi F, et al. Endometrial protection from tamoxifen-stimulated changes by a levonorgestrel-releasing intrauterine system: a randomised controlled trial. Lancet 2000;356:1711-1717.

24. World Health Organization. Depot-medroxyprogesterone acetate (DMPA) and risk of endometrial cancer. The WHO Collaborative Study of Neoplasia and Steroid Contraceptives. Int J Cancer 1991;49:186-190.
25. Lassise DL, Savitz DA, Hamman RF, Baron AE, Brinton LA, Levines RS. Invasive cervical cancer and intrauterine device use. Int J Epidemiol 1991;20:865-870.
26. Parazzini F, La Vecchia C, Negri E. Use of intrauterine device and risk of invasive cervical cancer. Int J Epidemiol 1992;21:1030-1031.
27. Fedele L, Bianchi S, Raffaelli R, Portuese A, Dorta M. Treatment of adenomyosis-associated menorrhagia with a levonorgestrel- releasing intrauterine device. Fertil Steril 1997;68:426-429.
28. Starczewski A, Iwanicki M. [Intrauterine therapy with levonorgestrel releasing IUD of women with hypermenorrhea secondary to uterine fibroids]. Ginekol Pol 2000;71:1221-1225.
29. Pakarinen P, Toivonen J, Luukkainen T. Therapeutic use of the LNG IUS, and counseling. Semin Reprod Med 2001;19:365-372.
30. Stewart A, Cummins C, Gold L, Jordan R, Phillips W. The effectiveness of the levonorgestrel-releasing intrauterine system in menorrhagia: a systematic review. BJOG 2001;108:74-86.
31. Zhang J, Feldblum PJ, Chi IC, Farr MG. Risk factors for copper T IUD expulsion: an epidemiologic analysis. Contraception 1992;46:427-433.
32. Bahamondes L, Diaz J, Marchi NM, Petta CA, Cristofoletti ML, Gomez G. Performance of copper intrauterine devices when inserted after an expulsion. Hum Reprod 1995;10:2917-2918.
33. Walsh T, Grimes D, Frezieres R, Nelson A, Bernstein L, Coulson A, et al. Randomised controlled trial of prophylactic antibiotics before insertion of intrauterine devices. IUD Study Group. Lancet 1998;351:1005-1008.
34. Farley TM, Rosenberg MJ, Rowe PJ, Chen JH, Meirik O. Intrauterine devices and pelvic inflammatory disease: an international perspective. Lancet 1992;339:785-788.
35. Grimes DA. Intrauterine device and upper-genital-tract infection. Lancet 2000;356:1013-1019.
36. Lee NC, Rubin GL, Ory HW, Burkman RT. Type of intrauterine device and the risk of pelvic inflammatory disease. Obstet Gynecol 1983;62:1-6.
37. Mishell DR Jr, Bell JH, Good RG, Moyer DL. The intrauterine device: a bacteriologic study of the endometrial cavity. Am J Obstet Gynecol 1966;96:119-126.
38. Grimes DA, Schulz KF. Prophylactic antibiotics for intrauterine device insertion: a meta-analysis of the randomized controlled trials. Contraception 1999;60:57-63.
39. Sawaya GF, Grady D, Kerlikowske K, Grimes DA. Antibiotics at the time of induced abortion: the case for universal prophylaxis based on a meta-analysis. Obstet Gynecol 1996;87:884-890.
40. Sinei SK, Schulz KF, Lamptey PR, Grimes DA, Mati JK, Rosenthal SM, et al. Preventing IUCD-related pelvic infection: the efficacy of prophylactic doxycycline at insertion. Br J Obstet Gynaecol 1990;97:412-419.
41. Kelaghan J, Rubin GL, Ory HW, Layde PM. Barrier-method contraceptives and pelvic inflammatory disease. JAMA 1982;248:184-187.
42. Vessey MP, Yeates D, Flavel R, McPherson K. Pelvic inflammatory disease and the intrauterine device: findings in a large cohort study. Br Med J (Clin Res Ed) 1981;282:855-857.
43. Buchan H, Villard-Mackintosh L, Vessey M, Yeates D, McPherson K. Epidemiology of pelvic inflammatory disease in parous women with special reference to intrauterine device use. Br J Obstet Gynaecol 1990;97:780-788.
44. Daling JR, Weiss NS, Metch BJ, Chow WH, Soderstrom RM, Moore DE, et al. Primary tubal infertility in relation to the use of an intrauterine device. N Engl J Med 1985;312:937-941.
45. Cramer DW, Schiff I, Schoenbaum SC, Gibson M, Belisle S, Albrecht B, et al. Tubal infertility and the intrauterine device. N Engl J Med 1985;312:941-947.
46. Wilson JC. A prospective New Zealand study of fertility after removal of copper intrauterine contraceptive devices for conception and because of complications: a four-year study. Am J Obstet Gynecol 1989;160:391-396.

47. Skjeldestad F, Bratt H. Fertility after complicated and non-complicated use of IUDs. A controlled prospective study. Adv Contracept 1988;4:179-184.
48. Hubacher D, Lara-Ricalde R, Taylor DJ, Guerra-Infante F, Guzman-Rodriguez R. Use of copper intrauterine devices and the risk of tubal infertility among nulligravid women. N Engl J Med 2001;345:561-567.
49. Gupta PK, Hollander DH, Frost JK. Actinomycetes in cervico-vaginal smears: an association with IUD usage. Acta Cytol 1976;20:295-297.
50. Lippes J. Pelvic actinomycosis: a review and preliminary look at prevalence. Am J Obstet Gynecol 1999;180:265-269.
51. World Health Organization. Improving access to quality care in family planning. Medical eligibility criteria for contraceptive use. 2nd edition. Geneva, Switzerland: World Health Organization, 2000.
52. Dardano KL, Burkman RT. The intrauterine contraceptive device: an often-forgotten and maligned method of contraception. Am J Obstet Gynecol 1999;181:1-5.
53. Thiery M. Pain relief at insertion and removal of an IUD: a simplified technique for paracervical block. Adv Contracept 1985;1:167-170.
54. Sinei SK, Morrison CS, Sekadde-Kigondu C, Allen M, Kokonya D. Complications of use of intrauterine devices among HIV-1-infected women. Lancet 1998;351:1238-1241.
55. Morrison CS, Sekadde-Kigondu C, Sinei SK, Weiner DH, Kwok C, Kokonya D. Is the intrauterine device appropriate contraception for HIV-1-infected women? BJOG 2001;108:748-790.
56. Richardson BA, Morrison CS, Sekadde-Kigondu C, Sinei SK, Overbaugh J, Panteleeff DD, et al. Effect of intrauterine device use on cervical shedding of HIV-1 DNA. AIDS 1999;13:2091-2097.
57. Durack DT. Prevention of infective endocarditis. N Engl J Med 1995;332:38-44.
58. Dajani AS, Taubert KA, Wilson W, Bolger AF, Bayer A, Ferrieri P, et al. Prevention of bacterial endocarditis. Recommendations by the American Heart Association. Circulation 1997;96:358-366.
59. Kjos SL, Ballagh SA, La Cour M, Xiang A, Mishell DR Jr. The copper T380A intrauterine device in women with type II diabetes mellitus. Obstet Gynecol 1994;84:1006-1009.
60. Skouby SO, Molsted-Pedersen L, Petersen KR. Contraception for women with diabetes: an update. Baillieres Clin Obstet Gynaecol 1991;5:493-503.
61. Kimmerle R, Heinemann L, Berger M. Intrauterine devices are safe and effective contraceptives for type I diabetic women. Diabetes Care 1995;18:1506-1507.
62. Petersen KR, Skouby SO, Jespersen J. Contraception guidance in women with pre-existing disturbances in carbohydrate metabolism. Eur J Contracept Reprod Health Care 1996;1:53-59.
63. Centers for Disease Control and Prevention. 1998 guidelines for the treatment of sexually transmitted diseases. MMWR 1998;47 (No. RR-1):1-116.
64. White MK, Ory HW, Rooks JB, Rochat RW. Intrauterine device termination rates and the menstrual cycle day of insertion. Obstet Gynecol 1980;55:220-224.
65. Grimes DA, Schulz KF, Stanwood N. Immediate post-abortal insertion of intrauterine devices. Cochrane Database Syst Rev 2000;2.
66. Grimes DA, Schulz K , van Vliet H, Stanwood N. Immediate post-partum insertion of intrauterine devices. Cochrane Database Syst Rev 2001;2.
67. Heartwell SF, Schlesselman S. Risk of uterine perforation among users of intrauterine devices. Obstet Gynecol 1983;61:31-36.
68. Chi IC, Potts M, Wilkens LR, Champion CB. Performance of the copper T-380A intrauterine device in breastfeeding women. Contraception 1989;39:603-618.
69. Chi IC, Wilkens LR, Champion CB, Machemer RE, Rivera R. Insertional pain and other IUD insertion-related rare events for breastfeeding and non-breastfeeding women—a decade's experience in developing countries. Adv Contracept 1989;5:101-119.
70. Hubacher D, Fortney J. Follow-up visits after IUD insertion. Are more better? J Reprod Med 1999;44:801-806.

71. Janowitz B, Hubacher D, Petrick T, Dighe N. Should the recommended number of IUD revisits be reduced? Stud Fam Plann 1994;25:362-367.
72. Stanback J, Grimes D. Can intrauterine device removals for bleeding or pain be predicted at a one-month follow-up visit? A multivariate analysis. Contraception 1998;58:357-360.
73. Ylikorkala O. Prostaglandin synthesis inhibitors in menorrhagia, intrauterine contraceptive device-induced side effects and endometriosis. Pharmacol Toxicol 1994;75 Suppl 2:86-88.
74. Kozman E, Collins P, Howard A, Akanmu T, Gibbs A, Frazer M. The effect of an intrauterine application of two percent lignocaine gel on pain perception during Vabra endometrial sampling: a randomised double-blind, placebo-controlled trial. BJOG 2001;108:87-90.
75. Trolice MP, Fishburne C Jr, McGrady S. Anesthetic efficacy of intrauterine lidocaine for endometrial biopsy: a randomized double-masked trial. Obstet Gynecol 2000;95:345-347.
76. Cicinelli E, Didonna T, Schonauer LM, Stragapede S, Falco N, Pansini N. Paracervical anesthesia for hysteroscopy and endometrial biopsy in postmenopausal women. A randomized, double-blind, placebo-controlled study. J Reprod Med 1998;43:1014-1018.
77. Gruber A, Rabinerson D, Kaplan B, Pardo J, Neri A. The missing forgotten intrauterine contraceptive device. Contraception 1996;54:117-119.
78. Adoni A, Ben Chetrit A. The management of intrauterine devices following uterine perforation. Contraception 1991;43:77-81.
79. Foreman H, Stadel BV, Schlesselman S. Intrauterine device usage and fetal loss. Obstet Gynecol 1981;58:669-677.
80. Hager WD, Eschenbach DA, Spence MR, Sweet RL. Criteria for diagnosis and grading of salpingitis. Obstet Gynecol 1983;61:113-114.
81. Hadgu A, Westrom L, Brooks CA, Reynolds GH, Thompson SE. Predicting acute pelvic inflammatory disease: a multivariate analysis. Am J Obstet Gynecol 1986;155:954-960.
82. Soderberg G, Lindgren S. Influence of an intrauterine device on the course of an acute salpingitis. Contraception 1981;24:137-143.

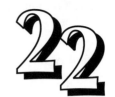

Female and Male Sterilization

Amy E. Pollack, MD, MPH
Charles S. Carignan, MD
Roy Jacobstein, MD, MPH

- A single decision and one simple surgical procedure provide permanent contraception.
- Sterilization is one of the safest, most effective, and most cost-effective contraceptive methods.
- Reversal of the sterilization procedure is expensive, requires either costly assisted reproductive technology (such as IVF) or highly technical major surgery, and results cannot be guaranteed.
- Contraceptive sterilization (female sterilization and vasectomy) has become one of the most widely used methods of family planning in the world in both developed and developing countries.

Healthy women may be fertile until about age 50 to 51; healthy men are fertile essentially throughout life. Because most couples have all the children they want well before the end of their reproductive lifespan, they will need effective contraception protection against unwanted pregnancies for many years.

Ideally, a couple should consider both vasectomy and female sterilization as options. They are comparable in effectiveness, and both are intended to be permanent. Vasectomy is simpler, safer, less expensive, and as effective as the currently available methods of female sterilization.

Better patient selection, improved anesthetic methods and patient monitoring, increased use of local anesthesia with light sedation, improved surgical techniques, better asepsis, and better trained personnel have contributed to the improved safety of sterilization over the past 20 years. Sterilization is the most prevalent contraceptive method in the United States today, and is used by 39% of contracepting fertile-aged couples.[1] The 1995 National Survey of Family Growth (NSFG) reported that 28% of all women 15 to 44 years of age currently practicing contraception relied on tubal sterilization.[2] An estimated 494,000 vasectomies were performed in the United States in 1995, for a rate of 9.9 procedures per 1,000 men aged 25 to 49, compared to 693,000 tubal sterilizations for a rate of 11.7 per 1,000 women aged 20 to 49.

There is no medical condition that would absolutely restrict a person's eligibility for sterilization. Some conditions and circumstances indicate that certain precautions should be taken.

MECHANISM OF ACTION

Sterilization for women involves cutting or mechanically blocking the fallopian tubes to prevent the sperm and egg from uniting.

Vasectomy is the male sterilization operation that blocks the vasa deferentia to prevent the passage of sperm into the ejaculated seminal fluid.

EFFECTIVENESS

FEMALE STERILIZATION

The risk of pregnancy following sterilization is lower than the risk associated with typical use of most temporary contraceptive methods during the first year. It is similar to the risk associated with some of the long-term methods such as the IUDs, injectable contraceptives, or implants. The Collaborative Review of Sterilization (CREST) study points to a first-year probability of pregnancy of 5.5 for every 1,000 procedures (Table 22-1) and a 10-year cumulative probability of 18.5 pregnancies for every 1,000 procedures.[3] Luteal phase pregnancies were not reported as failures in the CREST studies. According to the CREST report, sterilization failure is more likely if the woman is relatively young when the procedure is performed, because young women are more fertile than older women. Although the bipolar method was associated with a high probability of pregnancy, the CREST study was initiated early in the use of the device and many technical issues had yet to be learned. There are many different reasons for failure, some of which can be prevented[4]:

- Pregnancy at time of sterilization. Perform female sterilization in the follicular phase of the menstrual cycle to prevent luteal phase pregnancies, assure that the patient uses effective contraception until after the sterilization procedure, take a careful sexual history (use postcoital contraception when indicated). Perform pregnancy testing on the day of surgery.

- Occlusion method. Fistula formation is associated with electrocautery and spontaneous reanastomosis with suture methods. Clips are not as occlusive as other methods.

- Surgical error. Training of surgeons, good care of instruments, and accurate identification of tubes and proper placement of devices are key to limiting this problem.
- Equipment or device failure. Laparoscopic procedures and electrical and clip methods can fail.

Table 22-1 First-year probability of pregnancy* for sterilization, condoms, pills, IUDs, and implants

Method	Percentage of Women Experiencing an Unintended Pregnancy Within the First Year of Use		% of Women Continuing Use at One Year
	Typical Use	Perfect Use	
Condom			
Male	15	2	53
Female (Reality)	21	5	49
Pill - combined and minipill	8	0.3	68
IUD			
Paragard	0.8	0.6	78
Mirena	0.1	0.1	81
Norplant and Norplant2	0.5	0.5	84
Surgical Female Sterilization[a]	0.5	0.5	100
Male Sterilization	0.15	0.10	100

* See Table 9-2 for first-year probability of pregnancy for all methods.
[a] See also section on Transcervical Approach, under Internal Female Sterilization.

Because surgical skill can seldom be separated from the inherent effectiveness of the occlusion technique, current evidence makes it difficult to conclude one technique is superior to others. For surgeons well-trained in the techniques they perform, it is unlikely important differences in efficacy will occur among the recommended occlusion techniques described in this chapter. However, the literature does suggest guidance about which techniques will be more effective depending on pregnancy status and surgical approach. (See the section on Occlusion Techniques.)

VASECTOMY

Vasectomy is a very effective contraceptive method. Commonly quoted failure rates range from 0.1% to 0.4%, but rates as high as 3 to 5% have been reported. It is very difficult to interpret the published literature on vasectomy efficacy because of short-term follow-up, most of the studies are retrospective and anecdotal, and there is no standard definition of what constitutes a failure. Unfortunately, few studies of vasectomy clearly address the issue of pregnancy. Many studies report failures, but these are failures to eliminate sperm from the ejaculate rather than to prevent pregnancies. The relationship between sperm counts after vasectomy and the risk of pregnancy is not well understood. When pregnancy rates are reported, there is the complicating factor that pregnancies may not always be attributable to the men who underwent the vasectomy. True failure of the technique can result from spontaneous recanalization of the vas, division or occlusion of the wrong structure during surgery, and (rarely) a congenital duplication of the vas that went unnoticed during the procedure. It is clear, nevertheless, that pregnancy can occur long after the vasectomy procedure.[b]

These studies do not include pregnancies resulting from unprotected intercourse before the reproductive tract has been cleared of sperm.

COST

The cost of sterilization procedures varies greatly. Nevertheless, in a 1995 study, vasectomy was found to be the most cost-effective contraceptive method among the 15 methods available in the United States.[5] Female sterilization ranked in the top one-third of the most cost-effective methods at 5 years of use. Unequivocally, however, female sterilization is much more expensive than male sterilization unless performed at the time of cesarean section. Table 22-2 presents figures on the cost of sterilization in 2000 dollars.

Table 22-2 Cost of sterilization[6]

	Female Sterilization	Vasectomy
Public Sector	$1,200	$350
Private Sector	$2,500	$755

ADVANTAGES AND INDICATIONS
FEMALE STERILIZATION

Sterilization for women is a safe operative procedure. Reported fatality rates for the U.S. are between 1 to 2 per 100,000.[7] By contrast, the maternal mortality rate is 7.9 deaths per 100,000 live births.[8] The risk of death from hysterectomy for benign disease is estimated to be 5/100,000 to 25/100,000 in women aged 35 to 44. Laparoscopy is associated with a lower mortality than is minilaparotomy, although this difference may be related to biases of patient selection.[9] In the United States, laparoscopy is the most common form of interval sterilization, usually performed under general anesthesia.[10]

Sterilization can be performed without increasing the health risks during the immediate postpartum or postabortion periods. When immediate postpartum sterilization is performed by trained personnel using local

---

[b] Studies that report pregnancies are summarized in Chapter 31 on Contraceptive Efficacy, Table 31-16.

anesthesia, a small incision, and refined surgical technique, the normal postpartum stay is often 24 hours or less. Both laparoscopy and suprapubic minilaparotomy at 4 weeks or more after delivery can be performed on an outpatient basis using local anesthesia. (See Table 22-3 for a comparison of methods.)

Female sterilization is ideal for those persons who are certain they want no further children and need a reliable contraceptive method. Other advantages include the following:

- Permanence
- High effectiveness
- High acceptability
- Safety
- Quick Recovery
- Lack of significant long-term side effects
- Cost effectiveness
- No need to buy anything
- No need for partner compliance
- No need to interrupt lovemaking
- Privacy of choice

VASECTOMY

Vasectomy continues to be simpler, safer, less expensive, and as effective as female sterilization. When both female and male sterilization are acceptable, vasectomy would be the preferred surgical contraceptive method. The main advantages of vasectomy are as follows:

- Permanence
- High effectiveness
- High acceptability
- Safety
- Quick Recovery
- Lack of significant long-term side effects
- Cost effectiveness (most cost effective of all contraceptive methods)
- No need to buy anything
- No need for partner compliance
- No need to interrupt lovemaking
- Privacy of choice
- Removal of contraceptive burden from the woman

Table 22-3 Various occlusion methods and techniques (advantages and disadvantages)

Occlusion Method	Recommended Occlusion Techniques	Advantages	Disadvantages
Interval Female Sterilization			
Suprapubic Minilaparotomy	1. Pomeroy and Pritchard (Parkland) techniques 2. Silastic bands or Falope-rings 3. Hulka or Filshie clips	1. Local or general anesthesia 2. Incision site usually not visible (below pubic hairline)	1. Difficult technique if the woman is obese, the uterus immobile or the tubes have adhesions from infection or previous surgery 2. Recovery can be more painful than with laparoscopy
Laparoscopy	1. Silastic bands or Falope-rings 2. Unipolar electrocoagulation 3. Bipolar coagulation 4. Hulka or Filshie clips	1. Small incision with either single- or double-puncture technique 2. Less pain than from minilaparotomy 3. Low rate of complication 4. Short recovery time 5. Local or general anesthesia	1. Need for specialist with expensive and intense training 2. Other staff must be trained 3. Necessary equipment is often difficult to obtain and maintain 4. Need a fully equipped operating and recovery room
Vaginal Approach (rarely used in 2004)	1. Pomeroy or Fimbriectomy technique	1. Direct visualization of the pelvic organs 2. Less pain after procedure	1. In several countries, this approach found to be less safe and less effective 2. Infection is more common 3. Technique is difficult to learn and perform
Transcervical Approach	Devices such as Essure™	1. Performed under local anesthesia 2. No scars 3. Can be safely performed in procedure room setting	1. Long-term effectiveness not well known after 3 years 2. Requires initial 3-months of back-up contraception

(continued)

Table 22-3 Various occlusion methods and techniques (advantages and disadvantages)—*(cont'd)*

Occlusion Method	Recommended Occlusion Techniques	Advantages	Disadvantages
Transcervical Approach *(cont'd)*	No others proven safe or effective. Under investigation: Chemicals such as quinacrine or phenol	1. Nonsurgical approach 2. No scars 3. Able to be performed by lower-level staff	1. Still experimental techniques 2. Efficacy and safety rates unknown 3. Many questions yet to be answered
Postpartum Female Sterilization			
Subumbilical Minilaparotomy	1. Pomeroy technique 2. Pritchard (Parkland) technique	1. Convenience 2. Lower costs 3. Ease of surgery 4. Longer hospital stay (beyond that for a normal delivery) is not required	1. Use of occlusion rings or clips not indicated and more likely to fail if used 2. Electrocoagulation not indicated[12] 3. Counseling must be prior to labor to reduce risk of regret
Cesarean Section	1. Pomeroy technique 2. Pritchard technique 3. Irving technique	1. Convenience 2. Lower costs 3. Anatomy fully visible	1. Cesareans should not be performed solely to occlude the tubes 2. Counseling must be prior to labor to reduce risk of regret
Postabortion Sterilization	Suprapubic minilaparotomy Pomeroy or Pritchard procedures Laparoscopy 1. Silastic bands or Falope-rings 2. Unipolar coagulation 3. Bipolar coagulation 4. Hulka or Filshie clips	1. Convenience 2. Client motivation	1. Need for careful counseling (patients have a higher risk of regret following post-abortion sterilization) 2. May increase the amount of blood loss with abortion procedure

DISADVANTAGES AND CAUTIONS

FEMALE STERILIZATION

Female sterilization is not recommended for anyone who is not sure of her desire regarding future fertility. Considerations include the following:

- Permanence (although reversal is possible; it is expensive, requires either costly assisted reproductive technology (such as IVF) or highly technical major surgery, and results cannot be guaranteed.)
- Regret for decision (high among some groups of women, especially women who at the time of sterilization are in an unstable marriage, younger than 31, have no children or very young children, or make their decision to be sterilized during a time of financial crisis or for reasons related to a pregnancy)
- Technical difficulty of the procedure
- Need for surgeon, operating room (aseptic conditions), trained assistants, medications, surgical (or hysteroscopic) equipment
- Expense at the time of the procedure
- Higher probability of pregnancy being ectopic if method fails (even so, the likelihood of a sterilized woman having an ectopic is less than that of a non-sterilized woman)
- Lack of protection against sexually transmitted infections (STIs), including infection with the human immunodeficiency virus (HIV)

VASECTOMY

Vasectomy is not effective until all sperm in the reproductive tract are ejaculated. Complications such as bleeding or infection as well as failure, although infrequent, do occur. As a contraceptive method, vasectomy provides indirect protection from pregnancy for women. The major disadvantages of vasectomy are as follows:

- Reversal is difficult, and, though possible, it is expensive, requires a highly technical and major surgery, and its results cannot be guaranteed
- Regret for decision (high among some groups of men, for the same reasons that regret is high in some groups of women: being in an unstable marriage at the time of sterilization, being younger than 31, having no children or very young children, or making their decision to be sterilized during a time of financial crisis or for reasons related to a pregnancy)
- Need for trained physician, procedure room (aseptic conditions), trained assistants, medications, surgical equipment
- Expense at the time of the procedure
- Lack of protection against STIs, including infection with HIV

SPECIAL ISSUES
FEMALE STERILIZATION

Although very few studies have examined the relationship between breast cancer, endometrial cancer, or bone density and sterilization, none report an increased risk.[12-15]

Ovarian cancer. Several well-designed studies now provide increasing evidence that tubal sterilization has a protective effect against ovarian cancer.[16-18] Protective effects have been studied for at least 15 years after sterilization. New evidence suggests that women with BRCA1 mutations who have undergone tubal sterilization have a 60% lower risk of developing invasive ovarian cancer than those who have not.[19]

Breast cancer. The Cancer and Steroid Hormone (CASH) study, a case-control study of 4742 women, found no association between tubal sterilization and breast cancer.[14]

VASECTOMY

Sperm antibodies. Antisperm antibodies are found in 50–80% of men following vasectomy[20-22] as compared to only 8–21% in the general population.[23] The theoretical concern that these antibodies may have adverse health consequences has led to numerous studies, results of which have shown no evidence of any immunologic or other diseases related to the formation of antisperm antibodies after vasectomy.[24-27] Antisperm antibodies may play a role in decreased fertility after vasectomy reversal, although conflicting results have been reported. Some studies have shown decreased pregnancy rates due to antisperm antibodies and others have not.[28-31] Current consensus is that fertility following vasectomy reversal is only inhibited by high levels of antisperm antibodies.[32] In addition, the class of antibody may be more important than the antibody titers themselves, with IgA antibodies leading to greater fertility impairment than IgG antibodies.[33,34]

Prostate cancer. The incidence of prostate cancer is rising, and in the United States it is the most commonly diagnosed cancer among men.[35,36] Little is known about the etiology and pathogenesis of prostate cancer, and few risk factors have been identified. There has been concern about a possible association between vasectomy and prostate cancer. Since the mid-1980s, there have been over a dozen epidemiological studies of the risk of prostate cancer after vasectomy reported in the literature. Results have been difficult to interpret because of conflicting study findings, lack of a convincing biological mechanism for vasectomy causing prostate cancer, and generally weak associations when they have been found (for a review, see Bernal-Delgado, et al. 1998).[37] In addition, the potential for bias in some studies was high and likely led to an overestimation of any effect.[37] Based on the result of the published studies to date, there is little evidence for a causal association between vasectomy and prostate cancer.[38]

A panel of experts gathered by the U.S. National Institutes of Health in 1993 concluded that no change in the current practice of vasectomy was necessary nor should vasectomy reversal be done as a prostate cancer prevention measure.[39] Studies published after the expert panel report support these conclusions.[40–42]

PROVIDING SURGICAL CONTRACEPTION FOR FEMALES

Female sterilization involves ligation, mechanical occlusion with clips or rings, or electrocoagulation (Figure 22-1). The fallopian tubes are usually approached through the abdomen via a laparoscopic approach, a minilaparotomy incision, or via laparotomy at the time of a cesarean section or other abdominal surgery. The surgical approach through the vagina via colpotomy has been largely abandoned because of increased risks of infection and failure.

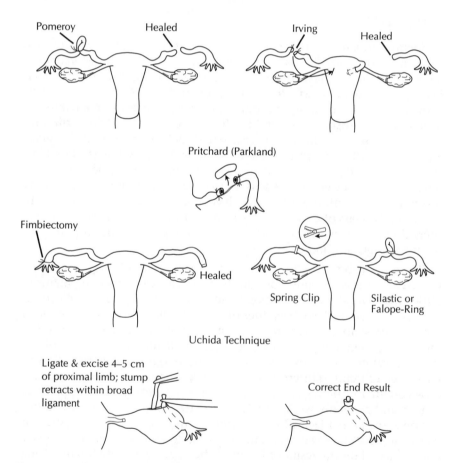

Figure 22-1 Tubal sterilization techniques

Occlusion method. The choice of occlusion method depends upon the provider's training, personal experience, and the availability of supplies. Data from the AAGL 1995 survey suggested that bipolar electrocoagulation was used for interval laparoscopic sterilization by 60% of respondents. Worldwide, the most common interval occlusion methods are Pomeroy ligation and the ring.[43]

In September 1996, the U.S. Food and Drug Administration approved the Filshie clip for use as a new contraceptive device in the United States. The Filshie clip is a good option for patients and clinicians because it is easier to use than other occlusion devices, destroys a minimal amount of the fallopian tube, and has high efficacy.[44] Small and designed to occlude the tube with minimal destruction, the device is made of titanium with a silicone rubber lining, which expands to keep the tube compressed as it flattens.[44,45]

Family Health International (FHI) conducted 11 studies of the Filshie clip at 43 sites in 10 countries. In two studies, the 12-month cumulative rate of pregnancy was 0.1% for the Filshie clip and 0.7% for the Wolf clip. Two studies comparing the Filshie clip and the tubal ring found the same 12-month cumulative rate of pregnancy for both methods (0.2%).[45] The Filshie clip may be less effective when used postpartum than when applied during interval sterilizations. In the single postpartum study conducted by FHI, the pregnancy rate at 24 months was 1.7% for the Filshie clip and 0.4% for the Pomeroy method. The Filshie clip compared favorably with other occlusion devices on safety issues. Studies do not support the routine application of multiple clips per tube.

Timing. The timing of female sterilization, whether postpartum or not, is very important for choosing the surgical approach, method of occlusion, presentation for counseling issues, use of staff and facilities, and organization of patient flow. Interval sterilization (at 4 or more weeks after delivery) is performed when the uterus is fully involuted.

The immediate postpartum period (within 48 hours of delivery) is the most common time for female sterilization in many countries and currently accounts for about half of all female sterilizations done annually in the United States.[46] This popularity is largely explained by the greater convenience, lower costs, ease of surgery, and more efficient use of health resources. A hospital stay beyond that for a normal delivery (24 hours or less in many hospitals) is usually not required. (See also Suprapubic Minilaparotomy.)

Immediate postpartum sterilization services should be an integral part of any maternity service. However, sterilization around the time of pregnancy can be associated with an increased risk of regret[47] and therefore these patients should be counseled carefully. Informed consent before delivery is also important. Many hospitals use a simple procedure room for postpartum sterilization, although the delivery suite or operating theater is most commonly used. Following a procedure performed using local anesthesia and light sedation, the woman is often able to walk back to her bed with assistance. Preoperative assessment is facilitated because her health status can usually be assessed from the delivery and prenatal records.

Tubal occlusion may be performed immediately after a first-trimester spontaneous or medically induced abortion as long as careful attention is given to counseling, informed choice, and medical contraindications.

INTERVAL FEMALE STERILIZATION

Suprapubic Minilaparotomy

Suprapubic minilaparotomy (also called microlaparotomy or MicroPfannenstiel) involves a 2 centimeter (cm) to 5 cm abdominal incision just above the pubic hairline, and use of instruments measuring 2 mm in diameter and less. Through this incision, the surgeon grasps the tubes and occludes them (Figure 22-2.) For many women, the incision lies within the hairline and so will not be visible. If the woman is obese, the uterus immobile, or the tubes have adhesions from infection or previous surgery, the minilaparotomy technique may be difficult. This technique requires mobility of the pelvic structures so that by manipulation of the uterus the tubes can be moved into the incision site and thus be easily accessible.

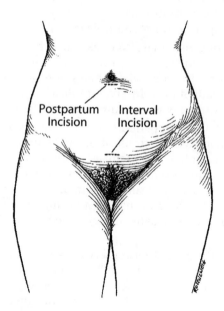

Postpartum
Incision

Interval
Incision

Figure 22-2 Minilaparotomy incision site and size

As part of screening, ask about pelvic disease, previous abdominal or pelvic surgery, diabetes mellitus, heart or lung disease, bleeding problems, allergies, and recent infections. Ascertain the date of last menstrual period and make certain the woman is not pregnant. (If the sterilization procedure is performed post-abortion or postpartum, make certain the client has no pregnancy-related problems, particularly anemia.) Examine the heart, lungs, abdomen, and general condition of the patient. Perform a pelvic exam, paying special attention to uterine position and mobility and presence of pelvic infection or masses. Laboratory evaluations usually include at least a hemoglobin measurement. Because sterilization is elective surgery, a postabortion procedure should be delayed if pregnancy-related complications could affect medical stability.

Procedure. The patient should empty her bladder by voiding or by catheterization immediately before the operation. Place the woman in the lithotomy position with a slight Trendelenburg position to move the pelvic viscera toward the upper abdomen. If the uterus is not already anteverted, elevate the uterus manually or with a uterine manipulator, also termed an elevator (Figure 22-3).

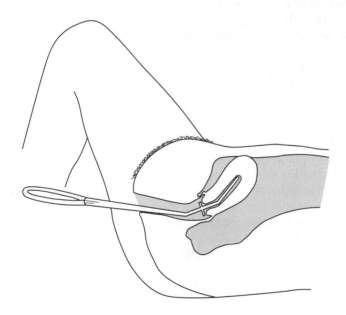

Source: Stewart et al. (1988).[50]

Figure 22-3 A metal elevator raises the uterus and moves it from side to side so that the uterus and tubes will be closer to the incision

Correct placement of the incision is essential to avoid injury. If the incision is too high, the tubes will be difficult to reach; if placed too low, the bladder may be incised. Significant anatomical variation occurs among patients; thus, take great care in entering the abdomen. Light sedation can be given preoperatively and local anesthesia used to infiltrate layer by layer (see the section on Anesthesia). When using local anesthesia, continue to communicate with the woman during the procedure to enhance the analgesic effect, reassure her, and when necessary, elicit her cooperation. Surgical manipulation should be slow and gentle. Often a tubal hook or small Babcock forceps facilitates lifting the fallopian tube from the abdomen. Identify the fimbria to ensure the structure is the tube and not the round ligament.

Use careful aseptic technique throughout. Achieve good hemostasis before closing the abdominal wound in layers. Growing evidence indicates it is unnecessary to suture the peritoneal layer because small peritoneal defects will heal without adhesions.[49] This principle applies as well to subumbilical minilaparotomy. EngenderHealth has published a training manual, *Minilaparotomy under Local Anaesthesia: A Curriculum for Doctors and Nurses*,[49] and an illustrated guide *Minilaparotomy for Female Sterilization: An Illustrated Guide for Service Providers*[50] that both describe this technique in greater detail.

Occlusion techniques. Occlusion options include the Pomeroy and Pritchard (Parkland) techniques, the Silastic or Falope-rings, the Spring clip (Hulka, Rocket, or Wolf clip), and the Filshie clip. The rings and clips require special applicators. Fimbriectomy and the Madlener procedures have been associated with higher failure rates and have no advantages over the Pomeroy and Pritchard techniques for routine cases. The Irving technique cannot be done through a minilaparotomy incision and is useful only after a cesarean section.

Laparoscopy

The laparoscopic approach to sterilization involves making a small incision and inserting an instrument to visualize the tubes so the surgeon can place rings (bands), apply clips, or use electrocoagulation. Use either a single- or double-puncture technique. With double-puncture techniques, the second puncture is used for manipulating the intra-abdominal organs and occluding the tubes (Figure 22-4). Using the single-puncture procedure, the operating instrument is passed through an opening beside the fiberoptic channel.

Because the incision is smaller than a minilaparotomy incision, this method is less painful, has a low rate of complications, a short recovery time, and leaves only a small scar. The same equipment and skills can be used for endoscopic diagnostic procedures.

Disadvantages of laparoscopic sterilizations include the need for a specialist with procedure-specific training, equipment that must be maintained, and a fully equipped operating room. Laparoscopic sterilization is not used in the immediate postpartum period.

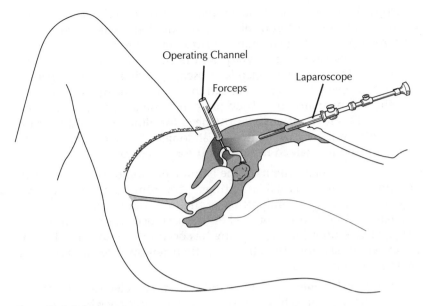

Figure 22-4 Laparoscopy

Procedure. Laparoscopic sterilizations can be performed under local or general anesthesia. (See the section on Anesthesia.) Clean the perineal area, the vagina, and the cervix. Scrub the abdominal site, especially the navel. Stabilize the cervix with a tenaculum and a uterine manipulator (Figure 22-5).

After making a small subumbilical incision, insert the Veress needle for insufflation. Apply upward traction on the abdomen. Advance the needle toward the pelvis, away from the great blood vessels. Place the patient in the Trendelenburg position and insufflate 1 to 3 liters of gas (the minimum needed for good visualization), using nitrous oxide (N_2O), carbon dioxide (CO_2), or room air. Withdraw the needle and advance the trocar toward the pelvis, away from the great vessels, as the abdominal wall is firmly elevated. Remove the trocar from its sleeve (cannula) and insert the

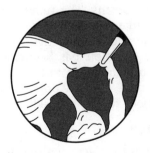

Figure 22-5 A laparoscopy instrument grasps one tube in preparation for cautery or application of a ring or clip

laparoscope. If you use the double-puncture procedure, make a second puncture under direct vision through the laparoscope. With single-puncture laparoscopy, insert the operating instruments through the operating channel of the laparoscope to grasp and occlude the tubes. Variations from this description include open laparoscopy, during which the peritoneal cavity is opened under visualization by the surgeon, similar to a subumbilical minilaparotomy. Then place a cannula for insertion of the laparoscope. This method obviates the need for blind entry of the sharp Veress needle and the trocar into the abdomen,[51-53] but requires more surgical time and has gained little support for general use.

If clips are used, place them on the isthmic portion of the tube at 1 to 2 cm from the uterus. Place Silastic rings 3 cm from the uterus. Perform electrocoagulation in the midportion of the tube away from other structures (Figure 22-5).[54] After both tubes are occluded, inspect the pelvic organs to ensure no injury or bleeding has occurred, remove the laparoscope, expel all gas from the abdomen; then remove the cannula, and suture the incision closed.

Occlusion techniques. Silastic bands, unipolar electrocoagulation, and Filshie clips appear to have similar short-term efficacy when correctly applied, although the ectopic pregnancy rate appears to be higher with electrocoagulation (bipolar and unipolar) in the longer term.[55] (See the section on Long-Term Complications.) A 10-year follow-up of unipolar and bipolar sterilization cases found higher pregnancy rates with bipolar cautery than with unipolar cautery.[3] These high pregnancy rates appear to be related to training and to technical problems with the instrumentation (e.g., incorrect wattage).[3,56,57] The Spring clip (Hulka, Rocket, or Wolf clip) has a lower force of compression than does the Filshie clip and requires precise placement at a 90-degree angle across the tube with the isthmic portion of the tube positioned at the hinged part of the jaws in order to avoid failures.

Vaginal Approach

The fallopian tubes can be reached through an incision high in the vagina (called a colpotomy) posterior to the cervix. This allows direct visualization of the pelvic organs. The tubes can also be reached and directly sutured and cut. In several countries, vaginal approaches have been found to be less safe and less effective than minilaparotomy and laparoscopic approaches. Infection has been more common, and the techniques are generally more difficult to learn and perform. Therefore, the vaginal approach should be used only for exceptional cases and performed in a well-equipped facility by a skilled surgeon.[43]

Transcervical Approach

Hysteroscopic techniques to inject occlusive agents into the tubes are still experimental. Also considered experimental are nonsurgical sterilization techniques using a chemical or other material to occlude the tubes through the cervix. Chemicals cause scarring at the proximal portion of the tube or cornua. Various agents, including quinacrine, a caustic agent that causes scarring, and liquid silicone, which hardens after placement, to form a plug, are under investigation for safety and efficacy.[58,59]

However, in November 2002, the U.S. FDA approved Essure, a soft, flexible, micro-insert device hysteroscopically placed in the proximal section of each fallopian tube (Figure 22-6). The device consists of two concentric metal coils. The outer coil anchors the device in the lumen. The inner coil's polyester fibers stimulate growth of fibrous tissue, which, over the subsequent few months occludes the tubes. By three months, 96% of women studied had both tubes occluded and by six months, 100% of women had both tubes occluded.[60]

Special training is needed for insertion of Essure, which can only be done as an interval procedure. Essure can be provided under local anesthesia and typically can be inserted in a physician's office or procedure room in 30 minutes. Essure was recently approved by PPFA for provision in some clinics. Placement may be difficult because of anatomical features or scarring. Since the procedure is not effective immediately, an alternate method of reliable contraception must be used until a hysterosalpingogram demonstrates that the device is correctly placed and the tubes are occluded. The procedure is irreversible through removal and microsurgical repair. IVF has not been used in patients with the device in place.

In the two clinical trials on which FDA approval was primarily based, which involved more than 700 patients, no pregnancies were reported in up to 24 months of use and the method was found to be highly acceptable.[60] In an Australian study of 108 women using the device for an average of 17 months, no intrauterine or ectopic pregnancies were reported.[61] As with other methods, Essure is not without risks, which include infection and uterine perforation. Because the device is in an introductory phase, long-term safety and efficacy have not been assessed.

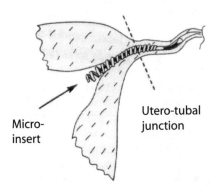

Micro-
insert

Utero-tubal
junction

Source: Kerin, Carignan & Cher (2001)[63] with permission.

Figure 22-6 Hysteroscopic placement of permanent birth control micro-insert within tubal lumen

Costs of the Essure procedure may be lower than with tubal sterilization because less infrastructure, fewer staff and less expensive equipment are needed to provide the method as an office-based procedure using local anesthesia.

Hysterectomy

Hysterectomy, whether performed through a vaginal or abdominal approach, carries a much higher risk of morbidity and mortality than other sterilization procedures. Hysterectomy should not be performed for contraceptive purposes alone.

POSTPARTUM AND POSTABORTION FEMALE STERILIZATION

Subumbilical Minilaparotomy

If minilaparotomy is performed at 10 or more hours after delivery, the risk of postpartum hemorrhage has passed, and the status of the baby can be assessed with some confidence.[62] (See Suprapubic Minilaparotomy for more on preoperative assessment.)

Procedure. Immediately after delivery, the uterus and tubes are high in the abdomen. A small 1.5 to 3 cm incision just below the umbilicus is usually adequate to reach the tubes. Local anesthesia with light sedation or analgesia is frequently sufficient because several of the more painful aspects of minilaparotomy are reduced or eliminated:

- The incision is smaller.
- Intra-abdominal manipulation of the tubes is less extensive.
- The lithotomy position is not used.
- The cervical tenaculum or uterine elevator are not required.

The fallopian tubes are easy to reach if the incision is gently moved over each tube by placing a hand on the side of the abdomen and moving the postpartum uterus.[49]

When a minilaparotomy is not feasible, sterilization should be delayed and provided as an interval procedure.

Occlusion techniques (Figure 22-1). The Pomeroy technique using plain catgut is an effective and safe approach and is the most widely used method to occlude the tubes in the immediate postpartum period. A 2-cm loop of tube in the midportion is ligated with plain catgut and then excised. The Pritchard (Parkland) technique avoids the approximation of the cut ends. The mesosalpinx is perforated in an avascular area; the tube is ligated in two places; and the intervening segment is excised.[62]

The fimbriectomy method of sterilization has gained less favor because it is less reversible, removes more tissue, has been associated with high pregnancy rates, and may cause more postoperative complications.

Electrocoagulation, the Falope-Ring, and the Spring clip (Hulka, Rocket, or Wolf clip) are not suitable or recommended for immediate postpartum application. The Filshie clip can be used with a special applicator.

Cesarean Section

Tubal occlusion can be readily accomplished during cesarean section. Cesarean section should not be performed solely to gain access for tubal sterilization. The Parkland procedure (Figure 22-1) is the method favored for use with cesarean section. It involves two individual sutures, use of chromic catgut suture, and excision of a small central tubal portion.[3] The Irving technique (which requires a wide surgical exposure for implanting the proximal end of the tube into the uterine wall and is thus possible with cesarean section) is a more complicated alternative.[62]

Postabortion Sterilization

A suprapubic minilaparotomy (incision somewhat higher than for a nonpregnant woman) or a laparoscopic approach may be used. The tubes will generally be less engorged and edematous than in the immediate postpartum period but will still require extra care during a minilaparotomy or a laparoscopy in which clips or Silastic rings are applied. (See the sections on Minilaparotomy and Laparoscopy Complications.)

Occlusion techniques may include the Pomeroy or Pritchard procedures with minilaparotomy. Failures with Silastic rings or Spring clips used in the postabortion period are of less concern than in the immediate postpartum period.

ANESTHESIA AND PAIN MANAGEMENT

General or regional anesthesia provided by trained personnel in appropriate settings is safe and is the most frequently used anesthesia for female sterilization procedures in the United States. A discussion of general anesthesia is beyond the scope of this text. The current trend today is toward outpatient-based surgery. Appropriate pain management can greatly improve the outcomes of such surgery, as well as increase patient's comfort. Local anesthesia with light sedation is generally sufficient to minimize the pain caused by sterilization procedures and offers safety advantages over general anesthesia, which can lead to compromised cardiorespiratory function.[7,63] Worldwide, local anesthesia is used for over 75% of sterilizations today. Although some U.S. providers use local anesthesia for sterilization,[63,64] general anesthesia for interval procedures and regional anesthesia (for postpartum procedures) are the most commonly used regimens.[10] Advantages of local anesthesia include lower complication rates, lower cost of the procedure, quicker recovery, better postoperative course with fewer or milder side-effects, and high acceptance by the patients. By not compromising the normal physiological control of vital functions, a high level of safety can be maintained. Both local and general anesthetic methods, however, need the attention of a trained professional who carefully monitors the patient and the drugs used. Avoid high doses of opioid (narcotic) analgesics and benzodiazepine (tranquilizer) sedatives that can compromise ventilation, sometimes dramatically, and may cause cardiovascular depression. The following regimen is suitable for minilaparotomy and, with modifications, laparoscopy. Doses given are for an adult with a body weight of 50 kilograms.

Premedication

Sedate the woman with diazepam (Valium) 10 milligrams (mg) p.o. about 30 to 60 minutes before the operation. Midazolam (Versed), a new short-acting parenteral benzodiazepine three to four times more potent than diazepam may be substituted. (Give 2.5 to 3 mg intramuscularly 1 hour preoperatively, or 1 to 2.5 mg intravenously in the operating room.)

Given in the Operating Room

1. Atropine 0.4 to 0.6 mg intravenously.
2. Meperidine (Demerol) 50 mg intravenously. Other opioid analgesics or ketamine can be substituted for meperidine. The intravenous doses, each of which give analgesia about equivalent to 50 mg meperidine, are listed in Table 22-4.[49]
3. Promethazine (Phenergan) 25 mg intravenously.
4. Lidocaine local anesthesia. Infiltrate the skin and subcutaneous tissues with 1% lidocaine (=lignocaine) (Xylocaine) 10 to 15 ml (without epinephrine). After opening the peritoneal cavity, 5 ml of 1% lidocaine may be flowed onto each tube and the uterus. During laparoscopy, this step is optional if the instrument does not permit lidocaine application. During double-puncture laparoscopy, the second site will also be infiltrated. The maximum safe dose of 1% lidocaine (without epinephrine) is 5 mg/kg body weight; for a woman weighing 50 kg the maximum safe dose is 250 mg or 25 ml of 1% lidocaine. If only 2% lidocaine is available, dilute to 1% with 0.9% sodium chloride only in order to better obtain adequate volume for local infiltration and to avoid exceeding the safe dose. Some surgeons will use sodium bicarbonate (1 cc of 8.4% sodium bicarbonate with 25 cc of 1% lidocaine) to decrease the burning sensation caused by the anesthesia infiltration in the subcutaneous space.

Table 22-4 Substitutes for meperidine anesthesia for female sterilization

Drug	Intravenous Dose	Analgesic Duration
Meperidine (Demerol)	50 mg*	2-3 hours
Fentanyl (Sublimaze)	0.05-0.06 mg*	30-60 minutes
Pentazocine (Talwin)	15-20 mg*	2-3 hours
Butorphanol (Stadol)	1 mg*	3-4 hours
Ketamine (Ketalar)	25-30 mg*	10-15 minutes

* Short acting—supplemental doses about one-third less than the initial ketamine dose may be given at 10-minute intervals as needed.

Monitor vital signs regularly during the operation and postoperatively until the woman is fully recovered and alert. EngenderHealth publications as well as the EngenderHealth training manuals, *Minilaparotomy under Local Anaesthesia: A Curriculum for Doctors and Nurses,* and *Minilaparotomy for Female Sterilization: An Illustrated Guide for Service Providers* describe anesthesia techniques and regimens in greater detail.

PROVIDING VASECTOMY

There is no medical reason that would absolutely restrict a man's eligibility for vasectomy. Some conditions and circumstances indicate that certain precautions should be taken or that the procedure should be delayed.[65] These include localized problems that make vasectomy more difficult to perform (such as inguinal hernia, large hydrocele or varicocele, cryptorchidism, and previous scrotal injury) or conditions that may be more likely to produce complications (such as diabetes, coagulation disorders, or AIDS). In cases of local skin infection, systemic infection, gastroenteritis, or filariasis, the vasectomy should be delayed until the condition is resolved. When an intrascrotal mass is present, the vasectomy should be delayed until the cause of the mass is determined.

In order to provide vasectomy, strictly adhere to technical guidelines for its provision.[66] During a preoperative history, take an inventory of past illnesses and surgeries, bleeding disorders, allergies (particularly to local anesthetics and pain medications), heart disease, kidney and bladder infection, diabetes, anemia, and STI. Evaluate the general health condition, including taking the pulse and blood pressure; assessing for local infections in the scrotal or inguinal area or inguinal hernia or previous surgery in the inguinal area; evaluating the scrotum for hydrocele or varicocele; and determining if the testicles are properly descended or are fixed in place. Assess the scrotal skin and subcutaneous tissues to see if there are factors that might affect a surgical procedure.

Laboratory examinations are not routinely performed, but should be available. If elements in the history or physical so indicate, obtain a lab test (e.g., liver function, bleeding and clotting time, etc.).

Clip the hair from around his scrotum and penis (if this was not already done at home). Shaving the scrotum is no longer recommended, as this significantly increases the chance of surgical-site infection. Strict adherence to good infection prevention practices is crucial for the safety of the procedure and essential to prevent both immediate and long-term infectious morbidity and mortality.

Wash the area with soap and water, just before surgery. Use an effective antiseptic (usually an iodophor such as povidone iodine) or a 4% chlorhexidine solution) to prep the scrotum, thighs, and perineum, then drape the area. Use aseptic technique to perform the procedure.

Both conventional and no-scalpel vasectomies are performed almost exclusively under local anesthesia only, using 1% lidocaine (lignocaine).

Pre-medication is not commonly used. Use of sedation, regional, or general anesthesia is rarely needed and unnecessarily increases the risk and the costs associated with the procedure.[67,68]

APPROACHES TO THE VAS

Regardless of the method of scrotal entry, the first step in the vasectomy is to identify and immobilize the vas through the skin of the scrotum. The second step is to deliver the vas. There are two approaches to delivering the vas: conventional vasectomy and no-scalpel vasectomy.

For conventional vasectomy, incise the skin and muscle overlying the vas, or open these with the no-scalpel method (see below). Through this small incision, isolate the vas and occlude with the preferred method (Figure 22-7 and 22-8). Perform the same procedure for the vas on the other side. Close the incisions with absorbable suture. Some surgeons use only a single midline incision, and some do not suture small skin incisions.[66,69] The patient should rest at least 15 minutes before he leaves.

A no-scalpel procedure is currently being used in many programs around the world, including in the United States. The no-scalpel vasectomy technique was developed in 1974 in China.[70,71] The surgical approach uses a different anesthetic technique and reaches the vas through a puncture in the scrotum rather than through a scalpel incision.[70] Thereafter, the surgical procedure is the same as the scalpel method. A detailed description can be found in EngenderHealth's Illustrated Guide for No-scalpel Vasectomy.

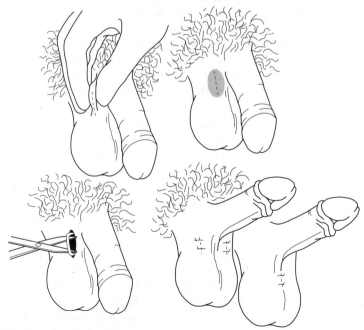

Figure 22-7 Sites of vasectomy incisions

No-scalpel vasectomy offers several advantages over the scalpel method: fewer complications, including infection and hematoma; less pain during the procedure and early follow-up period; and earlier resumption of sexual activity after surgery.[72-74]

This procedure employs two unique instruments. After local anesthetic is injected, creating a perivasal block, a specially designed ring forceps encircles and firmly secures the vas without penetrating the skin. The second instrument, a sharp-tipped dissecting forceps, punctures and stretches a small opening in the skin and vas sheath. The vas is lifted out and occluded, as with other vasectomy techniques. The same midline puncture site is used to deliver and occlude the other vas in an almost bloodless procedure. No sutures are needed to close the small wound (Figure 22-8).

Occlusion techniques. Once the vas has been delivered, it is then occluded using a variety of methods, including ligation with sutures, division, cautery, application of clips, excision of a segment of the vas, fascial interposition, or some combination of these. The same techniques are used to occlude the vas when using conventional or no-scalpel vasectomy. Ligation and excision of a section of the vas is the most widely used technique worldwide. Another popular occlusion technique is cautery— electrosurgical (electrical coagulation) or thermal. This is done by inserting a needle electrode or a cautery device into the vas lumen and desiccating the luminal mucosa of the vas to create a firm scar that will occlude the vas. Sometimes a segment of the vas is removed as well. Clips can be applied to the vas to compress a narrow segment and block the passage of sperm. After division of the vas, a clip is applied to both of the cut ends. Sometimes a segment of the vas is removed.

A modification performed by a few surgeons is to leave the testicular end of the vas open (open-ended vasectomy). This method appears to reduce the frequency of postoperative congestive epididymitis without increasing the rate of painful sperm granulomas.[69,75,76] Open-ended vasectomy may reduce postoperative complaints and success rates for reversal may also be higher. No studies on open-ended vasectomy and the success of reversal have been reported in the literature.

Data to support the superiority of any of these vas occlusion techniques had been lacking, but several recent studies have suggested that there are some differences in effectiveness among different occlusion techniques. Several studies found higher then expected failure rates for vasectomy by ligation (with suture or clips) and excision.[77-79] Results of a recent randomized clinical trial demonstrated that use of fascial interposition with ligation and excision significantly improves the effectiveness of vasectomy—ligation and excision without fascial interposition should no longer be recommended.[80,81]

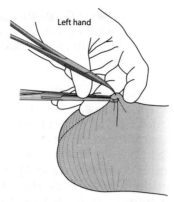

A. Inserting both tips of the dissecting forceps into the puncture site

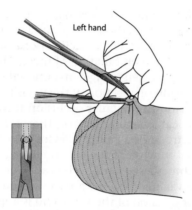

B. Spreading the tissues to make a skin opening twice the diameter of the vas

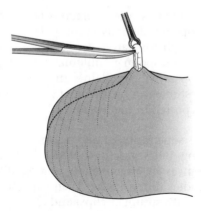

C. Grasping a partial thickness of the elevated vas

Source: Engenderhealth (2002) with permission.

Figure 22-8 No-scalpel vasectomy

COUNSELING FOR FEMALE STERILIZATION AND VASECTOMY

The goal of counseling is to guide clients to help them select a contraceptive method that they will use, that will be effective, that is most consistent with their reproductive intentions, and that will not have adverse effects. The permanence of sterilization methods is a significant consideration with respect to counseling. For some clients, reversals can be done but are expensive and require surgery or complex procedures; results are not guaranteed. Both female and male sterilization should be considered permanent. In the preoperative assessment, ensure the patient has been appropriately counseled and provided an informed consent for surgical sterilization. In addition, be certain she or he is counseled regarding the anesthetic method to be used.

REGRET AFTER STERILIZATION

In addition to failure, regret is the most significant potential long-term consequence of sterilization.

A variety of studies suggest regret rates anywhere from 0.9% to 26% for female sterilization.[47] Regret for vasectomy has been reported to be lower, most often reported as less than 5%.[82] Studies also show that the rate of regret increases over time and that up to 20% of women sterilized at a young age later regret this decision. Young age is the strongest predictor of regret that can be identified before female sterilization.[47,83] Regret following vasectomy is associated with marital instability at the time of vasectomy or age younger than 31 years, making the decision to have a vasectomy during a time of financial crisis or related to pregnancy, and having very young or no children at the time of vasectomy.[82,84,85] Identifying individuals at risk prior to sterilization is helpful, but in many cases, unpredictable life changes are the cause of regret.[82,86,87] Persons who are recently divorced or whose life circumstances are changing should receive individualized counseling. Postpartum sterilization is associated with an increased incidence of regret in many studies.[87–90] People who are poor (e.g., Medicaid clients) or of Hispanic origin also make up a disproportionate group of those who would wish a reversal procedure.[47]

SPECIFIC COUNSELING GUIDELINES FOR FEMALE AND/OR MALE STERILIZATION

The factors contributing to an individual's decision about female sterilization vary. Each woman needs to weigh the risks, benefits, effectiveness, and side effects of the various contraceptive options available to her, as well as her personal need to use a barrier method for protection against sexually transmitted infections, especially HIV/AIDS.

1. **Provide choices.** The clear answer is to provide clients with choices. New and old long-term contraceptive methods (e.g., injectables, IUDs, or implants) can be excellent methods for women who wish a highly effective, long-term method.

2. **Assess the client's understanding of the procedure.** In the United States, awareness of female sterilization is widespread, and one of the interviewer's tasks is to assure the individual correctly understands the procedure and has no misconceptions.

3. **Facilitate the decision-making process.** Give the client sufficient time to make a thoughtful, informed decision about a permanent method of contraception, especially women having immediate postpartum or postabortion (spontaneous or induced) sterilization. The woman should have decided she wants a permanent method well before delivery or a pregnancy-related event or procedure. Her decision may be unduly influenced by the emotional and physical stress produced by the pregnancy and related events. Postpartum clients have a higher rate of regret following sterilization than interval sterilization clients.[47]

4. Clients should be informed that sterilization (male and female) is not 100% successful, that failure occurs, even years after the procedure was performed.

5. Men should be advised that vasectomy is not immediately effective, that success should be confirmed by semen analysis if possible, and another contraceptive should be used until their provider says they can rely on the vasectomy alone for contraception.

POSTPARTUM COUNSELING GUIDELINES

Women who come to the hospital for the first time during labor may be counseled after delivery when they are free of the immediate stresses related to labor and delivery and are not under the influence of sedatives. If the baby is healthy and the woman clearly desires no more children, she may be a suitable candidate for sterilization. Husbands should also be brought into the discussion whenever possible; however, spousal consent should not be mandatory.

For postpartum clients, assure the patient has no medical problems such as eclampsia, postpartum hemorrhage, or endometritis that might contraindicate the sterilization surgical procedure.

Staff should be skilled in explaining and providing alternative contraceptive methods, such as the IUD, implants, or hormonal methods. Women should feel no pressure to decide upon sterilization because of the unavailability of alternative methods or lack of clinical skill to provide them. Moreover, interval sterilization services should be available so if uncertainty or any medical contraindication exists at the time, the procedure can be comfortably scheduled at four weeks or later after delivery.

If the procedure is delayed beyond 6 months after delivery and she is not fully or nearly fully breastfeeding and not amenorrheic, advise the woman to use an effective contraceptive method until the sterilization procedure.

POLICY/LEGAL ISSUES

Laws and regulations regarding sterilization procedures have undergone many changes over the last few decades. Be aware of rulings in counseling sterilization candidates:

- Pragmatically, ethically, and legally, strict adherence to informed choice and consent procedures is critical prior to sterilization.[91]
- Partner or spousal consent in the United States is not legally required.[92]
- Clients using federal or state funds for sterilization must be age 21 or older, mentally competent, and must wait 30 days after signing a consent before performance of a sterilization procedure.[36]

Arbitrary decisions by health professionals to restrict access to sterilization have been judged by courts in the United States to violate a woman's basic rights. Although these rulings were set to address the concerns of women seeking sterilization, the laws and regulations set forth apply equally to men seeking services for vasectomy.

The policy and legal status of providing sterilization for mentally challenged women and men remains a problem. Clear guidelines need to be established. Health care providers, policy makers, and the public should be informed of the ethical and legal issues involved in providing voluntary sterilization to those who may not be able to provide informed consent.

INFORMED CONSENT

Informed consent is the voluntary decision made by a person who has been fully informed regarding the surgical procedure and its consequences. Provide the information in a language the client can understand. Most informed consent documents cover the following important points:

- Type of operation, including risks and benefits
- Availability of alternative methods of family planning
- Inability to have children once sterilized
- Intended permanence of sterilization
- Possibility of reversal, but that it is expensive, requires complex procedures, and success cannot be guaranteed
- Possibility of failure (pregnancy, including ectopic pregnancy following female sterilization) after the procedure
- Option to decline sterilization without loss of medical or financial benefits

- Does not protect against sexually transmitted infections, including HIV/AIDS
- The client must always sign or mark the informed consent form. The surgeon or authorized representative must also sign the form. The authorized representative may be the person with the primary responsibility for counseling the client. Illiterate clients should mark the informed consent form with a thumbprint or "X"; a witness chosen by the client must also sign or mark the form. Preferably, the witness should be of the same sex as the client. The informed consent document should be readily understandable in the client's own language.

MANAGING PROBLEMS AND FOLLOW-UP
FEMALE STERILIZATION

Major complications from tubal sterilizations are uncommon and vary by study definition, occurring at levels that range from 1 to 3.5%.[93-95] The types of complications vary by the type of surgical procedure and anesthesia. Most of these complications can be prevented by careful screening, use of local anesthesia with light sedation, close monitoring of vital signs, good asepsis, and careful surgical technique. Infection prevention must always be a high priority.[96] The seriousness of complications can often be minimized by early recognition and aggressive management.

- Brisk bleeding from the engorged postpartum vessels can be avoided by gentle handling of the tubes.
- Postoperative hemorrhage can be avoided if ligatures around the tubes are secure to prevent slipping.
- Infections can be minimized by screening clients preoperatively and avoiding surgery on patients with prolonged ruptured membranes or evidence of current infection (with fever). Prophylactic antibiotics are usually given if the procedure is performed between the third and seventh postpartum day. If the procedure cannot be performed within 7 days after delivery, it is often advisable to wait until 4 to 6 weeks postpartum, primarily because of the technical difficulty of reaching the tubes.[62,97]

Laparoscopy Complications

Although complications from laparoscopy are not more common than from minilaparotomy, some are more severe.[7] The rate of laparoscopic complications is highly dependent on the level of surgical skill. To reduce complications, the operator should receive special training in laparoscopy. Surgeons performing fewer than 100 procedures per year have a much higher complication rate than more experienced surgeons.

The insufflation needle should have a blunt obturator (as does the Veress needle), and correct placement should be verified by aspiration, hanging drop, or pressure test.[97] Keep equipment in good working order;

keep the trocar sharp. When removing the cannula after all gas has been expelled, reinsert the laparoscope to the end of the cannula to prevent omentum or bowel from herniating into the abdominal wall defects as the cannula is removed.[97]

Anesthesia. Anesthesia-related complications can be aggravated by the gas-filled abdomen and the Trendelenburg position, especially if general anesthesia is used.

Instrument trauma and trauma of abdominal organs. Injury to intra-abdominal organs results either from accidental blunt or sharp trauma by surgical instruments or from electrical-thermal trauma.

Gentle use of all instruments on human tissues minimizes trauma. It is essential to determine the position of each organ or vessel during the surgery to avoid damage.

If injury occurs but is unrecognized, serious complications arise; prompt recognition is paramount. Unrecognized injuries have very high mortality rates due to the delay in recognition of intra-abdominal infection or hemorrhage.

Complications such as mesosalpingeal tears and transection of the tube can occur with ring application, which may require laparotomy to control bleeding. Sometimes an additional ring can be placed on each severed end of the tube for hemostasis.

Uterine perforation with the uterine elevator can usually be managed conservatively. Injuries to vessels, intestines, or other organs can occur with the insufflation needle or the trocar. General anesthesia back-up is necessary when doing laparoscopic sterilization procedures in order to manage rare complications of severe bleeding from a major vessel.

Bowel burns can occur from electrocoagulation, resulting in late perforation and peritonitis. Although bipolar electrocoagulation may carry less risk of burns than unipolar electrocoagulation, most international agencies discontinued support for electrocoagulation in the early 1980s. Most laparoscopic injuries are not related to the cautery (although electrical and technical changes can cause problems), but rather to the trocar or other surgical instruments.[98,99]

Minilaparotomy Complications

Wound infection. As with all surgical procedures, careful aseptic technique, proper skin preparation, sterilization of instruments, appropriate operating room technique, and diligent postoperative wound care decrease the likelihood of infection.

Uterine perforation with uterine elevator. Gentle use of all instruments on human tissues minimizes trauma. Determine the uterine position prior to inserting the elevator.

Bladder injury. This common surgical complication occurs because of the proximity of the bladder at the lower incision. Careful dissection and attention to landmarks assist in prevention.

Intestinal injury. Recognition of tissue layers and careful entry into the abdominal cavity help in prevention of injury. If injury is unrecognized, serious complications arise; therefore, prompt recognition is paramount.

LONG-TERM COMPLICATIONS

Ectopic pregnancy. Any time a woman shows signs of pregnancy following tubal sterilization, an ectopic pregnancy must be considered. In general, sterilization has an overall protective effect on the risk of ectopic pregnancy because of its protective effect against pregnancy overall. However, when a pregnancy does occur, the risk of ectopic pregnancy is significant. The 1996 CREST study stated that 32% of subsequent pregnancies were ectopic, and that risk was continuous and cumulative for the 10 years of follow-up.[3] This study and others indicate the lowest probability of ectopic pregnancy following unipolar coagulation and postpartum salpingectomy.[100-102]

Causes for ectopic pregnancy following sterilization include:

* Uteroperitoneal fistula after electrocoagulation (unipolar or bipolar)
* Inadequate coagulation after bipolar procedures
* Inadequate occlusion or fistula formation after the Pomeroy, clip, or ring procedure

Hormonal changes. The effect of tubal occlusion on hormonal feedback between the pituitary and ovaries has been extensively studied. While levels of luteinizing hormone (LH), follicle stimulating hormone (FSH), testosterone, and estrogen remain within the normal range, serum progesterone may decline.[27,103,104] Different conclusions have been reached by other investigators.[105,106]

Menstrual changes. For many years there has been controversy over the existence of a post-tubal ligation syndrome, referring to symptoms such as dysmenorrhea, heavy bleeding or spotting, and changes in cycle length or regularity. It has also been suggested that those methods of occlusion resulting in more extensive damage to the fallopian tubes may be more likely to cause subsequent changes in menstrual function. To date, however, the evidence does not consistently support this hypothesis.

Early studies reporting post sterilization menstrual function change failed to control for other factors leading to a change in menstrual function following sterilization such as pre-sterilization use of oral contraceptives and previous menstrual dysfunction. Most recent retrospective and prospective studies that account for these factors and others have found little or no difference in women before and after sterilization, or between sterilized women and nonsterilized controls for the first two years of follow up. Findings from reports that included follow up for more than two years appear to be less consistent. However recent CREST data suggest that at 5 years post sterilization when controlling for confounding variables, no significant difference in menstrual cycle change between cases and controls (women whose partners underwent vasectomy) can be described. The study found that women who underwent sterilization were no more likely than the control group to report persistent changes in their cycle length or inter-menstrual bleeding. However, they were more likely to have beneficial changes in their cycle including decreases in the amount of bleeding, the number of days of bleeding and menstrual pain. Although an increase in 'cycle irregularity' was reported in one study subset, this was considered likely due to chance. Method of tubal occlusion did not significantly impact findings.[107]

Laboratory studies of hormone levels have yielded little useful information on the post-ligation syndrome. Although many studies include control subjects, they do not measure the subject serum levels preoperatively in women undergoing sterilization. Studies that did measure such levels preoperatively found no changes following sterilization, but these involved only small numbers of women.[108,109] Further research needs to be conducted on this issue.

Psychological problems. Sterilized women have no more psychological problems than nonsterilized women.[57,110–112] A study of female marital sexuality found no detrimental long-term effects from female or male sterilization. Conversely, the study found an increase in coital frequency after 1 year among women who had undergone tubal sterilization as compared with women not planning sterilization.[113]

Sexuality. A CREST study to determine if interval tubal sterilization leads to a change in female sexual interest or pleasure found that interval tubal sterilization is unlikely to result in changed sexual interest or pleasure. Among those women with changes, the majority experienced positive sexual effects.[114]

Hysterectomy and other surgery. Several prospective studies report a concentrated increased risk of hysterectomy following female sterilization performed in women less than age 30.[115–117] There does not appear to be a biological basis for these surgeries. If sterilization does increase the incidence of hysterectomy or D&C, this must be considered an adverse outcome associated with sterilization.[118]

VASECTOMY

Vasectomy is a minor surgical procedure, and most postoperative complications of vasectomy are minor as well, usually subsiding within one or two weeks. The most frequent complaints after surgery are swelling of the scrotum, bruising, and pain. Minor bleeding under the skin is common. Some men experience tenderness or a dragging sensation in the scrotum for up to a week after vasectomy. A scrotal support, mild pain medication, and local application of ice are usually sufficient for treatment. Careful surgical technique, early recognition of a problem, and proper postoperative care and follow-up greatly reduce the risks of complications. Bleeding complications can be minimized by careful surgical technique and having men avoid strenuous activity for a day or two. Hemostasis (controlling any bleeding) during the operation can limit the likelihood of hematomas. Small noninfected hematomas may be managed with rest and analgesics; large, painful, or infected hematomas usually require surgical drainage. One of the main advantages of the no-scalpel method is a decreased rate of bleeding and infection complications.[72-74]

Infections are prevented by strict aseptic practices, using sterilized equipment, careful surgical technique, and keeping the incision clean. An infection should be treated with antibiotics and wet heat applied locally. Leakage of sperm from the occluded end of the vas can cause an inflammatory nodule (granuloma) that generally subsides spontaneously, although pain medication may be required. Only about 2% to 3% of cases are painful or significantly symptomatic. The rare granuloma that increases in size, is painful, and does not recede can be treated surgically. Back pressure in the occluded vas can cause congestive epididymitis, which usually subsides in a week with heat treatment and scrotal support.

Chronic pain in the testis after vasectomy has been reported by a small percentage of vasectomized men. While up to one-third of men have reported occasional testicular discomfort following vasectomy, only a small percentage of all vasectomized men (around 2%) said the pain had negatively impacted their life or that they regretted having had the vasectomy because of chronic pain.[119,120] Conservative therapy such as nonsteroidal anti-inflammatory drugs, sitz baths, antibiotics, or spermatic cord blocks is sufficient treatment in most cases. When this fails, there is some evidence that vasectomy reversal or denervation of the spermatic cord may be helpful.[121,122] Mortality due to vasectomy is extremely rare (Table 9-4).[123-125]

REVERSAL OF FEMALE STERILIZATION AND VASECTOMY

Sterilization should be considered permanent, but even with careful counseling, some women and men will request reversal following a divorce or remarriage, a child's death, or the desire for more children.[86,126] Emphasize the following points:

- Reversal requires major surgery or complicated procedures and special skills.
- Some clients are not appropriate candidates because of the way the sterilization was performed, because of the client's or partner's advanced age, or because of the partner's infertility.
- Fertility may not be restored, even when the patient is a good candidate and the surgery or procedure is performed by an experienced professional.
- Both reversal surgery and assisted reproductive technologies are very expensive for both male and female procedures.

- Surgery, especially major abdominal surgery, carries operative risks as well as risks due to anesthesia.
- Ectopic pregnancy is more common among pregnancies occurring after surgical reversal of female sterilization, ranging from 2 to 12.5%.[1]

If the woman wishes to have a reversal, a thorough evaluation of fertility should inform the choice of method to maximize success.

SUCCESS RATES FOR REVERSAL OF FEMALE STERILIZATION

Success rates based on intrauterine pregnancies after reversal surgery are highest for occlusion techniques that damage the smallest segment of tube. Higher success rates are generally achieved through the use of microsurgical techniques:

- Use of magnification (loupe, hood, or operating microscope)
- Accurate alignment of the fallopian tube segments and placement of sutures
- Constant irrigation of tissues to prevent drying
- Use of very fine suture and needles
- Microsurgical electrocautery to minimize bleeding
- Care to keep foreign materials from being left in the wound.

Women must consider any sterilization technique as permanent, even clips, because reversal is not always successful and reversal surgery will not be available to all who want it. For more and more women who are poor candidates for reversal surgery and who choose to avoid major abdominal surgery, in vitro fertilization (IVF) is usually an option.

SUCCESS RATES FOR REVERSAL OF VASECTOMY

Both macroscopic and microsurgical techniques have been used for vasectomy reversal. The current consensus is that the microsurgical techniques are more successful.[127–129] The percentage of men with sperm in the ejaculate ranges from 75% to 100% for microsurgical reversal.[28,127,130] However, presence of sperm should not be presented to men as the measure of success, since pregnancy is the desired outcome. Reported pregnancy rates are lower, ranging from 38% to 82%.[127,130,131] The time elapsed between the vasectomy and the reversal is a major factor in the success of reversal; the longer the interval between vasectomy and reversal, the less likely the man is to be fertile after the reversal. Reversal is usually more successful when done within 10 years after vasectomy. Pregnancy rates drop to less than 50% when reversal is performed more than 9 to 10 years after vasectomy.[28,127,131] Other factors that affect the success of vasectomy reversal include the skill of the surgeon, the type of vasectomy procedure originally performed, levels of antisperm antibodies, the age of the female partner, and partial obstruction of the vas after the reversal surgery that prevent movement of sperm through the vas.

Assisted reproduction technologies have been successful in vasectomized men who want children but do not want a vasectomy reversal or have had one or more unsuccessful reversal surgeries. Sperm can be retrieved from the epididymis or the testis and then used for intracytoplasmic sperm injection (ICSI). Pregnancy rates following ICSI with epididymal sperm and testicular sperm are reported to be between 25% and 36% and 17% and 36% respectively.[132] Similar to the case with vasectomy reversal, a negative correlation exists between pregnancy rates and time elapsed from the vasectomy until sperm aspiration and ICSI.[133,134]

Vasectomy reversal has been shown to be equally or more successful and less costly than ICSI following epididymal sperm aspiration.[135,136] Thus, surgical reversal appears to be a better first choice for vasectomized men who wish to have children.[137] This is the case even in men who are undergoing repeat vasectomy reversal surgery due to a previously failed reversal attempt.[138] Attempts to develop a plug, valve, or simple reversible vasectomy have not been successful.[85,139] Men must accept vasectomy as a permanent procedure even though improved microsurgical techniques have increased the chances of restoring fertility.

INSTRUCTIONS FOR FEMALE STERILIZATION AND VASECTOMY

FEMALE STERILIZATION

Preoperative Instructions

1. Be completely comfortable with your decision to use a surgical method for contraception. You must be certain you understand sterilization is permanent and that you desire a permanent method of contraception. Be certain all of your questions have been asked and answered. You can change your mind at any time before the procedure or can postpone the operation if you need more time to think about it.

2. Shower or bathe just before surgery. Pay particular attention to the area around the umbilicus (navel) and the pubic hair.

3. **Do not eat or drink** in the 8 hours before surgery.

4. Have someone accompany you on the day of surgery, if at all possible. This person should accompany you when you go home. You should plan to have someone with you for the first 24 hours following surgery.

5. **Rest for at least 24 hours** after the procedure and avoid heavy lifting for 1 week.

6. Be prepared for pain over the incision and occasional pelvic aching or discomfort. The pain is usually not severe and can be relieved with mild pain medications provided to you.

7. Plan a flexible schedule for the week after the sterilization. Some women recover less quickly than others from the effects of anesthesia and surgery.

8. Be certain to ask questions if you have them.

Postoperative Instructions

1. **Rest for 24 hours** following surgery. Resume normal activities as you gradually become more comfortable.

2. **Avoid intercourse for 1 week** and when you resume having intercourse, stop if it is uncomfortable.

3. **Avoid strenuous lifting for 1 week** to allow the incisions to heal.

4. Return to the clinic or contact the clinic or doctor promptly if you develop:

Condition:	Action:
Temperature: 100+ degrees Fahrenheit	Immediate contact with M.D. either by phone or for exam.
Fainting: Fainting spells	Contact M.D. by phone
Pain: Abdominal pain that is persistent, severe and/or increasing after 12 hours	Immediate contact with M.D. for exam.
Incision sites: Bleeding or spotting from incision sites	1. Put pressure and tape x 12 hours. 2. Keep clean with betadine or peroxide. 3. If condition continues or worsens, contact M.D.
Pus or discharge from incision sites	1. Clean with betadine or peroxide 2 times/day. 2. If condition continues or worsens, contact M.D.
Stitch in wound	It will eventually fall out (unless a permanent suture was put in place).

Postoperative Warning Signs

Caution

- Fever (greater than 100.4°F, 39°C)
- Dizziness with fainting
- Abdominal pain that is persistent or increasing
- Bleeding or fluid coming from the incision
- If you should ever get pregnant, you must be seen immediately

5. Take one or two analgesic tablets at 4- to 6-hour intervals if you need them for pain. (Do not use aspirin since it may promote bleeding.)

6. You may bathe 48 hours after surgery but avoid putting tension on the incision and do not rub or irritate the incision for 1 week. Dry the incision site after bathing.

7. Stitches will dissolve and do not require removal. (Note to provider: this instruction must be modified if nonabsorbable sutures such as silk are used.)

8. **Return to the clinic** 1 week after the procedure to make sure the healing process is normal.

9. If you think you are pregnant at any time in the future, return to the clinic immediately. Although pregnancy after female sterilization is rare, when it does occur, chances are increased that it will be outside the uterus (an ectopic pregnancy). This is a dangerous life-threatening condition and must be treated immediately.

10. You should know this method of birth control is permanent. Reversal surgery is possible under certain conditions, but it is expensive, requires highly technical and major surgery, and its results cannot be guaranteed.

VASECTOMY

Preoperative Instructions

1. Be completely sure of your decision to have a vasectomy. You must be certain you understand and desire the permanence of vasectomy. You can change your mind at any time before the operation.

2. Before surgery while you are home, use scissors to cut all hair from around the penis and scrotum to about 1/4-in. in length.

3. Shower or bathe, washing the penis and scrotum thoroughly to remove all loose hairs.

4. If possible, bring someone who can accompany you home after the procedure. Do not ride a bicycle and avoid walking long distances or using other transportation that may rub or put pressure on the scrotum.

5. **Plan to remain quiet for about 48 hours** following the vasectomy. A 48-hour rest is important to decrease the risk of complications.

Postoperative Instructions

1. Following the surgery, return home and rest for about 2 days. If possible, **keep an ice pack on the scrotum for at least 4 hours** to reduce the chances of swelling, bleeding, and discomfort. Wear a scrotal support for 2 days. (Jockey shorts will be adequate.) You may be able to resume your normal activities after 2 or 3 days.

2. **Avoid strenuous physical exercise for 1 week.** Strenuous exercise means hard physical exertion or lifting or straining that could bring pressure to the groin or scrotum.

3. Do not shower or bathe for the first 24 hours after the vasectomy.

4. The stitches will dissolve and do not have to be removed. (Note to provider: this instruction must be modified if nonabsorbable skin sutures, such as silk, are used or if no skin sutures are used.)

5. **You may resume sexual intercourse after 2 or 3 days** if you feel it would be comfortable; but remember, **you are not sterile immediately.** For many men, sperm will not be cleared from the tubes until after a minimum of 3 months. Until then, use condoms or another method of birth control to prevent pregnancy. The best way of finding out if you are sterile is to have the doctor look at your semen under a microscope after a minimum of 3 months.

6. If you have pain or discomfort, simple analgesics taken at intervals of 4 to 6 hours usually give adequate relief. (Note to provider: name and dose should be specified.)

7. It is important for you to know what is normal and what is abnormal following your surgery. You will probably have some pain and swelling in the scrotal region; the scrotum may be somewhat discolored. These conditions are normal and should not worry you. Occasionally, blood from a tiny blood vessel may escape into the scrotum at the time of surgery, and bleeding may continue. Notify your doctor or health worker if you have any of the following danger signals or if you notice any other unusual body changes:

Condition:	Action:
Temperature: 100+ degrees Fahrenheit	Contact with M.D. either by phone or for exam.
Pain: Unable to sleep or work	If unrelieved by analgesic, see a clinician.
Discharge: Pus or inflammation at incision site	Clean with betadine or peroxide. If redness in skin increases, contact M.D.
Bleeding: Bleeding from incision site	If after placing pressure on area for 10 minutes the bleeding continues, contact clinician for futher assessment.
Swelling: Greater than twice normal size	Contact M.D. by phone.
Nodules: Larger than a nickel (5 cent piece), pain and tenderness	Contact M.D. by phone.
Stitches: Extreme pulling sensation	Contact M.D. by phone.

8. You should know this method of birth control is permanent. Reversal surgery is possible under certain conditions, but it is expensive, requires highly technical and major surgery, and its results cannot be guaranteed.

References

1. Pati S, and Cullins V. Female sterilization—evidence. Obstet Gynecol Clin North Am. Update in Contraception. 2000;27(4):859-899.
2. MacKay AP, Kieke BA, Koonin LM, Beattie, K. Tubal sterilization in the United States 1994-1996. Fam Plann Perspect 2001;33(4):161-165.
3. Peterson HB, Xia Z, Hughes JM, Wilcox LS, Tylor LR, Trussell J. The risk of pregnancy after tubal sterilization: Findings from the U.S. Collaborative Review of Sterilization. Am J Obstet Gynecol 1996;174:1161-1170.
4. Soderstrom RM, Levy BS, Engel T. Reducing bipolar sterilization failures. Obstet Gynecol 1989;74:60-63.
5. Trussell J, Leveque JA, Koenig JD, London R, Borden S, Henneberry J, LaGuardia KD, Stewart F, Wilson TG, Wysocki S, Strauss M. The economic value of contraception: a comparison of 15 methods. Am J Public Health 1995;85:494-503.
6. AVSC International. Personal communication with Daria Teutonico, 2000.
7. Peterson HB, DeStefano F, Rubin GL, Greenspan JR, Lee NC, Ory HW. Deaths attributed to tubal sterilization in the United States, 1977 to 1981. Am J Obstet Gynecol 1983;146:131-136.
8. U.S. Bureau of the Census. Statistical abstract of the United States: 1992 (112th ed.) Washington DC, 1992.
9. Wingo PA, Huezo CM, Rubin GL, Ory HW, Peterson HB. The mortality risk associated with hysterectomy. Am J Obstet Gynecol 1985;152(7-1):803-808.
10. Westhoff C, Davis A. Tubal sterilization: Focus on the US experience. Fertil Steril 2000;73:913-922.
11. Chi I-c, Petta CA, McPheeters M. A review of safety, efficacy, pros and cons, and issues of puerperal tubal sterilization--an update. Adv Contracept 1995;11:187-206.
12. Castellsague, X, Thompson WD, Dubrow R. Tubal sterilization and the risk of endometrial cancer. Int J Cancer 1996;65:607.
13. Fox KM, Cummings SR. Is tubal ligation a risk factor for low bone density and increased risk of fracture? Am J Obstet Gynecol 1995;172:101.
14. Irwin KL, Lee NC, Peterson HB, et al. Hysterectomy, tubal sterilization, and the risk of breast cancer. Am J Epidemiol 1998;127:1192.
15. Kelsey JL, Livolsi VA, Holford TR, et al. A case-control study of cancer of the endometrium. Am J Epidemiol 116:333, 1982.
16. Greene A, Purdie D, Bain C, et al. Tubal sterilisation, hysterectomy and decreased risk of ovarian cancer: Survey of Women's Health Study Group. Int J Cancer 1997;71:948.
17. Hankinson SE, Hunter DJ, Colditz GA, et al. Tubal ligation, hysterectomy, and risk of ovarian cancer: A prospective study. 1993;JAMA 270:2813.
18. Miracle-McMahill HL, Calle EE, Kosinski AS, et al. Tubal ligation and fatal ovarian cancer in a large prospective cohort study. Am J Epidemiol 1997;145:349.
19. Narod SA, Sun P., Ghadirian P., Lynch, H., Isaacs, C., Garber, J., Weber, B., Karlan, B., Fishman, D., Rosen, B., Tung N., Neuhausen, S.L., and the Hereditary Ovarian Cancer Clinical Study Group. Tubal ligation and risk of ovarian cancer in carriers of BRCA1 or BRCA2 mutations: a case-control study. Lancet 2001;357(9267):1467.
20. Bernstein GS, Chopp R, Cosgrove M, Coulson A, Kiely W, Friou G, Korelitz J, Massey FJ, Mendez R, Mestman J. A controlled, prospective study of the effects of vasectomy. In: Lepow LH, Corzier R (eds). Vasectomy: immunologic and pathophysiologic effects in animals and man. New York: Academic Press, 1979:473-489.
21. Hellema HWJ, Rumke P. Sperm autoantibodies as a consequence of vasectomy: I. Within 1 year post-operation. Clin Experim Immunol 1978;31:18–29.
22. Lenzi A, Gandini L, Lombardo F. Antisperm antibody detection: 2. Clinical, biological, and statistical correlation between methods. Am J Reprod Immunol 1997;38:224–230.
23. Gubin DA, Dmochowski R, Kutteh WH. Multivariant analysis of men from infertile couples with and without antisperm antibodies. Am J Reprod Immunol 1998;39:157–160.

24. Petitti DB, Klein R, Kipp H, Kahn W, Siegelaub AB, Friedman GD. A survey of personal habits, symptoms of illness, and histories of disease in men with and without vasectomies. Am J Public Health 1982;72:476-480.
25. Goldacre MJ, Holford, TR, Vessey M. P. Cardiovascular disease and vasectomy: Findings from two epidemiologic studies. New England Journal of Medicine 1983;308(14):805–808.
26. Giovannucci E, Tosteson TD, Speizer FE, Vessey MP, Colditz GA. A long-term study of mortality in men who have undergone vasectomy. N Engl J Med 1992;326(21):1392-1398.
27. Massey FJ, Bernstein GS, O'Fallon WM, Schuman LM, Coulson AH, Crozier R, Mandel JS, Benjamin RB, Berendes HW, Chang PC. Vasectomy and health: results from a large cohort study. JAMA 1984;252:1023-1029.
28. Huang MK, Wu X, Fu C, Zou P, Gao X, Huang Q. Multiple factors affecting human repregnancy after microsurgical vasovasostomy. Reprod Contracept 1997;8:92–100.
29. Meinertz H, Linnet L, Fogh-Andersen P, Hjort T. Antisperm antibodies and fertility after vasovasostomy: a follow-up study of 216 men. Fert Steril 1990;54:315–321.
30. Newton RA. IgG antisperm antibodies attached to sperm do not correlate with infertility following vasovasostomy. Microsurgery 1998;9:278–280.
31. Thomas Jr, AJ, Pontes JE, Rose NR, Segal S, Pierce JM Jr. Microsurgical vasovasostomy: Immunologic consequences and subsequent fertility. Fertil Steril 1981;35:447–450.
32. Lea IA, Adoyo P, O'Rand MG. Autoimmunogenicity of the human sperm protein Sp17 in vasectomized men and identification of linear B cell epitopes. Fertil Steril 1997;67:355–361.
33. Parslow JM, Poulton TA, Besser GM, et al: The clinical relevance of classes of immunoglobulins on spermatozoa from infertile and vasovasostomized males. Fertil Steril 1985;43:621-627.
34. Hjort T. Antisperm antibodies. Antisperm antibodies and infertility: an unsolvable question? Hum Reprod 1999;14:2423-2426.
35. Hayes RB. Are dietary fat and vasectomy risk factors for prostate cancer? J Nat Cancer Inst 1995;87:629-630.
36. Levy IG, Gibbons, L, Collin JP, Perkins, D.G., Mao, Y. Prostate cancer trends in Canada: Rising incidence or increased detection. Can Med Assoc J 1993;149:617.
37. Bernal-Delgado E, Latour-Perez J, Pradas-Arnal F, Gomez-Lopez LI. The association between vasectomy and prostate cancer: A systematic review of the literature. Fertil Steril 1998;70:191–200.
38. Peterson HB, Howards SS. Vasectomy and prostate cancer: The evidence to date. Fertil Steril 1998;70:201–203.
39. Healy B. From the National Institutes of Health: does vasectomy cause prostate cancer? JAMA 1993;269:2620.
40. Cox, B. Sneyd MJ, Paul C, Delahunt B, Skegg DC. Vasectomy and risk of prostate cancer. JAMA 2002;287:3110-3115.
41. Stanford JL, Wicklund KG, McKnight B, Daling JR Brawer MK. Vasectomy and risk of prostate cancer. Cancer Epidemiology, Biomarkers & Prevention 1999;8:881-886.
42. Lynge E. Prostate cancer is not increased in men with vasectomy in Denmark. J Urol 2002;168:488-90.
43. World Health Organization. Female sterilization: A guide to provision in services, 1992.
44. Anonymous. Sterilization device to offer ease of use. Contracept Tech Update 1996;17:53-64.
45. Anonymous. Update on female sterilization. The Contraception Report 1996;7(3):13-14.
46. Haws JM, Pollack AE, Beattie KJ, et al. New data on sterilization in the United States. Invited presentation at a meeting convened by the NICHD, NIH, Bethesda, MD, June 1998.
47. Hills SD, Marchbanks PA, Tylor LR, et al: Poststerilization regret: Findings from the United States collaborative review of sterilization. Obstet Gynecol 1999;83:889.

48. Stewart FH, Guest F, Stewart GK, Hatcher RA. Understanding your body. New York: Bantam, 1987.
49. AVSC International. Minilaparotomy under local anaesthesia: a curriculum for doctors and nurses. Trainer's manual. New York: AVSC International, 1993.
50. EngenderHealth. Minilaparotomy for Female Sterilization: An Illustrated Guide for Service Providers. New York, NY: EngenderHealth, 2003.
51. Hasson HM. Open laparoscopy. Biomedical Bulletin, Association for Voluntary Surgical Contraception 1984;5(1).
52. Hasson HM. Open laparoscopy. In: Sciarra JJ (ed). Gynecology and obstetrics. Philadelphia PA: Harper & Row, 1982:44.
53. Penfield AJ. Female sterilization by minilaparotomy or open laparoscopy. Baltimore MD: Urban and Schwarzenberg, 1980.
54. Yoon IB. The Yoon Ring as compared with other sterilization methods. In: Phillips JM. Endoscopic female sterilization. Downey CA: The American Association of Gynecologic Laparoscopists, 1983.
55. Uribe-Ramirez LC, Camarena R, Hernandez F, Diaz-Garcia M. A retrospective analysis of surgical complications of four tuboocclusive techniques. In: Phillips JM (ed). Endoscopic female sterilization. Downey CA: The American Association of Gynecologic Laparoscopists, 1983.
56. Kwak Hyon-Mo. Laparoscopic sterilization: Korean experience, particularly ectopic pregnancy subsequent to female sterilization. Proceedings of the Pre-Congress Seminar of the XIth AUFOG Congress, Bangkok, Thailand, Dec. 1-4, 1987.
57. World Health Organization. Mental health and female sterilization: report of a WHO collaborative prospective study. J Biosoc Sci 1984;16:1-21.
58. Sokal, D., Hieu, D.T., Weiner, D.H., Vinh, D.Q., Vach, T.H., Hanenberg, R. Long-term follow-up after quinacrine sterilization in Vietnam. Part 1: interim efficacy analysis. Fertil Steril 2000;74(6):1084-1091.
59. Sokal, D., Hieu, D.T., Weiner, D.H., Vinh, D.Q., Vach, T.H., Hanenberg, R. Long-term follow-up after quinacrine sterilization in Vietnam. Part 2: interim safety analysis. Fertil Steril 2000;74(6):1092-1101.
60. U.S. Food and Drug Administration. FDA approves new female sterilization device. FDA Talk Paper. 2002;T02-41:1-2.
61. Kerin JF, Carignan CS, Cher D. The safety and effectiveness of a new hysteroscopic method for permanent birth control: results of the first Essure™ pbc clinical study. Austral NZ J Obstet Gynaecol 2001;41:364-370.
62. Pritchard JA, MacDonald PC, Grant NF. Williams obstetrics, 17th ed. Norwalk CT: Appleton- Century-Crofts, 1985: Chapter 40.
63. Peterson HB, Hulka JF, Spielman FJ, Lee S, Marchbanks PA. Local versus general anesthesia for laparoscopic sterilization: a randomized study. Obstet Gynecol 1987;70:903-908.
64. Poindexter AN III, Abdul-Malak M., Fast JE. Laparoscopic tubal sterilization under local anesthesia. Obstet Gynecol 1990;75:5.
65. World Health Organization. Improving access to quality care in family planning: medical eligibility criteria for contraceptive use. Second edition. Geneva:World Health Organization, 2000.
66. World Health Organization. Technical and managerial guidelines for vasectomy services. Geneva: World Health Organization, 1988.
67. Kendrick JS, Gonzales B, Huber DH, Grubb GS, Rubin GL. Complications of vasectomies in the United States, J Fam Pract 1987;25(3):245–281.
68. Kendrick JS, Rhodenhiser EP, Rubin GL, Greenspan JR. Characteristics of vasectomies performed in selected outpatient facilities in the United States, 1980. Journal of Reproductive Medicine 1985;30(12):936–938.
69. Alderman P. The lurking sperm: a review of failures in 8879 vasectomies performed by one physician. JAMA 1988;259:3142-3144.
70. EngenderHealth. No-scalpel vasectomy: an illustrated guide for surgeons. Third edition. New York NY: EngenderHealth, 2003.
71. Li SQ, Goldstein M, Zhu J, Huber D. The no-scalpel vasectomy. J Urol 1991;145:341-344.

72. Kumar V, Kaza RM, Singh I, Singhal S, Kumaran V. An evaluation of the no-scalpel vasectomy technique. BJU International 1999;83:283-284.
73. Skriver M, Skovsgaard F, Miskowiak J. Conventional or Li vasectomy: a questionnaire study. Br J Urol 1997;79:596–598.
74. Sokal D, Hieu DT, Weiner DH, Vinh DQ, Vach TH, Hanenberg R. Long-term follow-up after quinacrine sterilization in Vietnam. Part 2: interim safety analysis. Fertil Steril 2000;74(6):1092-1101.
75. Errey BB. Follow-up of 6014 open-ended vasectomy cases. Personal communication with Gary Stewart, Sept. 4, 1987.
76. Errey BB, Edwards IS. Open-ended vasectomy: an assessment. Fertil Steril 1986; 45(6):843-846.
77. Barone MA, Nazerali H, Cortes M, Chen-Mok M, Pollack AE, Sokal D. A prospective study of time and number of ejaculations to azoospermia after vasectomy by ligation and excision. J Urol. In press for Sept 2003.
78. Nazerali H, Thapa S, Hays M, Pathak LR, Pandey KR, Sokal DC. Vasectomy effectiveness in Nepal: a retrospective study. Contraception 2003;67:397-401.
79. Labrecque M, Nazerali H., Mondor M, Fortin V, Nasution M.: Effectiveness and complications associated with 2 vasectomy occlusion techniques. J Urol 2002;168:2495.
80. Sokal D, Irsula B, Hays M, Barone MA. Vasectomy with fascial interposition vs. ligation and excision alone: A randomized controlled trial. BMC Medicine 2004;2:6. Available http://www.biomedcentral.com/bmcmed.
81. Chen-Mok M, Bangdiwala SI, Dominik R, Hays M, Irsula B, Sokal DC: Termination of a randomized controlled trial of two vasectomy techniques. Control Clin Trials, 2003;24:78.
82. Shain RN. Psychosocial consequences of vasectomy in developed and developing countries. In: G.I. Zatuchni, et al. (eds). Male contraception: advances and future prospects. Philadelphia: Harper and Row, 1968:34-53.
83. Hardy E, Bahamondes L, Osis MJ, Costa RG, Faundes A. Risk factors for tubal sterilization regret, detectable before surgery. Contraception 1996,54:159-162.
84. Clarke L, Gregson S. Who has a vasectomy reversal? J Biosoc Sci 1986;18:253-259.
85. Howard G. Who asks for vasectomy reversal and why? BMJ 1982;285:490-492.
86. Wilcox LS, Chu SV and Peterson HB. Characteristics of women who considered or obtained tubal reanatomosis: results from a prospective study of tubal sterilization. Obstet Gynecol 1990;75:661-665.
87. Wilcox LS, Chu SY, Eaker ED, Zeger SL, Peterson HB. Risk factors for regret after tubal sterilization: 5 years of follow-up in a prospective study. Fertil Steril 1991; 55:927-933.
88. Chi I-c, Gates D, Thapa S. Performing tubal sterilizations during a women's postpartum hospitalization: a review of the United States and international experiences. Obstet Gynecol Surv 1992;47:71-79.
89. Pitaktepsombati P, Janowitz B. Sterilization acceptance and regret in Thailand. Contraception 1991;44:623-637.
90. Ramsay IN, Russell SA. Who requests reversal of female sterilization? A retrospective study from a Scottish unit. Scott Med J 1991;36:44-46.
91. Soderstrom R. Clinical Challenges: share warning information, court case teaches. Contra Technol Update 1981;2:8-9.
92. Coe vs. Bolton. United States District Court, Civil Action No. C-76-785-A. September 29, 1976 (N.D. Georgia).
93. Dominik R, Gates D, Sokal D, Cordero M, et al. Two randomized controlled trials comparing the Hulka and Filshie clips for tubal sterilization. Contraception 2000;62:169-175.
94. Sokal D, Gates D, Amatya R, Dominik R.Two randomized control trial comparing the tubal ring and Filschie clip for tubal sterilization. Fertil Steril 2000;74:523-533.
95. Jameison DJ, Hillis SD, Duerr A, Marchbanks PA, Costello C, Peterson HB. Complications of interval lap tubal sterilization: findings from the US collaborative review of sterilization. Obstet Gynecol 2000;96:997–1002.

96. Engender Health. Infection prevention: a reference booklet for healthcare providers, 2001.
97. World Federation of Health Agencies for the Advancement of Voluntary Surgical Contraception. Safe and voluntary surgical contraception. New York: World Federation of Health Agencies, 1988.
98. DiGiovanni M, Vasilenko P, Belsky D. Laparoscopic tubal sterilization. The potential for thermal bowel injury. J Repro Med 1990;35(10):951-954.
99. Li S, Zhu J. Ligation of vas deferens with clamping method under direct vision. Unpublished, 1984.
100. Family Health International, Obstetrics and Gynecology Devices Panel of the Department of Health and Human Services, Public Health Service, Food and Drug Administration meeting, February 26, 1996.
101. Holt VL, Chu J, Daling JR, et al. Tubal sterilization and subsequent ectopic pregnancy: A case-control study. JAMA 266:242,191.
102. Kjer JJ, Knudsen LB. Ectopic pregnancy subsequent to laparoscopic sterilization. Am J Obstet Gynecol 1989;160:1202.
103. Radwanska E, Berger G, Hammond J. Luteal deficiency among women with normal menstrual cycles, requesting reversal of tubal sterilization. Obstet Gynecol 1979;54:189-192.
104. Radwanska E, Headley SK, Dmowski P. Evaluation of ovarian function after tubal sterilization. J Repro Med 1982;27:376-384.
105. Alvarez-Sanchez F, Segal SJ, Brache V, Adejuwan CA, Leon P, Faundes A. Pituitary-ovarian function after tubal ligation. Fertil Steril 1981;36:606-609.
106. Corson SL, Levinson CJ, Batzer FR, Otis C. Hormonal levels following sterilization and hysterectomy. J Repro Med 1981;26(7):363-370.
107. Peterson HB, Jeng G, Folger SG, Hillis SA, Marchbanks PA Wilcox LS. The risk of menstrual abnormalities after tubal sterilization US CREST working group. NEJM 2000; 343:1681-1687.
108. Alvarez F, Faundes A, Brache V, Tejada AS, Segal S. Prospective study of the pituitary-ovarian function after tubal sterilization by the Pomeroy or Uchida techniques. Fertil Steril 1989;51:604-608.
109. Garza-Flores J et al. Assessment of luteal function after surgical tubal sterilization. Adv Contracept 1991;7:371-377.
110. Vessey M, Huggins G, Lawless M, McPherson K, Yeates D. Tubal sterilization: findings in a large prospective study. Br J Obstet Gynaecol 1983;90:203-209.
111. Wilcox LS, Martinez-Schnell V, Peterson HB, Ware JH, Hughes JM. Menstrual function after tubal sterilization. Am J Epidemiol 1992;135:1368-1381.
112. Bledin KD, Cooper JE, Mackenzie S, Brice B. Psychological sequelae of female sterilization: short-term outcome in a prospective controlled study. Psychol Med 1984;14:379-390.
113. Shain RN, Miller WB, Holden AE, Rosenthal M. Impact of tubal sterilization and vasectomy on female marital sexuality: results of a controlled longitudinal study. Am J Obstet Gynecol 1991;164:763-771.
114. Costello C, Hillis SD, Marchbanks PA, Jamieson DJ, Peterson HB. The effect of interval tubal sterilization on sexual interest and pleasure. U.S. Collaborative Review of Sterilization Working Group. Obstet Gynecol 2002;100:511-517.
115. Cohen MM. Long-term risk of hysterectomy after tubal sterilization. Am J Epidemiol 1987;125:410.
116. Goldhaber MK, Armstrong MA, Golditch IM, et al. Long-term risk of hysterectomy among 80,007 sterilized and comparison women at Kaiser Permanente. Am J Epidemiol 1993;138:508.
117. Stergachis A, Shy KK, Grothaus LC, Wagner EH, Hecht JA, Anderson G, Normand EH, Raboud J. Tubal sterilization and the long-term risk of hysterectomy. JAMA 1990;264:2893-2898.
118. Chi I-c. Is tubal sterilization associated with an increased risk of subsequent hysterectomy but a decreased risk of ovarian cancer? A review of recent literature. Adv Contr 1996;12:77-99.

119. McMahon AJ, Buckley J, Taylor A, Lloyd SN, Deane RF, Kirk D. Chronic testicular pain following vasectomy. Br J Urol 1992;69:188–191.

120. Choe JM, Kirkemo AK. Questionnaire-based outcomes study of non-oncological post-vasectomy complications. J Urol 1996;155:1284–1286.

121. Ahmed I, Rasheed S, White C, Shaikh NA. The incidence of post-vasectomy chronic testicular pain and the role of nerve stripping (denervation) of the spermatic cord in its management. Br J Urol 1997;79:269–270.

122. Myers SA, Mershon CE, Fuchs EF. Vasectomy reversal for treatment of the post-vasectomy pain syndrome. J Urol 1997;157:518–520.

123. Grimes DA, Satterthwaite AP, Rochat RW, Akhter N. Deaths from contraceptive sterilization in Bangladesh: rates, causes, and prevention. Obstetrics and Gynecology 1982;60:635–640.

124. Khairullah Z, Huber DH, Gonzales B. Declining mortality in international sterilization services. Intl J Gynecol Obstet 1992;39:41–50.

125. Khairullah Z, Huber DH, Gonzales B. Declining mortality in international sterilization services. International Journal of Gynecology and Obstetrics 1992;39:41–50.

126. Siegler AM, Hulka J, Peretz A. Reversibility of female sterilization. Fertil Steril 1985;43:499–510.

127. Belker AM, Thomas AJ, Jr., Fuchs EF, Konnak JW, Sharlip ID. Results of 1,469 microsurgical vasectomy reversals by the Vasovasostomy Study Group. J Urol 1991;145:505–511.

128. Fox M. Failed vasectomy reversal: is a further attempt worthwhile using microsurgery? Europ Urol 1997;31(4):436–440.

129. Belker AM. Evaluation of partial anastomotic obstruction after vasovasostomy and predictors of success after vasoepididymostomy. J Urol 1998;159:835–836.

130. Lee HY. Twenty-year experience with vasovasotomy. J Urol 1986;136: 413-415.

131. Takihara H. Treatment of obstructive azoospermia in male infertility—past, present, and future. Urology 1998;51:150–155.

132. Pollack AP, Barone MA. "Reversing vasectomy" In: J. Sciarra (ed). Gynecology and obstetrics. Vol. 6: Fertility regulation, psychosomatic problems, and human sexuality. Lippincott Williams & Wilkins. Philadelphia, 2000, chapter 48.

133. Borges E Jr, Rossi-Ferragut LM, Pasqualotto FF, Rocha CC, and Iaconelli A Jr. Different intervals between vasectomy and sperm retrieval interfere in the reproductive capacity from vasectomized men. J Assist Reprod Genet. 2003;20:33-37.

134. Abdelmassih V, Balmaceda JP, Tesarik J, Abdelmassih R, Nagy ZP. Relationship between time period after vasectomy and the reproductive capacity of sperm obtained by epididymal aspiration. Hum Reprod 2002;17:736-740.

135. Fuchs EF, Burt RA. Vasectomy reversal performed 15 years or more after vasectomy: correlation of pregnancy outcome with partner age and with pregnancy results of in vitro fertilization with intracytoplasmic sperm injection. Fertil Steril 2002;77:516-519.

136. Kolettis PN, Sabanegh ES, D'amico AM, Box L, Sebesta M, Burns JR. Outcomes for vasectomy reversal performed after obstructive intervals of at least 10 years. Urology 2002;60:885-888.

137. Kolettis PN, Thomas Jr AJ: Vasoepididymostomy for vasectomy reversal: A critical assessment in the era of intracytoplasmic sperm injection. J Urol 1997;158:467.

138. Donovan Jr JF, DiBaise M, Sparks AE et al: Comparison of microscopic epididymal sperm aspiration and intracytoplasmic sperm injection/in-vitro fertilization with repeat microscopic reconstruction following vasectomy: Is second attempt vas reversal worth the effort? Hum Reprod 1998;13:387.

139. Liskin L, Benoit E, Blackburn R. Vasectomy: new opportunities. Population Reports, Series D, No. 5. Baltimore, Johns Hopkins University, Population Information Program, March 1992.

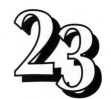

Postpartum Contraception and Lactation

Kathy I. Kennedy, DrPH
James Trussell, PhD

- Breastmilk is the ideal source of nutrition for infants and confers immunological protection against many infections. Family planning clinicians can play an important role in promoting breastfeeding.

- The Lactational Amenorrhea Method (LAM) is a highly effective, *temporary* method of contraception. To maintain effective protection against pregnancy, another method of contraception must be used as soon as menstruation resumes, the frequency or duration of breastfeeds is reduced, bottle feeds or regular food supplements are introduced, or the baby reaches 6 months of age.

- Other good contraceptive options for lactating women are (1) barrier methods, such as the male or female condom, which also confer protection against sexually transmitted infections; (2) progestin-only methods such as the minipill, Norplant or Depo-Provera; (3) the Copper T 380A intrauterine device (IUD) or the Levonorgestrel intrauterine system (LNg IUS); and (4) the permanent methods, male or female sterilization.

- The combined pill, patch, injectable, and vaginal ring are not good contraceptive options for lactating women because estrogen decreases milk supply.

- HIV can be transmitted through breastmilk. Therefore, in the United States, where safe alternatives to breastmilk are available, HIV-infected mothers are advised to avoid breastfeeding.

After childbirth, a woman soon becomes capable of becoming pregnant again since the postpartum period of infertility may be brief. Although the breastfeeding woman will have a longer period of infertility than will the nonbreastfeeding woman, her fertility usually returns during weaning, as the frequency of breastfeeds decreases. During weaning, the breastfeeding woman should use a contraceptive method so that she may breastfeed for as long as she chooses before becoming pregnant again. Fortunately, most family planning methods are compatible with breast-feeding, and the provider can play an important role in promoting both contraception and breastfeeding. In addition to helping to devise a post-partum plan for contraception, the provider can ensure that the new mother has several essential breastfeeding experiences and lessons while still in the hospital, prior to discharge after delivery (see Figure 23-1[1]). Breastmilk is the ideal source of nutrition for infants and confers immu-nological protection against many infections. Health experts around the globe have declared that all women should be enabled to breastfeed exclusively for 6 months,[2-4] to continue to breastfeed for 1 year[3,4] or 2 years or beyond,[2] and to have access to family planning information and services that allow them to sustain breastfeeding.[5]

POSTPARTUM INFERTILITY

During pregnancy, cyclic ovarian function is suspended. The corpus luteum, which arises from the ovulated follicle, secretes steroids, includ-ing estrogen and progesterone, that are essential in maintaining the early weeks of pregnancy. Later, steroids secreted by the placenta emerge to play a more dominant role in hormonal support of the pregnancy. Luteal and placental steroids suppress the mother's circulating levels of follicle stimulating hormone (FSH) and luteinizing hormone (LH) but more im-portantly disrupt their pulsatile release from her pituitary.[6] When the placenta is delivered, the inhibiting effects of estrogen and progesterone are removed so that levels of FSH and LH gradually rise and pulsatile release by the pituitary of FSH and LH returns.[7]

Most nonlactating women resume menses within 4 to 6 weeks of delivery, but about one-third of first cycles are anovulatory, and a high proportion of first ovulatory cycles have a deficient corpus luteum that secretes sub-normal amounts of steroids. In the second and third men-strual cycles, 15% are anovulatory and 25% of ovulatory cycles have luteal-phase defects. The first ovulation occurs on average 45 days postpartum, although few first ovulations are followed by normal luteal phases.[8] The duration of postpartum infertility is variable and unpredictable.

LACTATIONAL INFERTILITY

Lactation, or breastfeeding, further extends the period of infertility and depresses ovarian function.[9] Plasma levels of FSH return to normal follicular phase values by 4 to 8 weeks postpartum in breastfeeding women.[10] In contrast, pulsatile LH stimulation is depressed, in terms of the frequency or the amplitude of the LH pulse, in the majority of lactating women throughout most of the period of lactational amenorrhea.[11]

Evidence-based guidelines for breastfeeding management during the first 14 days

1. Help the mother begin breastfeeding as soon as possible after birth, ideally within the first 2 hours.

2. Help the mother choose a comfortable position. (Observe infant and mother for correct positioning and signs of correct latch-on and milk transfer.)

3. Facilitate rooming-in 24 hours a day.

4. Encourage the mother to give unrestricted breastfeeds 8 to 12 times every 24 hours.

5. Confirm that the parents know to respond to early cues that the infant is ready to suckle.

6. Confirm that the parents understand that the amount of milk removed from the breast determines the amount of milk produced.

7. Confirm that the parents know when and how to wake a sleepy infant.

8. Encourage the parents to avoid the use of pacifiers, artificial nipples, and supplements, unless medically indicated, until breastfeeding is well established. For most infants, this is after 4 to 6 weeks. Some infants never use pacifiers or bottles.

9. Observe at least one breastfeeding in each 8-hour period during the hospital stay and document the standard elements of a lactation assessment (such as mother-infant interaction, number of wet diapers, etc.).

10. Know the signs of ineffective breastfeeding (such as no audible swallowing during feedings, engorgement not relieved by feeding, etc.)

11. If effective breastfeeding (as demonstrated by milk transfer) is not observed within 24 hours initiate remedial measures (such as initiating pumping with a hospital grade pump, etc.).

12. Identify risk factors that can affect the infant's ability to breastfeed effectively (such as birth trauma, < 38 weeks' gestation, etc.). Provide the necessary feeding assistance and monitor closely.

13. Identify maternal risk factors for breastfeeding difficulty (such as breast surgery, medication use, etc.). Provide appropriate assistance and follow-up.

14. Identify maternal and infant contraindications to breastfeeding, such as HIV infection, chemotherapy, substance abuse, etc.

15. If it is medically indicated, provide supplementation with a method of feeding that does not compromise the infant's transition to the breast, such as using mother's own colostrum and milk, etc.

16. Confirm the parents' knowledge of appropriate and effective breastfeeding behaviors and elimination patterns and their understanding about how to manage common concerns.

17. Confirm that the parents have scheduled a follow-up visit with the infant's primary care provider within 2 to 3 days of hospital discharge.

18. Provide educational materials that are accurate, consistent, and appropriate to the mother's literacy and culture; include a list of available community resources for breastfeeding support.

19. Support continued breastfeeding during any re-hospitalization of mother or infant.

20. Discourage the distribution of sample packs that include infant feeding products or advertising.

21. Include family members or significant others in the breastfeeding education.

22. Provide anticipatory guidance for common problems that can interfere with continued breastfeeding.

Source: Adapted from and reprinted by permission from the International Lactation Consultant Association (1999).[1]

Figure 23-1 Evidence-based guidelines for breastfeeding management during the first 14 days

Nipple and areola sensitivity increases at birth.[12] Infant suckling stimulates the nerve endings in the nipple and areola. Nerve impulses are passed to the hypothalamus, stimulating the release of various hormones, including prolactin. Prolactin controls the rate of milk production but is not believed to play a major role in suppressing ovarian function.[13] Instead, suckling appears to disrupt the pulsatile release of gonadotropin releasing hormone (GnRH) by the hypothalamus,[10] perhaps by increasing hypothalamic β-endorphin production.[14] The interference with GnRH in turn averts the normal pulsatility of LH, which is required for follicle stimulation in the ovary. Small amounts of secreted estrogen at this time are insufficient to trigger an LH surge necessary to induce ovulation.[10,15]

Ovulation can occur even though the breastfeeding mother has not yet resumed menstruation. The probability that ovulation will precede the first menses increases over time, from 33% to 45% during the first 3 months postpartum, to 64% to 71% during months 4 through 12, to 87% to 100% after 12 months.[16,17] Only about 60% of ovulations preceding first menses have an adequate luteal phase,[17] which suggests that the contraceptive effect of breastfeeding may be partly due to inhibiting implantation of a fertilized egg. Clearly, lactational amenorrhea becomes increasingly unreliable as an indicator of infertility beyond 6 months postpartum.

Full or nearly full (unsupplemented) breastfeeding is associated with longer periods of lactational amenorrhea and infertility than supplemented breastfeeding. Frequent stimulation of the breast by around-the-clock suckling helps to maintain the cascade of neuroendocrine events that produces the contraceptive effect.[18] The breastfeeding characteristics that contribute significantly to delay the return of ovulation include a high feeding frequency, long duration of each feed, short interval between breastfeeds, and the presence of night feeds.[16,19] Milk production appears to be reduced far more by supplementary bottle feeds than by supplementary cup and spoon feeds.[16]

In summary:

- Full or nearly full breastfeeding (with no or limited food supplements) is associated with longer periods of lactational amenorrhea and infertility than is supplemented breastfeeding,

- Breastfeeding delays the resumption of ovulation and the return of menses,

- The longer a woman breastfeeds, the more likely menstruation will return while she continues to breastfeed,

- The longer the return of menses is delayed, the more likely ovulation will precede the first menses,

- Luteal phase insufficiency is frequent in ovulatory cycles that precede first menses, particularly in the first 6 months postpartum. Therefore, the contraceptive effect of breastfeeding may be partly due to inhibiting implantation of a fertilized egg.

CONTRACEPTIVE BENEFITS OF LACTATION

In traditional societies, and in developing countries, lactation plays a major role in prolonging birth intervals and thereby reducing fertility.[20–22] In developed countries, however, breastfeeding has a much smaller contraceptive impact because proportionately fewer infants are breastfed, and those who are breastfed are completely weaned at earlier ages. For example, in Indonesia, 96% of infants are breastfed, and those who are breastfed are not completely weaned until they are 2 years old on average.[23] In contrast, in the United States, only 1 in 2 infants is breastfed[24] and the mean and median times to complete weaning are only 23 weeks and 13 weeks, respectively.[25]

THE LACTATIONAL AMENORRHEA METHOD (LAM) OF CONTRACEPTION

Women who breastfeed can learn to make use of breastfeeding's natural contraceptive effect. If the woman feeds her infant only her breastmilk (or gives supplemental non-breastmilk feeds only to a minor extent) and has not experienced her first postpartum menses, then breastfeeding provides more than 98% protection from pregnancy in the first 6 months following a birth.[18,26,27] See Figures 23-2 and 23-3.[26] Four prospective clinical studies of the contraceptive effect of this Lactational Amenorrhea Method (LAM) demonstrated cumulative 6-month life-table perfect-use pregnancy rates of 0.5%, 0.6%, 1.0%, and 1.5% among women who relied solely on LAM.[28–31]

LAM requires "full or nearly full" breastfeeding because the infant who obtains nearly all nutritional requirements through breastfeeding is providing maximal suckling stimulation at the breast. As long as additional foods do not decrease this optimal amount of suckling, small amounts of supplementation should have little or no effect on the return of fertility. Thus, if LAM is to be used, supplements should be given only infrequently, in small amounts, and not by bottle. The only real challenge concerning the correct use of LAM is determining the allowable extent of supplementation to the infant's diet, if the mother wishes to supplement. Figure 23-2 defines different infant feeding patterns that can be helpful in determining whether the woman is fully or nearly fully breastfeeding.[26,32] Milk expression, such as by hand pump, is not a substitute for breastfeeding in terms of its fertility inhibiting effect. A study of LAM used by working women reported an elevated pregnancy rate (5.2%) indicating that frequent suckling, despite adequate milk production and full breastfeeding, is necessary to acquire the benefits of LAM.[33]

Experience with LAM in the United States is limited. Currently, only half of new mothers initiate breastfeeding, but it is unknown whether more women would breastfeed if they appreciated the contraceptive effect of lactation (or the other benefits of breastfeeding). Some U.S. women are already highly motivated to breastfeed, and they would be good candidates to use LAM as a temporary contraceptive option.[34] Women who choose to use LAM are basically choosing to fully or nearly fully breastfeed for at least some period (up to six months), so the choice to use LAM should be associated with the motivation to maintain good breastfeeding practices. In the United States, LAM probably is best delivered in the context of support for sound breastfeeding practices. Breastfeeding support (from the healthcare system, friends, employers) will facilitate full/nearly full breastfeeding, which will maximize the duration of amenorrhea[35] and the duration for which women can use LAM.

If a woman wishes to avoid becoming pregnant when LAM protection expires, then she must begin to use another contraceptive method at that time.[36,37] (See Figure 23-3.)

While pregnancy rates during lactational amenorrhea compare favorably with those for many other methods of contraception (see Table 9-2 in chapter 9 on Essentials of Contraception), even greater efficacy could be achieved by both breastfeeding and using an additional method of contraception.

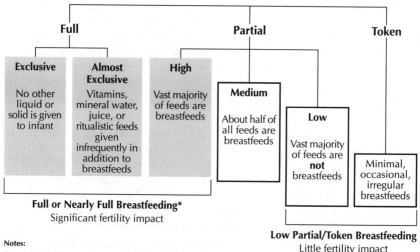

Notes:

*Intervals should not exceed 4 hours during the day or 6 hours at night, and supplementation should not exceed 5%-15% of all feeding episodes, preferably fewer. While the high-partial pattern is adequate for fertility suppression, the woman should be counseled that any supplementation or disruption of the breastfeeding pattern can increase the risk of fertility return.

Source: Labbok et al. (1994).

Figure 23-2 Schema for breastfeeding definition

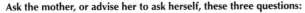

Ask the mother, or advise her to ask herself, these three questions:

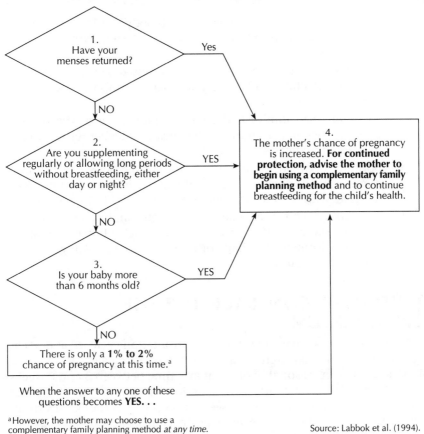

1.
Have your
menses returned?

Yes

NO

2.
Are you supplementing
regularly or allowing long periods
without breastfeeding, either
day or night?

YES

4.
The mother's chance of pregnancy
is increased. **For continued
protection, advise the mother to
begin using a complementary family
planning method** and to continue
breastfeeding for the child's health.

NO

3.
Is your baby more
than 6 months old?

YES

NO

There is only a **1% to 2%**
chance of pregnancy at this time.[a]

When the answer to any one of these
questions becomes **YES. . .**

[a] However, the mother may choose to use a
complementary family planning method *at any time.*

Source: Labbok et al. (1994).

Figure 23-3 LAM: lactational amenorrhea method

POSTPARTUM SEXUALITY

Most American couples resume sexual intercourse within several weeks of delivery. Among U.S. lactating women, 66% are sexually active in the first month postpartum and 88% are sexually active in the second month postpartum.[38] In small samples of breastfeeding Western women, monthly coital frequency in the second month postpartum averaged 2.4, increasing to 3.2 to 4.9 in the third postpartum month.[39]

Contraception is only one counseling issue for postpartum women. Women—and men—may experience reduced sexual feelings associated with bodily changes caused by pregnancy and delivery. Discussion of these bodily changes may help to alleviate a couple's anxiety:

- Tenderness in the perineum may make intercourse painful, especially if there has been an episiotomy.

- Reduced postpartum estrogen secretion may result in diminished vaginal lubrication.
- Most women experience a heavy and bloody lochial discharge for a couple of weeks postpartum. This may interfere with a woman's sexual feeling.
- Couples may find that the exhaustion caused by the around-the-clock responsibilities of being a new parent temporarily decreases sexual drive.
- Lactation may diminish the erotic significance of the breasts. Couples need to communicate feelings about whether sucking or touching the breasts is acceptable.
- Bonding between mother and child creates skills and commitment in the mother and trust and security in the infant but may interfere with the mother's emotional availability to her partner.
- Conversely, a birth (especially if planned) can be an exceedingly joyous experience that can enhance sexual intimacy. To some men and women, the shape or fullness of the lactating breast is particularly arousing.

NITIATING CONTRACEPTIVE USE POSTPARTUM

Traditionally, a postpartum follow-up consultation occurred at 6 weeks because the uterus had pretty much involuted and healed. However, a physical exam can reasonably occur at any time between 3 and 8 weeks postpartum. In terms of contraceptive service delivery, routine adherence to the 6-week convention does not seem appropriate. Although nearly all contraceptive methods can be used postpartum, the methods vary in terms of when in the postpartum period they can be initiated.[40–44] Six weeks is too late for non-breastfeeding mothers who wish to start using combined oral contraceptives, the patch, the vaginal ring, Lunelle, Norplant or Depo-Provera.[45] On the other hand, 3 weeks is too soon for inserting an IUD or fitting a diaphragm. The authors therefore advocate an individual approach to timing postpartum follow-up and contraceptive initiation.

Counseling for postpartum contraception should begin in the prenatal period.[46–48] Many methods can be provided at the time of delivery or during the hospital stay, such as IUDs, female sterilization and, for non-breastfeeding women, Norplant or Depo-Provera. However, plan in advance, preferably in the prenatal period, so informed choice is valid and method choice and initiation is uncomplicated, convenient, and cost-effective. One large study showed that one year pregnancy and contraceptive continuation rates were the same whether the women received family planning counseling before or after the delivery, with the exception of a significantly higher rate of sterilization among women counseled before delivery in one urban center.[49]

When the couple's method of choice cannot be initiated during the hospital stay after delivery, they can choose temporary methods such as LAM or the brief use of condoms and plan to initiate a longer-term method later. Schedule the first postpartum visit for the most logical time based on the longer-term method choice. For example, if a breastfeeding woman will be using progestin-only pills, schedule her follow-up visit at 6 weeks postpartum, with the plan for her to use condoms or LAM until that time. To help ensure success, provide a cycle of progestin-only pills (or a prescription) and a package of lubricated condoms at hospital discharge and instruct her about when to use each. Perhaps most importantly, the woman should be contacted 2 to 4 weeks after delivery to check on her postpartum recovery and to confirm and support her personal contraception plan.

If the couple has been unable to select a contraceptive method by the time of hospital discharge, the authors endorse the suggestion that a postpartum visit be scheduled for 3 weeks after delivery.[50]

The following considerations may prove useful when counseling and providing contraceptives to the postpartum woman, whether or not she is breastfeeding:

- Withdrawal may be a good method for couples in the postpartum period. Withdrawal is effective if used correctly and consistently. (See Table 9-2.)
- Postpartum endometritis is a serious complication. The risk of introducing bacteria into the uterus is elevated before cervical closure is complete. The condom may be a particularly attractive option for this reason.
- Episiotomies may still be tender. Fitting a woman for a cervical cap or diaphragm may cause discomfort.
- Avoid the diaphragm, cervical cap, and contraceptive sponge until six weeks after delivery. The diaphragm and cervical cap cannot be (re)fitted properly until that time. Moreover, the risk of toxic shock syndrome is increased when blood, including the postpartum lochia, is present.[51] (See Chapter 18.)
- The sponge and the cervical cap (though not the diaphragm) have much higher failure rates among women who have delivered a child than among women who have not, *even during perfect use.* (See Chapter 31.) Inform women about this substantial decrease in efficacy for parous women so they can make an informed choice of a contraceptive method.
- Postpartum abstinence, if practiced properly, is 100% effective in preventing pregnancy. It can, however, be notoriously difficult to maintain. Counsel women about other contraceptive methods should they desire to resume intercourse.

Copper intrauterine devices (IUDs) can be inserted postpartum, either (1) immediately after the expulsion of the placenta (immediate postpartum insertion), or (2) during the first week postpartum (delayed postpartum insertion), though preferably within 48 hours of delivery. Expulsion rates following postpartum insertion are higher than those following interval insertion, but they are lower for immediate than for delayed postpartum insertion.[52] Discuss this option before delivery to ensure that consent is fully informed. (See Chapter 21 on Intrauterine Devices.) If insertion is not performed within the first week postpartum, it should be delayed. Copper-T IUDs can be inserted with care at 4 to 6 weeks (but preferably 6 to 8 weeks) postpartum.[52] Some women experience mild uterine cramping when they breastfeed with an IUD in place, but the cramping does not usually interfere with lactation or with the effectiveness of the IUD. IUD insertion is less painful, and pain and bleeding removal rates are lower, for the lactating mother.[53,54] Although case reports and small studies have suggested that the risk of uterine perforation is higher among breastfeeding women, other, larger studies find no evidence of increased risk and low rates of perforation in both breastfeeding and nonbreastfeeding women.[53-56]

- Nevertheless, it seems prudent to exercise special care when inserting an IUD postpartum. An IUD can be inserted immediately after a cesarean delivery through the uterine incision.[42] Whether after a cesarean or a vaginal delivery, IUD insertion should be avoided when premature rupture of the membranes, prolonged labor, or fever has occurred, because of the elevated risk of infection.[52,55] Immediate postpartum insertion has not been associated with excessive bleeding or endometritis.[57]

- Vasectomy is an appropriate postpartum choice for couples who want a permanent method. As soon as the health of the mother and infant is determined to be sound, the vasectomy can be performed. If the woman is breastfeeding, a back-up method may not be needed while waiting for confirmation that the vasectomy has taken effect.[11,40] As with tubal ligation, vasectomy requires counseling and reflection under non-stressful circumstances,[47] preferably before delivery.

- Tubal ligation performed during the immediate postpartum period can be a more cost-effective and simpler technique than interval sterilization.[40] While tubal ligation is a highly effective method of contraception, a small risk of sterilization failure persists for at least a decade. However, partial salpingectomy performed postpartum carries the lowest known pregnancy risk of any female sterilization procedure.[58] Discuss immediate postpartum sterilization well before the delivery to help ensure that consent is fully informed.[47] Take great care that the woman is confident of this choice[59] since the timing of the procedure during the postpartum period is a risk factor for regret.[60] (See Chapter 22 on Male and Female Sterilization.) After a vaginal delivery, sterilization should be performed by minilaparotomy within 48 hours or else delayed for 4 to 6 weeks. After 48 hours, access to the tubes is reduced and the risk of infection increased.[47] Minilaparotomy can be performed up to 6 days postpartum,[43] but infection precautions must be taken and the procedure will likely be more difficult. Tubal ligation can be performed through the abdominal incision after a cesarean delivery. As with minilaparotomy after vaginal delivery, cesarean sterilization may need to be delayed in the case of complications, such as severe pre-eclampsia, eclampsia, premature rupture of the membranes, sepsis, fever, severe hemorrhage, uterine rupture or perforation.[43,61]

POSTPARTUM CONTRACEPTION FOR THE NONBREASTFEEDING WOMAN

If she wishes to avoid becoming pregnant, the nonbreastfeeding woman should begin using a contraceptive method immediately postpartum or at least by the beginning of the fourth postpartum week.[45] Most nonbreastfeeding mothers have few restrictions placed on which method of contraceptive they can choose. Nonetheless, a few guidelines—in addition to those given above—are warranted:

- Combined oral contraceptives (OCs) and the combined patch, injectable, and vaginal ring may be prescribed immediately postpartum. However, caution women not to use them until three weeks after delivery.[40,42,43] The risk of postpartum thrombophlebitis and thromboembolism is greatest just after delivery.[62] Delaying combined hormonal contraceptive use for at least two weeks tends to bypass the period of peak risk for postpartum thrombotic complications.[63]
- Caution women that it is difficult to practice fertility awareness before their cycles are reestablished and cyclic signs of fertility return.
- Suggest that lubricated condoms are a good option at least for the short period before the woman becomes better suited to her preferred method.
- Norplant can be inserted and Depo-Provera can be safely injected immediately postpartum. Discussion of these options before delivery will help to ensure that consent is fully informed.

POSTPARTUM CONTRACEPTION FOR THE BREASTFEEDING WOMAN

NONHORMONAL METHODS

General comments regarding contraceptive use among postpartum women are given above. In addition, the following considerations are relevant for women who are breastfeeding.

Tubal ligation can be performed immediately postpartum, although it can disrupt lactation if it requires general anesthesia or separation of mother and infant. Both problems can be minimized by performing the procedure with only regional or local anesthetic.[64] If tubal ligation does not occur while the mother is on the delivery table, breastfeeding should occur just before, and be delayed immediately after, anesthesia, to reduce the transfer of the anesthetic agent to the infant.[65,66]

Copper T 380A IUDs are also good choices for breastfeeding women. The copper on the Copper T does not affect the quantity or quality of breastmilk.[67] (See the following section on Hormonal Methods for information on the IUDs containing a progestin or progesterone.)

Spermicides and barrier methods have no effect on the ability to breastfeed. The lubricated condom is especially useful in the postpartum period because of increased vaginal dryness. Spermicides also may help offset dryness due to estrogen deficiency. In the United States, barrier methods are the most widely used contraceptive among lactating mothers in the first 6 months postpartum.[38] In animal studies, nonoxynol-9 is absorbed through the skin and secreted in breastmilk.[68] The question of whether nonoxynol-9 is secreted in breastmilk has not been completely evaluated in humans.

Lactational Amenorrhea Method (LAM) provides effective protection against pregnancy for up to six months postpartum. If continued protection is desired, another method of contraception must be introduced when the LAM criteria indicates a return to the risk of pregnancy. (See the detailed description of LAM earlier in this chapter.)

Fertility awareness methods can be difficult to use during the return of fertility which can extend for many cycles during lactation.[69] The couple needs to abstain for 2 weeks in order to establish a "basic infertile pattern" (BIP) of cervical mucus (and other) symptoms. Intercourse can then occur every other night unless/until there is some change in the BIP, in which case more abstinence is necessary.[70] The changing fertility symptoms after the first postpartum menses may be especially difficult for new users to identify, and may lead to an increased risk for unplanned pregnancy.[71]

Basal body temperature cannot be ascertained unless a woman has at least six hours of uninterrupted sleep. Thus, the woman who gets up in the night to care for her infant is precluded from using the temperature symptom to help determine her fertility status.

The rules for using the symptothermal method during breastfeeding have been found to detect the onset of true fertility extremely well. However, these same rules often necessitate many days of abstinence when there is virtually no risk of pregnancy.[72] LAM should be recommended to users of fertility awareness methods who are breastfeeding.[70] LAM can eliminate the requirements for abstinence for up to 6 months with no apparent additional risk of unplanned pregnancy.[73] The transition from LAM use to the use of a fertility awareness method begins with the establishment of a BIP.[70]

HORMONAL METHODS

The use of hormonal contraception by a lactating woman is an area of dispute among experts.[74] Since all steroids pass through the breastmilk to the infant, the World Health Organization and the International Planned Parenthood Federation do not consider hormonal methods of contraception to be the category of first choice for breastfeeding women.[44,75] Estrogen decreases the volume of milk.

Progestin-only contraceptives such as Norplant, the LNg IUS, the Progestasert IUD, Depo-Provera, and minipills do not have adverse effects on lactation, and some studies suggest they may even increase milk volume. They do not have adverse effects on child growth and development.[42,43,76-86] In addition, their contraceptive efficacy is high (see Table 9-2), and they are simple to use. Therefore, these methods are good options for lactating women who wish to postpone a subsequent pregnancy.

Experts recommend that breastfeeding women delay using these methods until 6 weeks after delivery.[40,42,43] This recommendation is based on the admittedly theoretical concern that early neonatal exposure to exogenous steroids, which have passed from the contraceptive into the milk, should be avoided if possible. The binding capacity of plasma is low, the neonatal liver is not well able to conjugate and oxidize drugs, and the immature kidneys are inefficient in excretion.[11,76] (However, the liver rapidly improves its ability to metabolize drugs, so the need to avoid exposure to exogenous steroids may be brief.[76]) Unable to be cleared from the infant's circulation, exogenous steroids or their metabolites may "compete with natural hormones for receptor sites in sex organs, brain or other tissues."[87] Experts issue their caution because animal literature has indicated long-term effects of inappropriate hormone exposure at critical postpartum periods.[87]

Although progestin-only contraceptives would probably have no adverse effects on lactation or infant health if used soon after delivery, little research has been conducted on their immediate postpartum use, since initiation prior to 6 weeks has been discouraged. A prudent approach would be to share information about the risks and benefits of early use with the client, and, if the client consents, to wait until breastfeeding has been well established before starting progestin-only pills, inserting Norplant capsules, or giving the Depo-Provera injection. However, if a breastfeeding woman requests Norplant insertion before leaving the hospital after delivery (especially if she plans to supplement the infant's diet relatively soon after delivery), and if there is some compelling reason to start the method early, then the real long-term contraceptive benefit of using this method seems likely to exceed the theoretical risks. Because the contraceptive benefit to the lactating woman in obtaining Depo-Provera immediately postpartum is smaller and the theoretical risks might be higher (because the hormonal levels are relatively high in the immediate post-injection days), a case would be less compelling for injecting Depo-Provera before breastfeeding is well established; a woman unlikely to return for a postpartum visit may be equally unlikely to return for a repeat injection. Discussion of these options before delivery will help to ensure that consent is fully informed.

Since the precipitous withdrawal of natural progesterone 2 to 3 days postpartum is the physiological trigger for lactogenesis,[88] receipt of a high dose of exogenous progestin (as with a Depo-Provera injection before the withdrawal) may interfere with the stimulus for milk synthesis. This reasoning argues for a delay in commencing progestin-only-contraception, especially injectable formulas, until the mature milk has come in.[89] If a woman wants to use Depo-Provera immediately, encourage her to remain in the hospital until her mature milk comes in. Some studies of Depo-Provera[86] and progestin-only pills (POPs), have found no overall deleterious effect of progestin on milk volume when begun as early as the first week postpartum,[90,91] suggesting that very early exposure to POCs is not always detrimental to lactogenesis. However, in these studies, progestin might have been initiated after the withdrawal of natural progesterone. In general, a reason for discontinuing use of Depo-Provera is that menstrual cyclicity is disrupted. Studies in China and Bolivia showed that breastfeeding women tolerate this side effect better, and their method continuation rates are higher.[92,93]

As with other progestin-only methods, the Progestasert IUD and the LNg IUS are not recommended for use by breastfeeding women until 6 weeks postpartum.[40,41,43]

Combined hormonal contraceptives (the combined pill, patch, injectable, and vaginal ring) generally should not be used by breastfeeding mothers. A reduction in milk supply is associated with the estrogen component in combined pills, even those with low-dose preparations.[94,95] Use of combined pills may alter the composition of breastmilk, although results vary among studies; most studies report declines in mineral content. Nevertheless, the available evidence suggests that use of combined pills while nursing does not directly harm infants.[95]

Just when combined hormonal contraceptives can be provided to lactating women remains a subject of disagreement. It would be ideal to avoid the use of combined hormonal methods entirely during breastfeeding especially since progestin-only methods are available.[96] The International Planned Parenthood Federation states that under normal circumstances combined hormonal contraceptives should not be used by breastfeeding women at all.[40] The World Health Organization (WHO) discourages the use of combined methods until at least 6 months postpartum.[43] Other experts recommend that only after non-estrogenic methods have been rejected through informed choice can combined hormonal contraceptives be started "after the first 8 to 12 weeks postpartum if she is still amenorrheic or whenever the service provider can be reasonably sure that the woman is not pregnant." [42]

When a woman's informed choice is to use combined hormonal contraception during breastfeeding, it seems prudent to caution her not to use it until 2 to 3 months after delivery, and if using the combined pill, to consume each pill at the beginning of the longest interval between breastfeeds.[97] There are several reasons for this delay in initiation:

- The longer combined hormonal method use is postponed, the better the ongoing establishment of the milk supply will be facilitated. Nevertheless, milk volume will still be reduced when the combined hormonal contraception is started.[94]
- The risk of postpartum thrombotic complications is highest just after delivery.[62] Women should avoid using any method containing estrogen for at least 3 weeks as a sensible health precaution.
- The lactating woman is usually at reduced risk of becoming pregnant, especially if she is amenorrheic and fully breastfeeding. Thus, she may opt to use LAM, or she can use condoms or other barrier methods for only a month or two, with efficacy enhanced by lactation itself.

There is no need for breastfeeding women using progestin-only pills to switch to combined pills during lactation. However, if it is the woman's informed choice to make this switch, it is best to do so after 6 months postpartum.[98]

EFFECTS OF HORMONAL CONTRACEPTION ON THE BREASTFED INFANT

Contraceptive steroids taken by the mother can be transferred to the nursing infant through breastmilk. The amounts, however, are small. Nevertheless, it is prudent to avoid exposing the neonate to exogenous steroids, which are not easily bound in plasma, conjugated by the liver or excreted, and may compete with natural hormones for receptor sites. Also, while concern about the possible effects on the liver, sex organs, and other tissues of the neonate or premature infant is theoretical, exposure should be avoided wherever possible.

- The dose of contraceptive ethinyl estradiol (about 10 nanograms per day) reaching the infant of a mother taking combined pills is comparable to the dose of the naturally occurring estradiol (from 6 to 12 ng per day depending on time of cycle) consumed by nursing infants of ovulatory mothers not taking combined pills.[63]
- The quantity of progestin transferred to mother's milk varies with the type of progestin. The 17-hydroxy compounds (such as medroxyprogesterone acetate) enter the milk at approximately the same level as is found in the mother's blood, whereas the 19-nor compounds (such as norgestrel and norethindrone) enter the milk at only one-tenth the level in the blood.[99]

Combined oral contraceptive use during lactation is not the only possible source of estrogen and progestin exposure for the infant. When a mother becomes pregnant and continues to breastfeed a prior infant, that child is exposed to estrogen and progesterone in the mother's milk. Dairy cattle may also be pregnant at the time that they are milked, so that cow's milk and infant formula made from it may have relatively high levels of estrogen and progesterone.

Although early studies of high-dose oral contraceptives did demonstrate some effect of hormones on nursing babies,[100] most of those reports were anecdotal and have not been corroborated in women using low-dose pills. One study of the male offspring of women who had used depot-medroxy-projesterone acetate (DMPA) found no effect on infant hormone regulation associated with breastfeeding exposure.[101] Although the short-term effects of absorbing contraceptive steroids through breastmilk appear minimal, the long-term consequences remain unstudied.[74,87]

B REASTFEEDING: ADVANTAGES TO THE INFANT

Mother's milk has both nutritional and anti-infective advantages for the infant.[102] The particular mixtures of protein, fat, carbohydrate, and trace elements change to meet the infant's evolving needs as breastfeeding proceeds from month to month.[103] Furthermore, breastfeeding may help to cement the psychological bond between mother and infant. This bonding may lead to better psychological and intellectual development, though the evidence is inconclusive.[104] Finally, the infant ingests host-resistant, humoral, and allergy prophylaxis factors. These are particularly concentrated in the colostrum, the high-protein fluid secreted in the first few days postpartum.

Breastfed infants have lower risk of respiratory and gastro-intestinal illness,[103–105] including neonatal necrotizing enterocolitis among pre-term infants[106] and sudden infant death syndrome.[107] Breastfed infants are less likely to develop allergies, including eczema, cow's milk allergy, and allergic rhinitis.[103] Whether breastmilk is protective or alternative diets are allergenic cannot be determined from the available evidence.[104] Asthma may be less common and less severe among children who were breastfed.[104] Other benefits include a decreased incidence of otitis media[103,104] and dental malocclusion and caries.[108] Preterm infants who consume mother's milk in the early weeks of life have higher IQ scores,[109] although the association may not be causal. The benefits of breastfeeding are by no means limited to infants in developing countries. All of the protective effects mentioned here have been demonstrated in children in industrialized nations.[105–107,110] Most medications taken by the breastfeeding mother are safe for the infant, and excellent references are available that distinguish those medications which may require an interruption of breastfeeding.[111,112] In the United States there are few contraindications to breastfeeding,[112] and maternal human immunodeficiency virus (HIV) infection is a notable exception.[113]

B REASTFEEDING AND HIV

The HIV, which causes acquired immune deficiency syndrome (AIDS), can be transmitted by an infected mother to her infant in utero, during childbirth, and through breastmilk. That HIV-1 can be transmitted by breastfeeding has been conclusively demonstrated by case reports, laboratory data, and epidemiologic studies,[114,115] such as prospective studies of mothers who were infected postnatally.[116] Rates of vertical transmission through all three routes combined average 25% to 30%, ranging from 13% to 43% in developing countries and from 14% to 25% in developed settings.[117] The majority of infants who are infected with HIV-1 acquire the infection in utero or during childbirth. The risk of perinatal transmission of HIV-2 is much lower than the risk of perinatal transmission of HIV-1.[118]

HIV-1 transmission via breastmilk probably is greater when the mother becomes infected postpartum than before delivery, because the maternal viral load is high during initial infection and because HIV in the milk is not yet neutralized by the anti-infective activities of the milk, such as inhibiting the binding of HIV-1 glycoproteins to CD4 molecules.[119–121] Although a meta-analysis attempted to quantify the risk of vertical transmission due only to breastfeeding,[122] the attributable risk of breastfeeding for HIV transmission according to time of maternal infection is not known with certainty.[115] Studies of mother-to-infant transmission of HIV according to breastfeeding status have produced widely varying results. The differences may be due to methodological limitations and differences among the studies, and to vast differences in the populations studied, such as women in sub-Saharan Africa versus central Europe. Confounding factors across such widely different environments and cultures are likely to differ as well.

The majority of infants who are breastfed by HIV-positive mothers do not become infected. Viral shedding into the milk is intermittent, and the persistence of HIV-specific antibodies in breastmilk confers some protection against transmission.[121] The duration of breastfeeding is not necessarily associated with HIV transmission[123] although some studies have found a substantial risk of late postnatal transmission via breastmilk.[114,115] These observations suggest that the anti-HIV factors present in breastmilk do provide some protection against HIV transmission during breastfeeding.

It is clear that breastfeeding can be a route for HIV transmission. It is also clear that breastmilk is normally protective (albeit to an unknown degree) against enveloped viruses such as HIV. However, since the consequence of HIV infection through breastfeeding is virtually always fatal for the infant, it would be important to avoid even a modest risk of infection (even though the exact magnitude of the risk through breastfeeding is not yet certain). Therefore, HIV-infected mothers *in the United States* should be counseled not to breastfeed or provide their milk to other infants.[112,113,124] In developing country settings where the risk of infant mortality from bottle feeding is high, women are advised to breastfeed regardless of their HIV status.[125]

B REASTFEEDING: EFFECTS ON THE MOTHER

Breastfeeding has a major protective effect against premenopausal cancers of the ovary, endometrium, and breast.[3,4,126-128] Breastmilk has a zero price and is always available at the right temperature, in contrast to infant formula. Breastfeeding also promotes emotional bonding between mother and infant. Finally, the breastfeeding mother experiences a rapid return of uterine tone. Oxytocin, which induces uterine contraction, is released from the posterior pituitary when the nipple is stimulated by suckling.

During lactation, the body's estrogen levels are very low, and vaginal lubrication may be less than usual and begin later during sexual intercourse. Vaginal lubrication improves when cycling resumes or when the frequency of breastfeeding declines. Nursing mothers have added requirements for calories, protein, calcium, and iron, as well as several vitamins and other micronutrients. The increased needs for specific nutrients can be provided by a well-balanced diet. Supplements are generally unnecessary unless the diet is deficient in one or more of these nutrients.[129,130]

I NSTRUCTIONS FOR AND INFORMATION ABOUT BREASTFEEDING

1. Congratulations! Enjoy your baby, rest, and keep in touch with your clinician.

2. Health experts concur that all women should be enabled to breastfeed, and to breastfeed exclusively for 6 months, and to continue supplemented breastfeeding for 12 to 24 months or longer.

3. **If you are not breastfeeding, begin using a contraceptive method before or at your first sexual encounter.** You can become pregnant before your first menstrual period after childbirth because ovulation can begin before menstruation.

4. **If you are breastfeeding and providing bottle supplements, begin using a contraceptive method as soon as your clinician advises based on the method you have chosen.**

5. **If you are breastfeeding and using the Lactational Amenorrhea Method (LAM) as a temporary method of contraception, breastfeed your baby on demand, avoid any bottle feeds, and**

provide any minimal supplements by cup or spoon. Begin using another method of contraception when you resume menstruation, when you reduce the frequency or duration of breastfeeds, when you introduce bottle feeds or regular food supplements, or when your baby turns six months old. (See Figures 23-2 and 23-3.)

6. **You can become pregnant while breastfeeding your baby,** although the risk is greatly reduced before your first menstrual period; in the first six months of amenorrhea when you feed your baby on demand, avoid any bottle feeds, and provide minimal supplements by cup or spoon, your risk of pregnancy will be about 2%, equivalent to or lower than the risk associated with many other contraceptive methods. Most U.S. women do not follow breastfeeding patterns that confer maximum protection against pregnancy. However, women who choose LAM may adopt breastfeeding behaviors that maximize both milk production and the duration of amenorrhea.

7. **Breastfeeding is a convenient, inexpensive, and nutritious way to feed your baby and it helps to protect the baby against infection, diarrhea, allergy, and sudden infant death syndrome. It also offers you protection against cancer of the breast, ovary, and uterus.**

8. **Neither intercourse nor menstruation affects the quality or quantity of your breastmilk. You do not need to stop breastfeeding because you start having intercourse again or start your period.** You can continue breastfeeding when you start using another contraceptive method.

9. **Lubricants, such as K-Y Jelly, spermicides, or saliva, may make intercourse easier after childbirth** because decreased estrogen production during breastfeeding diminishes vaginal lubrication.

10. **When you are nursing your child, your own nutrition is important.** Women can usually obtain all the calories and nutrients they need to breastfeed through their usual diet. There is no need to buy any special foods. Just eat a sensible, well-balanced diet, which is always a good idea.

11. **Avoid smoking.** Nursing women who smoke may transfer nicotine to their infant through their breastmilk. Nicotine is a poison that can harm the child. Inhaling smoke is also harmful to the baby. Smoking may also influence your ability to produce milk.

12. **Alcohol that you drink will be passed to your baby through breastmilk.** Your baby will have more difficulty metabolizing alcohol than you do, especially in the first few weeks after delivery. No good studies have been conducted to assess what level of alcohol

consumption is safe. Thus it seems prudent to drink only modest amounts of alcohol.

13. **If you are using any medications while breastfeeding, be sure to tell your physician.** You can breastfeed while using virtually all common drugs. However, for some medications you may need advice concerning the best timing for ingestion to decrease infant exposure.

14. **If you are infected with HIV, the virus that causes AIDS, you could transmit the virus to your baby through breastmilk.** For this reason, most experts recommend that you not breastfeed your baby.

15. **It is indeed possible to combine work and breastfeeding successfully,** yet any separation of mother from infant for more than a few hours can create challenges to breastfeeding. Working women (or any breastfeeding woman!) should be sure to locate a certified lactation consultant, preferably before delivery, who can help in the event of any difficulty, from engorgement to declining milk supply. Lactation consultants are highly trained to give advice on a broad spectrum of breastfeeding issues, including the storage and transport of expressed milk, and can often help you rent an electric breast pump if you need one. The headquarters of the International Lactation Consultants Association can help you locate a certified lactation consultant near you (Telephone: 919-787-5181; Website: http://www.ilca.org). (See also Chapter 11 on Selected Reproductive Health Resources.)

RESOURCE MATERIALS

International Lactation Consultant Association (ILCA): Evidence-based guidelines for breastfeeding management during the first fourteen days. Raleigh NC: ILCA, April 1999. Can be purchased at 919-787-5181 or http://www.ilca.org/.

REFERENCES

1. International Lactation Consultant Association (ILCA): Evidence-based guidelines for breastfeeding management during the first fourteen days. Raleigh NC: ILCA, April, 1999.
2. World Health Assembly. Infant and young child nutrition. Fifty-fourth World Health Assembly Resolution WHA54.2. WHO: Geneva, 18 May 2001. Available at http://www.who.int/gb/EB_WHA/PDF/WHA54/ea54r2.pdf. Accessed November 9, 2001.
3. American Academy of Pediatrics. Breastfeeding and the Use of Human Milk (RE9729). Pediatrics 1997;100:1035-1039.
4. U.S. Department of Health and Human Services, Office of Women's Health. Breastfeeding—HHS blueprint for action on breastfeeding. Washington DC: DHHS, 2000. Available at: http://www.4woman.gov/Breastfeeding/bluprntbk2.pdf. Accessed November 9, 2001.
5. UNICEF. Innocenti Declaration on the protection, promotion and support of breastfeeding. New York NY: UNICEF, 1990.

6. Hodgen GD, Itskovitz J. Recognition and maintenance of pregnancy. In: Knobil E, Neill JD, Ewing LL, Greenwald GS, Markert CL, Pfaff DW (eds). The physiology of reproduction. New York NY: Raven Press, 1988:1995-2021.

7. Willson JR. The puerperium. In: Willson JR, Carrington ER, Ledger WJ, Laros RK, Mattox JH (eds). Obstetrics and gynecology. St. Louis MO: CV Mosby Company, 1987:598-607.

8. Gray RH, Campbell OM, Zacur H, Labbok MH, MacRae SL. Postpartum return of ovarian activity in non-breastfeeding women monitored by urinary assays. J Clin Endocrinol Metab 1987;64:645-650.

9. McNeilly AS. Lactational control of reproduction. Reprod Fertil Dev 2001;13:583-590.

10. McNeilly AS. Neuroendocrine changes and fertility in breastfeeding women. Prog Brain Res 2001;133:207-214.

11. Díaz S, Croxatto HB. Contraception in lactating women. Curr Opin Obstet Gynecol. 1993;5:815-822.

12. Robinson JE, Short RV. Changes in breast sensitivity at puberty, during the menstrual cycle, and at parturition. Br Med J 1977;1:1188-1191.

13. Diaz S, Seron-Ferre M, Croxatto HB, Veldhuis J. Neuroendocrine mechanisms of lactational infertility in women. Biol Res 1995;28:155-163.

14. Gordon K, Renfree MB, Short RV, Clarke IJ. Hypothalamo-pituitary portal blood concentrations of β-endorphin during suckling in the ewe. J Reprod Fertil 1987;79:397-408.

15. McNeilly AS, Tay CCK, Glasier A. Physiological mechanisms underlying lactational amenorrhea. In: Human reproductive ecology: interactions of environment, fertility and behavior. New York NY: New York Academy of Sciences, 1994:145-155.

16. Campbell OMR, Gray RH. Characteristics and determinants of postpartum ovarian function in women in the United States. Am J Obstet Gynecol 1993;169:55-60.

17. Lewis PR, Brown JB, Renfree MB, Short RV. The resumption of ovulation and menstruation in a well-nourished population of women breastfeeding for an extended period of time. Fertil Steril 1991;55:529-536.

18. Kennedy KI, Rivera R, McNeilly AS. Consensus statement on the use of breastfeeding as a family planning method. Contraception 1989;39:477-496.

19. Gray RH, Campbell OM, Apelo R, Eslami SS, Zacur H, Ramos RM, Gehret JC, Labbok MH. Risk of ovulation during lactation. Lancet 1990;335:25-29.

20. Casterline JB, Singh S, Cleland J, Ashurst H. The proximate determinants of fertility. WFS Comparative Studies, Number 39. Voorburg, Netherlands: International Statistical Institute, 1984.

21. Thapa S, Short RV, Potts M. Breastfeeding, birth spacing and their effects on child survival. Nature 1988;335:679-682.

22. VanLandingham M, Trussell J, Grummer-Strawn L. Contraceptive and health benefits of breastfeeding: a review of the recent evidence. Int Fam Plann Perspect 1991;17:131-136.

23. Demographic and Health Surveys. Indonesia demographic and health survey 1997. Calverton MD: Macro International Inc., 1998.

24. Kennedy KI, Visness CM. A comparison of two U.S. surveys of infant feeding. J Hum Lact 1997;13:39-43.

25. Visness CM, Kennedy KI. Maternal employment and breast-feeding: findings from the 1988 National Maternal and Infant Health Survey. Am J Public Health 1997;87:945-950.

26. Labbok M, Cooney K, Coly S. Guidelines: breastfeeding, family planning, and the Lactational Amenorrhea Method—LAM. Washington DC: Institute for Reproductive Health, Georgetown University, 1994.

27. World Health Organization. The WHO multinational study of breastfeeding and lactational amenorrhea: III. Pregnancy during breastfeeding. Fertil Steril 1999;72:431-440.

28. Kazi A, Kennedy KI, Visness CM, Khan T. Effectiveness of the Lactational Amenorrhea Method in Pakistan. Fertil Steril 1995;64:717-723.

29. Labbok MH, Hight-Laukaran V, Peterson AE, Fletcher V, von Hertzen H, Van Look PFA. Multicenter study of the Lactational Amenorrhea Method (LAM): I. Efficacy, duration, and implications for clinical application. Contraception 1997;55:327-336.

30. Pérez A, Labbok MH, Queenan JT. Clinical study of the Lactational Amenorrhoea Method for family planning. Lancet 1992;339:968-970.

31. Ramos R, Kennedy KI, Visness CM. Effectiveness of lactational amenorrhea in prevention of pregnancy in Manila, the Philippines: non-comparative prospective trial. Br Med J 1996;313:909-912.

32. Labbok M, Krasovec K. Toward consistency in breastfeeding definitions. Stud Fam Plann 1990;21:226-230.

33. Valdés V, Labbok MH, Pugin E, Perez A. The efficacy of the lactational amenorrhea method (LAM) among working women. Contraception 2000;62:217-219.

34. Hight-Laukaran V, Labbok MH, Peterson AE, Fletcher V, von Hertzen H, Van Look PFA. Multicenter study of the Lactational Amenorrhea Method (LAM): II. Acceptability, utility, and policy implications. Contraception 1997;55:337-346.

35. Valdés V, Pérez A, Labbok M, Pugin E, Zambrano I, Catalan S. The impact of a hospital and clinic-based breastfeeding promotion programme in a middle class urban environment. J Trop Pediatr 1993;39:142-151.

36. Kennedy KI, Labbok MH, Van Look PFA. Consensus statement—Lactational Amenorrhea Method for family planning. Int J Gynaecol Obstet 1996;54:55-57.

37. Van Look PFA. Lactational Amenorrhoea Method for family planning. Br Med J 1996;313:893-894.

38. Ford K, Labbok M. Contraceptive usage during lactation in the United States: an update. Am J Public Health 1987;77:79-81.

39. Visness CM, Kennedy KI: The frequency of coitus during breastfeeding. Birth 1997;24:253-257.

40. International Planned Parenthood Federation (IPPF). IMAP Statement on breast feeding, fertility and post-partum contraception. IPPF Med Bull 1996;30:1-3.

41. Technical Guidance/Competence Working Group (TG/CWG). Recommendations for updating selected practices in contraceptive use. Volume II. Chapel Hill NC: Program for International Training in Health (INTRAH), School of Medicine, The University of North Carolina at Chapel Hill, 1997.

42. Technical Guidance Working Group (TGWG). Recommendations for updating selected practices in contraceptive use: results of a technical meeting. Volume I. Chapel Hill NC: Program for International Training in Health (INTRAH), School of Medicine, The University of North Carolina at Chapel Hill, 1994.

43. World Health Organization. Improving access to quality care in family planning—medical eligibility criteria for contraceptive use, second edition. Geneva, Switzerland: Reproductive Health and Research Division, World Health Organization, WHO/RHR/00.02, 2000. Available at http://www.who.int/reproductive-health/publications/RHR_00_2_medical_ eligibility_criteria_second_edition/. Accessed October 27, 2001.

44. World Health Organization. Selected practice recommendations for contraceptive use. Geneva, Switzerland: Reproductive Health and Research Division, World Health Organization WHO/RHR/02.07, 2002.

45. Guillebaud J. Postpartum contraception unnecessary before three weeks. Br Med J 1993;307:1560-1561.

46. Acheson LS, Danner SC. Postpartum care and breast-feeding. Prim Care 1993;20:729-747.

47. Association for Voluntary Surgical Contraception (AVSC). Safe and voluntary surgical contraception. New York NY: AVSC International, 1995.

48. Glasier AF, Logan J, McGlew TJ. Who gives advice about postpartum contraception? Contraception 1996;53:217-220.

49. Smith KB, van der Spuy ZM, Cheng L, Elton R, Glasier AF. Is postpartum contraceptive advice given antenatally of value? Contraception 2002;65:237-243.

50. Speroff L, Darney PD. A clinical guide for contraception (Second Edition). Baltimore MD: Williams and Wilkins, 1996.

51. Faich G, Pearson K, Fleming D, Sobel S, Anello C. Toxic shock syndrome and the vaginal contraceptive sponge. JAMA 1986;255:216-218.
52. O'Hanley K, Huber DH. Postpartum IUDs: keys for success. Contraception 1992;45:351-361.
53. Chi I, Potts M, Wilkens LR, Champion CB. Performance of the copper T-380A intrauterine device in breastfeeding women. Contraception 1989;39:603-618.
54. Farr G, Rivera R. Interactions between intrauterine contraceptive device use and breast-feeding status at time of intrauterine contraceptive device insertion: analysis of TCu-380A acceptors in developing countries. Am J Obstet Gynecol 1992;167:144-151.
55. Treiman K, Liskin L, Kols A, Reinhart W. IUDs—an update. Popul Reports 1995;22(5). Series B(6).
56. Andersson K, Ryde-Blomquist E, Lindell K, Odlind V, Milson I. Perforations with intrauterine devices: Report from a Swedish survey. Contraception 1998;57:251-255.
57. Welkovic S, Costa LOBF, Faúndes A, Ximenes RA, Costa CFF. Postpartum bleeding and infection after post-placental IUD insertion. Contraception 2001;63:155-158.
58. Peterson HB, Xia Z, Hughes JM, Wilcox LS, Tylor LR, Trussell J. The risk of pregnancy after tubal sterilization: findings from the U.S. Collaborative Review of Sterilization. Am J Obstet Gynecol 1996;174:1161-1170.
59. American College of Obstetricians and Gynecologists. Postpartum tubal sterilization. Int J Gynaecol Obstet 1992;39:244.
60. Wilcox LS, Chu SY, Eaker ED, Zeger SL, Peterson HB. Risk factors for regret after tubal sterilization: 5 years of follow-up in a prospective study. Fertil Steril 1991;55:927-933.
61. Chi IC, Thapa S. Postpartum tubal sterilization: an international perspective on some programmatic issues. J Biosoc Sci 1993;25:51-61.
62. World Health Organization Task Force on Oral Contraceptives. Contraception during the postpartum period and during lactation: the effects on women's health. Int J Gynaecol Obstet 1987;25(Suppl):13-26.
63. McGregor JA. Lactation and contraception. In: Neville MC, Neifert MR (eds). Lactation. Physiology, nutrition, and breast-feeding. New York NY: Plenum Press, 1983:405-421.
64. Labbok MH. Contraception during lactation: considerations in advising the individual and in formulating programme guidelines. J Biosoc Sci 1985;9(Suppl):55-66.
65. American Academy of Pediatrics Committee on Drugs. The transfer of drugs and other chemicals into human milk. Pediatrics 1994;93:137-150.
66. Burkman RT. Puerperium and breast-feeding. Curr Opin Obstet Gynecol 1993;5:683-687.
67. Wenof M, Aubert JM, Reyniak JV. Serum prolactin levels in short-term and long-term use of inert plastic and copper intrauterine devices. Contraception 1979;19:21-27.
68. Chvapil M, Eskelson CD, Stiffel V, Owen JA, Droegemueller W. Studies on nonoxynol-9. II. Intravaginal absorption, distribution, metabolism and excretion in rats and rabbits. Contraception 1980;22:325-339.
69. Howie PW. Natural regulation of fertility. Br Med Bull 1993;49:182-199.
70. Parenteau-Carreau S, Cooney KA. Breastfeeding, Lactational Amenorrhea Method, and natural family planning interface: teaching guide. Washington DC: Institute for Reproductive Health, Georgetown University, 1994.
71. Labbok MH, Stallings RY, Shah F, Pérez A, Klaus H, Jacobson M, Muruthi T. Ovulation method use during breastfeeding: is there increased risk of unplanned pregnancy? Am J Obstet Gynecol 1991;165:2031-2036.
72. Kennedy KI, Gross BA, Parenteau-Carreau S, Flynn AM, Brown JB, Visness CM. Breastfeeding and the symptothermal method. Stud Fam Plann 1995;26:107-115.
73. Kennedy KI, Parenteau-Carreau S, Flynn A, Gross B, Brown JB, Visness C. The natural family planning—Lactational Amenorrhea Method interface: observations from a prospective study of breastfeeding users of natural family planning. Am J Obstet Gynecol 1991;165:2020-2026.

74. Johansson E, Odlind V. The passage of exogenous hormones into breast milk—possible effects. Int J Gynaecol Obstet 1987;25(Suppl):111-114.
75. International Planned Parenthood Federation. IMAP statement on hormonal methods of contraception. IPPF Med Bull 2002;36:1-8.
76. Fraser IS. A review of the use of progestogen-only minipills for contraception during lactation. Reprod Fertil Dev 1991;3:245-254.
77. McCann MF, Potter LS. Progestin-only oral contraception—a comprehensive review. Contraception 1994;50:S1-S198.
78. World Health Organization. Progestogen-only contraceptives during lactation: I. Infant growth. Contraception 1994;50:35-53.
79. World Health Organization. Progestogen-only contraceptives during lactation: II. Infant development. Contraception 1994;50:55-68.
80. Sinchai W, Sethavanich S, Asavapiriyanont S, Sittipiyasakul V, Sirikanchanakul R, Udomkiatsakul P, Chantaeyoon P, Roybang K, Trakankamol J, Suti S, Parnraksa W. Effects of a progestin-only pill (Exluton) and an intrauterine device (Multiload Cu250) on breastfeeding. Adv Contracep 1995;11:143-155.
81. Coutinho EM, Athayde C, Dantas C, Hirsch C, Barbosa I. Use of a single implant of Elcometrine (ST-1435), a nonorally active progestin, as a long acting contraceptive for postpartum nursing women. Contraception 1999;59:115-122.
82. Reinprayoon D, Taneepanichskul S, Bunyavejchevin S, Thaithumyanon P, Punnahitananda S, Tosukhowong P, Machielsen C, van Beek A. Effects of the etonogestrel-releasing contraceptive implant (Implanon®) on parameters of breastfeeding compared to those of an intrauterine device. Contraception 2000;62:239-246.
83. Massai MR, Díaz S, Quinteros E, Reyes MV, Herreros C, Zepeda A, Croxatto HB, Moo-Young AJ. Contraceptive efficacy and clinical performance of Nestorone implants in postpartum women. Contraception 2001;64:369-376.
84. Schiappacasse V, Díaz S, Zepeda A, Alvarado R, Herreros C. Health and growth of infants breastfed by Norplant contraceptive implants users: a six-year follow-up study. Contraception 2002;66:57-65.
85. Curtis KM, Chrisman CE, Peterson HB. Contraception for women in selected circumstances. Obstet Gynecol 2002; 99:1100-1112.
86. Hannon PR, Duggan AK, Serwint JR, Vogelhut JW, Witter F, DeAngelis C. The influence of medroxyprogesterone on the duration of breast-feeding in mothers in an urban community. Arch Pediatr Adolesc Med 1997;151:490-496.
87. Harlap S. Exposure to contraceptive hormones through breast milk—are there long-term health and behavioral consequences? Int J Gynaecol Obstet 1987;25(Suppl):47-55.
88. Cowie AT, Forsyth IA, Hart IC. Hormonal control of lactation. Berlin, Germany: Springer-Verlag, 1980:164-165.
89. Kennedy KI, Short RV, Tully MR. Premature introduction of progestin-only contraceptive methods during lactation. Contraception 1997;55:347-350.
90. McCann MF, Moggia AV, Higgins JE, Potts M, Becker C. The effects of a progestin-only oral contraceptive (Levonorgestrel 0.03 mg) on breast-feeding. Contraception 1989;40:635-648.
91. Moggia AV, Harris GS, Dunson TR, Diaz R, Moggia MS, Ferrer MA, McMullen SL. A comparative study of a progestin-only oral contraceptive versus non-hormonal methods in lactating women in Buenos Aires, Argentina. Contraception 1991;44:31-43.
92. Danli S, Qingxiang S, and Guowei S. A multicentered clinical trial of the long-acting injectable contraceptive Depo Provera in Chinese women. Contraception 2000;62:15-18.
93. Hubacher D, Goco N, Gonzalez B, Taylor D. Factors affecting continuation rates of DMPA. Contraception 1999;60:345-351.
94. Tankeyoon M, Dusitsin N, Chalapati S, Koetsawang S, Saibiang S, Sas M, Gellen JJ, Ayeni O, Gray R, Pinol A, Zegers L. Effects of hormonal contraceptives on milk volume and infant growth. Contraception 1984;30:505-522.
95. Wharton C, Blackburn R. Lower-dose pills. Popul Rep 1988;16(3). Series A(7).

96. Guillebaud J. Contraception, your questions answered. New York NY: Churchill, 1993.
97. Erwin PC. To use or not to use combined hormonal oral contraceptives during lactation. Fam Plann Perspect 1994;26:26-30, 33.
98. Visness CM, Rivera R. Progestin-only pill use and pill switching during breastfeeding. Contraception 1995;51:279-281.
99. Toddywalla VS, Mehta S, Virkar KD, Saxena BN. Release of 19-nor-testosterone type of contraceptive steroids through different drug delivery systems into serum and breast milk of lactating women. Contraception 1980;21:217-223.
100. Curtis EM. Oral-contraceptive feminization of a normal male infant. Obstet Gynecol 1964;23:295-296.
101. Virutamasen P, Leepipatpaiboon S, Kriengsinyot R, Vichaidith P, Muia PN, Sekadde-Kigondu CB, Mati JKG, Forest MG, Dikkeschei LD, Wolthers BG, d'Arcangues C. Pharmacodynamic effects of depot-medroxyprogesterone acetate (DMPA) administered to lactating women on their male infants. Contraception 1996;54:153-157.
102. Heinig MJ, Dewey KG. Health Advantages of Breastfeeding for Infants: A Critical Review. Nutrition Research Reviews 1996;9:89-110.
103. McCann MF, Liskin LS, Piotrow PT, Rinehart W, Fox G. Breastfeeding, fertility and family planning. Popul Reports 1984;12(2). Series J(24).
104. Kovar MG, Serdula MK, Marks JS, Fraser DW. Review of the epidemiologic evidence for an association between infant feeding and infant health. Pediatrics 1984;74(4-Suppl):615-638.
105. Howie PW, Forsyth JS, Ogston SA, Clark A, Florey C du V. Protective effect of breast feeding against infection. Br Med J 1990;300:11-16.
106. Lucas A, Cole TJ. Breast milk and neonatal necrotising enterocolitis. Lancet 1990;336:1519-1523.
107. Woolridge MW, Phil D, Baum JD. Recent advances in breast feeding. Acta Paediatr Jpn 1993;35:1-12.
108. Labbok MH. Consequences of breastfeeding for mother and child. J Biosoc Sci 1985;9(Suppl):43-54.
109. Lucas A, Morley R, Cole TJ, Lister G, Leeson-Payne C. Breast milk and subsequent intelligence quotient in children born preterm. Lancet 1992;339:261-264.
110. Cunningham AS. Breastfeeding, bottlefeeding and illness: an annotated bibliography, 1986. In: Jelliffe DB, Jelliffe EFP (eds). Programmes to promote breastfeeding. Oxford, England: Oxford University Press, 1988:448-480.
111. American Academy of Pediatrics. The transfer of drugs and other chemicals into human milk. Pediatrics 2001;108:776-789.
112. Lawrence RA. A review of the medical benefits and contraindications to breastfeeding in the United States. Maternal and Child Health Technical Information Bulletin. Arlington VA: National Center for Education in Maternal and Child Health, 1997.
113. American Academy of Pediatrics. Human milk, breastfeeding and the transmission of Human Immunodeficiency Virus in the United States. Pediatrics 1995;96:977-979.
114. Ekpini ER, Wiktor SZ, Satten GA, Adjorlolo-Johnson GT, Sibailly TS, Ou CY, Karon JM, Brattegaard K, Whitaker JP, Gnaore E, De Cock KM, Greenberg AE. Late postnatal mother-to-child transmission of HIV-1 in Abidjan, Côte d'Ivoire. Lancet 1997;349:1054-1059.
115. Ruff AJ. Breastmilk, breastfeeding and transmission of viruses to the neonate. Semin Perinatol 1994;18:510-516.
116. Van de Perre P, Simonon A, Msellati P, Hitimana DG, Vaira D, Bazubagira A, Van Goethem C, Stevens AM, Karita E, Sondag-Thull D, Dabis F, Lepage P. Postnatal transmission of human immunodeficiency virus type I from mother to infant. N Engl J Med 1991;325:593-598.
117. Working Group on Mother-to-Child Transmission of HIV. Rates of mother-to-child transmission of HIV-1 in Africa, America, and Europe: results from 13 perinatal studies. J Acquir Immune Defic Syndr Hum Retrovirol 1995;8:506-510.

118. Adjorlolo-Johnson G, De Cock KM, Ekpini E, Vetter KM, Sibailly T, Brattegaard K, Yavo D, Doorly R, Whitaker JP, Kestens L, Ou C-Y, George JR, Gayle HD. Prospective comparison of mother-to-child transmission of HIV-1 and HIV-2 in Abidjan, Ivory Coast. JAMA 1994;272:462-466.
119. Bélec L, Bouquety JC, Georges AJ, Siopathis MR, Martin PMV. Antibodies to human immunodeficiency virus in the breast milk of healthy seropositive women. Pediatrics 1990;85:1022-1026.
120. Newburg DS, Viscidi RP, Ruff A, Yolken RH. A human milk factor inhibits binding of human immunodeficiency virus to the CD4 receptor. Pediatr Res 1992;31:22-28.
121. Van de Perre P, Simonon A, Hitimana DG, Dabis F, Msellati P, Mukamabano B, Butera JB, Van Goethem C, Karita E, Lepage P. Infective and anti-infective properties of breastmilk from HIV-1-infected women. Lancet 1993;341:914-918.
122. Dunn DT, Newell ML, Ades AE, Peckham CS. Risk of human immunodeficiency virus type 1 transmission through breastfeeding. Lancet 1992;340:585-588.
123. Guay LA, Hom DL, Mmiro F, Piwowar EM, Kabengera S, Parsons J, Ndugwa C, Marum L, Olness K, Kataaha P, Jackson JB. Detection of human immunodeficiency virus type 1 (HIV-1) DNA and p24 antigen in breast milk of HIV-1-infected Ugandan women and vertical transmission. Pediatrics 1996;98:438-444.
124. Centers for Disease Control (CDC). Recommendations for assisting in the prevention of perinatal transmission of human T-lymphotropic virus type III/lymphadenopathy-associated virus and acquired immunodeficiency syndrome. MMWR 1985;34:721-726, 731-732.
125. WHO Technical Consultation on Behalf of the UNFPA/UNICEF/WHO/UNAIDS Inter-Agency Task Team on Mother-to-Child Transmission of HIV. New Data on the Prevention of Mother-to-Child Transmission of HIV and their Policy Implications—Conclusions and Recommendations. Geneva, Switzerland: WHO/RHR/ 01.28, 2001. Available at http://www.who.int/reproductive-health/RTIs. Accessed October 27, 2001.
126. Eaton SB, Pike MC, Short RV, Lee NC, Trussell J, Hatcher RA, Wood JW, Worthman CM, Blurton Jones NG, Konner MJ, Hill KR, Bailey R, Hurtado AM. Women's reproductive cancers in evolutionary context. Q Rev Biol 1994;69:353-367.
127. Rosenblatt KA, Thomas DB. Prolonged lactation and endometrial cancer: WHO Collaborative Study of Neoplasia and Steroid Contraceptives. Int J Epidemiol 1995;24:499-503.
128. Speroff L, Glass RH, Kase NG. Clinical gynecologic endocrinology and infertility (Fifth Edition). Baltimore MD: Williams and Wilkins, 1994.
129. Institute of Medicine (IOM). Nutrition during lactation. Washington DC: National Academy Press, 1991.
130. Worthington-Roberts BS, Williams SR. Nutrition in pregnancy and lactation (Fifth Edition). St. Louis MO: Mosby-Year Book, Inc., 1993:340.

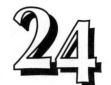

Contraceptive Research and Development

Felicia Stewart, MD
Henry L. Gabelnick, PhD

- Developing methods that women can use to protect against both pregnancy and sexually transmitted infections (STIs) including HIV/AIDS, especially methods that can be used with little or no effort required from a male partner, is a high priority for current contraceptive research.
- Research to develop systemic methods for men is ongoing, but the introduction of new options for men is likely to be at least 5 to 10 years away.
- Contraceptive research has the potential to provide improved technologies and also new thinking about regimens and requirements for service delivery. Methods with simpler rules for use and fewer obstacles to provider initiation could improve a user's ability to use contraceptives more effectively.
- Increased resources are needed for both public and private sectors in the field of contraception. New discoveries in biotechnology, genetics, immunology, and molecular biology have the potential to accelerate innovation; we urgently need methods that provide both pregnancy and STI, HIV/AIDS prevention.

CONTRACEPTIVE RESEARCH OVERVIEW

WHY IS CONTRACEPTIVE RESEARCH NEEDED?

In addition to the intuitive appeal of assuring the latest, best medications and technologies in all medical fields, the need for improvement in the field of contraception is clear from public health statistics. First, we urgently need methods that provide dual protection—against both unintended pregnancy and also sexually transmitted infections (STIs) including HIV/AIDS.[1] Worldwide, this is an imperative problem, but it is also very important for many couples in the United States. Second, the goal of assuring that all pregnancies are intended and planned for is still elusive.[2]

Although couples have a range of family planning methods available now, almost half of all pregnancies in the United States and worldwide are not intended. Many unintended pregnancies occur because the couple was not using a method at the time, but almost half—as many as 1.5 million annually in the United States—are "failures" that occur despite method use. A tiny minority of unintended pregnancies is attributable to technical failure of a method or to a decision not to use contraception for religious reasons; most instead reflect inconsistent or incorrect use of a method, or interruptions in use. Improving the way in which individuals use contraception will require improved education and access to family planning care, but improvements in technology can also play an important role.

Contraceptive research in the past focused on finding highly effective methods and on method safety. Newer research priorities include efforts to reduce side effects and develop methods that are easier and more appealing to use. For example, recent research has sought methods that have incidental beneficial effects such as such as clearer skin or reduced fluid retention. Ideal methods might even have a positive effect on the couple's sexual experience. Methods that are easier to use—simpler, with less to remember—potentially could improve effectiveness in actual use. Research to reduce obstacles to initiating and continuing a method, and to help providers adopt improved service delivery approaches more quickly, also provides the potential to help reduce unintended pregnancy. New thinking is needed in this field along with new technologies. The introduction of emergency contraception (EC), for example, has helped prompt a shift in both technology and services. The widening dissemination of EC may turn out to have had an unintended positive effect to the extent that providers and couples begin to understand and respond to contraceptive need as an urgent rather than "routine" medical issue. Reducing typical delays in initiation of contraception would result in a significant reduction in unintended pregnancy rates.

Medical problems and side effects are not a serious obstacle for most couples, but they are important for some. For example, women with serious chronic diseases that make use of hormonal products inappropriate have limited alternative options, as do women who experience unacceptable side effects when using hormonal products. Continued efforts to develop entirely new categories of contraceptives would help both of these groups and might have important advantages for other women as well.

The widening HIV pandemic and the role that STIs play in accelerating HIV spread make it an urgent priority to find methods that can reduce infection. There is also a parallel need for research to clarify how existing methods affect the risks for acquiring or transmitting infection—including effects on the immune system.[3] Research about the effects of current hormonal methods on infection risk has so far not had consistent results—either positive or negative. Hormone patterns, however, do alter immune system function in the reproductive tract. If some current hormone methods turn out to have undesirable effects on infection risk for some couples, then new methods based on other mechanisms of action will be desperately needed.

This chapter provides information practitioners can use in supporting or advocating for adequate research funding, and for educational presentations about the future of contraception. It also describes new methods available elsewhere, that are ready for imminent introduction or re-introduction in the United States, and that may become available in the next 5 to 10 years, especially new microbicide and barrier options. The chapter also reviews the status of male methods and immunocontraceptives, although the time horizon for these possibilities may be longer.

A BRIEF HISTORY OF CONTRACEPTIVE RESEARCH

Modern private-sector contraceptive research began in the 1950s and led to the first oral contraceptive pill (Enovid) approved by the FDA in 1960 and marketing of IUDs (Lippes Loop and Saf-T-Coil) in the early 1960s (see Table 24-1). At its peak in the late 1970s, significant investments in contraceptive research were being made by at least six large U.S. companies.[4]

Support for basic research prior to 1950, and continuing through the 1980s, was provided principally by three visionary foundations—Rockefeller, Mellon, and Ford—and was critical in establishing the basis for most of the methods available today. Public research funding began when the National Institute of Child Health and Human Development (NICHD) was established at the National Institute of Health (NIH) in 1963. Soon after, U.S. Agency for International Development (USAID) allocated additional research funding.

Private-sector involvement after 1970 declined, however, and focused on improvements in hormonal formulations. The level of public and foundation funding for research, after significant growth in the 1960s and early 1970s, also slowed in the 1980s.[5] By 1990, a U.S. Academy of Sciences report concluded that declining and sporadic funding from foundations and public sources and the decreased interest of most pharmaceutical companies threatened to reduce the pool of scientific personnel and resources for the field.[4] The committee noted that resource limitations would be likely to delay the application of new biotechnology, genetic engineering, and molecular biology discoveries that otherwise might provide significant advances in contraception.

Table 24-1 Method timeline: date of introduction and/or FDA approval *

1839	Condoms mass-produced by Goodyear (vulcanized rubber)
1925	Diaphragms manufactured in United States
1960	Enovid estrogen plus progestin oral contraceptive pill
1962	Lippes Loop licensed for use in public programs
1982	Contraceptive sponge (subsequently withdrawn in 1994)
1984	Cu T 380A copper-releasing intrauterine device
1988	Prentif cavity-rim cervical cap
1990	Norplant levonorgestrel 6-rod implant device
1992	Depo Provera 3-month progestin injectable
1994	Reality female condom
1996	Jadelle levonorgestrel 2-rod implant device (not marketed)
1998	Preven estrogen plus progestin emergency contraceptive
1999	Plan B progestin emergency contraceptive
2000	Lunelle estrogen plus progestin injectable (subsequently withdrawn from sale)
2000	Mifepristone antiprogestin for early abortion
2000	Mirena levonorgestrel-releasing intrauterine system
2002	Ortho Evra contraceptive patch
2002	Organon vaginal contraceptive ring
2002	Lea's Shield (not marketed)
2003	FemCap (not marketed)
2003	Essure transcervical permanent sterilization device
2004	Implanon etonogestrel single-rod implant (approved earlier) marketing expected

* Note: This table does not include the many oral contraceptive pill products introduced following the 1960 approval for Enovid, the first "pill." Pill development has provided major improvements, especially with gradual reduction in the hormone dose for both the estrogen and progestin components, and development and introduction of improved progestins. Intrauterine devices introduced after the Lippes Loop but no longer available also are not listed.

During the 1980s and 1990s, the increasing complexity of regulatory review for new drugs and devices along with concerns about product liability and public controversy in the field of contraception also had a detrimental effect on the development of new methods, especially in the United States.[6] Damaging litigation following the Dalkon shield scandal led to withdrawal of other IUDs from the market in the 1970's, and attacks against Norplant beginning in 1994 were followed by a dramatic decline in its sales.[7] Large companies were logically more reluctant to assume the financial risks involved in development of innovative approaches, and smaller companies lacked sufficient resources to do so. Initial development of new approaches, therefore, became increasingly dependent on public sector resources and research organizations.[8]

Development of a new drug or device is a long and costly process (see Table 24-2). Drug discovery and device invention typically involve many discarded possibilities before an option promising enough to warrant human studies is identified. Human studies require IND (Investigational New Drug) or IDE (Investigational Device Exemption) approval by the Food and Drug Administration (FDA), and applications must include a review of laboratory and toxicology testing in animals. For drugs, human studies are conducted in phases to assess safety (Phase I), effectiveness (Phase II), and extended safety and effectiveness in clinical use (Phase III). Research data from these studies provide the basis for a New Drug Application (NDA) to the FDA. If the product is approved, the data are the basis for product labeling, including dosing, instructions, and indications. When the NDA is approved, the company is entitled to sell and market the drug for the approved indications. FDA processes for reviewing applications for device approval (called PMA—Premarket Approval applications) are similar, although somewhat more complex.[4]

Table 24-2 The drug development process

Preclinical Development	
Concept & synthesis	
Production of sufficient drug quantity for research	
Formulation to provide suitable dose and administration route	
Preclinical Research	
Toxicology, safety and effectiveness (animals)	1–3 years
Investigational New Drug Application (IND) Filed	
Reviewed by FDA	30 days for FDA review*
FDA Acceptance permits research use for human subjects	
Clinical Research (human subjects)	
Phase 1 Fewer than 100 subjects to establish safety	6 mo–1 year
Phase 2 100 + human subjects to establish effectiveness	6 mo–2 years
Phase 3 Sufficient subject number (1000 +) to confirm safety, effectiveness, and dosage	1–4 years
New Drug Application (NDA) Filed	
Reviewed by FDA	2 mo–7 years for
FDA Approval for Marketing	FDA review*
Postmarketing Surveillance	
Adverse event reporting	
Additional studies as required in FDA Approval Decision	

Source: adapted from Mastroianni, 1990.[4]

* Review and decision by FDA staff, with recommendations to FDA from Advisory Committee.

Reviewing available information in 2004, the Institute of Medicine Committee on New Frontiers in Contraceptive Development concluded that development of a new drug takes 10 to 14 years, and involves an investment of $400 million to $800 million.[9] The investment in contraceptive research and development from all sectors is insufficient to develop more than just a handful of new possibilities. Although private sector companies are investing in research on drugs for conditions that primarily affect women, contraception is not a high priority. A 2001 survey of its members reported by PhRMA (the Pharmaceutical Research and Manufacturers of America) identified 358 new drugs in development for diseases that primarily affect women. Only 7 were contraceptives (the patch, the single rod implant, 3 new oral contraceptive pill formulations, a vaccine against hCG, and a microbicide). In contrast, this group included 82 new drugs for women's cancers, 52 arthritis drugs, 11 post-menopausal symptom drugs, and 36 new psychiatric drugs.[10] Contraceptive research clearly needs continued support for public funding.

Public funding for research through the NIH has increased significantly over the last decade. The total allocated for women's health issues has also increased: A review by ACOG in 2001 found that women's health accounted for 15.2% of the NIH budget in 2001, up from 14.2% in 1993. Of this total ($2.7 billion out of the total for NIH of $18.1 billion), about half is spent for heart disease and cancer research; approximately 10% ($270 million) is allocated to reproductive, maternal, child and adolescent health, including approximately $27 million for research on contraception in 2001.[11] Additional public funding for contraception is also provided through USAID. The public total, however, is modest in relation to the estimated development cost for even a single new product.

The urgent need for methods that women can use to protect against HIV/AIDS and STIs as well as pregnancy has infused the contraceptive development field with new vitality and some new resources. Although the primary sources of funding for this effort have been public sector and foundation grants, private sector organizations have begun to work in this area. The steady increase in contraceptive use in developing countries—a vast potential market for products estimated to include 2.5 billion women by the year 2025—along with the successful introduction of new products, including the hormone-releasing vaginal ring, the patch, and the levonorgestrel intrauterine system, has helped create renewed interest in contraceptive development at major pharmaceutical companies.

WHAT IS NEEDED?

More public funding. Along with all "women's health" issues, resources for contraceptive development research continues to lag behind research in other areas. Inadequate resources means the opportunity to apply major advances in immunology, genetics and molecular biology is delayed or lost, and is tragic because the human need is great. Contraceptive options that could dent unintended pregnancy would have a huge health impact—certainly comparable to that of a major heart disease or cancer breakthrough. Not everyone will develop these important diseases, but almost everyone does need effective contraception, and unintended pregnancy involves serious health risks for young people that translate to high losses in years of productive life.

Support for increased participation of private-sector companies. Courageous companies that work in this field should be applauded, and will be assisted by efforts to increase public awareness of the importance of this research area and to diminish controversy about family planning and reproductive health in national public policy. Commitment to adequate public funding of family planning services and supplies for low income couples in the United States and as part of international aid can also fortify private sector involvement in the field.

Development of innovative approaches is needed. In addition to methods that protect against both infection and pregnancy, investment is needed to insure that entirely new approaches can be pursued as well as improvements in existing hormonal methods.

CURRENT CONTRACEPTIVE RESEARCH

MICROBICIDES

Chemical barriers have been used for contraception in conjunction with cervical caps and diaphragms, and also alone as foams, suppositories, tablets, creams and gels. In addition to their spermicidal effect, currently marketed products—nonoxynol-9 (N-9) in the United States and similar detergents in other countries—also kill bacteria and viruses when tested in the laboratory. This microbicide effect led to the initial hope that existing products might also reduce infection risk in actual use. Contrary to the hope, however, research on the effect of N-9 spermicide use by women in a high infection risk group found higher HIV incidence with spermicide use than with use of a placebo.[12-14] Vaginal irritation caused by the N-9 may have compromised normal vaginal defenses against infection, leaving women more vulnerable.[15] Other available spermicide detergents also may cause irritation. Because of the potential harm, N-9 use is no longer recommended for women at high risk for HIV/AIDS and it also should not be used as a lubricant for rectal intercourse. Efforts to find methods to prevent infection have therefore turned to the task of finding entirely new microbicide options.[16]

The microbicide development challenge is to find an option that is effective in stopping bacterial or viral infection but does not cause irritation. Ideally, a product might even enhance natural infection defenses and/or protect against irritation. HIV or pathogen protection for many potential microbicide candidates identified so far is based on their ability to kill or inactivate HIV virus or pathogens. Alternatively, a microbicide could act by interfering with essential steps in the infection process such as cell attachment or entry, or replication of the pathogen. Most of the chemicals and compounds being studied also interfere with sperm fertility or kill sperm. In the future, a product that could safely prevent infection without impairing fertility would also be desirable. Demonstrating safety of use in conjunction with intended fertility, however, would be an even more formidable research challenge than demonstrating infection protection alone.

Research efforts over the last five years have identified several "promising" candidates, and several are already undergoing human safety studies (see Table 24-3). Clinical studies to demonstrate effectiveness and extended safety, however, will require several years so it is unlikely that a new microbicide could be ready for FDA approval before 2007. In the meantime, researchers are also re-assessing lubricants currently marketed for other purposes.[17] Lubrication in itself may be desirable because its use may decrease irritation and trauma during intercourse, which in turn may reduce infection risk.

Table 24-3 Microbicide Clinical Trials Planned, Ongoing, or Completed

Product / Company	Clinical Research: Ongoing or Completed	Planned
Acid buffers / enhancers of vaginal defenses		
Acidform, Global Microbicide Project	Phase 1	
BufferGel, Reprotect L.L.C.	Phase 1	Phase 2/3
Invisible Condom, Laval University	Phase 1	Phase 1/2
Lactobacillus Crispatus (CTV-05), Osel, Inc.	Phase 2	
Surfactant		
Benzalkonium Chloride (BZK), Biofem	Phase 1	
Savvy (C31G), Biosyn	Phase 1	Phase 2/3
Entry inhibitors		
Calanolide A, SRI International		Phase 1
Carragard (PC 515), Population Council	Phase 1, 2	Phase 3
Cellulose Sulfate (CS), Global Microbicide Project	Phase 1	
Emmelle (Dextrin02 Sulfate), Medical Research Council	Phase 1, 2	
Monoclonal Antibodies (C2F5, C2G12, C4E10), Polymun Scientific	Phase 1	
Polystyrene Sulfonate, Global Microbicide Project	Phase 1	
PRO 2000/5, Interneuron Pharmaceutical, Inc.	Phase 1, 2	
SPL 7013, Starpharma		Phase 1
Replication inhibitor		
Topical PMPA (Tenofovir), Gilead Sciences, Inc.		Phase 1
Other mechanism (uncharacterized)		
Praneem Polyherbal Vaginal Tablet, Indian Council of Medical Research		Phase 1

Source: adapted from Alliance for Microbicide Development, Clinical Trials Information Center Summary and Table of Microbicide Products in Development, May 2003; www.microbicide.org, accessed 9 July 2003.

It is also possible that the "microbicide" goal could be achieved with a product administered systemically. For example, pre-exposure treatment, or daily treatment, with a drug that could block infection or fortify immune defenses could be considered, as could an agent released continuously from a vaginal ring or barrier device that acted primarily or partially through a systemic effect. Drugs developed for HIV/AIDS treatment and for parasite therapy are being considered for this application.

Research related to microbicide development may also prove to have unanticipated long-term benefits. The microbicide effort has required a major investment in basic research about vaginal physiology, and the pathophysiology of HIV/AIDS and STI transmission. Advances are likely also to be helpful in combating common problems such as bacterial vaginosis, and have already produced some important findings. The complex vaginal ecosystem was previously little understood. It is a delicate system that can easily be disrupted by trauma or by chemical alteration. "Mildly" toxic exposures such as N-9 or a solution that is too acid or too alkaline can disrupt normal vaginal bacteria and impair normal defenses against infection. Use of "hygiene" products including douching seems likely to turn out to be a much more significant issue than previously recognized.

MECHANICAL BARRIER METHODS

Renewed attention has been directed to development of new mechanical barriers in parallel with the emphasis on microbicide development. A mechanical barrier may be helpful for use in conjunction with a new microbicide, and there is also some hope that a barrier may itself provide some protection against transmission of infection. Providing a physical shield for the cervix is a plausible strategy since cervical epithelium is an important infection target: it is the primary site for chlamydial infection, and also contains a rich supply of immune system cells that are the target for initial HIV uptake.[18] Studies in Zimbabwe and South Africa are planned to evaluate the effectiveness of a diaphragm used with one of the promising microbicide products in reducing HIV acquisition, and results should be available within the next 5 years.

The Today contraceptive sponge, previously marketed for more than a decade in the United States but not available since 1994, may return. This product contains N-9 in a small, soft pillow shaped device (see Chapter 18, Vaginal Barrier Devices). At the time of its withdrawal, the manufacturer explained that the investment required to meet FDA-mandated manufacturing equipment upgrades was not feasible. The product was purchased in 1999 by a new company that has periodically reaffirmed plans to reintroduce the product in the United States; the product is marketed in Canada. Other contraceptive sponge options, Protectaid, containing a lower concentration of N-9 along with benzalkonium chloride, and Pharmatex, containing benzalkonium chloride, are also available in Canada and in Europe, but are not FDA approved.

Two new vaginal barrier devices have been approved by the FDA, with marketing expected in the United States in the near future. Lea's Shield is a one-size, rounded, cup-shaped silicone device that incorporates a one-way valve to allow air to escape during placement and help provide suction to hold it in place against the cervix. FemCap is a cervical cap with a sailor's cap shape. It is made of silicone, and requires fitting to select one of three sizes. Both devices are intended for use with spermicide, but may also prove suitable for use with microbicide in the future.

Research is also ongoing to develop new, improved diaphragm and cap models. A one-size, flatter oval silicone device has been designed with the help of women volunteers who provided feedback during the design process about comfort and ease of use. Adaptation of the menstrual protection device, Instead, is also being explored to provide an inexpensive, disposable vaginal barrier that could be marketed with microbicide. Similarly, a small, soft transparent disposable silicone cervical cap called Oves, available in three sizes, was licensed in accordance with European Union regulations in 1997, and is available in France and in the United Kingdom.[19] This device might be appropriate for marketing together with a new microbicide. There is also research interest in evaluating a process for self-fitting for diaphragms, recognizing that a method that does not require provider fitting will be more feasible for wide adoption if the combination of a vaginal barrier and microbicide proves to be effective in helping reduce HIV/AIDS and STI transmission.

Development of new, female condom models is also ongoing. Prototypes based on incorporating a vaginal pouch in a bikini panty have been developed, as well as improved methods for inserting and stabilizing a condom designed to line the vagina only (similar to the Reality female condom). New male condom models are also being developed utilizing materials other than latex and providing a design that can be put in place before erection,[20] a less snug fit, or an alternative shape for the portion covering the glans and penis.

HORMONAL AND SYSTEMIC METHODS FOR WOMEN

Hormonal methods have been the mainstay of reversible contraception because of their safety and effectiveness. New developments have provided methods with a lower hormone dose, improved progestin options, and drug delivery that simplifies use. Several options used in other countries, however, are not available in the United States, including implants and injectables that have already received FDA approval and initial marketing here.

The low dose, 6-rod progestin-releasing implant—Norplant—was approved by the FDA in 1990. Sales of the product were stopped in 2000, and the company announced in 2002 that it did not plan to reintroduce the device. The improved, 2-rod version of this method—Jadelle—is currently marketed in Europe by Schering Oy of Finland. Jadelle has also been approved for sale in the United States, but the patent-holder in the United States, Wyeth, has not marketed it here. Another implant option, the single-rod Implanon, has been marketed in Europe for several years, and has FDA approval for marketing in the United States, but has not yet been introduced by the company. Implants gained a small but very appreciative user group because of their extremely high efficacy and use simplicity.

The combination estrogen and progestin injectable, Lunelle, had a history similar to that of Norplant. Although this method is marketed in many other countries, it was available only briefly in the United States, then voluntarily recalled by Pharmacia in 2002. It is not clear when or whether this option will again become available, although it too had a wider-than-expected, enthusiastic user adoption while it was marketed.

Research on hormonal methods has the potential to improve bleeding patterns for women using low-dose, progestin-only methods including implants. Implants are a very appealing approach because their efficacy is as good as or better than other long-term methods, including surgical sterilization, and their average continuation rate is higher than that with other reversible methods.[21] New progestins, such as nesterone, also have the potential for use in a hormone releasing vaginal ring, and might also provide incidental "side benefits" related to the characteristics of the progestin or a method with fewer undesirable side effects.

Development of hormone receptor blocking approaches might also provide new contraceptive options. The anti-progestin Mifepristone has been studied for use as an emergency contraceptive after unprotected intercourse, for low-dose, daily use and also for possible use as a once-a-month regimen. Such regimens can provide contraceptive protection, but have also caused menstrual disruption. Further basic research is ongoing to identify and evaluate other members of the anti-progestin family.[22]

In the future, systemic methods that do not disrupt normal hormone cycles may also be possible. A narrowly targeted method, for example, with effect only on zona pellucida binding of sperm, or factors essential for implantation, might provide effective contraception without the side effects related to hormone disruption. These approaches have the potential for development of methods that could be used monthly. Initial laboratory or animal research has identified two peptides, leukemia inhibitory factor (LIF) and perimplantation factor (PIF) that might be feasible targets for inhibition. The peptide leptin, better known for its role in regulation of hunger, may also play a role in implantation. Development of such options, however, will require more basic research and a better understanding of the molecular biology and biochemistry involved, so would be unlikely to reach clinical use within the next decade.

SYSTEMIC METHODS FOR MEN

Although one third of the world's couples rely on male methods (condoms, withdrawal, and vasectomy), development of systemic methods for men has been slow. Part of the reason is that male fertility physiology is a difficult challenge: sperm are continuously produced, with maturation and development over an interval of weeks, and part of the reason is that issues like adverse effects, side effects, acceptability, and affordability are a more powerful constraint now than they were in the 1950s when female systemic methods were devised. Three possible approaches include: (1) blocking hormonal support for testicular cell function by stopping pituitary LH and FSH, (2) interfering with seminiferous tubule function to stop sperm production, and (3) disrupting maturation, functioning, and/or transport of sperm after they are produced. Targeting the second or third approach would have significant advantages, but except for gossypol, no method has yet been developed sufficiently for clinical studies.[23] Current research has focused on the first option.

Suppression of testicular cells responsible for sperm development has the incidental effect of stopping testosterone production, and along with it libido and potency. Too much testosterone has unfavorable effects on lipids, acne, weight gain, and possibly also mood. Hormonal methods for men, therefore, must provide an ideal amount of testosterone to avoid these effects, but at the same time insure effective hormonal suppression of sperm production. Regimens most likely to become available first involve androgen (synthetic testosterone) administered along with a progestin sufficient to suppress LH, the normal pituitary stimulus for testicular cell hormone and sperm production.[8] Clinical (human) studies are ongoing to identify an optimal combination. Progestins under consideration include familiar progestins such as levonorgestrel, norethindrone enanthate, etonogestrel, and depot medroxyprogesterone acetate (DMPA). Providing sufficient testosterone has also been a development challenge because available testosterone products would require frequent administration (daily or weekly injections). Longer acting preparations such as testosterone undecanoate or testosterone pellets may provide a more feasible approach.[24]

Non-hormonal possibilities have been evaluated as systemic contraceptives for men. Gossypol, derived from cottonseed oil, has been used for clinical research extensively in China. Large studies there have found that it can provide effective sperm suppression without changing testosterone production or libido. Concern about reduced blood potassium levels reported in the initial studies for 10% of subjects, as well as irreversibility of the contraceptive effect in as many as 20% of users, reduced international interest in developing this method further. Subsequent Chinese research, however, found that the low potassium effect was related to the low level of potassium in the diets of study subjects, and a recent review concluded that additional potential for this approach should be explored.[25] Other non-hormonal options being considered for development are anti-cancer drugs such as lonidamine. These agents are known to reduce normal sperm production, and it may be possible to find a compound that has high effectiveness in reducing sperm but acceptable toxicity profile in other respects.

INTRAUTERINE DEVICES (IUDS)

Several improvements for existing intrauterine contraceptives are being investigated with the hope of reducing expulsion, reducing discomfort and cramping that some women experience, and providing an intrauterine option for women whose uterine depth is too small to accommodate current devices. A smaller version of the levonorgestrel-releasing intrauterine system, Mirena, is being tested for use in women at or after menopause. An IUD without a rigid frame, it is held in place instead by an anchoring knot implanted in the myometrium at the uterine fundus. GyneFix carries copper tubes on a string, and provides similar efficacy to the CuT, with (at least) five year duration. It has been approved for marketing in the European Union, and is also available in China and Indonesia.[26–28] The Belgian company that markets GyneFix is now developing a second frameless option, the FibroPlant-LNG. Instead of copper tubes, this model incorporates a levonorgestrel-releasing ethylene vinyl acetate hormone reservoir similar to that of the Mirena T-shaped intrauterine system.[29]

METHODS FOR STERILIZATION

In the United States and worldwide, sterilization surgery is one of the most widely used of all contraceptive options. Research to improve technologies for sterilization therefore has important promise for increasing safety and effectiveness for sterilization, as well as lower cost and simplification that would avoid the need for surgical facilities and general anesthesia. Several transcervical sterilization methods for women are being studied, in addition to the transcervical sterilization device, Essure, approved by the FDA in 2002. The Intratubal Ligation Device developed by BioMedical Engineering Solutions Inc. uses an adhesive-coated balloon and an O-ring to invaginate a section of the fallopian tube and create a sphincter with the O-ring. It is designed to be used with hysteroscopy equipment, or with blind transcervical placement of the catheter and device into the proximal portion of the tube. The Adiana transcervical sterilization system, and the Eclipse Permanent Contraceptive Device are small implants, placed through a transcervical catheter using hysteroscopy. Once in place the implanted device serves as a matrix for growth of tissue that occludes the tube within a few weeks. A reversible occlusion device is being developed by Berkeley Applied Science and Engineering. It utilizes a nickel-titanium stent, similar to materials already used for vascular implants, and is intended to be reversible by catheter insertion into the tube to change the device structure mechanically or electrically.

Transcervical insertion of a chemical or drug that causes tissue sclerosis is also being studied. Initial human research using a quinacrine solution was begun in the 1970s, but abandoned because of an unacceptably high failure rate, and deaths during insertion of the solution reported to the FDA. Subsequently, a pellet formulation of quinacrine was developed, and research initiated in several countries including Indonesia, Chile and Vietnam in the 1980s. Following reports of a cluster of cancers among women treated in Chile a larger follow-up study was undertaken which did confirm the cluster but found no other cases and concluded that there is no significant increase in cancer risk. A follow up study of women treated in Vietnam also found no increased incidence of cancer, but raised concerns about effectiveness of the method, and additional safety concerns. With concerns raised by women's health advocates as well as by the World Health Organization (WHO), the governments of Vietnam, Indonesia, and Chile halted quinacrine research, and the Swiss pellet manufacturer stopped providing the drug in 1998. Proponents for the method, however, have continued to work for development of this approach, and in 2001, a Phase I safety study to enroll up to 10 women in the United States was approved by the FDA and by the IRB for the university site involved.[10] Toxicology studies, meanwhile, are ongoing to provide the information that would now be necessary for FDA review and approval if this approach does prove to be safe and effective.

Erythromycin, an alternative agent with the potential to cause sufficient sclerosis to occlude the fallopian tubes, has been evaluated in animal and clinical studies. However, its efficacy in women was unacceptably low.

Research is also ongoing to improve sterilization methods for men. A device to provide a non-surgical vasectomy approach is being evaluated in animal studies. Ultrasound pulses are used with a vas clamp to cause localized heat sufficient to seal the vas while the overlying skin is shielded from heat by a cold balloon on the surface.

IMMUNOCONTRACEPTIVES

Development of a contraceptive vaccine has received considerable research attention. Theoretically, it might be possible to induce immune system reaction to a protein target in the reproductive system that could interrupt one or more essential fertility steps. A protein found only in reproductive events potentially could avoid the wider systemic effects of contraceptives that interrupt normal hormone patterns. For this reason, one of the most extensively studied targets has been human chorionic gonadotropin (hCG) which is released by the early embryo and placenta, and is necessary for maintaining pregnancy. Human clinical trials, however, found that frequent vaccine boosters were needed to maintain an antibody level high enough for contraceptive effectiveness. Also, researchers were concerned about possible immune cross reaction with hormones of similar structure normally produced by the pituitary gland.[8]

A vaccine targeting sperm antigens would also be theoretically feasible, and could potentially be used by both men and women. Research to identify targets has been undertaken for dozens of sperm proteins, but has not yet progressed to a stage ready for human studies. A male vaccine targeting pituitary FSH, to block sperm production without stopping testicular androgen production, has also been evaluated in animal research, as have vaccines based on combinations of different immunogens. Research has also been addressed to development of a vaccine that would produce both local mucosal immunity as well as a system (humoral) immune response. This approach could potentially use an oral or vaginal route of administration, rather than injection, and might also be feasible for inducing immunity against reproductive tract pathogens.[5]

The timeline to availability for a vaccine method is long. There has been little private sector interest in this approach, clinical studies to document safety, reversibility, and effectiveness will be long and difficult, and advocacy groups have not favored this approach because of possible misuse of a vaccine method.

THE 21ST CENTURY

Compared with the extraordinary advances in pharmaceuticals in other fields, progress in development of contraceptives has been modest. Most of the options now in wide use are variations of half-century-old hormonal suppression technology, and realistic possibilities for the next decade are not plentiful. Major innovations are not even apparent on the horizon. It would be a shame to be content with this slow pace when the need is so great, and the public health benefit to be gained so large. Surely this is a time for renewed effort and fortified resources—if not for ourselves, then for the billions of couples in less affluent nations whose lives would be so greatly improved.

REFERENCES

1. Potts M. The urgent need for a vaginal microbicide in the prevention of HIV transmission. Am J Public Health. Jun 1994;84(6):890-891.
2. Brown S, Eisenberg L, Editors. The best intentions: unintended pregnancy and the well-being of children and families. Washington, DC: National Academy Press; 1995.
3. Mostad SB, Overbaugh J, DeVange DM, et al. Hormonal contraception, vitamin A deficiency, and other risk factors for shedding of HIV-1 infected cells from the cervix and vagina. Lancet. Sep 27 1997;350(9082):922-927.
4. Mastroianni LJ, Donaldson PJ, Kane FJ, Jr., editors. Developing new contraceptives: obstacles and opportunities. Washington, D.C.: National Academy Press; 1990.
5. Harrison PF, Rosenfield A, editors. Contraceptive Research and Development: Looking to the Future. Washington, D.C.: National Academy Press; 1996.
6. Harrison PF, Rosenfield A. Research, introduction, and use: advancing from Norplant. Contraception. Dec 1998;58(6):323-334.
7. Johansson ED. The return of the pharmaceutical industry to the market of contraception. Steroids. Oct-Nov 2000;65(10-11):709-711.
8. Schwartz JL, Gabelnick HL. Current contraceptive research. Perspect Sex Reprod Health. Nov-Dec 2002;34(6):310-316.

9. Nass SJ, Strauss JF III, Editors. New Frontiers in contraceptive research: a blueprint for action. Washington, D.C.: National Academics Press, 2004.

10. Anonymous. New medicines in development for women. Washington, D.C.: Pharmaceutical Research and Manufacturers of America; October, 2001.

11. ACOG. Facts and figures: a closer look at women's health research. Washington, D.C. 2001.

12. Roddy RE, Zekeng L, Ryan KA, Tamoufe U, Weir SS, Wong EL. A controlled trial of nonoxynol-9 film to reduce male-to-female transmission of sexually transmitted diseases. N Engl J Med. Aug 20 1998;339(8):504-510.

13. Roddy RE, Zekeng L, Ryan KA, Tamoufe U, Tweedy KG. Effect of nonoxynol-9 gel on urogenital gonorrhea and chlamydial infection: a randomized controlled trial. Jama. Mar 6 2002;287(9):1117-1122.

14. Van Damme L, Ramjee G, Alary M, et al. Effectiveness of COL-1492, a nonoxynol-9 vaginal gel, on HIV-1 transmission in female sex workers: a randomised controlled trial. Lancet. Sep 28 2002;360(9338):971-977.

15. Roddy RE, Cordero M, Cordero C, Fortney JA. A dosing study of nonoxynol-9 and genital irritation. Int J STD AIDS. May-Jun 1993;4(3):165-170.

16. Richardson BA. Nonoxynol-9 as a vaginal microbicide for prevention of sexually transmitted infections: it's time to move on. Jama. Mar 6 2002;287(9):1171-1172.

17. Baron S, Poast J, Nguyen D, Cloyd MW. Practical prevention of vaginal and rectal transmission of HIV by adapting the oral defense: use of commercial lubricants. AIDS Res Hum Retroviruses. Jul 20 2001;17(11):997-1002.

18. Moench TR, Chipato T, Padian NS. Preventing disease by protecting the cervix: the unexplored promise of internal vaginal barrier devices. Aids. Sep 7 2001;15(13):1595-1602.

19. Roizen J, Richardson S, Tripp J, Hardwicke H, Lam TQ. Oves contraceptive cap: short-term acceptability, aspects of use and user satisfaction. J Fam Plann Reprod Health Care. Oct 2002;28(4):188-192.

20. Cook L, Nanda K, Taylor D. Randomized crossover trial comparing the eZ.on plastic condom and a latex condom. Contraception. Jan 2001;63(1):25-31.

21. Meirik O. Implantable contraceptives for women. Contraception. Jan 2002;65(1):1-2.

22. Van Look PF, von Hertzen H. Clinical uses of antiprogestogens. Human Reproduction Update. 1995;1(1):19-34.

23. Brady BM, Anderson RA. Advances in male contraception. Expert Opin Investig Drugs. Mar 2002;11(3):333-344.

24. Meriggiola MC, Costantino A, Cerpolini S. Recent advances in hormonal male contraception. Contraception. Apr 2002;65(4):269-272.

25. Coutinho EM. Gossypol: a contraceptive for men. Contraception. Apr 2002;65(4):259-263.

26. Wu S, Hu J, Wildemeersch D. Performance of the frameless GyneFix and the TCu380A IUDs in a 3-year multicenter, randomized, comparative trial in parous women. Contraception. Feb 2000;61(2):91-98.

27. Wildemeersch D, Cao X, Zhang W, et al. Efficacy of a mini version of the frameless GyneFix intrauterine system (IUS) with effective copper surface area of 200 mm2. dirk.wildemeersch@contrel.be. Contraception. Oct 2002;66(4):237-241.

28. Wildemeersch D, Batar I, Affandi B, et al. The 'frameless' intrauterine system for long-term, reversible contraception: a review of 15 years of clinical experience. J Obstet Gynaecol Res. Jun 2003;29(3):164-173.

29. Wildemeersch D, Schacht E, Wildemeersch P. Contraception and treatment in the perimenopause with a novel "frameless" intrauterine levonorgestrel-releasing drug delivery system: an extended pilot study. Contraception. Aug 2002;66(2):93-99.

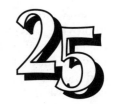

Preconception Care

Luella Klein, MD
Felicia Stewart, MD

- Steps to assure the best possible pregnancy outcome need to begin months and years beforehand.
- For some women, pregnancy is an important time for correct and consistent condom use. Every effort should be made to avoid primary Herpes 2 infection during pregnancy as well as acquisition of HIV, syphilis, gonorrhea, hepatitis, or chlamydia.
- Pregnancy affords an important opportunity to encourage women to adopt healthier behaviors. For example, the 22% of women who smoke and 20% who drink alcohol can improve their chances for a healthy baby by stopping (or reducing) these exposures.

Sometime during the reproductive years, most women wish to become pregnant and most men wish to become fathers. Optimal pregnancy outcomes for both mother and fetus depend on advance planning to provide the best environment for conception and pregnancy. All women and men need to know about pre-pregnancy health measures long before a pregnancy occurs. These measures include steps to protect future fertility and maintain good general health as well as steps needed when a woman contemplates pregnancy in the near future.

Prevention of reproductive tract infections before and during pregnancy is an important priority. Infections can cause infertility or ectopic pregnancy, and if present during pregnancy, pose multiple risks to mother, fetus, and neonate.

If pregnancy occurs accidentally, the opportunity to prepare is lost; this is one of the important health reasons for avoiding unintended pregnancy. In addition, a medical visit specifically for preconception care is recommended to assure systematic review of a medical history, completion of recommended screening tests and immunizations, and planning for pregnancy care.[1]

ESSENTIAL PRE-PREGNANCY INFORMATION FOR EVERYONE

Every family planning visit or routine periodic exam is an opportunity to provide preconception education and care. Ask each patient about plans for pregnancy in the future. Counsel about effective contraceptive use: how an optimal pregnancy outcome is correlated with its intendedness and the woman's ability to prepare in advance. Assess lifestyle and personal health risk factors. If appropriate, provide screening and offer preventive services. In addition to educating about the general pre-pregnancy health precautions (Table 25-1), check for diabetes in any woman with risk factors such as a family history of diabetes, obesity, or previous abnormal sugar levels during pregnancy. Diabetes is common and, often, unsuspected. Poor control of blood sugar during the very early weeks of pregnancy is associated with a marked increase in risk for fetal abnormality.[2]

Include pre-pregnancy education and preconception planning during routine visits. Some situations pose uniquely opportune "teachable moments," when education about optimal pregnancy is likely to be directly relevant to the patient:

- A negative pregnancy test result

- Diagnosis and management of a reproductive tract infection

- Identification of possible risk of infection with the human immunodeficiency virus (HIV)

- Diagnosis of a reproductive tract abnormality

- Identification of a substance abuse problem

- Diagnosis of a significant medical problem

In each of these situations, providing information about possible consequences and planning needed for optimal future pregnancy is an essential aspect of medical management.

Negative pregnancy test visits are a common and under-exploited opportunity for intervention. As many as one-quarter of all adolescent girls who conceive have had one or more visits to learn that their pregnancy test was negative.[3] Clearly, this is a group at high risk for unintended pregnancy. In these encounters, review how to successfully use contraception and provide basic education about health precautions needed before pregnancy. If the woman intends to become pregnant in the near future, a visit specifically for systematic preconception care is indicated.

Table 25-1 Pre-pregnancy health precautions

Avoid toxic exposure	Tobacco, alcohol, and illicit drugs are potentially toxic to fetal development; minimizing caffeine may also be reasonable. Avoid exposure to abdominal x-ray and to potentially toxic chemicals.
Take folic acid (prenatal vitamin)	To reduce the risk for neural tube defects such as spina bifida, beginning several months before pregnancy, take a vitamin that contains at least 400 micrograms (mcg) of folic acid (folate) every day.
Make healthy diet a top priority	Dieting for weight-loss is not recommended during pregnancy. Eat a well-balanced diet with fresh fruits and vegetables. Drink 3 glasses of milk daily to ensure a total of 1500 mg of calcium, or take calcium supplements to provide this amount. Avoid eating fish that may contain high levels of methyl mercury such as shark, swordfish, king mackerel, tilefish, and fish from non-commercial sources. Eat no more than 6 ounces of canned tuna per week, and no more than one serving of farm-raised salmon per month.
Discuss all medications with your clinician	Before taking any medication, discuss how it may affect your pregnancy. This includes prescription and non-prescription drugs such as pain remedies (ibuprofen) as well as herbal or other remedies. Avoid mega-dose anything, including vitamins.
Review your immunization status	Check to be sure your immunizations are up to date, especially rubella (German measles), chickenpox, Hepatitis B, and polio; if not, arrange for this at least 3 months before you want to become pregnant.
Review the medical and family histories for you and for the baby's father	If either of you has a family history of genetic abnormalities, counseling or testing may be helpful. If you have any serious medical problems, discuss them with your clinician before pregnancy. Make sure you do not have diabetes; if you do, careful management before and during early pregnancy reduces the risk of birth defects.
Avoid elevated body temperature or fever	Do what you can to avoid exposure to contagious illnesses like flu, or activities such as sauna, hot tubs, or prolonged physical exertion that might cause elevated core body temperature. Elevated temperature can increase the risk of abnormal fetal development.
Write down menstrual cycle dates	A record of the first day of each menstrual period will help your clinician determine your pregnancy due date accurately. This is especially important if tests are needed during pregnancy or if you need to have labor induced or a C-Section delivery.
Don't risk exposure to sexually transmitted infection (STI)	Avoid intercourse or use condoms carefully if there is any chance at all of STI exposure; infection such as herpes, syphilis, gonorrhea, chlamydia, or HIV/AIDS acquired during pregnancy is a very serious risk for the fetus. Get testing and treatment promptly if you have any possible STI symptoms.
Avoid toxoplasmosis and other uncommon infectious organisms	Acquiring toxoplasmosis infection during pregnancy is a serious risk for the fetus; avoid handling kitty litter (someone else should empty it every day) and wear gloves if you are handling soil outdoors. Also avoid eating raw meat or fish, or drinking unpasteurized milk.
Confirm pregnancy early	When you think you may be pregnant, have a pregnancy test and exam as soon as you can—within the first two weeks after missing your period if at all possible. If your period is abnormal or you have any pregnancy symptoms, get a test right away.

THE PRECONCEPTION CARE VISIT

A preconception care visit offers the patient a battery of services to prevent problems that could affect a pregnancy. Counseling can help a woman improve her lifestyle and health habits and consider the responsibilities of carrying a pregnancy. Counseling should also be directed toward helping the patient avoid an unintended pregnancy. Risk assessment identifies the woman at risk for a poor pregnancy outcome or for whom pregnancy will endanger her health. Screening tests reveal a mother's underlying medical and genetic conditions that may require medical intervention or may require her to make a decision about how to manage a pregnancy or whether to even attempt carrying a pregnancy. Request laboratory tests to determine the patient's blood group, Rh and antibody status, blood and platelet count, and fasting blood sugar and cholesterol levels. Finally, interventions can help a woman improve her health, adopt healthier lifestyle behaviors, identify health problems that indicate caution in undertaking aerobic exercise during pregnancy, and arrange necessary social and family support. Table 25-2 outlines the content of a preconception care visit.

Table 25-2 The preconception care visit

Action	Risk Reduction
Review contraceptive use	Prevent unintended pregnancy Decrease chance of abortion
Improve nutrition and fitness	Improve maternal health and well-being Decrease risk of low-birth weight infant
Advise smoking cessation (or at least a decrease in number of cigarettes smoked)	Decrease risk of pregnancy loss Increase birthweight Decrease risk of sudden infant death syndrome (SIDS)
Advise abstinence from alcohol (or at least a decrease in amount consumed)	Prevent fetal alcohol syndrome
Supplement with folic acid	Decrease risk of neural tube defects
Screen for HIV infection	Decrease perinatal transmission by giving anti-retroviral treatment Avoid transmission via breast milk
Screen for hepatitis B	Protect the neonate from infection by administering vaccine
Screen for other sexually transmissible infections	Protect maternal fertility Prevent fetal and neonatal infection
Immunize	Prevent vaccine-preventable diseases
Control diabetes	Decrease risk of congenital anomalies
Counsel about domestic violence	Prevent injuries
Screen for genetic diseases	Provide choices about pregnancy outcome
Review psychosocial status	Improve emotional support and well-being
Screen for bacterial vaginosis	Decrease risk of premature delivery by treating the infection with antibiotics

In addition to a preconception care visit, some couples need referral for more detailed evaluation and counseling by a genetics specialist or perinatologist. Arrange a referral well in advance to allow time for testing or planning for prenatal testing during the first trimester for persons with the following conditions:[2,4]

- The woman is age 35 or older.
- Either partner has had a child with a birth defect or cystic fibrosis.
- Either partner has a birth defect, genetic disorder, cystic fibrosis, chromosome abnormality, or has a family history of birth defects or genetic disorders.
- Either partner's ethnicity indicates risk for Tay Sachs disease (Ashkenazic Jewish, French Canadian), sickle cell anemia (black), or thalassemia (Mediterranean ancestry) if carrier status is not already known.
- Either partner has previously experienced three or more pregnancies ending in spontaneous abortion.
- The woman has a serious medical condition, or takes medication routinely.

FAMILY AND GENETIC CONDITIONS

Explore the patient's family history and the possibility of any genetic disorders. Chronic diseases such as hypertension or diabetes in a patient's family history frequently manifest during pregnancy.[2] Genetic disorders include congenital anomalies, mental retardation, Down syndrome, cystic fibrosis, Tay Sachs disease, phenylketonuria (PKU), muscular dystrophy, bleeding disorders, and sickle cell and thalassemia and other anemias. Screening and carrier testing are available for a number of disorders. Risks for chromosomal abnormality are strongly associated with age (Table 25-3), and many couples considering childbearing in the later reproductive years are very concerned about this issue. Prenatal testing is recommended for women who are age 35 or older at the time of delivery, and may also be reasonable when the father is age 55 or older.[2,4]

Table 25-3 Mother's age and risk for chromosome abnormalities

Maternal Age	Midtrimester		Term Liveborn	
	Down Syndrome	All Aneuploidies	Down Syndrome	All Aneuploidies
33	1 / 417	1 / 208	1 / 625	1 / 345
35	1 / 250	1 / 132	1 / 384	1 / 204
37	1 / 149	1 / 83	1 / 227	1 / 130
39	1 / 89	1 / 53	1 / 137	1 / 81
41	1 / 53	1 / 31	1 / 81	1 / 50
43	1 / 31	1 / 19	1 / 50	1 / 30
45	1 / 19	1 / 12	1 / 30	1 / 19

Source: adapted from ACOG (2001).[4]

REPRODUCTIVE AND OBSTETRIC HISTORY

Problems that occurred during the patient's past pregnancies can suggest interventions needed before or during pregnancy. Women who have had a low-birthweight infant will need focused counseling on how to improve birthweight of the next infant. Question women who have had a previous spontaneous abortion about risk factors. Women who previously delivered by cesarean section should be counseled regarding the advantages and disadvantages of a trial of labor instead of a scheduled elective cesarean delivery.

Teach the patient to record her menstrual dates, then review her pattern of menstrual cycles for evidence of ovulation. Ask whether she has ever tried to become pregnant before, and emphasize the need to use contraceptives effectively until she wants to conceive.

REPRODUCTIVE TRACT INFECTION

Some reproductive tract infections (RTIs) such as chlamydia and gonorrhea can cause pelvic inflammatory disease (PID) that can result in tubal damage, the most common cause of preventable infertility. (See Chapter 27 on Impaired Fertility.) Untreated or inadequately treated RTIs can infect a fetus; the risk for serious consequences is especially high if the infection is acquired during pregnancy. Syphilis, chlamydia, gonorrhea, HIV, hepatitis B, and genital herpes can lead to severe fetal, neonatal, and infant complications and fetal death. (See Table 8-3 in Chapter 8 on Reproductive Tract Infections.) Cervical and vaginal infections such as bacterial vaginosis can also affect fetal growth and risk for preterm delivery.[5,6]

Asymptomatic endometrial infection following vaginal, cervical, or pelvic infection may infect the amniotic sac after conception and cause preterm labor or preterm rupture of the membranes, resulting in preterm delivery.[5] Preterm delivery is the most important cause of infant mortality, cerebral palsy, and developmental problems. Appropriate antibiotic therapy given before or early in pregnancy might prevent conditions leading to preterm delivery. Unfortunately, studies of screening and treatment for asymptomatic bacterial vaginosis during pregnancy have not consistently demonstrated significant reduction in risk for preterm delivery,[7] and treatment given late in the pregnancy, or after the onset of premature labor or rupture of membranes, will usually not prevent preterm delivery due to infection.

Counseling for HIV infection should be a part of every preconception care evaluation. Be aware of the regulations in your state regarding HIV counseling and testing. Early identification of HIV infection is especially critical in relation to pregnancy. If the mother's positive HIV status is known, treatment with anti-retroviral drugs during pregnancy can reduce the risk of maternal-infant transmission by at least two thirds.[8,9] Because breast milk can also transmit the virus, advise HIV-infected women to avoid breastfeeding.

Women most at risk for an RTI are those who have had multiple sexual partners or a history of a prior RTI. Women under the age of 25 years have the highest incidence of sexually transmissible infections (STIs) and should be carefully screened.[10] Consistent, correct condom use is especially important for women who may be at risk for infection exposure during pregnancy, and for women with a partner who has known HSV or HIV infection. Viral suppression therapy for the infected male partner may also be considered to reduce the risk of transmission during pregnancy.[11,12]

IMMUNIZATIONS

Evaluate the patient's immunization status for diphtheria and tetanus, measles, mumps, rubella, varicella, hepatitis B, and polio. Bring her immunizations up to date before she becomes pregnant. Attenuated live viral immunizations such as measles, mumps, and rubella should not be administered to a pregnant woman. If a pregnant woman is inadvertently exposed to varicella vaccine, however, reassure her that that there have been no reports of birth defects related to the vaccine.[13,14]

Certain situations pose a special risk and call for other immunizations. Patients with pulmonary disease or other chronic problems would benefit from immunization against influenza and pneumococcus. Patients exposed to young children in day care centers, schools, or neonatal intensive care units could be at risk for rubella, cytomegalovirus, or herpes simplex. Patients exposed to cats may contract toxoplasmosis and should be tested and treated before becoming pregnant. Unfortunately, testing because of symptoms during pregnancy is of little or no value unless the woman has had previous negative test results or a low antibody titer, and a significant rise in titer can be documented.

PSYCHOSOCIAL AND LIFESTYLE BEHAVIORS

During pregnancy, some women feel motivated to adopt healthier behaviors. Others, however, find the natural stresses that occur during pregnancy make taking on new behaviors a more challenging undertaking. Therefore, the earlier before pregnancy a woman can practice a healthy lifestyle, the better.

Smoking. About one-fourth of women age 18 and older smoke.[15] Smoking during pregnancy increases bleeding during the pregnancy and the risk of spontaneous abortion. Mothers who smoke have infants with lower birthweights, more respiratory problems, and a higher incidence of hospital admissions compared with infants of mothers who do not smoke. They are also more likely to die of sudden infant death syndrome.

Alcohol and substance abuse. About 20% of pregnant women drink alcohol. Fetal alcohol syndrome, associated with heavy and binge drinking during pregnancy, results in mental retardation and malformations of the brain, face, and body. Because the spectrum of defects decreases as the amount of alcohol intake decreases, an effective intervention includes simply cutting back on consumption if the mother is unable to stop drinking entirely.[16]

Refer women who are pregnant and drug dependent for treatment. If appropriate, consider residential treatment. There is some evidence that residential treatment can significantly reduce drug use and rates for premature delivery, low birth weight, and infant deaths.[17]

Psychological problems. Refer patients for appropriate treatment if they suffer from depression, stress, anxiety, panic disorders, or other mental illness. Ask the patient about domestic violence, including verbal or psychological abuse. Domestic violence occurs during pregnancy and the immediate postpartum interval, affecting both the woman and her offspring.[18] Help the patient assess her own risk, arrange counseling and support, and make contingency plans to protect her safety.

Financial and social support. Pregnancy care is expensive, and without adequate insurance coverage, pregnancy and delivery can be financially devastating for a family, especially if the infant is premature or has a low birthweight. Review the patient's insurance coverage and provisions for maternity leave and childcare, and provide information about federal or state programs that may be able to offer help. Evaluate the patient's social and family networks and how supportive these are of a pregnancy. Encourage the patient to improve her relationships with family and friends.

NUTRITIONAL AND FITNESS STATUS

Record every patient's height, weight, and body mass index (BMI) to identify potential problems with obesity, poor weight gain, or eating disorders such as anorexia or bulimia. Ask about the patient's general nutritional patterns. A woman who is fasting or following an unusual diet or has pica needs counseling and education. Vegetarians will need dietary vigilance to assure they obtain adequate amounts of protein, calcium, and vitamins. Maintaining calcium balance during pregnancy demands a total daily intake of 1,500 mg. Although calcium supplementation had been suggested for prevention of eclampsia, as had the administration of aspirin, the potential promise of the initial smaller studies has not been confirmed in larger clinical trials.[19,20]

Folic acid deficiency is associated with an increased risk of neural tube defects (NTD).[21,22] Only half of all reproductive-aged women receive the recommended 400 mcg of folate from all sources.[23,24] Folic acid fortification of grain products became mandatory in 1998, and was expected to add 100 mcg of folic acid to the daily diet of the average person. To reach the recommended daily total, every woman contemplating pregnancy is also advised to take a daily folic acid supplement of at least 400 micrograms (mcg), and women at high risk for neural tube defects because of previous NTD-affected pregnancy or because they have spina bifida themselves, are advised to take 4,000 micrograms (mcg) daily before pregnancy and during the first trimester. Following fortification of the food supply and promulgation of recommendations for folic acid supplementation before and during pregnancy, the prevalence of NTDs decreased 20-30%.[23,24] Awareness among reproductive-age women also improved, but the proportion reporting that they took the recommended supplement in a 2002 March of Dimes survey was less than one third. Further education and prevention efforts are clearly needed.[24] Concerns have been raised about whether folic acid supplements might increase risks for spontaneous abortion. A study of 23,000 pregnancy outcomes in China, however, found no difference in the rates for spontaneous abortion for women who did and those who did not take folic acid supplements.[25]

Regular, moderate exercise is recommended for most pregnant women, including participation in sports other than scuba diving and those that involve high risk for falls or for abdominal trauma such as ice hockey, soccer, basketball, gymnastics, horseback riding, downhill skiing, and vigorous racquet sports. Exercise may be especially important for primary prevention of gestational diabetes for women who are obese. Women who should avoid aerobic exercise during pregnancy include those with significant heart or lung disease, incompetent cervix, multiple gestation, second- or third-trimester bleeding, placenta previa at 26 weeks or later, ruptured membranes, preeclampsia, or pregnancy-induced hypertension. Caution is also recommended for women with severe anemia, cardiac arrhythmia, chronic bronchitis, morbid obesity or underweight, poorly controlled type 1 diabetes, hypertension, seizure disorder, hyperthyroidism, intrauterine growth restriction in the current pregnancy, orthopedic limitation, history of extremely sedentary lifestyle, or heavy smoking. Exercise in supine position or motionless standing should also be avoided after the first trimester.[26]

MEDICAL CONDITIONS

Treat any underlying medical conditions. A healthy woman is more likely to have a healthy pregnancy. Evaluation will be needed if the patient has any serious, chronic condition including depression, heart disease, autoimmune disease, epilepsy, asthma, or renal disease.

Hypertension. Chronic hypertension is associated with intrauterine growth retardation, preeclampsia, and placental abruption, any of which may be life threatening to a fetus or newborn. Blood pressure should be controlled and the patient evaluated for end-organ damage of the cardiac, vascular, and renal systems. Review her antihypertensive medications, such as ACE inhibitors, which if continued can kill the fetus, and some diuretics, which can harm the fetus.

Diabetes. Congenital anomalies are more prevalent among offspring of insulin-dependent diabetic women. When blood sugar levels are controlled for 2 to 3 months before conception, the incidence of anomalies drops to levels found in the general population. Preconception care is especially important for diabetic women because cardiac and other anomalies occur during organogenesis in the first 7 to 8 weeks of pregnancy—the time many women first become aware they are pregnant.

Medication. Many medications can be detrimental to fetal development (Table 25-4). It is reasonable to avoid treatment with any medication that is not medically indicated. A woman who takes any drug for a significant chronic medical problem should consult with her clinician to determine whether the drug or dose needs to be altered during pregnancy. Category X drugs should be avoided for all women likely to become pregnant; category D drugs should also be avoided if at all possible; if continuing treatment is necessary for the woman's health, the lowest possible dose that is therapeutically effective should be used.[2]

Table 25-4 Common medications that may adversely affect fetal development

Isotretinoin (Accutane)	Diethylstilbestrol
Some antibiotics (including tetracycline, streptomycin, aminogylcosides, trimethoprim, triamterene)	Lindane (Kwell)
Some anticoagulants (dicumarol, warfarin)	Lithium
Some antiepileptics (including diphenylhydantoin, tridione, paramethadione, valproic acid, phenobarbital, primidone, phenytoin)	Meprobamate
Benzodiazepines (including Valium, Librium)	Podophyllin
Some cancer chemotherapeutics (including methotrexate, aminopterin)	Thalidomide
Chlorpropamide	Some thyroid drugs (propylthiouracil, iodide, methimazole)
Corticosteroids (including cream or ointment)	Tolbutamide

Note: Toxic effects depend on the drug, dose and timing of exposure. These drugs (as well as others) should be avoided during pregnancy unless treatment is medically necessary and no satisfactory alternative can be substituted.

Source: Adapted from Stewart et al. (1987).[27]

ENVIRONMENT AND WORK

Inquire about any hazards or exposure to teratogens, toxins, chemicals, or radiation at home or work. Also discuss work activities. If the woman's job requires prolonged standing or walking, or she has fatigue or stress, she should plan for careful follow-up throughout pregnancy to be certain that there is no indication of fetal growth retardation or symptoms of preterm labor.[28,29]

MALE PARTNER'S RISK FACTORS

Both men and women play critical roles in relation to pregnancy. Although studies of men's roles are limited, there is some evidence that paternal smoking, alcohol use, and illicit drug use may be associated with adverse pregnancy outcomes as well as impaired fertility and impaired sexual functioning.[2] The father's age is also a factor in the risk of congenital abnormalities. Men who become fathers after age 40 have a slightly higher risk of having offspring with autosomal abnormalities such as Marfan syndrome and achondroplasia, and there is some evidence that older paternal age is associated with an increased risk for Down syndrome independent of the mother's age.[2] Male exposure to toxic chemicals and drugs is associated with increased risk for infertility and pregnancy loss through spontaneous abortion.

PRENATAL CARE

One obvious advantage of preconception care is the opportunity to plan for and arrange prenatal care. Encourage the patient to schedule a pregnancy test and confirmation exam as early in pregnancy as possible, and to register early for prenatal care so she can take advantage of early prenatal testing and, if indicated, pregnancy ultrasound. Early care will also give her time to anticipate and complete chorionic villus sampling, amniocentesis, or other recommended tests. In addition, describe the symptoms and signs that may signal problems during early pregnancy: bleeding, spontaneous abortion, and ectopic pregnancy. (See Chapter 26 on Pregnancy Testing).

REFERENCES

1. ACOG. ACOG technical bulletin. Preconceptional care. Number 205—May 1995. American College of Obstetricians and Gynecologists. Int J Gynaecol Obstet 1995;50(2):201-207.
2. Cefalo R, Moos, M-K. Preconceptional health care: a practical guide. 2nd ed. St. Louis, MO: Mosby-Year Book, Inc.; 1995.
3. Zabin LS, Emerson MR, Ringers PA, Sedivy V. Adolescents with negative pregnancy test results. An accessible at-risk group. JAMA 1996;275(2):113-117.
4. ACOG. ACOG Practice Bulletin. Clinical Management Guidelines for Obstetrician-Gynecologists. Prenatal diagnosis of fetal chromosomal abnormalities: Am Coll Obstet Gyn, May 2001.
5. McGregor JA, French JI, Parker R, Draper D, Patterson E, Jones W, Thorsgard K, McFee J. Prevention of premature birth by screening and treatment for common genital tract infections: results of a prospective controlled evaluation [see comments]. Am J Obstet Gynecol 1995;173(1):157-167.
6. Koumans E, Kendrick J. Preventing adverse sequelae of bacterial vaginosis: a public health program and research agenda. Sex Transm Dis 2001;28(5):292-297.
7. Lamont RF, Duncan SL, Mandal D, Basset P. Intravaginal clindamycin to reduce preterm birth in women with abnormal genital tract flora. Obstet Gynecol Survey 2003;101(3):516-522.
8. CDC. Zidovudine for the prevention of HIV transmission from mother to infant. MMWR 1994;43(16):285-287.

9. Connor EM, Sperling RS, Gelber R, Kiselev P, Scott G, O'Sullivan MJ, VanDyke R, Bey M, Shearer W, Jacobsen RL. Reduction of maternal-infant transmission of human immunodeficiency virus type 1 with zidovudine treatment. Pediatric AIDS Clinical Trials Group Protocol 076 Study Group. N Engl J Med 1994;331(18): 1173-1180.

10. Cates W Jr, Holmes KK. Sexually transmitted diseases. Public health & preventive medicine. 14th ed. Stamford, CT: Appleton & Lange; 1998.

11. Barnabas RV, Carabin H, Garnett GP. The potential role of suppressive therapy for sex partners in the prevention of neonatal herpes: a health economic analysis. Sex Transm Infect 2002;78(6):425-429.

12. Casper C, Wald A. Condom use and the prevention of genital herpes acquisition. Herpes 2002;9(1):10-14.

13. Shields KE, Galil K, Seward J, Sharrar RG, Cordero JF, Slater E. Varicella vaccine exposure during pregnancy: data from the first 5 years of the pregnancy registry. Obstet Gynecol 2001;98(1):14-19.

14. CDC. General Recommendations on Immunization. Recommendations of the Advisory Committee on Immunization Practices (ACIP) and the American Academy of Family Physicians (AAFP). MMWR 2002;51(RR02;01):1-36.

15. CDC. State and territory-specific prevalence of current cigarette smoking among adults, 2001, and changes in prevalence of current and same day smoking, United States, 1996-2001. MMWR 2003;52(14):303-309.

16. Braun S. New experiments underscore warnings on maternal drinking. Science 1996;273(5276):738-739.

17. Anonymous. Benefits of residential substance abuse treatment for pregnant and parenting women. Bethesda, Md: Center for Substance Abuse Treatment, Department of Health and Human Services; 2001.

18. Gazmararian JA, Lazorick S, Spitz AM, Ballard TJ, Saltzman LE, Marks JS. Prevalence of violence against pregnant women [published erratum appears in JAMA 1997 Apr 9;277(14):1125]. JAMA 1996;275(24):1915-1920.

19. Levine RJ, Hauth JC, Curet LB, et al. Trial of calcium to prevent preeclampsia [see comments]. N Engl J Med 1997;337(2):69-76.

20. Roberts JM. Prevention or early treatment of preeclampsia. N Engl J Med 1997;337(2):124-125.

21. CDC. Recommendations for the use of folic acid to reduce the number of cases of spina bifida and other neural tube defects. MMWR 1992;41(RR-14):1-7.

22. Schwarz RH, Johnston RB, Jr. Folic acid supplementation—when and how. Obstet Gynecol 1996;88(5):886-887.

23. Honein MA, Paulozzi LJ, Mathews TJ, Erickson JD, Wong LY. Impact of folic acid fortification of the US food supply on the occurrence of neural tube defects. JAMA 2001;285(23):2981-2986.

24. Erickson JD. Folic acid and prevention of spina bifida and anencephaly. 10 years after the U.S. Public Health Service recommendation. MMWR Recomm Rep. Sep 13 2002;51(RR-13):1-3.

25. Gindler J, Li Z, Berry RJ, et al. Folic acid supplements during pregnancy and risk of miscarriage. Jiaxing City Collaborative Project on Neural Tube Defect Prevention. Lancet. 2001;358(9284):796-800.

26. ACOG Committee on Obstetric Practice. Committee opinion #267: exercise during pregnancy and the postpartum period. Obstet Gynecol 2002;99(1):171-173.

27. Stewart F, Guest F, Stewart G, Hatcher R. Understanding your body: the concerned woman's guide to gynecology and health. New York: Bantam Books, 1987.

28. Gabbe SG, Turner LP. Reproductive hazards of the American lifestyle: work during pregnancy [see comments]. Am J Obstet Gynecol 1997;176(4):826-832.

29. Luke B, Avni M, Min L, Misiunas R. Work and pregnancy: the role of fatigue and the "second shift" on antenatal morbidity. Am J Obstet Gynecol 1999;181(5 Pt 1):1172-1179.

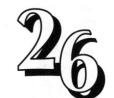

Pregnancy Testing and Management of Early Pregnancy

Felicia Stewart, MD

- Providing immediate scheduling for a pregnancy confirmation exam, as soon as the woman suspects she may be pregnant, is an essential family planning service.

- With early pregnancy diagnosis, a woman planning to continue her pregnancy can begin prenatal precautions and medical care during the early, most vulnerable stages of fetal development.

- A woman considering abortion will have time for adequate counseling and decision making. Abortion can be performed when it is safest—early in pregnancy. A woman considering medical abortion will be able to arrange for care within the first 9 weeks following her last normal menstrual period, when this option is possible.

- Early pregnancy diagnosis helps ensure that ectopic pregnancy can be detected early. Early detection reduces the risk of life-threatening ectopic pregnancy complications. Early diagnosis and treatment are more likely to preserve the affected fallopian tube.

Early pregnancy diagnosis is an essential part of every family planning program. Screening very early in pregnancy can avert serious complications and provide the pregnant woman with an opportunity to learn about precautions needed during pregnancy and prenatal care resources, or about options for abortion care. Early evaluation also provides an opportunity to screen for infection with the human immunodeficiency virus (HIV). Nonjudgmental, supportive counseling and information are also important, including accurate and specific referral options for abortion, adoption services, and prenatal care.

Inexpensive pregnancy test kits, sensitive enough to provide accurate results as early as 1 week after implantation, are widely available and simple to use. Thus, there is no reason to impose an arbitrary delay in pregnancy evaluation based on the date of the woman's last menstrual period. Clinical assessment and pregnancy testing should be offered as soon as the patient seeks these services. Prompt evaluation and referral are critical if the woman wishes to consider medical abortion (see Chapter 28 on Abortion), which is provided only during the very early weeks of pregnancy—the first 63 days following the woman's last normal menstrual period. Pregnancy is not likely to be suspected or confirmed before day 28, when the woman's next period is due. That means the interval for pregnancy confirmation and referral is short—only 35 days. Delay in scheduling a visit is obviously not wise.

PREGNANCY EVALUATION

Clinical evaluation for a woman who may be pregnant should include a review of pertinent history and symptoms, a laboratory test to detect human chorionic gonadotropin (hCG), and a pelvic exam. In most though not all cases, the last menstrual period date provides an accurate estimate of gestational age. A pelvic exam can confirm pregnancy test results and correlate uterine enlargement with menstrual dates. The pelvic exam may also be helpful in identifying the possibility of abnormal pregnancy. Pregnancy diagnosis has several goals:

1. Determine whether or not the woman is pregnant.

2. Identify possible problems that require further evaluation and/or emergency intervention, such as ectopic gestation or threatened abortion.

3. Assess gestation length accurately (in days or weeks).

4. Help the patient make and implement her own plans for prenatal care or abortion.

5. Screen for chlamydia and bacterial vaginosis and provide testing and treatment if indicated. Screening for gonorrhea is also indicated if the woman is at high risk because of high community prevalence or exposure to multiple partners. Screen even if the patient is considering abortion, because these infections are statistically associated with an increased risk of post-abortal infection. Whether or not treatment reduces risk is not clear, but annual chlamydia screening is recommended for all women less than 25 years of age and for those at risk for sexually transmitted infection; bacterial vaginosis testing requires only an office wet smear.

History and symptoms. The most common sign that prompts a woman to seek pregnancy evaluation is an overdue menstrual period. Often the woman herself suspects pregnancy or has reason to believe that she could be pregnant. A particularly useful question to ask is simply: Do you think you are pregnant now? An unusually light or mistimed period may mean fertilization actually occurred before the last menstrual period (LMP), and for this reason, the date of the previous menstrual period (PMP) should be determined. The date when pregnancy symptoms began can help corroborate fertilization date. Breast tenderness and nipple sensitivity typically begin 1 to 2 weeks after fertilization; fatigue, nausea, and urinary frequency at about 2 weeks. Bleeding, spotting, or lower abdominal pain may signal ectopic gestation or threatened spontaneous abortion. Note that women who have had a previous ectopic pregnancy may seek evaluation slightly earlier in pregnancy than do women experiencing a first ectopic pregnancy, so are less likely to have experienced abonormal bleeding or spotting that could indicate possible ectopic location with the current pregnancy.[1] However, an episode of light bleeding can occur in the early weeks of a normal, continuing pregnancy.

Physical examination. Cervical softening, blurring of the cervico-uterine angle, and uterine softening are early signs of pregnancy, appearing within the first 2 to 3 weeks after implantation. If the uterine size does not correspond to the estimated length of gestation based on last menstrual period, consider possible reasons for the discrepancy (Table 26-1). Ultrasound evaluation often is helpful in this situation.

Table 26-1 Possible reasons for discrepancy between uterine size and menstrual dates

Uterus Smaller Than Expected	Uterus Larger Than Expected
Fertilization later than dates suggest	Fertilization earlier than dates suggest
Ectopic pregnancy	Uterine leiomyomata (fibroids)
Incomplete or missed, spontaneous abortion	Twin gestation
Error in pregnancy test	Uterine anomaly
	Hydatidiform mole

PREGNANCY TEST BIOLOGY

Pregnancy tests detect hCG in a pregnant woman's urine or serum. Correctly interpreting pregnancy test results, however, is not entirely straightforward because:

1. hCG levels change drastically over the course of pregnancy (Figure 26-1).

2. Both positive and negative test results must be interpreted in relation to the sensitivity, specificity, and characteristics of the particular test being used and the clinical evaluation findings, including ultrasound examination when appropriate.

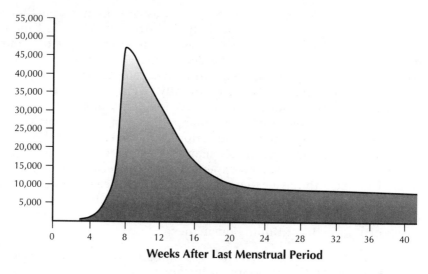

Source: Braunstein et al. (1976) with permission.

Figure 26-1 hCG levels during normal pregnancy

hCG LEVELS DURING PREGNANCY

When the blastocyst implants in the endometrium, the proliferation of trophoblastic cells initiates placental development and rapidly increasing hCG production. hCG can be detected in the woman's serum at low levels as early as 7 to 9 days after ovulation, very soon after implantation occurs. During the first 3 weeks after implantation (the first six weeks dated from the woman's last normal menses), the hCG level in normal pregnancy doubles approximately every 1-1/2 to 2 days so that the serum level reaches 50 to 250 mIU/ml by the time of the first missed menstrual period (Figure 26-2). hCG reaches a peak approximately 60 to 70 days after fertilization and then decreases.

In abnormal pregnancies, hCG levels often increase abnormally. Elevated levels are normal with a multiple gestation, reflecting the increased placental mass. Extremely high hCG production, with hCG levels as high as a million mIU/ml, can occur with molar pregnancy (hydatidiform mole or gestational trophoblastic disease). Such very high levels can be documented with a quantitative serum hCG test. Abnormally low hCG levels often occur before a spontaneous abortion or with an ectopic pregnancy. On the other hand, low levels may simply indicate that a normal pregnancy is earlier in gestation than menstrual dates suggest. For example, if ovulation had been delayed slightly in the preceding cycle, fertilization could have actually occurred on cycle day 21 or later. Ovulation occurring later than expected is not unusual, especially if the woman discontinued oral contraceptives in the previous menstrual cycle.

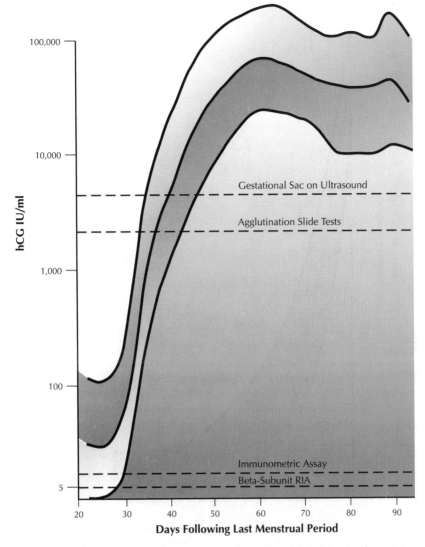

Source: Braunstein et al. (1978) with permission.

Figure 26-2 hCG levels in early pregnancy

hCG LEVELS AFTER PREGNANCY

After a pregnancy is terminated by delivery or abortion, blood and urine hCG levels gradually decrease (Figure 26-3). The initial decrease is quite rapid, so that an hCG level after 2 weeks should be less than 1% of the level at the time the pregnancy is terminated.[2] Following full-term delivery, the level will have dropped to less than 50 mIU within 2

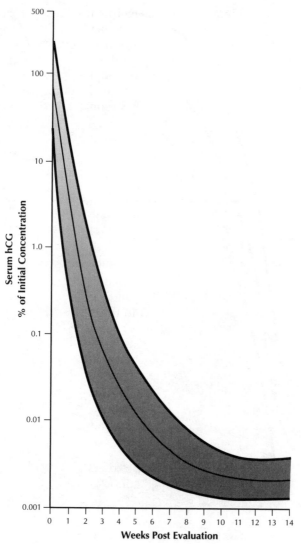

Source: Braunstein (1983) with permission.

Figure 26-3 hCG disappearance after pregnancy

weeks, and hCG will be undetectable after 3 to 4 weeks. In the case of first-trimester abortion, however, initial hCG levels may be much higher. If the abortion occurs at 8 to 10 weeks of gestation when hCG may be as high as 150,000 mIU, then 2 weeks after abortion the hCG levels may still be 1,500 mIU, high enough that all pregnancy tests will still be positive. hCG is likely to be detectable by sensitive tests, including commonly-used office urine test kits, for as long as 60 days after first-trimester abortion.[3] If continuing intrauterine pregnancy, retained placenta fragments, or ectopic pregnancy are possibilities, consider obtaining serial quantitative hCG levels to track an upward or downward trend. If hCG is clearing normally from the bloodstream, the hCG level should decline steadily with a half-time of disappearance of no more than 24 to 48 hours. A more prolonged plateau level or slower decline may occur as an ectopic or abnormal pregnancy spontaneously resolves.

HORMONE STRUCTURE AND PREGNANCY TEST DESIGN

hCG is closely related in molecular structure to the pituitary hormones LH (luteinizing hormone), FSH (follicle stimulating hormone), and TSH (thyroid stimulating hormone). Each is composed of two subunits: an alpha and a beta subunit. The alpha subunits of LH, FSH, TSH, and hCG are virtually identical. Therefore, only a test that selectively identifies the beta subunit of hCG or its unique molecular conformation is specific for hCG.

Two-site, immunometric kits commonly used for office or home tests are specific for hCG, and so is the beta subunit radioimmunoassay used for quantitative serum hCG determination in the laboratory. Most agglutination inhibition slide tests, however, detect whole hCG rather than the beta subunit and therefore show at least some cross-reactivity with other hormones, especially LH. Because they are so inexpensive and simple to use, slide tests nevertheless may be an appropriate option in certain circumstances. Other, older test methods including tube tests and radioreceptor assays are no longer needed.

PREGNANCY TEST OPTIONS

Pregnancy testing has been revolutionized with the development of monoclonal antibody techniques. Many monoclonal test kits, as well as old agglutination slide tests, are available so that the array of options is extensive. Test kits suitable for use in the family planning clinic or clinician's office are shown in Table 26-2.

OFFICE AND HOME URINE IMMUNOMETRIC TESTS

Immunometric tests exploit technology that has made possible the inexpensive production of pure antibody in large quantities. Immunometric tests for pregnancy are based on the ELISA (enzyme-linked immunosorbent assay) assay design; they are sometimes called "two-site" or sandwich tests and require two different antibodies. One antibody captures the beta subunit of hCG; the other antibody is conjugated to an enzyme that provides a color change. Because immunometric tests are specific for the beta subunit of hCG, cross-reaction with other hormones is not a problem. Some test kits, which may also be suitable for clinic use, are available without prescription for home use.

Table 26-2 Commonly used clinic and office pregnancy tests

Immunometric Tests: Specific for beta hCG, no LH, FSH, or TSH cross-reaction. Reliably detect pregnancy 7 to 10 days after fertilization, approximately one week before the next period is due. Cost $0.68 to $4.25**

Name (Manufacturer)	Sensitivity (mlU/ml)*	Time Required	# Steps/ Specimen
Acceava hCG (ThermoBioStar)	25	5 Min	1 Step/Urine***
Acceava hCG Combo (ThermoBioStar)	10	4–7 Min	1 Step/Urine or Serum***
Assure hCG (Conception Technologies)	20	1–5 Min	1-Step/Urine
CARDS QS+ hCG (Quidel)	10 in serum 20 in urine	3–5 Min	1 Step/Urine or Serum***
Clearview Easy HCG, Prevue HCG Stick or Cassette, (Wampole)	25	3–4 Min	1 Step/Urine or Serum***
Clearview hCG II	25	3 Min	1-Step/Urine
Confirm hCG One Step Urine (Mainline Technology)	25	3–5 Min	1 Step/Urine
Double-Check (Bio-Medical Products)	25	2–5 Min	1 Step/Urine
EX hCG Pregancy Test (Biomerica)		5 Min	1-Step/Urine
Fortel Ultra (Biomerica)	10	1–5 Min	1 Step/Urine
Icon 25 hCG	25	3 Min urine 5 Min serum	1 Step/Urine or Serum***
Icon II HCG (Beckman Coulter)	20 urine 10 serum	3 Min urine 5 Min serum	1 Step/Urine or Serum***
Immuno/hCG Detector, Stix & Cassette (Immunostics)	20	3–5 Min	1-Step/Urine
One Step dBest Strip and Cassette (Ameritek)	20 10	3 Min 3–5 Min	1 Step/Urine 1 Step/Urine
One-Step Urine Dip Stick Pregnancy Test (Biotron)	20	2 Min	1 Step/Urine
OSOM hCG Strip or Cassette (Wyntek)	25	1 Min	1 Step/Urine
ProPhase Plus (Arlington Scientific)	25	4–30 Min	1 Step /Urine
ProStrip HCG, ProPhase Combo S/U (Arlington Scientific)	25	4 Min	1 Step/Urine or Serum***
QuickCard hCG, Quick Card hCG Combo (Med Gyn)	25	5 Min	1 Step/Urine or Serum***
QuickCard Pro, QuickStick Pro, Quick Check PLUS, Quickstream (IPAS)	25	5 Min	1 Step/Urine or Serum***
Quick Vue One Step hCG (Quidel)	25	3–5 Min	1-Step/Urine
Quick Vue Semi-Q hCG Combo (Quidel)	25	3–5 Min	1-Step/Urine

(continued)

Table 26-2 Commonly used clinic and office pregnancy tests—*(cont'd)*

Name (Manufacturer)	Sensitivity (mIU/ml)*	Time Required	# Steps/ Specimen
Rapid Vue hCG (Quidel)	25	3 Min	1-Step/Urine
SAS Pregnancy Strip, SAS One-Step, SAS Ultra HCG Kit (S.A. Scientific)	25, 20 urine 10 serum	4 Min, 4 Min 7 Min	2 Step/Urine or Serum***
Status HCG (Wampole)	15	3–10 Min	1-Step/Urine or Serum
SureStep HCG, SureStep HCG Combo (Conception Technologies)	20	1–5 Min	1 Step/Urine, 1 Step Urine or Serum
Yes/No Pregnancy Test (Bantex)	25	2 Min	1 Step/Urine
dBest hCG Test Strip and Cassette (Ameritek)	2,000	5 Min	1 Step/Urine

Agglutination Inhibition Slide Tests: Immunocept-d Polyclonal and UCG-Slide use antibody that reacts to whole hCG, not specific for beta hCG; cross-reaction with LH, FSH, and TSH is possible. All require urine specimen, and all are CLIA moderate complexity. Cost $1.26–$3.50**

Name (Manufacturer)	Sensitivity (mIU/ml)*	Time Required	# Steps/ Specimen
Immuno/cept-direct Monoclonal (Immunostics Inc)	200	2 Min	Urine
Immuno/cept-d Monoclonal (Immunostics Inc)	500	2 Min	Urine
Immuno/cept-d Polyclonal (Immunostics Inc)	1,000	2 Min	Urine
UCG-Slide (Wampole)	2,000	2 Min	Urine
UCG-Beta Slide Monoclonal II (Wampole)	500	2 Min	Urine
Immuno/pregnacol (Immunostics Inc)	200		Urine

Source: Manufacturers' product literature (2002, 2003, 2004).

* Sensitivity specified as the lower limit of reliable hCG detection in product literature. Test results may be positive at lower hCG levels in some cases.

** Bulk or nonprofit agency discount purchase may reduce costs significantly.

*** Urine tests are CLIA waived; serum tests and latex inhibition tests are moderate complexity.

Specificity and sensitivity. Immunometric tests provide accurate qualitative (yes/no) results with hCG levels as low as 5 to 50 mIU/ml, depending on the specific test kit. With a urine test kit with a sensitivity of 25 mIU/ml, results are positive for some women as early as 3 to 4 days after implantation (10 days after fertilization); test results are positive for 98% of women within 7 days after implantation.[4]

For both office and home immunometric tests, the expected accuracy of detection is based on extrapolating a "next menses due date" from the timing of the first day of the woman's last normal menstrual period. Predicting accurately when a menstrual period *should* be due is not a simple task. Women's cycle lengths vary from month to month as well as from individual to individual. If ovulation is delayed for some reason, a test on the day the woman thought her period was due could easily be "falsely" negative because the cycle events—implantation, and subsequent rising production of hCG—are all a week or two behind schedule.[5] In this situation, a test repeated a week or two later will be positive. A study of hCG levels during the first few weeks of pregnancy found that as many as 10% of pregnancies might be missed with a test done on cycle day 28.[6] One researcher also found that sensitivity and accuracy varied for different test kit brands.[45]

Uses. Immunometric tests can be used to confirm pregnancy, or to "rule out" the diagnosis of pregnancy. These tests are appropriate for screening prior to procedures such as biopsy or x-ray, or prior to prescribing a drug that would be contraindicated during pregnancy. They are also appropriate in screening for possible ectopic pregnancy. Only 1% of patients with ectopic pregnancy would be missed (falsely negative) with a urine test sensitivity of 50 mIU/ml.[2] Immunometric urine tests are CLIA waived.

QUANTITATIVE BETA hCG RADIOIMMUNOASSAY (RIA) OR IMMUNOMETRIC ASSAY

Use of a quantitative hCG RIA or immunometric "blood test" as a qualitative (yes/no) pregnancy test does not have any advantage over immunometric urine tests. Immunometric urine kits are equally specific for hCG and provide sensitivity that is completely satisfactory for clinical evaluation, with immediate results, and at much lower cost.

Specificity and sensitivity. Radioimmunoassay (RIA) or two-site immunometric assays provide accurate quantitative results with hCG levels as low as 5 mIU/ml; they can detect pregnancy reliably as soon as implantation occurs, about 7 days after fertilization. Tests are usually performed in batches because of expense; test processing requires 1 to 2 hours.

Uses. Serum hCG tests can provide a quantitative result; serial test specimens can be used to check doubling time or disappearance time when ectopic pregnancy, impending spontaneous abortion, or possible retained placental fragments are being evaluated. Very high levels can be documented to confirm the diagnosis of molar pregnancy. Be sure to specify quantitative beta hCG when ordering this test. Also, serial tests should all be ordered from the same laboratory to avoid possible confusion about assay standardization differences between laboratories.

AGGLUTINATION INHIBITION SLIDE TESTS

Inexpensive agglutination inhibition slide tests, widely used for the last 20 years, depend on binding of hCG in the patient's urine with an anti-hCG antibody in the test solution. Binding of the test antibody prevents clumping (agglutination) of latex particles in the test solution.

Specificity. Because antibodies used in most slide tests are not specific for the beta subunit of hCG, cross-reactions are possible. To minimize problems of cross-reaction with LH, FSH, or TSH, slide-test sensitivity is set so that high levels of hCG are required to give a positive test result. A cross-reaction, therefore, is unlikely to be a source of clinical confusion. However, a test specimen obtained during the brief surge of LH just before ovulation or during the perimenopausal years may cause false positive results in a slide pregnancy test because of LH cross-reaction. Cross-reactivity with TSH is unlikely because its level is normally quite low.

Uses. Slide tests are inexpensive, easy to perform, and appropriate for confirming pregnancy at and after the sixth week of gestation. hCG levels early in pregnancy (the first month after implantation) may be below the level detected by latex agglutination slide pregnancy tests. (In rare cases, the hCG level later in pregnancy (after 16 to 20 weeks) may also decline below the sensitivity for these tests.) Slide agglutination tests are not appropriate to "rule out" pregnancy because early pregnancy, ectopic pregnancy, and impending spontaneous abortion may be missed. If the initial agglutination test is negative, a more sensitive test should be used (see Immunometric Tests), or the test should be repeated a few days later. Agglutination tests also can be used to help document disappearance of hCG after induced aspiration or medical abortion. Although inexpensive and simple to use, slide tests are classified "moderate" complexity by CLIA, so billing and reimbursement for slide tests is not permitted unless the provider is CLIA certified.

HOME PREGNANCY TESTING

Home pregnancy test kits offer the advantages of privacy, anonymity, and convenience. Moreover, they are popular. In a national survey, approximately 33% of pregnant women reported using them.[7] In another survey, 17% of college women reported that they had used a home test at least once. Most women chose home testing because results can be obtained quickly and confidentially.[8] Because home pregnancy tests are easily accessible, a woman may identify pregnancy early and thus be more able to be an active manager of her own health care.

Accuracy. Unfortunately, the accuracy of home tests in actual use may not be ideal. In one study of three commonly used home kits,[9] the predictive value was only 84% for positive home test results and 62% for negative results. Another researcher found that when test kits were used by non-technical personnel, results did not agree with standard laboratory test results in approximately 10% of 200 samples tested.[10] Test accuracy can be affected by the techniques and experience of the user, and by the user's ability to follow the test instructions precisely.[11] The most common error with home pregnancy tests is a negative result that occurs because the test was performed too early in pregnancy. An incorrect result could mislead a woman, causing her to delay in getting a clinical evaluation.

Uses. If a home test result is positive, clinical evaluation is needed to confirm the pregnancy, determine the length of gestation, and identify any possible risk for ectopic or abnormal pregnancy. If the home test result is negative, clinical evaluation also may be needed to determine the cause of menstrual delay or of the other symptoms that have prompted the test, especially if the woman does not resume normal menses soon. In either case, a second pregnancy test is likely to be indicated, so that the cost of the home kit may be an unnecessary expense. On the other hand, positive results may prompt a woman to seek pregnancy confirmation earlier than she otherwise might, and also to change her lifestyle earlier than were she to wait for a clinical evaluation.

AVOIDING PREGNANCY TEST INTERPRETATION ERRORS

If pregnancy test results do not agree with other clinical signs, consider the possible reasons for the discrepancy. Plan appropriate follow-up or further evaluation to protect the patient against possible consequences of an incorrect test result:

1. Any test result can be wrong. Laboratory errors do occur, including specimen mix-up and incorrectly performed test procedures. For accurate results, instructions for the kit must be followed meticulously and timed with a stopwatch. Use control solutions to verify accuracy. Observe test-kit expiration dates.

2. Know exactly what kind of pregnancy test was performed, and what sensitivity the test has. Without this information, it is not possible to assess the clinical significance of a negative result or to evaluate the possibility of a false positive result.

3. Send all serial specimens for quantitative beta hCG assays to the same laboratory. Results of quantitative immunoassay performed by different laboratories may not be comparable because of differences between immunoassay kits and standards used by different manufacturers. Some laboratories record hCG levels in metric units; these can be roughly converted to mIU by multiplying the metric results by 5.2 (10 ng/ml = 52 mIU at the Second International Standard for hCG). Results should be multiplied by 2 for comparison to the First International Standard Preparation for hCG, which is identical to the Third International Standard. Know what standard your laboratory uses.

4. Do not base clinical management on the results of a home pregnancy test. Although home kits have excellent theoretical accuracy, their use even by trained personnel may not reliably provide the

sensitivity or specificity needed for optimal clinical management.[9,10,12] Be careful about accepting the results of a pregnancy test performed in another facility, especially if critical clinical situations such as ectopic pregnancy are possible.

5. False negative results are common with agglutination inhibition tests. False negative results frequently occur because the test is performed too early or too late in pregnancy. Abnormal pregnancy, urine that is too dilute, and medication that interferes with test result may all be responsible. Use an immunometric test (Table 26-1) to "rule out" pregnancy.

6. False negative results are rare with immunometric tests but can occur if test procedures are performed incorrectly (such as excessive rinsing) or if the test reader has red-green color blindness.[13] An immunometric test also may be negative if the test is performed too early in the cycle, before implantation occurs. In this situation, the result is a "true" negative, which could be misleading if not repeated a few days later. Elevated lipids, high immunoglobulin levels, and low serum protein associated with severe kidney disease also can interfere with a test assay. If a false negative result is suspected, order a quantitative beta subunit radioimmunoassay.

7. False positive pregnancy test results are not common, but they can cause perplexing dilemmas:
   - False positive results with an immunometric test are very rare, but laboratory error is always possible. An "accurate" false positive result could occur if the woman has had treatment involving hCG injection within the preceding 14 days, and faint false positive results have been reported with urine sample contaminated by blood or recent use of Chinese herbal medication.[14] If a false positive result is suspected, obtain a quantitative beta subunit radioimmunoassay. To rule out a false positive serum hCG test, test the urine for hCG. If the urine is positive, the serum test is not falsely positive.
   - If an agglutination inhibition slide test is positive, but the uterus is not enlarged, perform a confirmatory immunometric test. The positive result could be caused by LH cross-reaction, in which case the immunometric test will be negative because it is specific for beta hCG.
   - Agglutination slide tests also can yield false positive results because of protein or blood in the urine specimen. Consider obtaining a confirmatory immunometric test if the urine specimen shows 1+ proteinuria or more. An immunometric test is likely to give an accurate (negative) result. When a positive pregnancy test is not confirmed by the presence of a pregnancy in the uterus, do not assume the test result is false. Seriously consider the possibility of an ectopic pregnancy.

8. In very rare cases, pregnancy test results are positive even though the patient is not pregnant because hCG actually is present, originating from a source other than pregnancy. hCG levels persist after a recent pregnancy or after hCG treatment. Low levels of hCG (5mIU to 30 mIU) may be associated with tumors of the pancreas, ovaries, breast, and many other sites.[15] Some normal postmenopausal women also have low levels of circulating hCG-like substance, of pituitary origin.[2]

9. For follow-up after molar pregnancy or choriocarcinoma, use immunometric quantitative hCG tests. The hCG protein produced by tumor cells may be abnormal and in some cases may be missed by other test methods. If persistent hCG levels are found, the condition must be managed by an expert, and hCG levels in both blood and urine should be checked, because false-positive blood results are possible.[16,17]

MANAGING PROBLEMS IN EARLY PREGNANCY

Consider the possibility of spontaneous abortion or ectopic pregnancy whenever a woman in the reproductive years has symptoms such as abdominal pain, abnormal bleeding, or irregular or missed menstrual periods. The patient's history, as well as her own assessment of pregnancy risk, may be helpful. For example, in a study of women undergoing evaluation at a hospital emergency department, 63% of the women who thought they might be pregnant, were pregnant. A sensitive pregnancy test, however, is a prudent precaution to take, no matter what the woman's history indicates. In the previously cited study, 10% of women who reported a normal last menstrual period, and stated that there was no chance they could be pregnant, were nevertheless found to be pregnant.[18]

No matter what the cause or diagnosis, Rh screening is a standard recommendation for any woman with bleeding in pregnancy. The risk of Rh sensitization resulting from bleeding in early pregnancy is low, and during the early days of development before fetal blood cells are present, the risk should be negligible or absent. The available research to document risk, however, is limited and is based primarily on studies to detect the presence of fetal cells in maternal blood detected by Kleihauer-Betke (KB) test rather than later development of maternal Rh(D) antibodies. Positive KB test results have been reported for non-bleeding women both before and after abortion with gestation as early as 5-6 weeks.[19] Because the risks associated with Rh testing and treatment are low, this approach has been widely accepted as a wise precaution in the U.S. even though the risk of sensitization is also low. Although Rh prophylaxis is recommended in the UK following first trimester induced abortion or diagnosis of ectopic gestation, it is no longer recommended at the time of complete spontaneous miscarriage during the first 12 weeks of pregnancy unless the bleeding is heavy, recurrent or associated with abdominal pain.[20] A blood count also is indicated at the time of initial evaluation. The results may help assess the cumulative extent of bleeding and may provide an important baseline for later comparison if internal hemorrhage is suspected.

Abnormal bleeding, cramping, and abdominal pain can occur with threatened abortion, complete or incomplete spontaneous abortion, and ectopic pregnancy. However, these symptoms also can occur in an early pregnancy that subsequently progresses to a normal outcome. When these symptoms occur, perform an evaluation immediately: exclude the presence of ectopic pregnancy and arrange appropriate care for possible spontaneous abortion.

POSSIBLE ECTOPIC PREGNANCY

A woman who has clinical evidence of possible ruptured ectopic pregnancy, such as hypotension and/or postural hypotension, severe abdominal pain, guarding, or rebound tenderness requires immediate referral for emergency management where surgery is available if needed. An immunometric urine pregnancy test is almost certain to be positive (false negative rate is less than 1%)[2] but agglutination inhibition tests are not sensitive enough to detect the lower hCG levels associated with ectopic gestation in about 50% of cases.[21] Because intervention should not be delayed, further nonsurgical evaluation is not prudent.

More commonly, the clinician considers the possibility of ectopic pregnancy because the woman has less serious and nonspecific symptoms such as bleeding in early pregnancy, uterine enlargement that does not correlate with dates (uterus is too small), or early vacuum abortion that has failed to recover identifiable placental tissue from the uterine cavity. Often the patient is completely asymptomatic. These situations allow time for further outpatient evaluation if the patient is willing and able to monitor her own symptoms carefully. While evaluation is pending, the patient must be warned to watch for ectopic pregnancy danger signs (Table 26-3) and to return immediately for emergency care if danger signs occur. Further steps in evaluation might include the following:

1. **Quantitative beta hCG assay.** Although test results probably will not be available until the next day, an initial level can be compared with the beta hCG level 2 days (48 hours) later if diagnosis is still uncertain. A decline of 50% to 60% or more favors the diagnosis of normal hCG disappearance after spontaneous or induced abortion, or after spontaneous resolution of an ectopic pregnancy.[22] A level of 1,000 mIU or less provides some reassurance about the safety of outpatient management, because life-threatening intra-abdominal hemorrhage is rare with ectopic pregnancy at such an early stage of pregnancy; hemorrhage risk, however, may also depend on the ectopic location involved.[23] As many as 10% of women with a ruptured ectopic pregnancy may have a serum hCG

Table 26-3 Early pregnancy danger signs

Possible Ectopic Pregnancy
Sudden intense pain, or persistent pain, or cramping in the lower abdomen, usually localized to one side or the other
Irregular bleeding or spotting with abdominal pain when period is late or after an abnormally light period
Fainting or dizziness persisting more than a few seconds. These may be signs of internal bleeding. (Internal bleeding is not necessarily associated with vaginal bleeding.)

Possible Miscarriage
Late last period and bleeding is now heavy, possibly with clots or clumps of tissue; cramping more severe than usual
Period is prolonged and heavy—5 to 7 days of "heaviest" days
Abdominal pain or fever

Contact your clinician immediately or go to a hospital emergency room if you develop any of these signs.

Source: Stewart et al. (1987).

level less than 100 mIU/ml[24] and clinically significant internal bleeding has been reported even at levels below the 25 mIU/ml sensitivity of immunometric tests.

2. **Pathology phone report.** If an abortion has been performed, request a microscopic tissue evaluation and a report by phone. The pathologist may be able to identify placental villi and confirm intrauterine pregnancy, in which case the likelihood of simultaneous ectopic pregnancy is extremely remote.

3. **Vacuum aspiration.** If the patient does not want to continue the pregnancy, vacuum aspiration can ascertain whether pregnancy tissue is present in the uterus. Placental villi identified in the specimen evacuated can rule out an ectopic pregnancy.[25]

4. **Ultrasound evaluation.** Pelvic ultrasound should be able to detect a fetal pole with cardiac activity inside the uterus by the 7th to 8th week of gestation dated from last menstrual period. The use of vaginal probe ultrasound moves this threshold forward by 7 to 10 days. With a vaginal probe, it is possible in some cases to detect a tiny gestational sac of 1 mm to 3 mm in size in the uterus as early as 30 days after ovulation, when hCG is 900 mIU/ml or less.[26] With good abdominal ultrasound equipment and technique, a gestational sac should definitely be detected when the beta hCG is 1,800 mIU (by 5 to 6 weeks of gestation). A vaginal probe should detect a gestational sac when hCG is 1,000 mIU (by 4½ to 5 weeks of gestation).[27] A distinct yolk sac provides definitive confirmation of intrauterine pregnancy and should

be visible with vaginal probe ultrasound at about 5½ weeks of gestation.[28]

Unfortunately, a sac-like ultrasound appearance, called a "pseudogestational sac," can occur in conjunction with ectopic pregnancy in as many as 10% of cases.[29] The other ultrasound signs of possible ectopic pregnancy, such as poorly defined adnexal mass and cul de sac fluid, are not specific enough for conclusive diagnosis. However, the diagnosis of ectopic pregnancy can be made conclusively if a gestational sac and fetal heartbeat are detected outside of the uterine cavity. The differential diagnosis usually includes intrauterine gestation earlier than menstrual dates would suggest, complete or incomplete spontaneous abortion, or pregnancy with a corpus luteum cyst. Unless intrauterine gestation can be identified with certainty or an extrauterine gestation is visible, ultrasound results do not provide a definite diagnosis.

If after completing these three diagnostic steps ectopic pregnancy cannot be excluded, arrange for additional evaluation. Refer immediately if the patient becomes symptomatic during the process of evaluation. Laparoscopy may be needed to ascertain the diagnosis.

In some cases, close observation alone may be an option: when beta hCG is low and declining, the patient remains asymptomatic, and the size of the ectopic pregnancy is small. Spontaneous resolution of an ectopic pregnancy by resorption occurs in as many as 70% to 80% of such cases.[23,30] In this situation, the beta hCG will decline slowly to zero. Fertility after expectant management was found to be similar in one study of 180 women seeking subsequent pregnancy.[31] Alternatively, some centers treat asymptomatic, early ectopic pregnancy with methotrexate,[32,33] to induce dissolution of trophoblast tissue. Success rates reported with a single or multiple dose treatment with methotrexate, 50 mg per square meter of body-surface area, range from 85% to 95%.[33-35] If gestation is early, it also may be possible to evacuate the pregnancy through an incision in the fallopian tube wall during laparoscopic or abdominal surgery; this approach has been recommended for the patient who would like to preserve her future fertility.[21] Unlike salpingectomy or salpingo-oophorectomy, salpingostomy does conserve the fallopian tube involved. Future fertility, however, may not be better if the contralateral tube is normal, and there is a 5% to 8% risk that the ectopic pregnancy will persist following this conservative surgery.[36]

Early diagnosis is very important in ectopic pregnancy. Although early diagnosis and intervention have helped to reduce ectopic pregnancy mortality,[37] ectopic pregnancy is the leading cause of pregnancy-related death during the first trimester, and the incidence is significant—approximately 2% of all pregnancies in 1992.[38] Also, early diagnosis allows more time for conservative management, which may help to preserve the woman's future fertility.

POSSIBLE SPONTANEOUS ABORTION

Approximately 15% of confirmed, early pregnancies end in spontaneous abortion; the proportion is even higher if pregnancy losses are counted during the first 2 weeks of gestation, before the menstrual period is overdue and pregnancy is likely to be recognized. Missed abortion is also fairly common, but is unlikely to cause symptoms that would prompt the woman to seek care. Often the diagnosis is not suspected until prenatal exams reveal that uterine enlargement is not keeping pace with pregnancy dates, or an ultrasound evaluation fails to detect an expected fetal pole or cardiac activity at an appropriate time.

In some cases the diagnosis of spontaneous abortion may be made on the basis of a pelvic examination. If the cervix is dilated and products of conception are visible in the cervix or vagina, then abortion is inevitable. An ultrasound evaluation may help determine whether the uterine cavity is already empty. In other cases, the diagnosis is suspected on the basis of abnormal bleeding or ultrasound findings. Once the possibility of ectopic pregnancy is excluded, if the woman's bleeding is not heavy, then uterine evacuation may not be necessary. One study of "expectant management" found that most women with a diagnosis of incomplete spontaneous abortion preferred this option to surgical evacuation, and that 81% had a successful outcome without surgical intervention.[39]

If bleeding and cramping are severe, vacuum aspiration can empty the uterus; aspiration is indicated if bleeding is so heavy that it is life-threatening. This is a situation where use of manual vacuum aspiration equipment in the office or emergency room may offer a simple and effective approach, with local paracervical block to provide appropriate pain relief. Alternatively, treatment with misoprostol could also be considered.[40-42] (See Chapter 28 on Abortion.)

If the pregnancy is wanted and the condition is not life-threatening, then intervention can be delayed while further evaluation is undertaken to determine whether the pregnancy may be viable. Serial quantitative beta hCG levels and an ultrasound evaluation are likely to document the diagnosis (see section on Possible Ectopic Pregnancy). When the pregnancy is desired, take time for a careful and thorough evaluation. Intervention on the basis of an initial exam or ultrasound will seem abrupt and shocking as the woman first begins to acknowledge the possibility of her loss and grief.

COUNSELING OBJECTIVES WITH PREGNANCY DIAGNOSIS

The issues surrounding personal fertility are complex, and a pregnancy diagnosis visit should provide the client an opportunity to clarify and articulate her feelings. Before beginning the physical exam and testing, find out what the woman hopes her result will be. When presenting the test results, elicit the client's reaction and allow time for her to express her feelings. Assess the woman's support system. Provide referrals if the patient feels counseling would be helpful. This is especially important if her own support system is not adequate. Emphasize that no decision based on the test results need be made that day. Encourage the woman to talk with her partner, family, or friends. Outline all the options available.

- If the client is pregnant and plans to continue her pregnancy, review precautions for optimal pregnancy (see Chapter 25 on Preconception Care) and be certain she has an appropriate resource for prenatal care. Remind her about danger signs of possible problems in pregnancy (Table 26-3).

- If the client plans to continue her pregnancy, but does not want to parent the child, refer her to a resource that can help with adoption.

- If the client is pregnant but does not plan to continue her pregnancy, refer her for abortion services. In this case, the sooner the decision is made and acted upon, the safer the procedure will be.

- If the client is not pregnant and wishes she were, counsel her about her own fertility. (See Chapter 27 on Impaired Fertility.) If appropriate, refer her for fertility evaluation and help. Remind her about precautions for optimal pregnancy and about taking a daily vitamin that includes folic acid 0.4 mg before and during pregnancy.[43,44] (See Chapter 25 on Preconception Care.)

- If the client is not pregnant, plans to continue being sexually active, and is happy with the negative test result, then birth control counseling is appropriate. A pregnancy scare can be a good bridge from risk-taking to effective, ongoing contraceptive use.

- If the client is not clear how she feels about the test result, positive or negative, consider referral for counseling. Appropriate pregnancy counseling services are likely to be available through a local abortion facility. Be sure that pregnancy counseling referral resources you recommend have been carefully evaluated. Anti-abortion groups advertise pregnancy counseling services in some communities; these agencies do not provide the nonjudgmental environment that your clients are entitled to have in making a personal decision about pregnancy. A woman who is not pregnant, but who has ambivalent feelings about pregnancy, may want to consider working with a mental health professional to clarify her feelings.

REFERENCES

1. Spandorfer SD, Barnhart KT. Role of previous ectopic pregnancy in altering the presentation of suspected ectopic pregnancy. J Reprod Med. Mar 2003;48(3):133-136.
2. Braunstein G. hCG testing: a clinical guide for the stesting of human chrionic gonadotropin. Abbott Park, IL: Abbott Diagnostics; 1992.

3. Marrs RP, Kletzky OA, Howard WF, Mishell DR, Jr. Disappearance of human chorionic gonadotropin and resumption of ovulation following abortion. Am J Obstet Gynecol 1979;135(6):731-736.
4. Chard T. Pregnancy tests: a review. Hum Reprod 1992;7(5):701-710.
5. Wilcox AJ, Baird DD, Dunson D, McChesney R, Weinberg CR. Natural limits of pregnancy testing in relation to the expected menstrual period. JAMA 2001; 286(14):1759-1761.
6. Wilcox AJ, Dunson DB, Weinberg CR, Trussell J, Baird DD. Likelihood of conception with a single act of intercourse: providing benchmark rates for assessment of post-coital contraceptives. Contraception 2001;63(4):211-215.
7. Jeng LL, Moore RM, Jr., Kaczmarek RG, Placek PJ, Bright RA. How frequently are home pregnancy tests used? Results from the 1988 National Maternal and Infant Health Survey. Birth. 1991;18(1):11-13.
8. Coons SJ, Churchill L, Brinkman ML. The use of pregnancy test kits by college students. J Am Coll Health 1990;38(4):171-175.
9. Doshi ML. Accuracy of consumer performed in-home tests for early pregnancy detection. A J Publ Health 1986;76(5):512-514.
10. Hicks JM, Iosefsohn M. Reliability of home pregnancy-test kits in the hands of laypersons. N Engl J Med 1989;320(5):320-321.
11. Lee C, Hart LL. Accuracy of home pregnancy tests. DICP. 1990;24(7-8):712-713.
12. Latman NS, Bruot BC. Evaluation of home pregnancy test kits. Biomedical Instrumentation and Technology. 1989;23(2):144-149.
13. Bluestein D. Monoclonal antibody pregnancy tests. American Family Physician. 1988;38(1):197-204.
14. IPAS. Pregnancy test trouble shooting guide. Product Literature. Chapel Hill, North Carolina: IPAS, 300 Market Street Suite 200; 2003.
15. Bandi ZL, Schoen I, Waters M. An algorithm for testing and reporting serum choriogonadotropin at clinically significant decision levels with use of "pregnancy test" reagents. Clin Chem 1989;35(4):545-551.
16. Rotmensch S, Cole LA. False diagnosis and needless therapy of presumed malignant disease in women with false-positive human chorionic gonadotropin concentrations. Lancet. 2000;355(9205):712-715.
17. Cole LA, Shahabi S, Butler SA, et al. Utility of commonly used commercial human chorionic gonadotropin immunoassays in the diagnosis and management of trophoblastic diseases. Clin Chem 2001;47(2):308-315.
18. Ramoska EA, Sacchetti AD, Nepp M. Reliability of patient history in determining the possibility of pregnancy. Ann Emerg Med 1989;18(1):48-50.
19. Jabara S BK. Is Rh immune globulin needed in early first-trimester abortion? A review. Am J Obstet Gynecol. 2003;188(3):623-627.
20. Weinberg L. Use of anti-D immunoglobulin in the treatment of threatened miscarriage in the accident and emergency department. Emerg Med J. 2001;18:444-447.
21. ACOG. Ectopic pregnancy: The American College of Obstetricians and Gynecologists; March 1989. 126.
22. Dart RG, Mitterando J, Dart LM. Rate of change of serial beta-human chorionic gonadotropin values as a predictor of ectopic pregnancy in patients with indeterminate transvaginal ultrasound findings. Ann Emerg Med 1999;34(6):703-710.
23. Leach RE, Ory SJ. Modern management of ectopic pregnancy. J Reprod Med 1989;34(5):324-338.
24. Saxon D, Falcone T, Mascha EJ, Marino T, Yao M, Tulandi T. A study of ruptured tubal ectopic pregnancy. Obstet Gynecol 1997;90(1):46-49.
25. Dart R, Dart L, Mitchell P, O'Rourke N. The utility of a dilatation and evacuation procedure in patients with symptoms suggestive of ectopic pregnancy and indeterminate transvaginal ultrasonography. Acad Emerg Med 1999;6(10):1024-1029.
26. Cacciatore B, Tiitinen A, Stenman UH, Ylöstalo P. Normal early pregnancy: serum hCG levels and vaginal ultrasonography findings. Br J Obstet Gynaecol 1990; 97(10):899-903.

27. Deutchman M. Advances in the diagnosis of first-trimester pregnancy problems. Am Fam Phys 1991;44(5 Suppl):15S-30S.
28. Stampone C, Nicotra M, Muttinelli C, Cosmi EV. Transvaginal sonography of the yolk sac in normal and abnormal pregnancy. J Clin Ultrasound. Jan 1996;24(1):3-9.
29. Thorsen MK, Lawson TL, Aiman EJ, et al. Diagnosis of ectopic pregnancy: endovaginal vs transabdominal sonography. Am J Roentgen 1990;155(2):307-310.
30. Banerjee S, Aslam N, Woelfer B, Lawrence A, Elson J, Jurkovic D. Expectant management of early pregnancies of unknown location: a prospective evaluation of methods to predict spontaneous resolution of pregnancy. Bri J Obstet Gynaecol 2001; 108(2):158-163.
31. Strobelt N, Mariani E, Ferrari L, Trio D, Tiezzi A, Ghidini A. Fertility after ectopic pregnancy. Effects of surgery and expectant management. Journal of Reproductive Medicine. 2000;45(10):803-807.
32. Stovall TG, Ling FW. Single-dose methotrexate: an expanded clinical trial. Am J Obstet Gynecol 1993;168(6 Pt 1):1759-1762.
33. Lipscomb GH, Stovall TG, Ling FW. Nonsurgical treatment of ectopic pregnancy. N Engl J Med 2000;343(18):1325-1329.
34. el-Lamie IK, Shehata NA, Kamel HA. Intramuscular methotrexate for tubal pregnancy. J Reprod Med. Feb 2002;47(2):144-150.
35. Barnhart KT GG, Ashby R, Sammel M. The medical management of ectopic pregnancy: a meta-analysis comparing "single dose" and "multidose" regimens. Obstet Gynecol. 2003;101(4):778-784.
36. Rulin MC. Is salpingostomy the surgical treatment of choice for unruptured tubal pregnancy? Obstet Gynecol 1995;86(6):1010-1013.
37. Centers for Disease Control and Prevention. Ectopic pregnancy—United States, 1988-1989. MMWR 1992;41(32):591-594.
38. Centers for Disease Control and Prevention. Ectopic pregnancy—United States, 1990-1992. MMWR 1995;44(3):46-48.
39. Luise C, Jermy K, May C, Costello G, Collins WP, Bourne TH. Outcome of expectant management of spontaneous first trimester miscarriage: observational study. BMJ Apr 13 2002;324(7342):873-875.
40. Cahill DJ. Managing spontaneous first trimester miscarriage. BMJ (Clinical Research Ed.) 2001;322(7298):1315-1316.
41. Weeks A, Alia G. Ultrasonography may have role in assessing spontaneous miscarriage. BMJ (Clinical Research Ed.) 2001;323(7314):694.
42. Pandian Z, Ashok P, Templeton A. The treatment of incomplete miscarriage with oral misoprostol. BJOG 2001;108(2):213-214.
43. Centers for Disease Control and Prevention. Recommendations for the use of folic acid to reduce the number of cases of spina bifida and other neural tube defects. MMWR 1992;41(RR-14):1-7.
44. Erickson JD. Folic acid and prevention of spina bifida and anencephaly. 10 years after the U.S. Public Health Service recommendation. MMWR Recomm Rep. Sep 13 2002;51(RR-13):1-3.

LATE REFERENCE

45. Cole LA, Khanlian SA, Sutton JM, Davies S, Rayburn WF. Accuracy of home pregnancy tests at the time of missed menses. Am J Obs Gyn 2004;190:100-105.

Impaired Fertility

Anita L. Nelson, MD
John R. Marshall, MD

- Maintaining a couple's ability to become pregnant until the man and woman reach their desired family size is a principal goal of reproductive health care providers.
- The first task in reproductive health care is to help individuals establish a reproductive life plan.
- The second task involves obtaining the information and skills necessary to attain such a plan.
- Basic education and fertility assessment can take place in the primary reproductive health care setting; couples who require more extensive assessment and treatment should be referred.

Providing contraception and treating impaired infertility are complimentary aspects of family planning. Contraception gives women time not only to space their pregnancies, but also to prepare for pregnancy in advance (preconceptional care) to optimize both maternal and infant outcomes—physical, psychological and, perhaps, even financial. Similarly, the evaluation and treatment of infertility directly enable couples to prepare for pregnancy. One interesting outcome of comprehensive infertility treatment is that each member of the couple generally gains a greater understanding of his or her own reproductive processes and becomes a more effective contraceptive user in the long run.

According to the American College of Obstetricians and Gynecologists, "The goals of an infertility evaluation are to provide a rational, organized approach to diagnosis, to present an accurate assessment of progress and prognosis during the evaluation, and to offer emotional and psychologic support."[1]

DEFINITIONS

On average, 80% to 85% of couples trying to become pregnant will conceive in 1 year, and an additional 5% to 10% will conceive in the second year. A couple is formally diagnosed as infertile if the man and woman have not conceived despite having had unprotected vaginal intercourse for 12 months without using contraception. However, the infertility work-up (see below) may be initiated before 12 months of "trying" if at least one partner has obvious fertility challenges (e.g., oligomenorrhea, ejaculatory dysfunction) or if there is a premium on time (e.g., a woman is in her late 30s or early 40s).

Primary infertility is the diagnosis when the couple has never conceived. *Secondary infertility* is the term used for couples that have previously conceived but have not conceived now despite at least 12 months of unprotected intercourse.

PROBABILITY OF PREGNANCY

About 10% to 15% of U.S. couples are infertile: they do not conceive after 1 year of unprotected intercourse. This fact can be confusing when applied to individual couples, some of whom are infertile, and some of whom are fertile. For the average *fertile* couple, the probability of conception is about 20% each cycle, which means that there is an 80% probability that conception will not occur. Multiplying that 80% probability by the 13 cycles in a year determines that only 5% of fertile couples will still not have conceived by the end of 1 year; the other 95% of fertile couples will have conceived by 1 year.[2] With more time, the number of couples who have not conceived decreases spontaneously, even without intervention. Couples with pregnancy potential but with a lower per-cycle fertility rate (subfertility) will have lower cumulative pregnancy rates for a given period of time. For example, it might take 18 months for them to achieve the same cumulative pregnancy rate that the more fertile couple achieved in 12 months.

Those who are not pregnant after 1 year of trying fall into three groups: normal but unlucky, subfertile, or sterile. We must recognize that the 12-month rule is arbitrary and that some couples may be labeled as being infertile when they are not. However, because many men and women carefully plan their careers and lives as parents, often delaying parenthood, they may not tolerate undue delays in conception. Therefore, evaluation and targeted interventions are often started before the rules of probabilities have had a chance to reveal all fertile couples. (This observation reminds us of the importance of using a placebo control group for comparison whenever new infertility therapies are being tested. The standard these new interventions must meet is not that they produce any pregnancies, but that they produce more pregnancies than would occur without any intervention.)

Because the fertile couples conceive and drop out of the group still trying to become pregnant, the longer couples have been infertile, the greater the likelihood that they are either infertile or sterile, and the lower the likelihood that they will ultimately conceive. This is illustrated in Table 27-1. However, the prognosis is not as bad as it first appears. Although the fecundity of a couple that has been infertile for 5 years is only 0.04 (i.e., 20% of normal), 37% of these couples will conceive within the next 12 months.[3]

Table 27-1 Incidence of conception over time among non-sterile couples with mean fecundability of 0.2 (pregnancy rate = 20% per month)

No. Months Without Conception	Proportion (%) Couples Not Yet Conceived	Mean Fecundability of Couples Not Yet Having Conceived	Proportion (%) Couples Who Will Conceive Within 12 Months Among Couples Not Yet Having Conceived
0	100	0.20	86
6	32	0.14	77
12	14	0.11	69
24	4	0.08	57
36	2	0.06	48
48	1	0.05	42
60	0.6	0.04	37

Source: Mishell D. (1997).

REQUIREMENTS FOR FERTILITY

An efficient approach to the work up of the infertile couple begins with an understanding of the requirements for fertility. There are requirements that relate exclusively to the woman, those that relate exclusively to the man, and the remaining requirements that relate to the couple. About 20% of couples will have no identifiable cause of infertility; they are classified as having idiopathic or unexplained infertility. Among couples who have an identifiable cause of infertility, 40% are related to male factors, 40% to female factors, and 20% to both male and female factors.

Requirements for Female Fertility

- Reasonably good health and nutrition to permit ovulatory cycling and support of a pregnancy
- Functioning reproductive anatomy and physiology

    — An introitus and vagina that permit penile entry

    — A vagina capable of capturing sperm

    — A patent cervix with cervical mucus that periodically permits passage of sperm into the upper genital tract

    — Ovulatory cycling with follicle extrusion

— Fallopian tubes that permit the sperm and ovum to fertilize and to facilitate migration of the conceptus into the uterus

— A uterus capable of permitting implantation and developing and sustaining the conceptus to maturity

— Adequate hormonal status to maintain pregnancy

• Normal immunologic responses to accommodate sperm, fertilization, and fetal health

• Absence of genetic causes of recurrent losses (e.g., balanced translocations, etc.)

Requirements for Male Fertility

• Normal spermatogenesis of functional sperm and a functioning ductal system

• Ability to transmit the sperm into the woman's vagina

— Ability to maintain an erection until coital ejaculation

— Ability to achieve a normal ejaculation within the vaginal vault

Requirements for a Couple's Fertility

• Ability and desire for sexual functions

— Intravaginal, penile coital activity

— Correct timing of intercourse within a woman's cycle

INFERTILITY EVALUATION OVERVIEW

The major identifiable causes of infertility are listed in Table 27-2 and Table 27-3. Unfortunately, these lists are not particularly helpful in the clinical evaluation of the patient. Consolidating these causes under the following five functional headings simplifies the evaluation process:

Category	% Cases Attributed To
1. Sperm	30–40%
2. Eggs and ovulation	10–15%
3. Transport	
Cervical mucus	10–15%
Tube/peritoneum	30–40%
4. Uterus	< 1%
5. Time	< 5%

Table 27-2 Causes of infertility in men

Endocrine disorders
    Hypothalamic dysfunction (Kallman's)
    Pituitary dysfunction (tumor, radiation, surgery)
    Hyperprolactinemia (drug, tumor)
    Exogenous androgens
    Thyroid disease
    Adrenal hyperplasia

Causes manifesting abnormal spermatogenesis
    History of mumps orchitis
    Chemical, radiation, or heat exposure
    Varicocele
    Cryptorchidism

Causes manifesting abnormal sperm motility
    Varicocele
    Antisperm antibodies
    Idiopathic

Sexual dysfunction
    Retrograde ejaculation
    Impotence
    Decreased libido

Idiopathic

Table 27-3 Causes of infertility in women

Causes resulting in an absence of ovulation or inadequate corpus luteum function
    Extremes of body mass index (BMI)
    Hypothalamic dysfunction
    Pituitary insufficiency (congenital, tumor, trauma)
    Hyperprolactinemia (tumor, drug, empty sella)
    Gonadal dysgenesis
    Premature ovarian failure
    Resistant oocytes
    Thyroid dysfunction (hyper- or hypo-)
    Androgen excess

Causes manifest in the uterus, tubes, or peritoneum
    DES exposure in utero
    Effects of prior surgical treatment of the cervix (cryotherapy, cone biopsy)
    Chronic cervicitis
    Hostile or inadequate cervical mucus
    Residual effects of acute salpingo-oophoritis
    Endometriosis
    Congenital anomalies
    Intrauterine synechiae (Asherman's syndrome)
    Prior tubal sterilization

Idiopathic

THE INITIAL DIAGNOSTIC EVALUATION

The initial evaluation has two focuses: routine preconceptional care (see Chapter 25 on Preconceptional Care) and workup to identify the cause of the infertility. The initial evaluation should involve both the man and the woman. In most instances, the woman will present for evaluation, so the evaluation will begin with her. However, because the evaluation of the male is so important and less complex, it should be completed before the woman undergoes any expensive or invasive tests.

INITIAL EVALUATION OF THE MAN

The initial evaluation of the man is a semen analysis. Because infertility so frequently results from the combination of both male and female factors, perform a semen analysis even if the woman has an obvious, treatable problem (such as anovulation), because treating her for a few cycles is not in her best interest when her partner may have a problem that leaves little or no possibility of conception. A history of having previously fathered children should not preclude performance of a semen analysis.

The semen analysis provides information about the quality of the sperm and the ejaculation process (that it is not retrograde). Customary standards for what is considered normal, which were first determined about 30 years ago,[4a] include the following ranges:

Volume: 2.0–6.0 cc

Count: > 20 million/ml

Motility: > 50% with forward progression

Morphology: > 30% normal with oval heads, acrosomal caps and single tails

White blood cells: < 1 million/ml

A recent study of semen analysis (using strict criteria for sperm morphology) classified the semen into three groups: fertile, indeterminate, and subfertile (see Table 27-4). Sperm concentration, motility, and morphology are each important. Morphology appears to be slightly but significantly more discriminating than either of the other two. If a single parameter is subfertile, the odds ratio for infertility is between 2 and 3. If two parameters are in the subfertile range, the odds ratio for infertility is between 5.5 and 7.2. If all three are in the subfertile range, the odds ratio for infertility is 15.8.[4b]

If the results of the semen analysis fall within the fertile range, no additional evaluation of the sperm is required. If the results do not fall within the fertile range, repeat the semen analysis. If the results persistently fall in the subfertile range, conduct a further evaluation to identify a treatable cause of the abnormality. If there is any question about the male contribution to infertility, ask about childhood illnesses and developmental health, systemic medical conditions, a history of surgeries or sexually transmitted infections (STI), as well as gonadal exposure to toxins, including heat. Physical finding of hypospadias, testicular irregularities, varicocele, or vas deferens abnormalities may warrant further work-up.[5]

Occasionally, cultural proscriptions preclude collection of a specimen. In those cases, a postcoital test (see below) may be helpful.

Table 27-4 Fertile, indeterminate, and subfertile ranges for sperm measurements

Variable	Semen Measurement		
	Concentration (10⁶/ml)	Motility (%)	Morphology (% normal)
Fertile range	> 48.0	> 63	> 12
Indeterminate range	13.5–48.0	32–63	9–12
Odds Ratio (95% CI)	1.5 (1.2 – 1.8)	1.7 (1.5 – 2.2)	1.8 (1.4 – 2.4)
Subfertile range	< 13.5	< 32	< 9
Odds Ratio (95% CI)	5.3 (3.3 – 8.3)	5.6 (3.5 – 8.3)	3.8 (3.0 – 5.0)

Source: Guzick D, et al. (2001).

INITIAL EVALUATION OF THE WOMAN

The initial infertility evaluation of the woman includes a history, a physical examination, and laboratory evaluation. The history can be very informative and can guide laboratory testing. Critical elements include a detailed menstrual history, including a history of dysmenorrhea, abdominal surgery, STIs (especially pelvic inflammatory disease, or PID), fertility with different partners, outcomes of any pregnancies, duration of unprotected intercourse, and coital activity (type, frequency, and timing in relation to the menstrual cycle).

- **Menstrual cycle factors.** Chronic anovulation can be diagnosed if the woman's cycles are longer than 35 days or if she has fewer than 8 spontaneous cycles a year. It is important to learn if she has moliminal symptoms that suggest ovulatory cycling (such as bloating, breast tenderness, or lower back pain that precede her menses, which indicate that ovulation probably occurred).

- **Endocrinologic factors.** Obesity commonly leads to anovulation. Noting her weight at different ages (especially if she ever had monthly cycles) can help pinpoint the role that excessive weight may have played in the etiology of her infertility. Similarly, thyroid dysfunction and other endocrine problems can affect fertility.

- **Tubal factors.** Suspect tubal factors if the woman has regular monthly menses (especially if she experiences Mittelschmerz or moliminal symptoms) but has a history of chronic pelvic pain, endometriosis, PID, or cervical infections.

- **Uterine factors.** Suspect endometrial scarring if a woman has had amenorrhea following a dilation and curettage (D&C) procedure.
- **Cervical factors.** Consider cervical factors if she has a history of having had a cone biopsy, LEEP, or a cervical laceration at childbirth or with D&C, etc.

The physical examination can be very targeted. Except for women with primary amenorrhea (see Chapter 6 on Menstrual Problems and Common Gynecologic Concerns) or women with indications of genetic conditions that can cause infertility (such as Turner's syndrome or premature ovarian failure), the examination of obviously healthy women includes inspection for hyperandrogenism (acne, hirsutism, etc.), a thyroid exam, a breast exam, and a careful and complete pelvic exam. During the pelvic exam, pay attention to the presence of any anatomical anomalies such as vaginal septa, uterine or ovarian masses, or fixed pelvic structures. Initial laboratory studies are listed in Table 27-5.

Table 27-5 Initial laboratory studies for evaluating fertility

All patients	Complete blood count
	Urinalysis
	Chlamydia trachomatis antibody titer
	Cervical cytology (if last exam > 1 yr)
If > 35 yrs of age	FSH on cycle day 3 or clomiphene challenge tests
If anovulatory	TSH, prolactin (especially if spontaneous galactorrhea)
If amenorrheic	FSH, E2 (interpret only after 14 days)
If obese	Post glucola serum glucose
If hirsute	Total or free testosterone, DHEAS, 17-hydroxyprogesterone

The presence of antibodies to *Chlamydia trachomatis* is correlated with the presence of tubal adhesions or obstruction.[6] Follicle stimulating hormone (FSH) levels greater than 12 mIU/ml but especially greater than 20 mIU/ml when measured on cycle day 3 are associated with very low pregnancy rates, even with sophisticated interventions. Early studies showed that no fertilizations occurred with aspirated eggs incubated with sperm when the woman's FSH was greater than 24 mIU/ml.[7,8] Thyroid stimulating hormone (TSH) and prolactin measurements are most informative if the woman is anovulatory.[9]

FURTHER EVALUATION OF THE WOMAN

Further evaluation is determined by the problems identified by the initial work-up. Many tests have been described; not all are useful. For a test to be useful, it must identify an abnormality, which, when treated, results in improved fecundability. Not all of these tests meet this criterion. Available tests are listed in Table 27-6.

Table 27-6 Tests for further evaluation of the woman

To evaluate and document ovulation/anovulation or to time intercourse
Progestin withdrawal test
Menstrual calendar
Basal body temperature (BBT) graphic recording
Urinary concentration of luteinizing hormone (LH)
Serum progesterone in mid-luteal phase

To identify tubal function and other pelvic abnormalities
Hysterosalpingogram (focuses on endometrial cavity and tubal structures)
Laparoscopy (can identify pelvic masses, adhesions, endometriosis or other visible pelvic pathology; tubal patency can also be determined by intraoperative dye injection)

To identify uterine abnormalities
Pelvic ultrasound (fibroids and other pelvic masses)
Sonohysterography (endometrial polyps, septa, submucosal fibroids, other endometrial surface anomalies)
Hysteroscopy (same as sonohysterography, but provides direct visualization)
Hysterosalpingogram (HSG)

Tests with limited or no value in modern infertility evaluation
Postcoital tests—except if used to determine if ejaculation is intravaginal or to assess sperm if semen analysis not permitted
Antisperm antibodies
Bacteriologic cultures of the cervix or endometrium
Hamster egg sperm penetration test (unless male factor requires)
Luteal phase endometrial biopsy

Basal body temperature (BBT) graphic recording. The BBT graphically records the basal temperature (obtained immediately upon awakening) using a special thermometer with an expanded scale. (See Chapter 15 on Fertility Awareness Methods.) The dip in the BBT usually occurs 1 to 3 days prior to ovulation. The BBT is difficult to interpret when used prospectively to predict ovulation; however, it can be used retrospectively to estimate when in the cycle ovulation has occurred. This estimate can be used to anticipate when ovulation is likely to occur in future cycles and to time coitus. Luteal phase levels of progesterone raise the BBT about 0.7° F for about 12 to 13 days, unless pregnancy ensues, in which case the elevation persists. A new BBT graph is started with each menses. Only about 80% of women have interpretable BBT patterns. Because the BBT chart also provides a place for recording coitus and other significant reproductive events, it can replace the menstrual calendar (see below).

Hysterosalpingogram (HSG). The HSG demonstrates intrauterine anatomy and tubal patency. Radio-opaque dye is injected through the cervix and its flow through the endometrial cavity and through the fallopian tube is examined by serial X-ray imaging. Tubal patency is demonstrated by the presence of crescent-shaped shadows of dye pooling at the end of the fimbria in the intraperitoneal space between loops of bowel.

All women need antibiotic prophylaxis with this invasive test. To avoid causing ectopic pregnancies, the HSG should be performed during the follicular phase of the cycle. Patients with a history of prior salpingitis, intraperitoneal surgery, symptoms consistent with endometriosis, or laboratory evidence of elevated *Chlamydia trachomatis* antibodies should have the procedure performed early in their infertility work-up. It has been suggested that there may be some therapeutic value to this test. Unfortunately, the HSG demonstrates only tubal patency, not tubal function, and it does not reliably demonstrate peritoneal adhesions.

Hysteroscopy. Hysteroscopy is the endoscopic examination of the uterine cavity. It can identify uterine septa, endometrial polyps, and submucosal fibroids, which may prevent implantation and can cause pregnancy loss in the first trimester.

Laparoscopy. Laparoscopy provides visualization of the peritoneal surface of the tubes, ovaries and pelvic peritoneum and can confirm the presence of adhesions, endometriosis and, with chromotubation (injection of dye into the uterus under pressure and observation of dye passage out the fimbria), tubal patency or occlusion. During the laparoscopic procedure, the adhesions can be excised, which can be therapeutic.

Menstrual calendar. The menstrual calendar records on a horizontal graph the important reproductive events of the month. It provides a visual display of the menstrual cycle interval, timing of coitus, and occurrence of premenstrual molimina. The calendar is helpful in determining the timing of the mid-luteal progesterone testing (see the following).

Mid-luteal phase serum progesterone. This test can substantiate both ovulation and the adequacy of corpus luteum function. Timing of the test is critical; the sample should be drawn about 7 days prior to the onset of the next menses. Because the day of onset of the next menses is never certain, the sample should be drawn 5 to 7 days after the BBT shift or 7 days after the urinary LH rise. (It is sometimes erroneously called a "day 21 progesterone" and is blindly drawn 21 days after the onset of the last menses.) Concentrations of 3 to 5 ng/ml indicate that ovulation has occurred; most ovulatory cycles associated with pregnancy will have mid-luteal progesterone levels of 10 ng/ml or greater.[10] If the value is less than 3 ng/ml, plot the value on the menstrual calendar or BBT graph in order to see if the specimen was drawn at the correct time of the cycle. The test can be repeated in the same cycle if there is a chance that it may have been drawn too early for interpretation.

Pelvic ultrasound. Pelvic ultrasound can identify fibroids, ovarian or tubal cysts, and some uterine anomalies. The test is indicated by the presence of a pelvic mass.

Progestin withdrawal test. For women with chronic anovulation and delayed menses, medroxyprogesterone acetate, 5 mg/day, is given orally for 5 to 10 days. Uterine bleeding after the withdrawal of the progestin clearly demonstrates that the woman has cervical patency, prior estrogen exposure, and a responsive endometrium (see Gynecologic Problems chapter).

Ovulation kits. Home urinary ovulation kits, available over-the-counter, can detect the ovulatory LH surge. The kits can anticipate ovulation in about 90% of women. Tests based on saliva concentrations have also received FDA approval. Ovum release generally occurs 36 hours after the initiation of the LH rise and 24 hours after the peak. Women should time intercourse directly after a positive urinary test, because fertilization is more likely to take place if intercourse precedes ovulation.[11]

Sonohysterography. Sonohysterography starts with a transvaginal real-time ultrasound. After the initial assessment of the pelvis, a small catheter is placed just inside the endometrial cavity, and a small balloon inflated to occlude the internal os. Then, a few tablespoons of sterile fluid are introduced into the endometrium to separate the walls and allow for real-time ultrasonographic visualization of intrauterine abnormalities such as polyps, submucosal fibroids, or septa.

D EVELOPING DIAGNOSES: INTEGRATING TEST RESULTS

The most efficient use of infertility tests is determined by the results of the initial evaluation. The questions listed below are organized into the five functional categories of infertility.

Sperm

1. Does the male ejaculate contain an adequate number of normal, motile sperm?
   - Answered by the semen analysis.

2. If no, is the cause treatable?
   - Answered by the subsequent work-up, usually performed by a urologist or andrologist.

Eggs and Ovulation

1. Does the woman have eggs?
   - Ovarian follicles ("eggs") are the source of endogenous estradiol, which can cause the signs listed below. These signs give evidence of the presence of "eggs":
     — The presence of secondary sexual characteristics proves that she had eggs, at least at the time of puberty.
     — Recent episodic uterine bleeding indicates recent prior endometrial stimulation by estrogen.
     — Even if there has been no recent spontaneous bleeding, bleeding following withdrawal of progestin indicates presence of eggs (but no ovulation).
     — An FSH level less than 20 mIU/ml indicates the presence of eggs.
     — A cycle-day-3 level of FSH less than 10 mIU/ml demonstrates that eggs are capable of being stimulated.

2. If the woman has eggs, does she ovulate regularly?

- A careful and detailed menstrual history often provides evidence of the presence of ovulation, although the absence of these findings does not indicate the absence of ovulation. The presence of the following are associated with ovulation in greater than 93% of cases:[12]
  — Episodic uterine bleeding occurs every 28 to 32 days.
  — The bleeding episodes are all similar, last 3 to 5 days, peak flow occurs within the first 12 hours, and both the beginning and the end have little, if any, spotting.
  — Premenstrual molimina (symptoms or signs that regularly precede menses).
- If menses are regular but the history suggests that they are not ovulatory, ovulation can be confirmed by either the BBT or a mid-luteal phase progesterone measurement (7 days prior to next menses).
- If menses are irregular or infrequent, assume they are anovulatory and that ovulation induction will be necessary if there is no underlying, correctable medical cause of amenorrhea (e.g., hypothyroidism, hyperprolactinemia).

3. If the woman ovulates regularly, does the corpus luteum function normally?

- Adequate corpus luteum function is confirmed by a mid-luteal progesterone value of 10 ng/ml or more.

Transport

1. Does the woman have a vagina?

- Confirmed by history and physical exam.

2. Are the sperm being ejaculated into the vagina in proximity to the cervix?

- Confirmed by finding sperm in the cervical mucus at postcoital test, if necessary.

3. Is the cervical mucus hospitable to the sperm? This question arises only in cases of significant cervical damage, generally from procedures such as LEEP or cone biopsy.

- Evaluated by post coital test.

4. Do the sperm move through the cervix, uterus, and tube to meet the ovum?

- Cervical stenosis is eliminated as an issue if the woman has menstrual bleeding.
- Other potential barriers to sperm motion are either measured by other tests (semen analysis) and cervical infection tests or cannot be assessed by currently available tests.

- Tubal patency can be demonstrated by HSG or dye injection during laparoscopy; however, there are no tests of tubal function.

5. Does fertilization take place?
   - Although not directly observable, problems with fertilization may be suspected in cases of endometriosis or when sperm fail specialized tests (hamster egg penetration test).

6. Does the conceptus move down the tube into the uterus?
   - Tubal patency is documented by HSG or laparoscopic dye injection test.

7. Are there other peritoneal causes of infertility (e.g., endometriosis)?
   - If there are any indications that endometriosis may be present, laparoscopy can provide a definitive diagnosis, staging, and an opportunity for therapy.[13,14]

Uterus

1. Is a uterus present?
   - A history of any prior menstrual or menstrual-like bleeding indicates the presence of a uterus.
   - In the absence of spontaneous bleeding, a uterus can be documented by pelvic exam, ultrasound, or presence of bleeding after administration of estrogen and progestin.

2. Is the endometrial cavity of appropriate size and shape?
   - Endometrial cavity size and shape is most easily determined by sonohysterography. Hysteroscopy also examines the endometrial cavity. HSG is usually reserved for cases in which tubal patency needs to be established.

3. Is the endometrium appropriately responsive to the estrogen and progesterone produced by the ovary?
   - The presence of normal menses demonstrates that the endometrium is responsive to hormonal stimulation. Historically, a mid-luteal phase endometrial biopsy had been used to detect a short luteal phase (less than 10 days) and an inadequate luteal phase (endometrial biopsy more than 2 days out of phase with the menstrual cycle day counting backward from 28, the day before the onset of menses). However, there is little persuasive evidence that infertility presumably due to either of these conditions is improved by treatment. Thus, there is little indication for such a biopsy.

Time

1. How many months has the couple been trying to conceive?
2. How many of those months were months in which ovulation occurred?

3. In how many of those months in which ovulation occurred was coitus timed such that sperm were present at the time of ovulation?

- The coital activity calendar compared to BBT or urinary LH tests will provide answers to these questions.

PROGNOSIS

Every infertile person should be given clear, accurate estimates of his or her prognosis. Studies show that although many women want to actively participate in fertility treatment decisions, they lack the information necessary to making informed choices.[15] Because many couples are seeking pregnancy relatively late in their reproductive lives, prognosis becomes of great importance. These couples have only a relatively few ovulations remaining, and their fecundity decreases with each passing month. Moreover, older couples face more obstacles in the adoption process. Prognosis is determined by the therapy applied and the underlying cause(s) of the infertility.

DESCRIPTION OF AVAILABLE THERAPIES

Infertility therapy has been revolutionized by new techniques for treatment, such as ovulation induction and the assisted reproductive technologies—intra-uterine insemination (IUI), in vitro fertilization (IVF), gamete intra-fallopian transfer (GIFT), zygote intra-fallopian transfer (ZIFT), and intra-cytoplasmic sperm injection (ICSI).

OVULATION INDUCTION TECHNIQUES

An early step in the work-up of anovulatory infertility treatment is to assess whether obesity is a contributing factor. Recommend that obese, anovulatory women lose weight. Regardless of their prior menstrual histories, women whose anovulation has been associated with weight gain can often resume ovulatory cycling after losing as little as 10% to 15% of their body weight.[16,17] Weight loss also has the advantage of reducing the risk these women face for gestational diabetes, should they conceive.

All medications used to induce ovulation provide increased gonadotropin stimulation of the ovaries to promote follicular maturation and ovulation. Increasing the dose can provide controlled hyperstimulation with maturation and release of multiple oocytes, which can increase fecundity, but which also increases the risks of multifetal pregnancy or ovarian hyperstimulation syndrome.

Clomiphene citrate. Clomiphene citrate is the drug that is most commonly prescribed for ovulation induction. It is an antiestrogen that competitively binds to estrogen receptors in the hypothalamus. With those receptors blocked, the hypothalamus senses a drop in circulating estrogen levels and increases GnRH pulses, which triggers FSH and LH release and induces follicular maturation and ovulation. Clomiphene is most effective in patients who have normal gonadotropin levels, oligo-ovulation or anovulation, and withdrawal bleeding following a progestin challenge. Clomiphene treatment, given orally for 5 days early in the cycle starting at low doses (e.g., 50 mg per day) induces ovulation in 70% of such patients. If the treatment is successful, ovulation usually occurs spontaneously on the 12th or 13th day following the start of the clomiphene. Sperm are made available just prior to ovulation by either normal vaginal coitus or by IUI. If ovulation does not occur, doses are increased each month up to a limit of 150 to 200 mg each day until ovulation is induced. Anovulatory women who are responsive to clomiphene citrate should be treated for at least 6 cycles, but the treatment should probably be limited to a maximum of 12 cycles. In the absence of other causes of infertility, pregnancy rates among women who take clomiphene are comparable to those among women who have spontaneous ovulations. Ovulation induction with clomiphene is associated with a modest increase in the occurrence of multiple pregnancy (8%) and ovarian cysts (>1%).[18] For women who do not respond to low-dose clomiphene citrate, many newer protocols call for pretreating with oral contraceptive pills or GnRH agonists during or in the cycle prior to clomiphene use, particularly if higher dosages of clomiphene are not appropriate.

Metformin. Women with polycystic ovary syndrome (PCOS) who fail therapy with low-dose clomiphene citrate have markedly higher rates of ovulation and pregnancy when metformin is introduced.[19] The optimal niche for this insulin-sensitizing drug is being defined.[20] Most specialists use this as first-line therapy for women with both PCOS and documented insulin resistance; others also use it in heavier women with PCOS; and others use it for virtually every woman with PCOS.

Gonadotropins and GnRH. Gonadotropins, such as FSH (with or without LH), provide direct stimulation to the ovaries. This therapy is best suited to patients who are not responsive to clomiphene. The gonadotropins are given by daily injection. Ovarian response is monitored by measuring serum estrogen daily and ultrasound. When the follicles are in the right size range (~16 mm), ovulation will be induced with an injection of hCG, the LH surrogate. If too many follicles are stimulated, no hCG will be given. Sperm are provided just prior to ovulation by either normal vaginal coitus or by IUI. In women who have no other causes of infertility, pregnancy rates are about the same as those in women with spontaneous ovulations. Even with close monitoring, multiple pregnancy rates are increased (20% of cases), as is the risk of ovarian cysts (1% to 3%).

Pulsatile GnRH administered by infusion pump also stimulates the pituitary to release FSH and LH. Patient selection, monitoring, and effectiveness are similar to gonadotropin therapy; however, the rate of high order multiple pregnancies may be lower.[21,22]

Both gonadotropins and pulsatile GnRH are used to promote the maturation of oocytes to be used in IVF, GIFT, ZIFT, or for intra-cytoplasmic sperm injection (ICIS), as discussed in the following section.

ASSISTED REPRODUCTIVE TECHNOLOGIES

Intrauterine insemination (IUI). IUI is the insemination, directly into the endometrial cavity, of washed and concentrated sperm, which can come from either the husband or a donor. Recent evidence suggests that washing the sperm with platelet activating factor may increase effectiveness.[23]

IUI with controlled hyperstimulation. IUI used in conjunction with ovulation induction improves fecundity in almost all clinical situations.[24] Two recent studies examining determinants of success[25,26] found that the overall pregnancy rate was 10% to 15% per cycle, with most pregnancies occurring within the first 3 to 4 cycles. Determinants of success were the number of follicles ovulated and the motility and morphology of the sperm in the ejaculate. Factors such as older female age, a diagnosis of endometriosis or tubal factor, duration of infertility, and number of cycles previously treated without pregnancy were associated with less success.

In-vitro fertilization (IVF). IVF is the process whereby oocytes, usually matured by controlled gonadotropin hyperstimulation, are aspirated from the ovary under ultrasonic guidance or laparoscopy and further matured and artificially fertilized in the laboratory. Following fertilization and development for 2 to 4 days (morula stage), the zygotes are transferred to the endometrial cavity via a catheter inserted through the cervix. Because of the gonadotropin stimulation, multiple oocytes are usually harvested. In order to diminish the likelihood of multiple pregnancies, no more than 3 or 4 fertilized eggs are placed in the endometrial cavity. Extra zygotes can be cryo-preserved for later transfer. If the subfertile woman is older than 35 to 39 years, most programs will require that she accept oocytes from a younger donor.

Gamete intrafallopian transfer (GIFT). Oocytes are matured and aspirated from the ovary, as in IVF. Sperm from the partner is washed and concentrated. Both oocytes and sperm are then placed directly into the fallopian tube where fertilization takes place. This method is used in women with no tubal damage.

Zygote intra-fallopian transfer (ZIFT). ZIFT uses the early steps of IVF; however, immediately following fertilization, the zygotes are placed into the fallopian tube to mature (with IVF, the zygotes are placed into the endometrial cavity during the morula stage). This method is also used in women with no tubal damage.

Intra-cytoplasmic sperm injection (ICSI). ICSI is useful when sperm are not able to penetrate the egg and fertilize it in vivo. Oocytes are matured and aspirated from the ovary as in IVF. Using micro-manipulative instruments under microscopic visualization, fertilization is accomplished by introduction of a single washed sperm into the cytoplasm of the oocyte. Following development to the morula stage, the zygote is transferred to the endometrial cavity as in IVF, although ZIFT is also possible.

TARGETED THERAPIES FOR INFERTILITY

Today, virtually all therapy is targeted toward overcoming the five categories of etiology: 1) male infertility, 2) ovulation disorders, 3) tubal abnormalities, 4) endometriosis, and 5) unexplained infertility. It is important to identify the cause of the infertility according to these categories. Success rates have been compared across many techniques,[27] but these rates are dependent upon the quality and experience of the provider. Adoption is an option that should be discussed with all couples, as should the psychological stresses that can arise in conjunction with infertility and its treatment.

TREATMENT OF MALE INFERTILITY

Azospermia (no sperm) in men with inadequate gonadotrophin levels can be treated with injections of FSH and LH. Men who have had a surgical sterilization can attempt to have the vas reanastomosed. Oligospermia or abnormalities of sperm form or motility due to varicocele can sometimes be improved by repair of the varicocele. Men whose sperm are unable to fertilize the egg can be offered ICSI.

However, most male infertility will require treatment using donor sperm, either alone or mixed with the male's sperm. Because of the potential for transmission of human immunodeficiency virus (HIV), virtually all donor semen is frozen pending the results of serial HIV testing. Most donor semen comes from large, commercial frozen-semen banks that can provide HIV-negative semen matched for the donor's physical characteristics and with a known ability to fertilize. Fecundity is about 10% per cycle using thawed donor semen placed in the vagina.[28] Intrauterine placement (IUI) is more effective than vaginal or endocervical placement of semen, and two IUIs performed just prior to ovulation are more effective than one.[29]

TREATMENT OF FEMALE INFERTILITY

Treatment of infertility caused by anovulation. Medical treatment of ovulation disorders is induction of ovulation. Therapy selection depends on whether the women is overweight, normal weight, or slender. For obese women, weight loss is the first line of treatment.[30] Once they have reduced their weight, the first medication for anovulatory women who have withdrawal bleeding with progestin challenge is clomiphene. For women with PCOS, treatment with insulin sensitizing agents such as metformin has been shown to be very effective both in lowering testosterone levels and in inducing ovulation, especially if they have insulin resistance. Metformin is often used for women who have not responded to clomiphene induction, either as a single agent or in combination with low-dose clomiphene.[31,32] Slender anovulatory women with low estrogen levels or endogenous gonadotrophins and estrogen and who do not withdraw to progestin challenges respond better to gonadotropin injections or pulsatile GnRH therapies. Laparoscopic ovarian drilling using diathermy or laser is a new therapy that appears to be as effective as gonadotropin therapy in some PCOS patients who have not responded to clomiphene.[33]

Treatment of infertility caused by tubal abnormalities. The most effective treatment of infertility caused by tubal abnormalities is IVF, which bypasses the tubal abnormality. Older surgical techniques for tuboplasty are less effective than IVF, except in cases of tubal ligation reversal. To increase intrauterine pregnancy rates, some experts recommend combining salpingectomy and IVF in cases of tubal damage due PID or endometriosis.

Treatment of infertility associated with endometriosis. Conservative management is often recommended for Stage I and II (mild to moderate) endometriosis because there is no clear evidence that intervention improves pregnancy rates for this degree of endometriosis.[34] A meta-analysis of large-scale studies has shown that none of the available medical therapies resulted in greater fertility than placebo, and many may delay fertility.[35] If conservative management is not successful, infertility associated with minimal/mild endometriosis is best treated by laparoscopic ablation of the endometriosis implants followed by IUI with controlled hyperstimulation.[13,14] A sobering note is that only one pregnancy will occur in every 7.7 women treated.[36] IVF has a role only if simpler therapy is unsuccessful. The preferred treatment of infertility associated with severe endometriosis is surgical ablation followed by IVF. There are no randomized trials to support this recommendation; however, the pregnancy rates in untreated advanced (Stage III, IV) endometriosis approach zero, and case reports of pregnancies after surgical repair suggest a benefit.

TREATMENT OF UNEXPLAINED INFERTILITY

After a trial of conservative management to rule out simple subfertility, the preferred treatment of unexplained infertility is IUI with controlled hyperstimulation.[37,38] ICSI is not superior to IVF.[39] The roles of empirical use of clomiphene with or without IUI in the treatment of unexplained infertility is debatable and present data are inconclusive.[18]

OTHER OPTIONS: ADOPTION

Many couples faced with infertility choose to adopt. Licensed adoption agencies may or may not allow communication between the birth parents and adopting parents, and they generally involve a longer wait than independent adoptions. Couples may seek the help of providers who have contact with women with unwanted pregnancies. Attorneys, clergy, friends, and independent adoption centers can also aid in matching couples with birth parents. Adopting children from other countries, older children, or children with special needs may minimize the waiting period. Present these options to infertile clients, along with referrals to adoption resources.

THE EMOTIONAL ASPECTS OF COPING WITH INFERTILITY EVALUATION AND THERAPY

Many couples who seek help for infertility eventually do achieve pregnancy, often in the course of the preliminary investigation. However, some couples will eventually confront the reality of childlessness. The impact of permanent infertility, coupled with the stresses of fertility evaluation and treatment, may damage a couple's relationship or an individual's self-concept. Normal reactions to the diagnosis of infertility include processes similar to other grieving processes: surprise, denial, isolation, anger, guilt, sorrow, and, finally, resolution. Frustration, isolation, depression, and prolonged stress are also common. Couples suffer a loss of privacy, a disruption of spontaneity, and the stresses that accompany performance on demand. The monthly menses is a painful mark of yet another cycle of failure.[40] Remember how disruptive infertility diagnosis and treatment can be for couples. Recognize also that stress may affect the success of fertility treatments.[41] Take an active and complementary role in helping infertile couples to cope:

- Refer couples for psychological counseling if their depression appears serious.
- Refer couples to infertility networks and support groups specifically designed to help people with infertility problems.
- Remain sensitive to heightened vulnerability of infertility patients.

REFERENCES

1. American College of Obstetricians and Gynecologists: Infertility (ACOG Technical Bulletin). Washington, DC, ACOG, 1989.
2. Hull M, Glazener C, Kelly J, et al. Population study of causes, treatment, and outcome of infertility. BMJ 1985;291:1693-1697.
3. Lobo RA, Mishell DR Jr, Paulsen RJ, Shoupe D. Mishell's Textbook of infertility, contraception, and reproductive endocrinology, 4th Edition. Malden MA: Blackwell Science, 1997. Adapted from Leridon H, Spira A. Problems in measuring the effectiveness of infertility therapy. Fertil Steril 1984;41:580-586.
4a. World Health Organization. Laboratory manual for the examination of human semen and sperm-cervical mucus interaction. Cambridge UK: Cambridge University Press, 1992.
4b. Guzick D, Overstreet J, Factor-Litvak P, et al. Sperm morphology, motility and concentration in fertile and infertile men. N Engl J Med 2001;345:1388-1393.
5. AUA and ASRM. Report on optimal evaluation of the infertile male. Baltimore MD and Birmingham AL: American Urological Association and American Society for Reproductive Medicine, 2001.

6. Dabeekausen Y, Evers J, Land J, Stals F. Chlamydia trachomatis antibody testing is more accurate than hysterosalpingography in predicting tubal factor infertility. Fertil Steril 1994;61:833-837.

7. Toner J, Philput C, Jones G, Muasher S. Basal follicle-stimulating hormone level is a better predictor of in vitro fertilization performance than age. Fertil Steril 1991;55:784-791.

8. van Montfrans JM, Hoek A, van Hooff MH, de Koning CH, Tonch N, Lambalk CB. Predictive value of basal follicle-stimulating hormone concentrations in a general subfertility population. Fertil Steril. 2000;74:97-103.

9. Mishell D. Evaluation of the infertile couple. In Lobo RA, Paulsen RJ, eds. Mishell's Textbook of infertility, contraception, and reproductive endocrinology, 4th Edition. Malden MA: Blackwell Science, 1997, p. 500.

10. Abdulla U, Diver MJ, Hipkin LJ, Davis JC. Plasma progesterone levels as an index of ovulation. Br J Obstet Gynaecol. 1983;90:543-548.

11. Schwartz D, Mayaux MJ, Martin-Boyce A, Czyglik F, David G. Donor insemination: conception rate according to cycle day in a series of 821 cycles with a single insemination. Fertil Steril. 1979;31:226-229.

12. Magyar D, et al. Regular menstrual cycles and premenstrual molimina as indicators of ovulation. Obstet Gynecol 1979; 53: 411-414.

13. Adamson GD. Treatment of endometriosis-associated infertility. Semin Reprod Endocrinol. 1997;15:263-271.

14. Ledger WL. Endometriosis and infertility: an integrated approach. Int J Gynaecol Obstet. 1999;64 Suppl 1:S33-40.

15. Stewart DE, Rosen B, Irvine J, Ritvo P, Shapiro H, Murphy J, Thomas J, Robinson GE, Neuman J, Deber R. The disconnect: infertility patients' information and the role they wish to play in decision making. Medscape Womens Health. 2001;6(4):1.

16. Kiddy DS, Hamilton-Fairley D, Bush A, Short F, Anyaoku V, Reed MJ, Franks S. Improvement in endocrine and ovarian function during dietary treatment of obese women with polycystic ovary syndrome. Clin Endocrinol (Oxf). 1992;36:105-111.

17. Pasquali R, Casimirri F, Vicennati V. Weight control and its beneficial effect on fertility in women with obesity and polycystic ovary syndrome. Hum Reprod. 1997;12 Suppl 1:82-87.

18. Nasseri S, Ledger WL. Clomiphene citrate in the twenty-first century. Hum Fertil (Camb) 2001;4:145-151.

19. Vandermolen DT, Ratts VS, Evans WS, Stovall DW, Kauma SW, Nestler JE. Metformin increases the ovulatory rate and pregnancy rate from clomiphene citrate in patients with polycystic ovary syndrome who are resistant to clomiphene citrate alone. Fertil Steril. 2001;75:310-315.

20. Barbieri RL. Metformin for the treatment of polycystic ovary syndrome. Obstet Gynecol. 2003;101:785-793.

21. Filicori M, Flamigni C, Dellai P, et al. Treatment of anovulation with pulsatile gonadotropin-releasing hormone: prognostic factors and clinical results in 600 cycles. J Clin Endocrinol Metab 1994;79:1215–1220.

22. Martin KA, Hall JE, Adams JM, Crowley WF Jr. Comparison of exogenous gonadotropins and pulsatile gonadotropin-releasing hormone for induction of ovulation in hypogonadotropic amenorrhea. J Clin Endocrinol Metab 1993;77:125–129.

23. Wild MD, Roudebush WE. Platelet-activating factor improves intrauterine insemination outcome. Am J Obstet Gynecol 2001;184:1064-1065.

24. Cohlen BJ, Vandekerckhove P, te Velde ER, Habbema JDF. Timed intercourse versus intra-uterine insemination with or without ovarian hyperstimulation for subfertility in men. In: The Cochrane Library, Issue 4, 1999. Oxford: Update Software. Search date 1996/1997; primary sources Medline; Embase; DDFU; Biosis; SciSearch; handsearching; and conference abstracts.

25. Montanaro GM, [need other authors' names] et al. Stepwise regression analysis to study male and female factors impacting on pregnancy rate in an intrauterine insemination programme. Andrologia 2001;33:135-141.

26. Nuojua-Huttunen S, Tomas C, Bloigu R, Tuomivaara L, Martikainen H. Intrauterine insemination treatment in subfertility: an analysis of factors affecting outcome. Hum Reprod 1999;14:698-703.
27. Duckitt K. Infertility and subfertility. In Clinical Evidence. London: BMJ Publishing Group, 2001:5:1279-1302.
28. Cooke ID. Donor insemination – timing and insemination method. In: Templeton A, Cooke ID, O'Brien PMS, eds. 35th RCOG Study Group evidence-based fertility treatment. London: RCOG Press, 1998.
29. Cohlen BJ, Vandekerckhove P, te Velde ER, Habbema JDF. Timed intercourse versus intra-uterine insemination with or without ovarian hyperstimulation for subfertility in men. In: The Cochrane Library, Issue 4, 1999. Oxford: Update Software. Search date 1996/1997; primary sources Medline; Embase; DDFU; Biosis; SciSearch; handsearching; and conference abstracts.
30. Pasquali R, Antenucci D, Casimirri F, Venturoli S, Paradisi R, Fabbri R, Balestra V, Melchionda N, Barbara L. Clinical and hormonal characteristics of obese amenorrheic hyperandrogenic women before and after weight loss. J Clin Endocrinol Metab. 1989;68:173-179.
31. Nestler JE. Role of hyperinsulinemia in the pathogenesis of the polycystic ovary syndrome, and its clinical implications. Semin Reprod Endocrinol. 1997;15:111-122.
32. Ehrmann DA. Insulin-lowering therapeutic modalities for polycystic ovary syndrome. Endocrinol Metab Clin North Am. 1999;28:423-438, viii.
33. Farquhar C, Vandekerckhove P, Lilfford R. Laparoscopic "drilling" by diathermy or laser for ovulation induction in anovulatory polycystic ovary syndrome (Cochrane Review). Cochrane Database Syst Rev 2001;4:CD001122.
34. Parazzini F. Ablation of lesions or no treatment in minimal-mild endometriosis in infertile women: a randomized trial. Gruppo Italiano per lo Studio dell'Endometriosi. Hum Reprod. 1999;14:1332-1334.
35. Hughes E, Fedorkow D, Collins J, Vandekerckhove P. Ovulation suppression for endometriosis. Cochrane Database Syst Rev. 2000;(2):CD000155.
36. Olive DL, Pritts EA. Treatment of endometriosis. N Engl J Med. 2001;345:266-275.
37. Hughes EG. The effectiveness of ovulation induction and intrauterine insemination in the treatment of persistent infertility: a meta-analysis. Hum Reprod 1997;12:1865-1872.
38. Singh M, et al. Superovulation and intrauterine insemination in cases of treated mild pelvic disease. J Assist Reprod Genet 2001;18:26-29.
39. Ruiz A, et al. The role of in vitro fertilization and intracytoplasmic sperm injection in couples with unexplained infertility after failed intrauterine insemination. Fertil Steril 1997;68:171-173.
40. Greil AL. Infertility and psychological distress: a critical review of the literature. Soc Sci Med. 1997;45:1679-1704.
41. Klonoff-Cohen H, Chu E, Natarajan L, Sieber W. A prospective study of stress among women undergoing in vitro fertilization or gamete intrafallopian transfer. Fertil Steril. 2001;76:675-687.

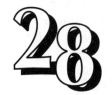

Abortion

Felicia H. Stewart, MD
Charlotte Ellertson, PhD, MPA
Willard Cates Jr., MD, MPH

- Legally induced abortion is safer than continuing a pregnancy to term.

- Approximately 88% of all abortions in the United States are performed during the first trimester; more than half are performed at or before 9 weeks following the woman's last normal menstrual period.

- Medication methods (most commonly mifepristone followed by misoprostol) are effective and safe options for women seeking abortion during the first 9 weeks following a normal menstrual period.

- Regard as urgent any request a woman makes for pregnancy confirmation and provide her with information about all her options, including prompt referral if she plans to consider abortion.

Women who wish to prevent pregnancy have a number of contraceptive options; none of the available methods, however, is perfect, even when used consistently and correctly. In addition, circumstances change, so some women who initially intend to become pregnant may later find themselves facing an unwanted pregnancy. Other women must decide what to do about a pregnancy resulting from coerced sex. To have real control over fertility, women need access to the full range of contraception and abortion options; they deserve to make their decisions without feeling judged or disparaged. A woman's decision to terminate her pregnancy is based on her unique situation; it is not appropriate or logical to treat abortion as a regrettable human "failure." Approximately 40% of U.S. women have had at least one abortion by the time they reach age 40.[1]

Aspiration is a venerable, safe, and effective method for women seeking abortion during the first trimester. Medication abortion is now an accepted option for use during the first 63 days (9 weeks) following the first day of a woman's last menstrual period (LMP), and is becoming widely available in the United States and internationally. For abortion after the first trimester, the most common method for abortion in the U.S. is dilation and evacuation (D&E), preceded by cervical dilation or preparation using osmotic cervical dilators or misoprostol. Medical induction using mifepristone and misoprostol or another prostaglandin is also possible for abortion after the first trimester, but it has been used less widely in the United States than in the United Kingdom.

In the past, many clinicians recommended that abortion not be scheduled before 7 weeks following a woman's LMP, because studies from the early 1970s found slightly higher rates of incomplete abortion when procedures were performed that early in pregnancy. Because pregnancy tests available during that era could not reliably detect pregnancy until about 6 weeks dated from LMP, and ultrasound was not yet available, clinicians providing abortion had no simple way to determine in advance of an early aspiration procedure whether a woman might have an incomplete spontaneous abortion, a missed abortion, or a possible ectopic pregnancy. When an attempted aspiration did not yield appropriate tissue, it may have been attributed to one of those problems—thus misleading the clinician and resulting in an incomplete procedure or continuing pregnancy. Today, highly sensitive pregnancy tests and ultrasound make it possible to avoid the confusion.

Contemporary studies provide evidence that vacuum aspiration abortion can safely be performed as soon as pregnancy is diagnosed,[2] so there is no longer any reason to recommend a routine delay for either pregnancy confirmation or abortion scheduling. Several excellent reviews describe the various clinical abortion techniques in more detail.[3-8] This chapter provides an overview for clinicians who offer early pregnancy confirmation, evaluate and refer women for abortion services, or wish to consider expanding their scope of practice to include early abortion care.

LEGAL STATUS OF ABORTION

Before 1970, legal abortion was not widely available in the United States. Beginning in 1968, however, several large states on the East and West coasts enacted more "liberal" laws allowing abortion under many circumstances. On January 22, 1973, the U.S. Supreme Court decided two landmark cases—*Roe v. Wade* [410 U.S. 113 (1973)] and *Doe v. Bolton* [410 U.S. 179 (1973)]—that legalized abortion nationwide. In brief, these decisions established the following "trimester framework":

1. In the first trimester, the abortion decision and procedure must be left to the judgment of the pregnant woman and her physician. States have little scope to interfere.

2. In the second trimester, each state may choose to regulate abortion procedures in ways that are reasonably related to the pregnant woman's health.

3. In the third trimester, when a fetus is already viable, the state may choose to promote its interest in potential human life by limiting, or

even prohibiting, abortion. It may not, however, impose restrictions that interfere with the life or health of the pregnant woman.

Since *Roe v. Wade*, induced abortion has become one of the most commonly performed procedures in the United States, although numerous and varied pieces of legislation to reduce access to abortion services have been introduced at the local, state, and national levels.[9] Attempts to pass a sweeping constitutional amendment overturning Roe *v.* Wade failed resoundingly in 1983. Since then, abortion opponents have concentrated on limiting abortion services in a piecemeal fashion[10,11] and on eliminating Medicaid funding for abortion. A landmark ruling for this approach was the 1992 Supreme Court decision in *Planned Parenthood of Southeastern Pennsylvania v. Casey* [505 U.S. 833 (1992)] that states could restrict early-abortion services as long as such restrictions do not impose an "undue burden" on a woman's ability to choose abortion. Specifically, the Court upheld waiting periods, counseling requirements, parental involvement provisions, and hospitalization requirements. Since the early 1990s, state legislatures have considered hundreds of bills intended to constrain providers and limit access for women seeking abortion care.

The 1993 Freedom of Access to Clinic Entrance (FACE) Act provided some protection for clinics and providers from harassment and violence directed against them.[12] Nearly all facilities affected by violence remain open, but the cumulative intimidation has contributed to a climate that discourages some clinicians from providing abortions.

PUBLIC HEALTH IMPACT OF LEGAL ABORTION

The *Roe v. Wade* decision ushered in a new era in women's health, producing immediate public health benefits: plummeting rates of abortion complications and deaths because fewer women underwent illegal abortion and legal abortion was more readily available closer to home, earlier in pregnancy, and at lower cost.[13] Abortion practices became safer after studies revealed that vacuum aspiration was safer than sharp curettage, local anesthesia was safer than general anesthesia, abortions performed in freestanding clinics were safer than those performed in hospitals, and D&E was safer than labor induction for early second-trimester abortions. In the midst of strident debate over the abortion issue, the foundation of objective public health data has helped guide, or at least inform, judicial rulings, and legislative actions.

CHARACTERISTICS OF WOMEN OBTAINING ABORTIONS

Legal abortion statistics are reported by 46 states (excluding Alaska, California, New Hampshire, and Oklahoma) to the Centers for Disease Control and Prevention (CDC), and also have been studied through independent surveys. Between 1972 and 1990, the number of reported abortions increased gradually (Table 28-1). Most of the increase occurred between 1972 and 1980, with reported legal abortions rising from about 600,000 to 1.3 million per year.[14] During the 1980s, the number of reported legal abortions and the legal abortion rate (procedures per 1,000 women ages 15 to 44) remained remarkably stable, varying each year by less than 5%. After peaking in 1990 at 1.4 million, the number of abortions reported to the CDC decreased to 861,789 in 1999. This decline, however, in part reflects CDC's 1997 decision to stop including the estimated rates for non-reporting states, including California, which accounted for 23% of the 1997 total.[15] Historically, the number of legal abortions reported by CDC has been 15% lower than the estimated number based on independent surveys by the Alan Guttmacher Institute (AGI).[16] With data from its 13th national survey, AGI estimated that the number of abortions performed in 2000 was 1.31 million—having declined from a peak of 1.61 million in 1990.[17]

More than half (58%) of all reported abortions occur during the first 9 weeks following LMP, and 88% are performed in the first trimester. The proportion of pregnancies that end in elective abortion is highest for women who are young, poor, unmarried, and non-white; over 40; or with three or more previous live births.[15] (See Table 28-1.) Most of the women are unmarried (78%); most (61%) have had one or more previous live births.[15] Younger women tend to obtain abortions later in pregnancy than do older women. More than 90% of women obtain the procedure in their state of residence.

DECIDING TO TERMINATE A PREGNANCY

The decision about whether to continue a pregnancy may begin before a woman knows for certain she is pregnant. Encourage women who suspect they are pregnant to seek pregnancy confirmation and evaluation as soon as they recognize the symptoms of pregnancy, including delayed menses. Regardless of whether a woman chooses to terminate her pregnancy or to continue it, a delay in confirming pregnancy can have adverse health consequences for the following reasons:[18]

- Delays the initiation of pregnancy precautions and prenatal care
- May reduce the woman's opportunity to obtain early termination
- Increases the risks of complications if the woman chooses abortion
- May limit the woman's options for abortion methods

Provide a supportive, nonjudgmental setting so the woman can explore her feelings concerning pregnancy, abortion, her partner, her future life plans, and her ability to provide for a child at present and in the future. Ambivalence is common, and for many women the decision is complicated. Basic factual information and discussion will meet the counseling needs of most women; some clients may need more extensive education, evaluation, or counseling and assurance to ensure they are making an informed decision without coercion. (See Chapter 10 on Education and

Counseling.) If your clinic or medical practice does not offer comprehensive services, refer patients to agencies providing services such as financial assistance, further counseling, first- and second-trimester abortions, prenatal care, and adoption.

Table 28-1 Characteristics of women who obtained legal abortions—United States, selected years, 1972 to 1999

Characteristics	1972 %	1980 %	1990 %	1995 %	1999 %
Residence					
In-state	56.2	92.6	91.8	91.5	91.2
Out-of-state	43.8	7.4	8.2	8.5	8.8
Age (years)					
≤19	32.6	29.2	22.4	20.1	19.2
20–24	32.5	35.5	33.2	32.5	32.2
≥25	34.9	35.3	44.4	47.4	46.6
Race					
White	77.0	69.9	64.8	59.6	56.2
Black and other	23.0	30.1	35.2	35.0	37.3
Marital status					
Married	29.7	23.1	21.7	19.7	19.2
Unmarried	70.3	76.9	78.3	80.3	80.8
Weeks' gestation					
≤8	34.0	51.7	51.6	54.0	57.6
9–10	30.7	26.2	25.3	23.1	20.2
11–12	17.5	12.3	11.7	10.9	10.2
13–15	8.4	5.1	6.4	6.3	6.2
16–20	8.2	3.9	4.0	4.3	4.3
≥21	1.3	0.9	1.0	1.4	1.5
Total legal abortions (estimate for all states)	586,760	1,297,606	1,429,577	1,267,415	not estimated
Total reported legal abortions (excluding AK, CA, NH, OK)				908,243	861,789

Source: Elam-Evans, LD (2002).[15]

SELECTING A METHOD OF ABORTION

The main factor guiding which abortion methods are possible is the duration of pregnancy (Figure 28-1). During the first 9 weeks of gestation (dated from LMP), both medication abortion and aspiration may be options. For women obtaining abortions at later gestational ages, the options are typically more limited. The patient will need information about the abortion procedures available; how they are done; their safety, success rates, risks, costs, and time required; and follow-up care. The woman may want her partner or other supportive persons involved in the counseling, but she will still need a chance to talk privately with you so you can be sure that her decision is not coerced.

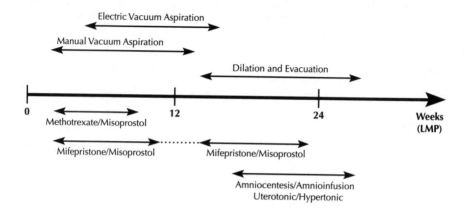

Figure 28-1 Options for terminating pregnancy, by length of pregnancy

In helping the early-abortion client decide between medication and aspiration methods, explain the important advantages and disadvantages of each (Table 28-2). The main advantages of aspiration are its speed and certainty and the option for general anesthesia. The drawbacks are the procedure's invasiveness and the small risk of uterine perforation and infection. By contrast, medication abortion advantages include women's perceptions that it is more "natural" and private and that it allows women a more active role in their abortions.[19] The disadvantages of medication methods are the length of time required (several days, or in the case of methotrexate abortion, possibly longer) for the abortion to occur, lower level of predictability, possibility of substantial cramping, and heavier bleeding, although the amounts are rarely clinically significant. Research from Europe and Canada suggests that over half of eligible women select medication methods.[20-22] The proportion of eligible women choosing medication abortion has increased gradually in countries where it is available,[23] including the United States (Figure 28-2).

Table 28-2 Advantages and disadvantages of early abortion methods

	Medication	Vacuum Aspiration
Advantages	Usually avoids surgery and anesthesia	Quicker
	More natural, like menses	More certain
	Less painful	Woman can be less involved
	Woman can be more in control, more involved	General anesthesia can be used
Disadvantages	Waiting, uncertainty	Invasive
	Bleeding, cramping, nausea	Small risk of uterine or cervical injury, or infection
	Extra clinic visit, longer time interval	

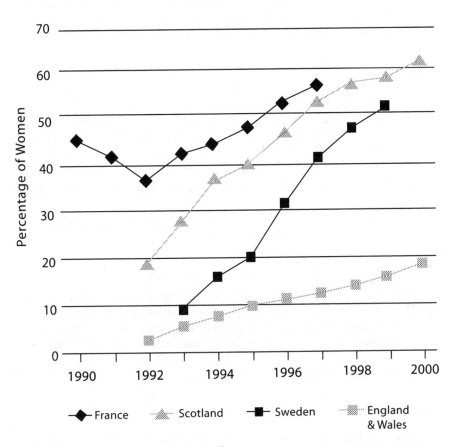

Source: Jones RK, et al. (2002).[23]

Figure 28-2 Percentage of women eligible for early medical abortion who were prescribed
mifepristone, four European countries, 1990-2000

PRE-ABORTION PROCEDURES

The goals in providing a pregnancy confirmation examination are
as follows:

- Determine whether the woman is pregnant.
- Identify possible problems that require further evaluation and/or
  emergency intervention, such as ectopic gestation or threatened
  abortion.
- Assess gestation length accurately (in days or weeks).
- Help the patient make and implement her plans for prenatal care
  or abortion.

- If the patient is considering abortion, screen as appropriate for infection and identify medical or gynecologic conditions that might influence the choice of appropriate abortion options.

HISTORY

- Recent menstrual history
- Prior obstetric and gynecologic history, including previous surgery involving the cervix or uterus, (e.g., conization of the cervix, cesarean delivery, history of leiomyomata [fibroids]) and any complications of previous abortions
- Contraceptive history, including current IUD wear, and future contraceptive plans
- Allergies to local anesthetics, analgesics, antibiotics, anti-progestins, prostaglandins, and other drugs
- Current drug use (legal, illicit, or over-the-counter) including anti-coagulants or systemic corticosteroids
- Acute or chronic illnesses (including asthma, inflammatory bowel disease, seizure disorder, cardiac valvular disease, hemorrhagic disorder, porphyria, or adrenal failure) that might require more evaluation, adjunctive therapy, or special care in the performance of the abortion or that might preclude one or more methods of abortion

CLINICAL EXAM

Perform a brief physical exam that includes vital signs and a pelvic exam or ultrasound to assess uterine size and position and to estimate gestation (independent of the history). Determine the presence of any abnormality that might indicate the need for further evaluation or influence the selection of a procedure: for example, does the medical history suggest possible heart or respiratory disease or do pelvic exam findings suggest the presence of uterine leiomyomata and adnexal masses? An ultrasound evaluation may help assess the duration of pregnancy and may be necessary if pelvic exam findings are not clear or if you suspect an adnexal mass or ectopic pregnancy.

LABORATORY TESTS

Recommended laboratory screening includes the following procedures:

- Urine pregnancy test* (unless pregnancy already has been confirmed by ultrasound)
- Hemoglobin or hematocrit if indicated. Offer iron supplementation to anemic women (hemoglobin <10g/dl or hematocrit <30%).

- Rho(D) determination[**]
- Screening for reproductive tract infection as appropriate. If chlamydia, gonorrhea, or bacterial vaginosis is suspected or identified, initiate treatment prior to abortion if possible.

---

[*] A serum pregnancy test is logical only when serial, quantitative hCG levels are needed to monitor a possible ectopic pregnancy or to evaluate a missed or incomplete spontaneous abortion. For confirming pregnancy, a urine pregnancy test is simple, inexpensive, and fast (results are available immediately), with sensitivity and specificity equal to serum test results. (See Pregnancy Testing, Chapter 26.)

[**] If the woman will be referred to another site for abortion care, referral can be scheduled with Rh results pending. Rh determination may be deferred if it is routinely provided as part of the abortion service.

FIRST-TRIMESTER ASPIRATION ABORTION

Introduced in the United States in 1967, aspiration (suction or vacuum curettage) rapidly became the most widely used abortion procedure,[14,24] so that by 1999, 96% of abortions in the nation were performed by aspiration.[15] A safe and simple way to empty the uterus completely and quickly with minimal cervical dilation, aspiration is most safely, and most commonly, performed using local anesthesia or a combination of mild intravenous sedation with local anesthesia. General anesthesia also can be used, but it increases slightly the risk of complications and involves a longer post-operative recovery time.

As the first step in an aspiration procedure, perform a bimanual examination to determine the uterine size and position. Next, insert a speculum and cleanse the cervix with an antimicrobial solution swab. Administer a local anesthetic such as 0.5% to 1% lidocaine amide (limiting the amount to less than 2 milligrams per pound) to the cervix to reduce pain. While the patient's cervix is anesthetized, place a tenaculum to keep the cervix stabilized. Using Pratt or Denniston dilators, gently dilate the cervix. Alternatively, an osmotic dilator placed up to 24 hours before, or misoprostol administered 3 to 4 hours before the procedure, can be used to establish needed dilation or minimize the need for additional mechanical dilation. (See the section on Adjunctive techniques.) In early pregnancy, little or no dilation may be needed; typically, the aspiration cannula diameter needed corresponds to the pregnancy week in millimeters (5 mm for pregnancy at 5 weeks, etc.). Through the dilated cervix, insert a cannula connected to a vacuum source (either an electric vacuum pump or a manual vacuum syringe) into the uterine cavity. The cannula, moved gently throughout the uterine cavity, evacuates the products of conception. When the uterus feels empty, examine the removed tissue to confirm that the pregnancy was intrauterine rather than ectopic and that the evacuation was complete. Tissue examination may also identify an abnormal pregnancy such as hydatidiform mole or incomplete spontaneous pregnancy loss. Tissue evaluation is facilitated by suspending products of conception in saline or white vinegar and checking with backlighting.

Aspiration with local anesthesia can safely and appropriately be provided in a medical office setting equipped with the same emergency back-up equipment and supplies needed to provide injectable medications (drugs and resuscitation equipment to manage allergic reaction, seizure, or cardiac arrest). In addition, the facility should have available medication to treat uterine atony and a plan for transfer to a surgical facility if a woman needs an evaluation for uterine perforation.

FIRST-TRIMESTER MEDICATION ABORTION

Medication options for early first-trimester abortion are currently available in the United States for abortion during the first 9 weeks (63 days) dated from the first day of the LMP.

Mifepristone

Mifepristone (formerly known as RU 486) was approved by the U.S. Food and Drug Administration (FDA) in September 2000 and is sold in the United States under the brand name Mifeprex. Widely used for early abortion in several European countries for more than 15 years,[29-32] it has been shown to be safe, effective, and acceptable in developing countries as well.[33-35] The combination of mifepristone and misoprostol for early abortion has been used safely by millions of women around the world. The same medications also can be used for second trimester abortion (see the section on Second Trimester Medical Methods). The regimen may also be effective for abortion performed between 9 and 12 weeks of gestation, but this use may prove to be inappropriate for women who are not hospitalized during the pregnancy expulsion. If hospitalization would be necessary for medication options, aspiration abortion is a quicker and less costly alternative.

Mifepristone is a 19-norsteroid with a high affinity for progesterone receptors. The drug blocks the action of progesterone—necessary to establish and maintain placental attachment—and also binds to glucocorticoid receptors and (to a lesser extent) androgen receptors. Mifepristone also stimulates synthesis of prostaglandins by cells of the early decidua. In addition to its use for inducing abortion, mifepristone (at a low dose) has been investigated as an emergency contraceptive, as well as for other indications including treatment of uterine leiomyomata, severe psychotic depression, and certain brain tumors.

Methotrexate

Methotrexate can be used to terminate both early pregnancy (during the first 7 weeks dated from the first day of the LMP) and early ectopic pregnancy.[22,36-38] It is marketed for treatment of severe psoriasis and choriocarcinoma and has been used widely for treatment of arthritis.

Regimens for early abortion and ectopic pregnancy are not included in the labeling for methotrexate, but protocols for early abortion reported in several clinical trials,[36,38,40] and the drug's use in ectopic pregnancy is based on published evidence accumulated over more than 20 years (see Chapter 27, Pregnancy Testing and Management of Early Pregnancy).[39]

Misoprostol

Both mifepristone and methotrexate are used in regimens that provide the prostaglandin E_1 analogue misoprostol, sold as Cytotec in the United States, to augment uterine contractions. Misoprostol produces cervical softening and dilation and stimulates uterine contractions; it is a widely available, inexpensive medication marketed for prevention of gastro intestinal ulcer disease.

Misoprostol can also be used alone to induce abortion, and a variety of regimens have been studied. This option is not generally recommended in the United States because reported effectiveness has been less consistent than regimens involving mifepristone or methotrexate.[41] It is more widely used as a "blackmarket" method in countries where legal abortion is not available.[42]

Misoprostol is a prostaglandin analog that acts directly on the uterus and cervix to soften and dilate the cervix and stimulate uterine contractions. It also can cause systemic prostaglandin effects, including nausea, vomiting, diarrhea, and temporary elevation of body temperature—side effects that women commonly report with all medical abortion regimens.

Uterine sensitivity to misoprostol increases with gestation: a higher and more sustained level (misoprostol 800 mcg administered vaginally) is required to induce abortion during the first trimester; while a much lower dose (misoprostol 25 to 50 mcg administered buccally) can induce labor in the third trimester. Uterine sensitivity increases through the second trimester, so lower doses may be sufficient later in the second trimester.[41] Misoprostol's effect also depends on the route of administration. An oral dose (swallowed) results in a more rapid, intense effect with more intense side effects, while a vaginal, buccal, or sublingual dose is absorbed more slowly, with fewer side effects and a less intense but more sustained uterine effect.

Research results for a variety of early abortion regimens using misoprostol alone have been reported;[41,57,58] most involve multiple doses. Studies of 800 mcg misoprostol administered vaginally up to 63 days following the LMP and repeated at 24-hour intervals for a total of three doses if abortion has not already occurred, have reported 92% effectiveness in inducing complete abortion.[59,60]

Anecdotal evidence suggests that some women in the United States are using misoprostol to induce abortion.[61] As word spreads through informal information networks, the practice may grow, and women may present for follow-up treatment after self-administration. Clinicians need to be aware of this use and to know how to provide or refer women for follow-up care, if needed.

Mifepristone and misoprostol regimens

Although use of mifepristone alone results in abortion in some cases, the addition of misoprostol increases efficacy. The research that the FDA reviewed for approval of mifepristone was based on the original French regimen, developed more than a decade ago, which specified 600 mg of mifepristone followed by misoprostol, 400 mcg orally. Subsequent research has shown that a lower dose of mifepristone, 200 mg, is equally effective,[43-45] and that misoprostol at a dose of 800 mcg self-administered vaginally at home is more effective than the original oral route and dose, has fewer side effects, is more convenient and private for women, and eliminates one medical visit.[6,44,46-51] The evidence-based regimen also provides flexibility about timing misoprostol 1, 2 or 3 days after mifepristone,[50] with excellent efficacy through at least 63 days of gestation.[47,48] (See Table 28-3).

Table 28-3 Comparison of Mifepristone Regimens

	FDA-approved Regimen	Evidenced-based Regimen
Recommended gestational age	49 days or less following LMP	63 days or less following LMP
Mifepristone dose	600 mg orally	200 mg orally
Misoprostol dose	400 mcg orally Administered during second office visit	800 mcg vaginally Supplied during first office visit Administered at home
Misoprostol timing	48 hours after mifepristone	24 to 72 hours after mifepristone*
Follow-up office visit	Day 14	Day 4 to 8
Minimum office visits	3	2
Approximate cost to patient	$270 for mifepristone $2 for misoprostol 3 office visits	$90 for mifepristone $4 for misoprostol 2 office visits
Advantages		Comparable efficacy to mifepristone 600 mg dose Treatment through 63 days LMP Decreased side effects Decreased time to expulsion Misoprostol self-administered at home 24 to 72 hours after mifepristone Lower cost

Source: Stewart FH, et al. (2001).[6]

* The 24- to 72-hour misoprostol treatment time frame has been studied only in women ≤ 56 days LMP.

Labeling for mifepristone describes the original regimen, so patients receiving the evidence-based regimen need to be informed that their treatment is based on newer evidence rather than FDA-approved label instructions. Many providers, including clinics affiliated with the Planned Parenthood Federation of America and the National Abortion Federation, have adopted the evidence-based regimen.[52,53]

Methotrexate and misoprostol regimens

Methotrexate stops cell division by blocking folic acid metabolism, proliferating trophoblastic tissue, and fetal cell division. Used in combination with misoprostol, it is 94% to 96% successful in terminating early pregnancy through 7 weeks (49 days) of gestation dated from the LMP.[22,38,54]

Several methotrexate-misoprostol protocols are currently used. At the first visit, the woman receives either 50 mg methotrexate per square meter of body surface, or a standard dose of 50 to 75 mg. Methotrexate can be administered intramuscularly in the gluteal muscle or given orally,[55] mixed with orange juice to disguise the taste. Three to 7 days after methotrexate treatment, misoprostol 800 mcg is inserted vaginally. Although some protocols have instructed the woman to moisten the misoprostol before insertion, subsequent research has shown that this practice does not improve efficacy.[56] Some protocols call for a second dose of misoprostol if bleeding has not begun within 24 hours of the initial misoprostol dose.

The woman returns for a follow-up visit 3 to 7 days after the initial misoprostol administration. If complete abortion is not confirmed by bimanual vaginal examination or vaginal ultrasound, or if her hCG level has not declined by at least 50%, she may be offered an additional dose of misoprostol or a vacuum aspiration. For those accepting an additional misoprostol dose, weekly follow-up is scheduled for a month or longer, if the woman opts to keep waiting for abortion to be completed without intervention. If the viable pregnancy persists for 2 weeks after treatment, aspiration abortion is recommended.

PROVIDING FIRST-TRIMESTER MEDICATION ABORTION

Assessing pregnancy accurately, identifying possible ectopic pregnancy, and assuring the availability of appropriate management are capabilities essential for any clinician who provides care for reproductive age women who may be pregnant. These capabilities are needed when a woman with any pregnancy presents for evaluation or experiences early pregnancy problems, such as bleeding, or bleeding and pain, that could indicate ectopic pregnancy or impending spontaneous abortion.

Providing medical abortion does not require specialized facilities; a typical medical office with space for private consultation, physical exam, equipment and medication for handling a medication allergic reaction, and arrangements or facilities for a urine pregnancy test and Rh typing is sufficient. In addition, you need to plan for emergency back-up and/or referral, 24-hour telephone emergency accessibility, and staff training. Practical issues to be considered also include state requirements, if any, specific to the provision of abortion services. Several organizations can provide additional information about these issues, including the National Abortion Federation (see www.prochoice.org).

A woman undergoing medication abortion needs detailed information about the regimen chosen, clear instructions about what to expect (timing of events, amount of bleeding, pregnancy tissue and embryonic tissue she may see, and possible emotions she may experience), how to use pain medication, warning signs and possible complications (see Table 28-4), and what to do if she has questions or needs help with a possible problem. She should also understand that she may need an aspiration procedure if the medical abortion is incomplete or unsuccessful. Approximately 1% to 4% of women using a mifepristone and misoprostol regimen will require vacuum aspiration for these reasons.[54,62]

If the woman will be using the misoprostol at home, she should be instructed to use the tablets when she can rest afterward, drink fluids to avoid feeling dizzy when rising, eat lightly because of the possibility of nausea or vomiting, insert the tablets deep into the vagina with clean fingers, and expect cramping and bleeding to begin within the next 2 to 4 hours.

In the United States, mifepristone is sold directly only to prescribers who agree to provide each patient with a Medication Guide supplied by the manufacturer, report any adverse events, and affirm that they are able to assess accurately the duration of pregnancy, diagnose ectopic pregnancy, and provide or arrange for any necessary surgical intervention. Note that the provider agreement does not require that clinicians prescribing mifepristone personally provide ultrasound evaluation or surgical intervention. Information and forms necessary to enroll as a mifepristone provider are available at the manufacturer's website, www.earlyoptionpill.com.

Table 28-4 Warning signs after abortion

- Fever (temperature of 100.4° F or more) that is sustained, or begins later than 6 to 8 hours after misoprostol
- Chills
- Abdominal pain, cramping, or backache (severe)
- Tenderness (to pressure) in the abdomen
- Prolonged or heavy bleeding (more than 2 soaked pads per hour for 2 hours)
- Foul vaginal discharge
- Delay (6 weeks or more) in resuming menstrual periods

Clinical Management

No matter which drug combination or regimen is used, women undergoing medication abortion are likely to experience cramping and bleeding; these are expected effects, rather than side effects. Women typically describe the experience as similar to spontaneous abortion in early pregnancy. In most cases, pain can be managed with aspirin or acetaminophen (Tylenol), a non-steroidal anti-inflammatory such as ibuprofen, or acetaminophen with codeine phosphate (300 mg/30 mg).[62] Non-steroidal anti-inflammatory agents such as ibuprofen do not interfere with the effectiveness of misoprostol.[63]

Although bleeding may seem abundant to those experiencing it, the amount of bleeding is rarely clinically significant. One study of mifepristone used with a vaginal prostaglandin to treat women through 63 days dated from the LMP found that median blood loss was only about 75 mls[64] compared with the 50 mls typically lost during menses or the nearly 500 mls typically given in a blood donation. The range of bleeding, however, can extend up to several hundred milliliters and is significantly correlated to length of gestation. Bleeding and spotting duration is also variable. Women in a U.S. study of mifepristone with misoprostol reported bleeding for a median of 13 days.[65]

Heavy bleeding, if the woman experiences it, typically occurs while the abortion is happening, and persists for 1 to 4 hours.[65] No evaluation or treatment is needed unless bleeding soaks two or more large pads per hour for two consecutive hours. Some clinicians treat excessive bleeding with an ergot alkaloid such as methylergonovine maleate (Methergine) before resorting to aspiration. Bleeding significant enough to require aspiration is rare and is most likely to occur 1 to 3 weeks after the woman has taken the medications. Approximately 1% of women experience uterine bleeding that requires vacuum aspiration; about 0.1% require transfusion.[45,65]

Side effects common with all medical abortion regimens include nausea, headache, vomiting, diarrhea, dizziness, fever, and chills. These side effects are also the systemic effects of misoprostol and subside within a few hours as the medication clears from the body. Temperature elevation (100.4° F or more) that is sustained, or begins later than 6 to 8 hours after misoprostol administration, however, should prompt a clinical assessment.

SECOND-TRIMESTER ABORTION

Dilation and evacuation (D&E) procedures are used for almost all second trimester abortion procedures in the United States. Although D&E requires surgical expertise, it is safer than older methods for medical induction[25] and does not involve a prolonged hospital stay. Only 0.2% of abortions reported to the CDC in 1999 were intrauterine instillation procedures—the second trimester medical induction approach commonly used in the 1970s and 1980s.[15] Instillation methods used in the past involved amnioinfusion to "instill" hypertonic saline or urea into the amniotic fluid, augmented by uterotonic drugs such as pitocin or prostaglandin to strengthen uterine contractions. In addition, osmotic cervical dilators were often placed before or at the time of the amnioinfusion to hasten cervical dilation and decrease the risk for cervical laceration.

Newer approaches to medical induction utilize mifepristone and misoprostol. This alternative is recommended by the Royal College of Obstetricians and Gynaecologists (RCOG) in the United Kingdom for abortion at 15 weeks and beyond in settings where specialized skills for D&E are not available.[66] The regimens recommended by RCOG include mifepristone 200 mg orally, followed 36 to 48 hours later by misoprostol 800 mcg vaginally, then misoprostol 400 mcg orally every 3 hours to a maximum of 4 oral doses.[66] Success rates as high as 97% have been reported for second trimester (13-21 weeks amenorrhea) abortion utilizing mifepristone and misoprostol.[67]

SECOND-TRIMESTER DILATION AND EVACUATION (D&E)

D&E, which combines vacuum aspiration with use of forceps,[25] is widely available for procedures performed between 13 and 16 weeks' gestation, and experts use this method through 20 or more weeks. An accurate estimate of the gestational age is crucial; intraoperative sonography may be used. The cervix requires more dilation for a D&E than for a first trimester aspiration, because the products of conception in the second trimester are larger. Pre-operative cervical dilation using osmotic dilators, or with misoprostol, is usually required as part of the D&E process. Steps in the procedure are similar to those described for aspiration above. After administering a cervical anesthesia or general anesthetic, remove the osmotic dilators. Use mechanical dilators if additional dilation of the cervix is needed. A large vacuum cannula, and other instruments as needed, are then used to evacuate the fetus and placenta from the uterus.

ADJUNCTIVE TECHNIQUES

Several adjunctive techniques are commonly used for second-trimester abortions and can be used for first-trimester aspiration abortion.

Osmotic dilators. Dried seaweed of the genus Laminaria is highly hygroscopic (absorbs water and expands) and can, over a period of time, dilate the cervix. Synthetic hygroscopic dilators—Lamicel, a magnesium sulfate-impregnated sponge or Dilapan, a polyacrylonitrile rod—produce faster cervical dilation than laminaria, although Lamicel is not as effective when wide dilation is needed. Osmotic dilators are effective and relatively painless, and they decrease the risk of cervical laceration or perforation.[7,25] Place osmotic dilators (one or two for procedures through 14 to 16 weeks; more for later procedures) the day before aspiration or D&E, or

2 to 4 hours beforehand for a one-day procedure using Lamicel or laminaria. Several serial insertions of an increasing number of dilators may be used for procedures later in gestation. Place the dilators so they extend through the endocervical canal and dilate both the internal os and the external os. Following placement of laminaria, most of the cervical expansion occurs by 6 hours, but maximum dilation occurs in 12 to 24 hours; dilation occurs in a shorter interval with use of Dilapan or Lamicel.

Misoprostol. Treatment with oral, buccal or vaginal misoprostol administered 2 or more hours prior to aspiration abortion or D&E causes cervical softening and dilation (called ripening) that can reduce or eliminate the need for additional mechanical dilation. Various regimens have been evaluated. For example, good results have been reported with use of misoprostol, 400 mcg administered vaginally 3 to 4 hours prior or sublingually 2 hours prior to first trimester aspiration,[26,27] and misoprostol, 600 mcg administered buccally 2 to 4 hours prior to second trimester D&E.[28] "Optimal" regimens, however, are not yet well defined, and this approach has the potential problem of inducing abortion (not just cervical preparation), so it may not be satisfactory for home administration. Also, side effects including nausea, vomiting, diarrhea, and fever can occur with misoprostol; rare cases of uterine rupture, most in women who had a scar from a previous uterine surgery, have been reported following misoprostol use in the second trimester.

Oxytocin or vasopressin. These agents strengthen uterine contractility and constrict blood vessels. They may be used intravenously or as part of the cervical anesthetic to reduce the amount of bleeding.

CAUTIONS AND PRECAUTIONS

There are no evidence-based contraindications to abortion, although severe anemia and hypotension are considered reasons for caution with any abortion procedure. Some medical conditions or problems may influence the decision about which method of abortion or clinical setting would be safest for the woman. No data are available about use of medical abortion regimens while breastfeeding.

Although the teratogenicity of mifepristone may not be of concern, it must be considered when methotrexate is used, or when either is used in combination with misoprostol. Fetal abnormalities have been reported in association with misoprostol exposure. Medication abortion options, therefore, should be used only when the woman is certain that she does not want to be pregnant, and aspiration should be considered if attempted medication abortion is unsuccessful.[6]

Contraindications to use of mifepristone

- Confirmed or suspected ectopic pregnancy or undiagnosed adnexal mass (methotrexate may be used)
- IUD in place (must be removed before treatment)

- Adrenal failure
- Current long-term systemic corticosteroid therapy
- History of allergy to mifepristone
- Hemorrhagic disorder or current anti-coagulant therapy
- Inherited porphyria

Contraindications to use of methotrexate

- Chronic renal or hepatic disease

  Note: Women should discontinue using vitamins containing folate for one week after taking methotrexate.

Contraindications to use of misoprostol

- Allergy to misoprostol or other prostaglandins
- Uncontrolled seizure disorder
- Acute inflammatory bowel disease

PREVENTING ABORTION COMPLICATIONS

Compared with childbirth, as well as with other surgical procedures, legal abortion is remarkably safe.[18] In the two largest studies of legally induced abortions reported to date, the rate of major complications is less than 1 in 200 cases.[5,68] Abortions are safer when performed early in pregnancy and clinicians in the community responsible for emergency care are well informed about abortion and about appropriate management of rare but potentially serious problems. Because teenagers tend to have abortions later in gestation than do adult women, they as a group experience more complications. Adjusted for length of gestation, however, teenagers have fewer complications than do older women.[69] Also influencing the risk of complication is the abortion method: dilation and evacuation, for example, is significantly safer than instillation procedures for pregnancies 13 to 20 weeks post LMP.[25]

Abortion-related problems are less likely under these conditions:

- The pregnancy is early.
- The woman is healthy.
- The woman does not have bacterial vaginosis, gonorrhea or chlamydial infection of the cervix.
- The woman understands the warning signs for potential postabortal problems.
- Prompt follow-up care is available on a 24-hour basis.
- Antibiotics are given to all aspiration patients.
- Osmotic dilators are used when appropriate.
- Local anesthesia is used in preference to general anesthesia.
- The uterus is carefully and completely emptied.

- The clinician carefully examines the aspirated tissue following an aspiration procedure to rule out the possibility of a molar or ectopic pregnancy.
- Rho(D) immune globulin (RhoGAM) is given to D-negative women.

Providing antibiotics to all patients can reduce infection complications following aspiration abortion.[70] A common regimen is 100 mg of doxycycline, taken twice a day for 3 to 7 days. Many providers wait until after the procedure to begin the antibiotics because of the problem of nausea and vomiting. Although some providers use additional antibiotic prophylaxis for women who may be at increased risk for subacute bacterial endocarditis, neither the American College of Obstetricians and Gynecologists nor the American Heart Association recommend preoperative endocarditis prophylaxis for uninfected therapeutic abortion procedures.[71,72]

A woman's risk of dying from a legal abortion decreased significantly between 1972 and 1990, and abortion deaths are now very rare.[24] In 1972, the case fatality rate was 4.1 deaths per 100,000 legal abortions. By 1990, the rate had declined over 90% to 0.3 deaths per 100,000 procedures. (The CDC has not estimated national case fatality rates for recent years because the lack of data for four nonreporting states means that an appropriate denominator for the rate is unknown.[15]) Legal-abortion mortality is related to the age and general health of the woman, the length of gestation, and the type of procedure used. Serious but unrelated health problems at the time of abortion, complications from general anesthesia, and pulmonary embolism are important contributors to abortion mortality.[73]

MEDICATION ABORTION COMPLICATIONS

Medical abortion using mifepristone has proven safe and effective. A review of the reports from the 108 Planned Parenthood sites that provided mifepristone during the first year found a 99.5% efficacy in terminating pregnancy and only 18 reports of adverse events among 8,799 patients—a rate of 0.02.[74] Adverse events included the following:

- Allergic reaction (hives)
- Ruptured cornual ectopic pregnancy, not diagnosed on ultrasound, treated surgically
- Vomiting and severe bleeding treated with rehydration and aspiration
- Endometritis (2 cases) requiring intravenous antibiotic treatment
- Heavy bleeding (6 cases) requiring emergency room care
- Heavy bleeding (5 cases) requiring transfusion and vacuum aspiration

The cases of heavy bleeding that required transfusion were not related to immediate, catastrophic hemorrhage but rather to persistent, ongoing bleeding that required treatment between 10 days and 4 weeks following the medication regimen.[74] Patients and providers, therefore, need to be aware that ongoing bleeding should be evaluated even if the findings appeared "normal" on the follow-up exam.

Serious adverse events reported to the manufacturer following early medical abortion using mifepristone were summarized 18 months after approval of the drug in a "Dear Health Care Provider" letter,[75] and in a review article based on the experience of an estimated 80,000 women treated during that time.[76] These included two fatalities—one caused by hemorrhage from a ruptured ectopic pregnancy and the other by systemic bacterial infection—as well as a second serious infection and a non-fatal myocardial infarction occurring in a 21-year-old woman 3 days following use of mifepristone and misoprostol. One additional infection death occurred in 2003. Although a causal relationship to the use of mifepristone was not established for these adverse events, providers were reminded to be aware of the possibility of unrecognized ectopic pregnancy or infection throughout the treatment period. In all three cases, more knowledgeable and prompt management might have made a difference in the outcome. False reassurance based on an incorrect ultrasound confirmation of intrauterine pregnancy may have delayed the patient's recognition of her ectopic pregnancy symptoms, and pain incorrectly attributed to the expected effects of abortion medications may have delayed diagnosis and treatment for infection. The total number of U.S. women treated with mifepristone regimens during this interval is not known, but was estimated to be more than 100,000 within the first 24 months after approval,[77] and at least 200,000 by the end of 2003.[78]

MANAGING POSTABORTION COMPLICATIONS

Take seriously any complaint or problem after an abortion procedure. Inform all abortion patients about warning signs to watch for (see Table 28-4), and tell them how to contact you in case of questions or a possible problem. Prompt recognition and management can be critical in preventing a serious outcome.

Immediate and short-term complications.

Abortion complications, while not common, include the following immediate and short-term problems. Minimize adverse health outcomes by prompt detection and appropriate treatment.

Infection. Infection rates reported in U.S. studies following first trimester aspiration abortion range from 0.1% to 1.3% and are lower for medication abortion.[7] Rates are slightly higher, 0.4% to 2.0%, following second trimester aspiration or induction.[7] Minimize the risk of postabortal infection by screening for and treating bacterial vaginosis, gonorrhea, and chlamydia before the abortion; by emptying the uterus completely; and by administering prophylactic antibiotics in conjunction with vacuum aspiration abortion. Persistent cramping, abdominal pain, fever, discharge, malaise, and pelvic discomfort are possible symptoms of infection. Advise women to seek help immediately if any warning symptoms develop after the procedure (see Warning Signs after Abortion). If you suspect the presence of retained products of conception, initiate antibiotics and arrange for vacuum aspiration to remove them. If the infection has extended beyond the uterus, hospitalize the woman and administer parenteral antibiotics.

Intrauterine blood clots. Intrauterine blood clots can occur immediately or as long as 5 days after an aspiration abortion; their presence is manifested by severe cramping and pain. The syndrome, sometimes called "postabortal" or "redo" syndrome, is uncommon—occurring after approximately 0.02% of first-trimester vacuum aspiration abortion procedures[7]—and is diagnosed by a pelvic exam finding of a large, tense, and tender uterus with little or no bleeding from the cervix. A simple vacuum aspiration remedies the problem; pain and cramping resolve within a few minutes.

Incomplete abortion. When part of the fetal or decidual tissue remains in the uterus, the abortion procedure is "incomplete." This problem occurs following approximately 0.3% to 2% of aspiration procedures[7] and 1.4% of medication abortion procedures.[79] Retained tissue is likely to cause continued bleeding and cramping that prompt the woman to seek care. Treatment with misoprostol or vacuum aspiration is appropriate.

Continuing pregnancy. In rare cases, an attempt to terminate pregnancy fails altogether (about 0.03% to 0.05% of aspiration procedures[7] and 0.5% to 1% of early medication abortions).[7,68,74] A woman with a continuing pregnancy may have ongoing symptoms of pregnancy and a soft or enlarged uterus. Ultrasound or a low-sensitivity pregnancy test may be helpful in identifying this problem. Aspiration to terminate the pregnancy is appropriate treatment. If the aspiration is not successful, consider the possibility of an abnormal uterus (e.g., bicornuate or cavity distorted by fibroids), in which case ultrasound guidance during aspiration may be helpful; also consider the possibility of unsuspected ectopic pregnancy.

Ongoing pregnancy after failed medication or aspiration abortion potentially involves an increased risk for fetal malformation, so the woman should be encouraged to consider carefully before deciding to continue the pregnancy to term. There is no evidence that exposure to mifepristone is associated with an increased risk for fetal abnormality, but other medical abortion drugs and aspiration may pose risks. Injury to the fetus during the attempted aspiration could, for example, cause limb defects. Case reports have linked methotrexate to limb defects and misoprostol to congenital abnormalities including limb defects, skull defects, and Möbius sequence.[80,81] Whether or not these cases reflect a true causal relationship is not known, and the magnitude of risk, if any, is also unknown because the prevalence of exposure to the drugs involved (methotrexate and misoprostol) is not known.

Cervical, uterine, or abdominal organ trauma. Cervical tears can occur with mechanical dilation; in most cases, management involves only pressure and observation or suture. Similarly, a small midline uterine perforation can safely be managed with careful observation for 2 to 4 hours, and hospitalization may not be necessary if there is no evidence of internal bleeding, abdominal pain, or rebound tenderness. More severe cervical or uterine trauma, and perforation with damage to nearby abdominal vessels or other organs, are rare—reported rates range from 0.009 % to 0.2%.[7] Depending on their severity, these complications may require exploratory surgery to identify and repair the uterus or abdominal organ injury, or even hysterectomy. The risk for trauma is reduced when osmotic dilators or misoprostol are used for cervical preparation, thereby avoiding the need for forceful mechanical cervical dilation. Perforation risk may also be reduced by avoiding the use of a uterine sound as part of aspiration abortion, by avoiding a "routine check" of the uterine cavity with a sharp curet,[7] and by using local rather than general anesthesia.

Uterine rupture has been reported with use of misoprostol for induction of labor at term and in conjunction with other uterotonic agents in second-trimester medical abortion. This catastrophic complication is very rare; an incidence estimate based on 14 cases reported in the United States is 2 ruptures per 100,000 second-trimester induction procedures; the incidence may be higher for women who have had a previous cesarean section delivery.[41]

Bleeding. Regardless of whether they have undergone medication or aspiration methods, almost all women have at least some bleeding during and after an abortion. The absence of bleeding is a warning sign that merits evaluation to be sure that pregnancy has been terminated. Typically, bleeding persists for at least several days, with light bleeding or spotting continuing for as long as 2 to 4 weeks.

Promptly evaluate the source of bleeding that is very heavy (more than 2 large pads soaked per hour for 2 consecutive hours) or heavy bleeding that continues longer than a few days. Problem bleeding may be caused by retained decidua or fetal tissue, which may require aspiration. Heavy bleeding that immediately follows the aspiration procedure may be managed with uterotonic agents or a repeat aspiration. After medical abortion, approximately 1% of women require aspiration or curettage to stop bleeding, and in rare cases, transfusion (0.1%).[64,65,82]

OVERALL HEALTH EFFECTS AND LONG-TERM COMPLICATIONS

Once pregnant, a woman can decide to terminate or continue her pregnancy. One key question with regard to long-term effects is whether a woman who decides to terminate her pregnancy faces greater risk of future adverse outcomes than she would were she to decide to continue the pregnancy. Because the immediate risks of death and of serious medical complications are so much lower for abortion than for full-term pregnancy, the *overall* health risks are much lower for abortion. The risk of pregnancy-related death was 13.2 per 100,000 live births in 1999,[83] and nearly 43% of women who give birth have some kind of maternal morbidity (including cesarean delivery).[84] The risk of death related to abortion is less than 1 in 100,000 cases,[15] and serious morbidity risk is less than 1%.[7]

Women appropriately ask about possible long-term health effects. Public debate about long-term effects has been used as a rationale for limiting women's access to legal abortion services. Several thoughtful and reassuring reviews of this topic have been published, including the conclusion by Surgeon General Everett Koop in 1989 that he found no evidence of medical or psychological harm. The evidence is summarized in Paul's *Clinician's Guide to Medical and Surgical Abortion.*[7] As new research findings are published, pay attention to the quality of study design and the criteria for determining causality. Conclusions in three key areas are briefly summarized below.

FUTURE REPRODUCTIVE HEALTH AND FERTILITY

First-trimester aspiration abortion is not associated with a measurable increased risk for subsequent fertility impairment and does not increase the woman's risk for spontaneous abortion, preterm delivery, or having a low birth–weight infant.[85] Subsequent fertility outcomes following medication abortion have not been reported, but the fact that medication abortion is less invasive than aspiration and has fewer infection complications provides reassurance.

Studies of ectopic pregnancy risk following first-trimester aspiration have been less conclusive, but none have found a statistically significant association. An increased risk for spontaneous abortion and preterm or low birthweight delivery has been reported for abortion with dilation and sharp curettage (D&C) and may be associated with a second-trimester D&E.[7]

PSYCHIATRIC PROBLEMS

Major psychiatric problems following abortion are rare.[32,86] Studies of psychiatric hospitalization rates have found that the incidence of serious psychiatric illness is approximately 10% after a birth, but less than 1% following induced abortion.[7] Transient feelings of stress or sadness may follow what is sometimes a difficult decision to terminate a pregnancy.[87] By contrast, feelings of relief are also common. Although "abortion trauma syndrome" has been described in materials distributed by lay groups, there is no such syndrome defined in peer-reviewed scientific literature or in the professional diagnostic codes. The characteristics described—such as persistent guilt and sadness—are conclusions of self-selected groups of women, in some cases linked to religious groups. If incapacitating dysphoric emotional responses were common, however, this association would be evident because abortion is a very common procedure.

BREAST CANCER

The question of whether induced abortion has any effect on subsequent breast cancer risk has received intense scrutiny. Full-term pregnancy has a dichotomous influence on breast tissue: during early pregnancy there is an increase in growth of breast tissue due to the stimulus of estrogens; later in pregnancy, differentiation of mammary tissue occurs. The differentiation effect is apparently related to a decrease in a future risk for breast cancer among women who have at least one full-term pregnancy.[88] Epidemiologic research on this topic is complex because of study design problems that could lead to spurious association. For example, ascertainment bias is a particular hazard, because the sensitive nature of abortion can affect a woman's willingness to report a previous experience, and several epidemiology studies have reported an apparent increase in risk. The most comprehensive analysis of induced abortion and breast cancer to date, based on the Danish population-based experience, found no association between induced abortion and breast cancer.[89] Also, the National Cancer Institute's (NCI) board of scientific advisers has reviewed and accepted the recommendations of an NCI expert workshop convened in February 2003, which reviewed the available research and concluded that there is no evidence of a true association between induced abortion and subsequent breast cancer risk.[90]

ROUTINE POSTABORTION CARE AND CONTRACEPTION

Fertility returns quickly following abortion. Ovulation, and with it the possibility of another pregnancy, may occur as soon as 10 days after abortion. Helping a woman initiate an effective method of contraception is an essential task in providing abortion care, and should not be deferred to a follow-up visit. If the unplanned pregnancy occurred while the woman was using a contraceptive, help her identify any personal or situational factors that may have contributed to the contraceptive failure. Also, explain the availability of emergency contraception and provide a supply she can have on hand at home in case of future need.

The woman may start a hormonal method of contraception immediately after an aspiration abortion or as soon as she wishes after using abortion medications. Many providers initiate the hormonal method the same day, or any time within the first 7 days for oral contraceptives and injectables, or any time within the first 5 days for the patch or ring. An IUD can safely be inserted at the conclusion of an aspiration procedure or at the time abortion is confirmed following medical abortion. If the woman anticipates that she will need contraception, there is no reason to delay—even if she will temporarily be abstaining from intercourse following aspiration.

REFERENCES

1. Henshaw SK. Unintended pregnancy in the United States. Fam Plann Perspect 1998;30(1):24-29, 46.
2. Edwards J, Carson SA. New technologies permit safe abortion at less than six weeks' gestation and provide timely detection of ectopic gestation. Am J Obstet Gynecol 1997;176(5):1101-1106.
3. Baird DT, Grimes DA, VanLook PFA. Modern methods of inducing abortion. Oxford; Cambridge, Mass.: Blackwell Science; 1995.
4. Darney P, Morbuch P, Korn A. Protocols on office gynecology surgery. London, UK: Blackwell Science; 1996.
5. Grimes DA. Management of abortion. In: Te Linde RW, Thompson JD, Rock JA, eds. Te Linde's operative gynecology. 8th ed. Philadelphia: Lippincott-Raven; 1997.
6. Stewart FH, Wells ES, Flinn SK, Weitz TA. Early medical abortion: issues for practice. San Francisco, CA: University of California, San Francisco Center for Reproductive Health Research & Policy; 2001.
7. Paul M. A Clinician's guide to medical and surgical abortion. New York: Churchill Livingstone; 1999.
8. American College of Obstetricians and Gynecologists (ACOG). Medical Management of Abortion: American College of Obstetricians and Gynecologists; 2001.
9. Cates W, Jr., Grimes DA, Hogue LL. Justice Blackmun and legal abortion—a besieged legacy to women's reproductive health. Am J Public Health. Sep 1995; 85(9):1204-1206.
10. Annas GJ. The Supreme Court, liberty, and abortion. N Engl J Med 1992;327(9): 651-654.
11. Cates W, Jr., Gold J, Selik RM. Regulation of abortion services—for better or worse? N Engl J Med 1979;301(13):720-723.
12. Grimes DA, Forrest JD, Kirkman AL, Radford B. An epidemic of antiabortion violence in the United States. Am J Obstet Gynecol 1991;165(5 Pt 1):1263-1268.
13. Cates W, Jr., Grimes DA, Schulz KF. The public health impact of legal abortion: 30 years later. Perspect Sex Reprod Health 2003;35(1):25-28.
14. Centers for Disease Control (CDC). Abortion surveillance: preliminary analysis— United States, 1994. MMWR 1997;45:1123-1127.
15. Elam-Evans LD, Strauss LT, Herndon J, Parker WY, Whitehead S, Berg CJ. Abortion surveillance—United States, 1999. MMWR Surveill Summ. Nov 29 2002;51(9):1-9, 11-28.
16. Henshaw SK, Van Vort J. Abortion services in the United States, 1991 and 1992. Fam Plann Perspect 1994;26(3):100-106, 112.
17. Finer LB, Henshaw SK. Abortion incidence and services in the United States in 2000. Perspect Sex Reprod Health 2003;35(1):6-15.
18. Cates W, Jr. Legal abortion: the public health record. Science. Mar 26 1982;215 (4540):1586-1590.
19. Winikoff B. Acceptability of medical abortion in early pregnancy. Fam Plann Perspect 1995;27(4):142-148, 185.
20. Blayo C. L'Evolution du Recours à L'Avortement en France Depuis 1976. Population. 1995;50(3):779-810.
21. Cameron ST, Glasier AF, Logan J, Benton L, Baird DT. Impact of the introduction of new medical methods on therapeutic abortions at the Royal Infirmary of Edinburgh. Br J Obstet Gynaecol 1996;103(12):1222-1229.
22. Wiebe ER. Abortion induced with methotrexate and misoprostol. Can Med Assoc J 1996;154(2):165-170.

23. Jones RK, Henshaw SK. Mifepristone for early medical abortion: experiences in France, Great Britain and Sweden. Perspect Sex Reprod Health 2002;34(3):154-161.
24. Koonin LM, Smith JC, Ramick M, Green CA. Abortion surveillance—United States, 1992. MMWR Surveill Summ 1996;45(3):1-36.
25. Grimes DA, Schulz KF, Cates W, Jr., Tyler CW, Jr. Mid-trimester abortion by dilation and evacuation: a safe and practical alternative. N Engl J Med 1977; 296(20):1141-1145.
26. Ashok PW, Flett GM, Templeton A. Mifepristone versus vaginally administered misoprostol for cervical priming before first-trimester termination of pregnancy: a randomized, controlled study. Am J Obstet Gynecol 2000;183(4):998-1002.
27. Vimala N, Mittal S, Kumar S. Sublingual misoprostol for preabortion cervical ripening in first-trimester pregnancy termination. Contraception 2003;67(4):295-297.
28. Todd CS, Soler M, Castleman L, Rogers MK, Blumenthal PD. Buccal misoprostol as cervical preparation for second trimester pregnancy termination. Contraception 2002;65(6):415-418.
29. Aubeny E, Peyron R, Turpin CL, Renault M, Targosz V, Silvestre L, Ulmann A, Baulieu EE. Termination of early pregnancy (up to 63 days of amenorrhea) with mifepristone and increasing doses of misoprostol [corrected]. Int J Fertil Menopausal Stud 1995;40 Suppl 2:85-91.
30. Peyron R, Aubeny E, Targosz V, Silvestre L, Renault M, Elkik F, Leclerc P, Ulmann A, Baulieu EE. Early termination of pregnancy with mifepristone (RU 486) and the orally active prostaglandin misoprostol. N Engl J Med 1993;328(21):1509-1513.
31. Silvestre L, Dubois C, Renault M, Rezvani Y, Baulieu EE, Ulmann A. Voluntary interruption of pregnancy with mifepristone (RU 486) and a prostaglandin analogue. A large-scale French experience. N Engl J Med 1990;322(10):645-648.
32. Urquhart DR, Templeton AA. Psychiatric morbidity and acceptability following medical and surgical methods of induced abortion. Br J Obstet Gynaecol 1991; 98(4):396-399.
33. Winikoff B, Sivin I, Coyaji KJ, Cabezas E, Xiao B, Gu S, Du MK, Krishna UR, Eschen A, Ellertson C. Safety, efficacy, and acceptability of medical abortion in China, Cuba, and India: a comparative trial of mifepristone-misoprostol versus surgical abortion. Am J Obstet Gynecol 1997;176(2):431-437.
34. Ngoc NTN, Winikoff B, Clark S, Ellertson C, Am KN, Hieu DT, Elul B. Safety, efficacy and acceptability of mifepristone-misoprostol medical abortion in Vietnam. Intl Fam Plann Perspect 1999; 25(1):10-14,33.
35. Coyaji K, Elul B, Krishna U, Otiv S, Ambardekar S, Bopardikar A, Raote, V, Ellerston C, Winikoff B. Mifepristone abortion outside the urban research hospital setting in India. Lancet 13 2001;357(9250):120-122.
36. Creinin MD, Darney PD. Methotrexate and misoprostol for early abortion. Contraception 1993;48(4):339-348.
37. Creinin MD, Park M. Acceptability of medical abortion with methotrexate and misoprostol. Contraception 1995;52(1):41-44.
38. Hausknecht RU. Methotrexate and misoprostol to terminate early pregnancy. N Engl J Med 1995;333(9):537-540.
39. Lipscomb GH, Stovall TG, Ling FW. Nonsurgical treatment of ectopic pregnancy. N Engl J Med 2000;343(18):1325-1329.
40. Schaff EA, Eisinger SH, Franks P, Kim SS. Combined methotrexate and misoprostol for early induced abortion. Arch Fam Med 1995;4(9):774-779.
41. Goldberg AB, Greenberg MB, Darney PD. Misoprostol and pregnancy. N Engl J Med 2001;344(1):38-47.
42. Coelho HL, Teixeira AC, Santos AP, et al. Misoprostol and illegal abortion in Fortaleza, Brazil. Lancet 1993;341(8855):1261-1263.
43. Creinin MD, Pymar HC, Schwartz JL. Mifepristone 100 mg in abortion regimens. Obstet Gynecol 2001;98(3):434-439.
44. Schaff EA, Eisinger SH, Stadalius LS, Franks P, Gore BZ, Poppema S. Low-dose mifepristone 200 mg and vaginal misoprostol for abortion. Contraception 1999; 59(1):1-6.

45. World Health Organisation Task Force on Post-ovulatory Methods of Fertility Regulation. Termination of pregnancy with reduced doses of mifepristone. Br Med J 1993;307(6903):532-537.
46. World Health Organisation Task Force on Post-ovulatory Methods of Fertility Regulation. Comparison of two doses of mifepristone in combination with misoprostol for early medical abortion: a randomised trial. Br J Obstet Gynaecol 2000; 107(4):524-530.
47. El-Refaey H, Rajasekar D, Abdalla M, Calder L, Templeton A. Induction of abortion with mifepristone (RU 486) and oral or vaginal misoprostol. N Engl J Med 1995;332(15):983-987.
48. El-Refaey H, Templeton A. Early induction of abortion by a combination of oral mifepristone and misoprostol administered by the vaginal route. Contraception 1994;49(2):111-114.
49. Schaff EA, Stadalius LS, Eisinger SH, Franks P. Vaginal misoprostol administered at home after mifepristone (RU486) for abortion. J Fam Pract 1997;44(4):353-360.
50. Schaff EA, Fielding SL, Westhoff C, et al. Vaginal misoprostol administered 1, 2, or 3 days after mifepristone for early medical abortion: A randomized trial. J Am Med Assoc 2000;284(15):1948-1953.
51. Ellertson C, Elul B, Winikoff B. Can women use medical abortion without medical supervision? Reprod Health Matters 1997(9):149-161.
52. National Abortion Federation. Clinical policy guidelines. Washington, D.C.: National Abortion Federation; 2003.
53. Anonymous. News from the National Medical Committee. Mife matters: a publication of the PPFA/CAPS Medical Abortion Training Program, 2002: 1.
54. Kahn JG, Becker BJ, MacIsaa L, et al. The efficacy of medical abortion: a meta-analysis. Contraception 2000;61(1):29-40.
55. Wiebe ER. Oral methotrexate compared with injected methotrexate when used with misoprostol for abortion. Am J Obstet Gynecol 1999;181(1):149-152.
56. Creinin MD, Carbonell JL, Schwartz JL, Varela L, Tanda R. A randomized trial of the effect of moistening misoprostol before vaginal administration when used with methotrexate for abortion. Contraception 1999;59(1):11-16.
57. Jain JK, Harwood B, Meckstroth KR, Mishell DR. Early pregnancy termination with vaginal misoprostol combined with loperamide and acetaminophen prophylaxis. Contraception 2001;63(4):217-221.
58. Koopersmith TB, Mishell DR, Jr. The use of misoprostol for termination of early pregnancy. Contraception 1996;53(4):238-242.
59. Esteve JL, Varela L, Velazco A, Tanda R, Cabezas E, Sanchez C. Early abortion with 800 micrograms of misoprostol by the vaginal route. Contraception 1999;59(4): 219-225.
60. Pymar HC, Creinin MD. Alternatives to mifepristone regimens for medical abortion. Am J Obstet Gynecol 2000;183(2 Suppl):S54-64.
61. Rosing MA, Archbald CD. The knowledge, acceptability, and use of misoprostol for self-induced medical abortion in an urban US population. J Am Med Womens Assoc. 2000;55(3 Suppl):183-185.
62. Kruse B, Poppema S, Creinin MD, Paul M. Management of side effects and complications in medical abortion. Am J Obstet Gynecol 2000;183(2 Suppl):S65-75.
63. Creinin MD, Shulman T. Effect of nonsteroidal anti-inflammatory drugs on the action of misoprostol in a regimen for early abortion. Contraception 1997;56(3): 165-168.
64. Rodger MW, Baird DT. Blood loss following induction of early abortion using mifepristone (RU 486) and a prostaglandin analogue (gemeprost). Contraception 1989;40(4):439-447.
65. Spitz IM, Bardin CW, Benton L, Robbins A. Early pregnancy termination with mifepristone and misoprostol in the United States. N Engl J Med 1998;338(18): 1241-1247.
66. Royal College of Obstetricians and Gynaecologists. The care of women requesting induced abortion. London: Guideline Development Group; 2000.

67. Ashok PW, Templeton A. Nonsurgical mid-trimester termination of pregnancy: a review of 500 consecutive cases. Br J Obstet Gynaecol 1999;106(7):706-710.
68. Hakim-Elahi E, Tovell HM, Burnhill MS. Complications of first-trimester abortion: a report of 170,000 cases. Obstet Gynecol 1990;76(1):129-135.
69. Cates W, Jr., Schulz KF, Grimes DA. The risks associated with teenage abortion. N Engl J Med 1983;309(11):621-624.
70. Sawaya GF, Grady D, Kerlikowske K, Grimes DA. Antibiotics at the time of induced abortion: the case for universal prophylaxis based on a meta-analysis. Obstet Gynecol 1996;87(5 Pt 2):884-890.
71. ACOG. ACOG Practice Bulletin. Antibiotic prophylaxis for gynecologic procedures. Washington, DC: American College of Obstetricians and Gynecologists; 2001;23.
72. Dajani AS, Taubert KA, Wilson W, Bolger AF, Bayer A, Ferrieri P, Gewitz MH, Shulman ST, Nouri S, Newberger JW, Hutto C, Pallasch TJ, Gage TW, Levison ME, Peter G, Zuccaro G Jr. Prevention of bacterial endocarditis. Recommendations by the American Heart Association. JAMA 1997;277(22):1794-1801.
73. Lawson HW, Frye A, Atrash HK, Smith JC, Shulman HB, Ramick M. Abortion mortality, United States, 1972 through 1987. Am J Obstet Gynecol 1994;171(5): 1365-1372.
74. Anonymous. A publication of the PPFA/CAPS Medical Abortion Training Program. What we've learned about mifepristone in almost 9,000 patients. MifeMatters. Vol 1; 2002:8.
75. Danco Laboratories LLC. New Safety Information. Danco Laboratories [FDA website www.fda.gov/cder/drug/infopage/mifepristone]. Accessed May 30, 2003.
76. Hausknecht R. Mifepristone and misoprostol for early medical abortion: 18 months experience in the United States. Contraception 2003;67:463-465.
77. Danco Laboratories LLC. Press Release: More than 100,000 U.S. women have chosen mifeprex for their non-surgical abortion. New York; September 24, 2002.
78. Danco Laboratories LLC., Website, Information for Health Care Professionals, http://www.earlyoptionpill.com/hcp_what.php3, accessed 15 February 2004.
79. Ashok PW, Penney GC, Flett GM, Templeton A. An effective regimen for early medical abortion: a report of 2000 consecutive cases. Hum Reprod 1998;13(1O): 2962-2965.
80. Wiebe ER. Abortion induced with methotrexate and misoprostol. CMAJ. Jan 15 1996;154(2):165-170.
81. Fonseca W, Alencar AJ, Mota FS, Coelho HL. Misoprostol and congenital malformations. Lancet 1991;338(8758):56.
82. Allen RH, Westhoff C, De Nonno L, Fielding SL, Schaff EA. Curettage after mifepristone-induced abortion: frequency, timing, and indications. Obstet Gynecol 2001;98(1):101-106.
83. Chang J, Elam-Evans LD, Berg CJ, et al. Pregnancy-related mortality surveillance— United States, 1991-1999. MMWR 2003;52(SS02):1-14.
84. Danel I, Berg C, Johnson CH, Atrash H. Magnitude of maternal morbidity during labor and delivery: United States, 1993-1997. Am J Public Health 2003;93(4):631-634.
85. Hogue CJ, Cates W, Jr., Tietze C. The effects of induced abortion on subsequent reproduction. Epidemiol Rev. 1982;4:66-94.
86. Stotland NL. The myth of the abortion trauma syndrome. JAMA 1992;268(15): 2078-2079.
87. Adler NE, David HP, Major BN, Roth SH, Russo NF, Wyatt GE. Psychological responses after abortion. Science 1990;248(4951):41-44.
88. Michels KB, Willett WC. Does induced or spontaneous abortion affect the risk of breast cancer? Epidemiology 1996;7(5):521-528.
89. Melbye M, Wohlfahrt J, Olsen JH, et al. Induced abortion and the risk of breast cancer. N Engl J Med 1997;336(2):81-85.
90. Couzin J. CANCER RISK: Review rules out abortion-cancer link. Science 2003; 299(5612):1498b-.

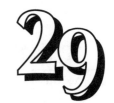

Adolescent Sexual Behavior, Pregnancy, and Childbearing

James Trussell, PhD
Sarah Brown, MSPH
Carol Hogue, PhD

- In 1997, 1 of every 9 women aged 15 to 19 years in the United States became pregnant. This proportion has dropped by 20% since 1990. This decline primarily reflects increasing proportions using effective contraception.

- Rates for both pregnancy and birth among teens in the United States are very high when compared with those in other developed countries, although rates of sexual activity are similar.

- Recent research suggests that the consequences of teenage childbearing are not as deleterious as has been claimed, but they nevertheless damage life chances for mother and child.

- While everyone agrees that teenage pregnancy is a problem, no consensus about a solution exists.

- Adolescents with a negative pregnancy test are an accessible but neglected target group for intervention.

In 1997, the latest year for which data are available, 1 in 9 women aged 15 to 19 in the United States became pregnant. Consequently, about 1.0 million pregnancies occurred to those in this age group. Another 46 thousand pregnancies occurred among women aged 14 and younger. (See Table 29-1.)[1,2] In 1999, the most recent year for which data are available, 1 in 20 women aged 15 to 19 years gave birth.[3] Of all births in the United States in 1999, 12% occurred to women younger than 20.[3] In 1999, 1 in 48 men aged 15 to 19 years fathered a child.[3] The sheer magnitude of these statistics has generated widespread public concern. The overwhelming consensus is that adolescent pregnancy is a serious problem and that public policies and programs should be implemented to reduce its incidence and ameliorate its consequences.

Table 29-1 Pregnancies, births, and abortions to adolescents (numbers in thousands): United States, 1997

Age Group	Pregnancies	Births	Abortions
15-19	1,001	483	254
<20	1,047	493	264
<15	46	10	10
15-17	432	180	98
18-19	569	303	156

Sources: Births—Ventura et al. (1999).[2]
Abortions and pregnancies—Henshaw (2001).[1]

Note:

The sum of births, induced abortions and spontaneous abortions among women aged *a* will not equal pregnancies to women aged *a*, because women are older when their pregnancies are resolved than when they are conceived. There are more births and induced abortions resulting from pregnancies to women under age 20 than there are births and induced abortions to women under age 20.

This consensus, however, offers little guidance for formulating public policy because the reasons for concern vary widely. Some view the problem primarily as a health issue, others as a moral issue, and yet others as an economic issue.

- Many object to adolescents having sex, simply because they are too young.

- Others would draw an important distinction between those who are married and those who are not. Some believe that sex among unmarried persons is unwise or immoral. Most pregnant adolescents aged 15 to 19 and virtually all those aged 14 and younger are unmarried at the time their pregnancy is resolved. Nearly 97% of births to women aged 14 and younger and 79% of births to women aged 15 to 19 occur out of wedlock.[3]

- Others would differentiate pregnancies that are intended from those that are not; 8 in 10 adolescent pregnancies are unintended.[4]

- Some, including many family planning clinicians, are particularly troubled by the large number of abortions obtained by adolescents: about 264 thousand in 1997.

- Still others view a birth to an adolescent as a tragedy, reasoning that giving birth at an early age not only seriously damages the young woman's life chances and limits her options, but also creates a suboptimal environment for the child. In 1999, 485 thousand births occurred to women under 20 years of age: 9 thousand to women under 15, 164 thousand to women aged 15 to 17, and 312 thousand to women aged 18 to 19.[3] Only 1 in 3 births to women aged 15 to 19 is intended.[5] Among births to women aged 15 to 17, 1 in 4 is fathered by a male 6 or more years older.[6]

- Most observers are particularly concerned about pregnancy, abortion, or childbearing among the poor or the very young. In 1997, 10 thousand births occurred and 10 thousand abortions were performed among women aged less than 15; another 180 thousand births occurred and 98 thousand abortions were performed among women aged 15 to 17. (See Table 29-1.) In the 1995 National Survey of Family Growth (NSFG), 55% of women aged 15 to 19 who had given birth in the previous year were at or below the poverty level, and 29% were between 101% and 250% of the poverty level.[7] In 1999, 79% of women aged 15 to 19 who gave birth were unmarried.[3]

We have identified four categories of arguments supporting public intervention to "solve" the adolescent pregnancy problem, each suggesting different intervention strategies and target groups:

Chastity promotion. Unmarried persons, especially young persons, should not engage in sexual intercourse. Our society places far too much emphasis on sex, especially in the media, and public institutions, especially the schools, have abandoned the teaching of traditional values. The solution, therefore, is a vigorous campaign to promote chastity among the unmarried. Because other strategies to reduce adolescent pregnancy (e.g., increasing the availability of contraceptive and abortion services) are thought to have the undesirable, if unintended, effect of "legitimizing" and perhaps even increasing sexual activity, they are unacceptable. The target group is very large. Almost 96% of women aged 15 to 19 have never married[8] and only 51% of these are still virgins.[9] Likewise, more than 98% of men aged 15 to 19 have never married,[8] of whom only 45% are still virgins.[9]

Pregnancy prevention. Campaigns with the sole aim of promoting chastity have not proven effective. Because such large proportions of adolescents are sexually active, it is prudent to provide young people accurate information on reproductive biology and contraception. Such information is an essential component of family life education, whose primary goal should be to promote rational and informed decision-making about sexuality. Nevertheless, providing information will not reduce pregnancy rates unless contraceptive services are also widely available. Preventing pregnancy should reduce the incidence of adolescent childbearing and abortion. The target groups are the sexually active and those about to become sexually active.

Pregnancy support and abortion services. While preventing pregnancies is an important goal, this objective will not be met in the short run.

Even if high-quality sex education and contraceptive services were universally available, some adolescents would nevertheless become pregnant. Many of them do not always plan their lives carefully. Moreover, typical contraceptive failure rates, even among more mature women, are not low (see Chapter 31 on Contraceptive Efficacy). Therefore, abortion services and programs to ameliorate the adverse consequences of adolescent childbearing must be available, particularly for the poor, who both suffer the consequences to a greater extent and generate more public costs. The target group here is much smaller, consisting of abortion services for whatever fraction of the 1 million pregnant teenagers who do not wish to carry their pregnancy to term (at least the 3 in 10 who actually obtain abortions) and ameliorative programs for the remainder.

Social Restructuring. Teenage childbearing is not the problem it appears to be; it is instead the symptom of the major underlying fundamental problem of poverty, an indicator of the extent to which many young people have been excluded from the American dream.[10] The target group is the poor and near-poor, and what is required is a fundamental restructuring of society so that young women no longer feel that they have nothing to lose by having a child at an early age. Because the problems faced by these youth are so many and so extensive, real solutions—such as better schools, safer neighborhoods, access to health care, and decent jobs for their mothers and fathers—would be very costly (and therefore very unlikely). Nevertheless, providing contraceptive and abortion services enables many poor teens to avoid childbearing.

These arguments are not mutually exclusive, and even those persons generally in agreement with one of them may not concur with all the points. Nevertheless, even this simple categorization shows the considerable discrepancies among the solutions advocated by those who view sex, those who view pregnancy, and those who view childbearing (particularly among the poor) as the main aspect of this problem and others who view teen pregnancy and childbearing not as the problem but only as a symptom. Conflict also exists (by no means limited to adolescents) about the use of abortion as a remedy for an unintended pregnancy. We return later in this chapter for further discussion of intervention strategies. Before doing so, we examine trends and levels of adolescent pregnancy in the United States, contrast the U.S. experience with that in other countries, analyze the determinants of adolescent pregnancy, examine the incidence of sexually transmitted infections (STIs) among adolescents, and analyze the consequences of adolescent childbearing.

LEVELS AND TRENDS IN ABORTION, BIRTH, AND PREGNANCY RATES

Pregnancies can end in births, induced abortions, or spontaneous abortions. Data for the United States are available for only the first two outcomes; spontaneous abortions must be estimated. In 1997 (the latest year for which estimates are available), 2% of females aged 14 became pregnant. This proportion rose steadily with age (Figure 29-1)[1,2] to reach 16% of women aged 18 and 19. The fraction of pregnancies ending in an induced abortion was virtually constant with age (about 32%).

Birth rates among women aged 15 to 19 declined steadily from 1970 to 1978, rose slightly thereafter, began to decline again in 1983 falling to a low in 1986, and rose very sharply in 1988 to a peak in 1991 and declined steadily thereafter, reaching a record low in 1999.[2] (See Figure 29-2.)[1,3,11] In contrast, *abortion rates* rose steadily from 1973 (the year abortion was legalized) to 1979, remained relatively constant through 1988, and declined thereafter, reaching a level in 1997 not observed since 1974.[1] *Pregnancy rates* rose slowly but steadily from 1973 to 1981, remained relatively constant through 1985, fell in 1986 to 1987, set successive record highs in 1988, 1989, and 1990, and dropped steadily after 1991, reaching a record low in 1997.[1] Between 1988 and 1995, the teen pregnancy rate declined from 131 to 116 per 1000 women; 75% of this decline is attributable to more effective contraception and 25% to increased abstinence.[12] (See also the section on Sexual Behavior.)

Teenage pregnancy rates among blacks are almost 3 times as high as those among whites (210 per 1,000 non-Hispanic black women versus 75 per 1,000 non-Hispanic white women aged 15 to 19 in 1997); pregnancy rates among Hispanics (193 per 1,000 women in 1997) are nearly as high as those among blacks.[1] Because blacks are more likely than whites to abort a pregnancy, the differential in birth rates is somewhat reduced: 91 births per 1,000 non-Hispanic black women versus 36 per 1,000 non-Hispanic white women aged 15 to 19 in 1997.[2] Hispanic teenagers are less likely to have an abortion than are blacks or whites. Consequently, the birth rate among 15 to 19 year-old Hispanics (97 per 1,000 women in 1997) is 2.7 times that for non-Hispanic whites and 7% higher than that for non-Hispanic blacks.[2] These racial and ethnic differentials are probably due in large part to differences in standards of living and in perceived life chances.

COMPARISON WITH EXPERIENCE IN OTHER COUNTRIES

Birth rates among women aged 15 to 19 are higher in the United States than in other developed countries.[13] (See Figure 29-3.)[13] Teenage birth rates in the United States are 4 times those in the countries of the European Union.[13] Likewise, pregnancy rates are higher in the United States than in four other countries (Canada, France, Great Britain, and Sweden) examined in a cross-national comparison. Why is the experience in the United States so different? For the five-country study, the difference

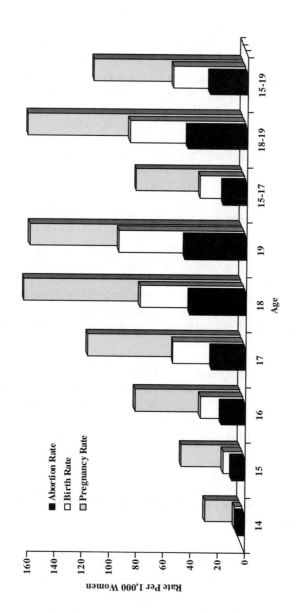

Figure 29-1 Abortions, births and pregnancies per 1,000 women aged 14–19, by age, United States, 1997

Sources: Birth rates—Ventura et al. (1999).[2]
Abortion and pregnancy rates—Henshaw (2001).[1]

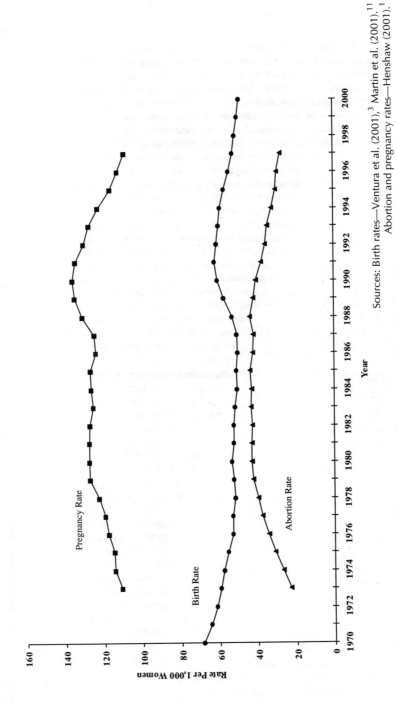

Sources: Birth rates—Ventura et al. (2001).[11] Martin et al. (2001).[3]
Abortion and pregnancy rates—Henshaw (2001).[1]

Figure 29-2 Abortions, births and pregnancies per 1,000 women aged 15–19, United States, 1970–1999

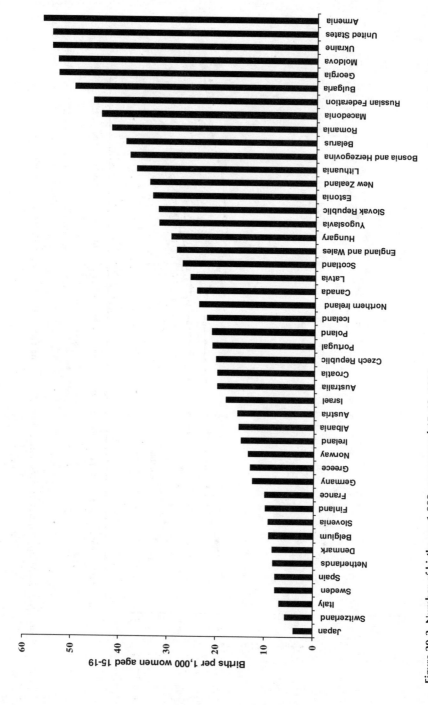

Source: Singh and Darroch (2000).[13]

Figure 29-3 Number of births per 1,000 women aged 15–19, 1990s

in pregnancy rates was not due to cross-national variations in proportions married, since the same qualitative conclusions would be obtained if comparisons were limited to the unmarried.[14] Part of the difference is attributable to the very high teenage pregnancy rates among U.S. blacks, but pregnancy rates for U.S. whites are still much higher than those for women in the other countries. The proportions of teenagers ever having had sexual intercourse are similar, so higher pregnancy rates in the United States are not caused by more prevalent sexual experience.

The reason for higher pregnancy rates in the United States is that American teenagers are less likely to use contraceptives, or less likely to use them effectively.[14] Lower proportions of teenage women in the United States use contraceptives regularly than do teenage women in the other four countries. Among users, a smaller fraction relies on the most efficient methods, particularly the pill and long-acting hormonal methods. Despite the evidence that the pill is a good pregnancy-prevention method for sexually active adolescents (and almost all women), public perceptions in the United States are heavily influenced by myth (particularly about cancer, future fecundity, and other side-effects). In a 2000 survey of teens, 39% of those aged 12 to 14 and an identical percentage of those aged 15 to 17 stated that it is unhealthy for girls to use the pill.[15]

Sexuality education in Sweden is compulsory and is taught in the schools at all grade levels. Information on contraception is provided, and its effectiveness is enhanced by a close link between the schools and adolescent family planning clinics. No other country approaches this level of implementation.[14] (In the Netherlands, where teenage pregnancy rates are lowest, sexuality education begins at an early age and is an ongoing lifelong process involving a variety of approaches and media; teen magazines and television programming are sexually explicit, focusing on real problems and feelings.)[16]

Four factors that inhibit use of contraceptives among sexually active adolescents in the United States are largely absent in Canada, France, Great Britain, and Sweden: (1) a political culture at odds with the reality of the adolescent world,[17] (2) large pockets of deep poverty, (3) little public support and expectations for the transition to adult economic roles, and (4) poor access to contraceptive services and supplies.[14]

Unrealistic political culture. One segment of the population judges many types of sexual activity, particularly sexual relations among unmarried persons, to be immoral, or at best unwise, and argues that availability of contraception and abortion causes teens to have sex and should therefore be vigorously opposed. Concern about the morality of sex, while by no means absent, has far less impact on public policy in the other countries. In Sweden, public policies recognize that sex is a healthy and normal part of life, not only for adults but also for adolescents. At the same time, there is a strong public emphasis on personal responsibility for reproductive behavior.[18] In short, adolescent sex is publicly accepted as normal but adolescent pregnancy and childbearing are not. The top public health official in these countries would never be fired, as was the Surgeon General of the United States, for suggesting that masturbation is a normal element of adolescent development and might delay the onset of intercourse. The political culture in this country hinders not only public provision of contraception but also frank public discussion about many sexual matters.[17] This political culture is all the more problematic because messages extolling sexuality are so pervasive in the mass media, while messages promoting healthy and responsible sexuality, including the use of contraception, are rare. Thus, while the "Just say No" message of the social conservatives is overwhelmed by the reality of sexual permissiveness, an effective countervailing force promoting contraceptive use is absent.

Pockets of deep poverty. The unequal distribution of income and the existence of a semi-permanent underclass in the United States guarantee that many poor adolescents will perceive that they are not sacrificing a bright future by having a child. In the other countries, the state redistributes income to a far greater extent. Moreover, public education, health care delivery, and other social services are more centrally controlled, thereby enabling the establishment of *national* policies far less subject to the influence of parochial interest groups.

Transition to adulthood. In the other four countries, youth tend to receive more societal assistance for this transition: vocational education and training, help in finding work, and unemployment benefits. As well as smoothing the transition from school to work, these efforts convey the powerful message that there are rewards for fitting into expected social roles. Moreover, there is far more social support for parenting in the other countries. In the United States, paid maternity leave is rare or of short duration, and child benefits are available only to the poor. In the other countries, working mothers (and sometimes fathers) are guaranteed paid parental leave and other benefits. Although parental leave and other family support policies, especially in France and Sweden, are quite generous, they offer little incentive for young women to have children because the benefits are tied to prior salary levels. These policies reinforce social norms that parenting is best postponed until careers have been established and offer young people the incentive to delay childbearing.

Access to contraception. Contraceptive supplies and services are more widely available, free of charge or at low cost, to adolescents in Sweden, France, Canada, and Great Britain. In contrast, a substantial segment of teenagers (and their families) in the United States have no health insurance; and those with health insurance may not be covered for contraceptive supplies or services or may fear that using insurance for contraception may result in loss of confidentiality, since most would be covered under their parents' policy.[14]

DETERMINANTS OF ADOLESCENT PREGNANCY

Although each year 1 in 9 women aged 15 to 19 becomes pregnant, 8 in 9 do not. Of those who do, 3 in 10 carry the pregnancy to term. A common opinion, expressed in popular books,[19] is that many adolescents perceive (however incorrectly) having a child as an attractive alternative to their current situation. They may, for example, be bored in school or have conflicts with parents. Undoubtedly, some do believe that a child is a ticket to independence or to a better life and act accordingly. Overwhelming evidence, however, shows that most unmarried adolescents who become pregnant do not intend to do so.[5,20,21] Nevertheless, intention is seldom adequately characterized by a sharp yes-or-no dichotomy. Therefore, even though few teenagers *intend* to become pregnant out-of-wedlock, the strength of the motivation of the rest to *avoid* pregnancy varies considerably.[22] The motivation to avoid pregnancy is governed in part by a young woman's perception of the benefits of deferring parenthood. This perception is strongly influenced by both her present circumstances and her belief in her future life chances. For many disadvantaged youth, the benefits of postponed parenthood must seem remote indeed.

SEXUAL BEHAVIOR

Why do unmarried adolescents become pregnant? The proximate cause is obviously vaginal sexual intercourse. In 1995, 49% of never-married women aged 15 to 19 had ever had sexual intercourse. See Table 29-2 for data by race/ethnicity.[9] The data from the 1995 NSFG reveal that by their 13th birthday 3% of never-married females have become sexually active.[9] The proportions rise to 8%, 19%, 32%, 47%, 59%, and 70% by the 14th, 15th, 16th, 17th, 18th, and 19th birthdays, respectively.[9] See Figure 29-4 for percentages by race.[9] In 1995, there was a decline, for the first time since 1971, in the proportion of never-married women ages 15 to 19 who had experienced sexual intercourse (30% in 1971, 41% in 1976, 43% in 1982, 51% in 1988, and 49% in 1995).[9] This increase in abstinence accounts for 25% of the decline in teen pregnancy rates between 1988 and 1995. Not all intercourse is consensual. Among women aged 15 to 19 in 1995 who had ever had intercourse, 25% had been forced to have intercourse at least once, 51% of these before age 15.[5]

Information on adolescent males is much more limited. Data from the 1988 and 1995 National Surveys of Adolescent Males (NSAM) show that the percentage of never-married males aged 15 to 19 who had ever had intercourse declined over this time period, from 60% to 55%.[9] There were declines in every single-year age group, with the overall decline attributable solely to a decline among whites. See Table 29-2 for data by race/ethnicity.[9] The data from the 1995 NSAM reveal that by their 13th birthday 4% of never-married males have become sexually active.[9] The

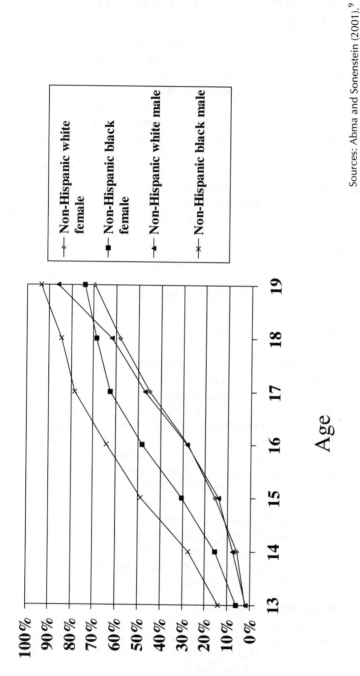

Non-Hispanic white female

Non-Hispanic black female

Non-Hispanic white male

Non-Hispanic black male

Age

100%
90%
80%
70%
60%
50%
40%
30%
20%
10%
0%

13 14 15 16 17 18 19

Sources: Abma and Sonenstein (2001).[9]
Females: 1995 National Survey of Family Growth
Males: 1995 National Survey of Adolescent Males

Figure 29-4 Percent of never-married females and males who have had sexual intercourse before reaching selected ages, by race, United States, 1995

proportions rise to 11%, 21%, 35%, 53%, 65%, and 84% by the 14th, 15th, 16th, 17th, 18th, and 19th birthdays, respectively.[9] See Figure 29-4 for percentages by race.[9]

Table 29-2 Percent of never-married males and females who had had sexual intercourse: United States, 1995

Sex and Age	Total	Race/ethnicity		
		Non-Hispanic White	Non-Hispanic Black	Hispanic
Females				
15-19	49.3	48.5	59.3	52.7
15-17	38.0	35.6	48.9	49.0
18-19	68.0	68.0	77.1	59.0
Males				
15-19	55.2	49.5	80.4	60.9
15-17	43.1	34.8	75.4	49.7
18-19	75.4	74.7	89.0	78.6

Source: Abma and Sonenstein (2001).[9]
Females: 1995 National Survey of Family Growth
Males: 1995 National Survey of Adolescent Males

CONTRACEPTIVE USE

Among teenage women who were currently exposed to the risk of unintended pregnancy in 1995, 19% were using no method (the same as in 1988 but substantially lower than the 30% in 1982) while 35% (down from 47% in 1988 and 44% in 1982) and 30% (up from 27% in 1988 and 15% in 1982) were relying on the pill and condom, respectively.[5,23] In addition, 8% were using the injectable and 2% the implant. Among teenage women surveyed in 1995, 77% reported use of a contraceptive at first premarital intercourse: 70% used the condom and 8% used the pill (5% used both pill and condom).[9] Among teenage men surveyed in 1995, 76% reported use of a contraceptive at first premarital intercourse: 69% used the condom and 10% relied on the pill (7% used both pill and condom).[9]

Increasing the effective practice of contraception is difficult in part because all currently available contraceptives require the type of abstract thinking about the future that many teens have not developed. Hence, a new contraceptive that could be used to induce menses at the end of cycles during which intercourse occurred (thereby reducing the importance of planning ahead), had few side-effects, was relatively inexpensive, and did not require a visit to a physician could reduce adolescent pregnancy significantly. A technological solution is unlikely, however, because (1) such a method would be considered to be an abortifacient and therefore not eligible for federal research and development support and (2) drug companies generally do not believe that developing new contraceptives is profitable.[24,25] Nevertheless, more effective promotion of currently available emergency contraception (Chapter 12) could significantly reduce unintended pregnancies among teens.[26]

Another problem is that the most effective methods for preventing pregnancy do not reduce the risk of acquiring STIs. As discussed more fully below, adolescents are at especially great risk for STIs. Promoting condom use is sound public health policy. Nevertheless, some health practitioners fear that it will be difficult to convince teens to use both pills and condoms. Others are concerned that if teens switch from pills to condoms then the pregnancy rate will consequently rise.

SEXUALITY EDUCATION

In a 1999 national survey, 3 in 4 teens in public secondary schools in grades 7 through 12 reported that they had received sexuality education in school.[27] Even among that group, large fractions said that they wanted more information on specific topics: how to talk with a partner about contraception and STIs (46%), how to use condoms (30%), how to use and where to get contraception other than condoms (40%), how to deal with emotional issues and consequences of being sexually active (46%), how to get tested for human immunodeficiency virus (HIV) and other STIs (51%).

Sexuality education in secondary public schools is increasingly focused on abstinence and is less likely to offer comprehensive instruction on contraception. In 1999, 23% of secondary school sexuality education teachers taught abstinence as the only way to prevent pregnancy and STIs, compared with 2% who did so in 1998.[28] In contrast, 49% of parents think that sexuality education should include contraception and safer sex in grades 7 and 8 and 88% of parents think this information should be covered in grades 9 through 12.[27]

In the fifth and sixth grades, about half of public schools do little to prepare students for puberty, much less for dealing with decisions regarding sexual activity. About half of teachers report that one of their top three problems in teaching sexuality education is pressure from the community, parents, or school administrators.[29]

Opposition to teaching comprehensive sexuality education is based on the concern that providing such information legitimizes and normalizes adolescent sex and promotes promiscuity. Rigorous evaluations, however, confirm that neither HIV nor sexuality education hastens the onset of sexual intercourse, increases the frequency of intercourse, or increases the number of sex partners. To the contrary, several studies have found that such programs can actually delay the onset of intercourse, reduce the frequency of intercourse, or reduce the number of partners. Some programs have been shown to delay the onset of intercourse and increase condom and other contraceptive use, thereby reducing the rate of unprotected intercourse.[30,31]

SEXUALLY TRANSMITTED INFECTIONS AMONG ADOLESCENTS

Most public attention to the consequences of teenage sexual behavior is focused on only one outcome: pregnancy. Much less attention is devoted to a second outcome: STIs. The incidence of STIs among adolescents increased rapidly during the 1960s and 1970s. In the 1980s and 1990s, despite the increase in awareness of STIs caused by HIV prevention messages, rates of genital infections in adolescents stayed at high levels.[32] Two-thirds of all STI cases occur among persons under 25 years of age, and one-quarter among teenagers.[33]

Between 1985 and 1999, reported gonorrhea infection rates declined among both male and female teens, but the overall incidence still remained very high.[34,35] In 1999, 738 per 100,000 females and 341 per 100,000 males aged 15 to 19 were reported to be infected. Most clinical investigations find that rates of chlamydia are at least double those of gonorrhea. In 1999, 232 thousand cases of chlamydia and 104 thousand cases of gonorrhea were reported among teens.[33] The number of visits of teenage women to office-based fee-for-service practices for genital herpes infections increased from 15 thousand in 1966 to an estimated 100 thousand in 1995. The number of visits for genital warts caused by the human papillomavirus (HPV) increased from 50 thousand in 1966 to an estimated 200 thousand in 1995 among teenage women. Perhaps 10 times as many sexually active women have asymptomatic cervical HPV infection. By the end of the teenage years, about 4% of whites and 17% of blacks have been infected with herpes simplex virus type 2.[32]

By the end of June 2000, 2,759 persons in the United States under the age of 20 had been reported to be infected with HIV, and an additional 1,691 persons with AIDS had been infected with HIV through sexual contact. Given the long latency period from infection with HIV to the development of AIDS, a considerable fraction of the 16,769 persons reported with AIDS at ages 20-24 who had been infected through sexual contact must have been infected while still teenagers.[36]

The epidemiology of STI transmission is the same among adolescents as among adults: unprotected intercourse with multiple partners is risky. Data from the 1995 NSFG and 1995 NSAM show that among the 38% of unmarried females and the 38% of never-married males aged 15 to 19 who had experienced sexual intercourse during the past 3 months, 22% of females and 19% of males had had 2 or more partners during that time period. In 1995, 64% of never-married teenage males and 32% of never-married teenage females reported condom use at last intercourse in the three months prior to the survey.[9] This difference is also found in the CDC's Youth Risk Behavior Surveillance System. In the 1999 national survey of students in grades 9 through 12, among those who had had sexual intercourse in the 3 months preceding the survey, 66% of males but only 51% of females reported using a condom at last intercourse.[37] It is difficult to resolve the discrepancy between these two statistics. Plausible explanations are that males overreport use of condoms because they know that it is the socially responsible answer, or females underreport condom use when a condom is used as an adjunct to a regular method of contraception. Regardless of the answer, condom use seems to have increased among adolescents. The most plausible explanation for this increase is greater awareness of STIs, primarily HIV. Nevertheless, the disturbing fact remains that large fractions of adolescents at risk of acquiring STIs do not use condoms.

CONSEQUENCES OF ADOLESCENT CHILDBEARING

In 1968, Art Campbell summarized the prevailing view about the consequences of teenage childbearing with the famous quote, "The girl who has an illegitimate child at the age of 16 suddenly has 90 percent of her life's script written for her. . . Her life choices are few, and most of them are bad."[38] *Risking the Future*, the 1987 report of the National Research Council, concluded that "women who become parents as teenagers are at greater risk of social and economic disadvantage throughout their lives than those who delay childbearing until their twenties."[39] And President Clinton echoed this conclusion in his 1995 State of the Union address when he declared that teenage pregnancy is "our most serious social problem."[40]

In sharp contrast, recent research suggests that the consequences of teenage childbearing are not as deleterious as has long been claimed. The reason is that most studies have simply compared outcomes in two groups of women: those who had a birth at an early age and those who did not.

The greatest analytical problem is determining whether the adverse conditions frequently observed among adolescent mothers are causally related to age at childbirth. Many studies fail to control for both maternal age and other factors correlated with age at first birth, such as socioeconomic status. Thus the adverse consequences of early childbearing per se are frequently overstated. An even more serious analytical problem arises because adolescents are able to select (or at least affect) whether they become pregnant or whether they will bear a child. Investigators can never study the consequences of adolescent childbearing by conducting a rigorous randomized trial. However, they can try to ensure that adolescent mothers are compared with a control group that is as similar as possible with respect to measurable background variables at an early age, such as achievement, aptitude, motivation, and socioeconomic status. One innovative methodological approach controls for a similar family environment by comparing the experiences of pairs of sisters, one of whom gave birth as a teenager and the other of whom did not. Another compares the experiences of teenage mothers who gave birth to twins to those who gave birth to singletons; those who give birth to twins experience a truly exogenous unplanned birth.

HEALTH CONSEQUENCES

Several studies have found that adolescents receiving good prenatal care exhibit pregnancy outcomes that are no worse than those of other women.[41] The problem, of course, is that adolescents, especially the very young, are much less likely to receive any prenatal care or, if they do, are more likely to initiate it later in the pregnancy.[3] The reasons for such behavior include not recognizing the pregnancy or desiring to conceal it, not realizing that prenatal care is valuable or available, and not being able to afford it.

The relation between poor birth outcome and maternal age may, however, not be entirely attributable to the effects of prenatal care. This question was examined among white women giving birth to their first singleton child in Utah. Even in the lowest-risk group—married women whose educational attainment was appropriate for their age and who obtained adequate prenatal care—babies of mothers under 18 years of age were 1.9 times as likely to be premature, 1.7 times as likely to weigh less than 2500 grams, and 1.3 times as likely to be small for gestational age as babies of women aged 20 to 24. Risks to babies of mothers aged 18 and 19 were lower, but still elevated.[42] These results suggest that even under optimal circumstances, young maternal age is still related to poor birth outcomes. The study design, however, only partly controls for family background.

When family background characteristics of mothers are controlled by comparing the health of children of sisters who gave birth at different ages, the effects of teen childbearing are mixed and modest.[43] For both blacks and whites, comparisons within sister-pairs (one who had a child as a teenager and one who did not) revealed fewer adverse effects for infants than did traditional cross-section comparisons. Generally, the differentials for whites were narrowed and for blacks were eliminated or even reversed. Compared with their sisters who first gave birth at older ages, black teen mothers were no more likely to smoke during pregnancy or to have low-birthweight babies and no less likely to breastfeed their infants or to bring them to clinics for well-baby visits. The situation was generally the opposite among whites. Further analyses that control for family-specific endowments suggest that the biological effect of having a birth at younger ages is to increase birthweight marginally.[44]

One positive health consequence of teenage childbearing has been identified. The risk of breast cancer increases with the age at which a woman delivers her first full-term child. A woman who bears a child before the age of 18 faces about one-third the risk of a woman whose first birth occurs after the age of 35.[45]

Comparisons of the children of sisters have also been used to examine the effects of teenage motherhood on child development.[46] For a cross-sectional sample in which the effects of family background are not controlled, the children of women who had first births after age 19 scored consistently better on measures of child development than children of teen mothers. But in the sisters comparison, children of teen mothers did no worse than their first cousins whose mothers had first births after age 19. Other U.S. and British studies show that cognitive development of the child is influenced by the age of the mother even after the effects of background variables have been controlled. Children of young mothers fare less well, though the difference is small. In contrast, the results for the social and emotional development of the child are rather inconclusive. In all these studies, however, maternal age proved to have much less influence than did the socioeconomic variables.[41,47]

SOCIOECONOMIC CONSEQUENCES

Analysis of data from three national surveys replicates findings from previous studies demonstrating that teenage childbearing leads to substantial long-term socioeconomic disadvantage when those who have births as teens are compared with all those who do not. This finding holds even when the effects of some background characteristics such as mother's and father's education and respondent's upbringing in a single parent family are controlled.[48] However, these conventional controls may not adequately make the two groups (teen mothers versus others) similar enough that the estimated effect of a teen birth can be interpreted as a causal effect. When the comparison group is confined to the sisters (who did not have births as teenagers) of the teenage mothers, a different conclusion emerges. In two of the three surveys, standard comparisons seriously overstate the costs of teenage childbearing. In the third survey, the methodology based on sister comparisons leads to the same conclusion as the conventional methodology that controls for several background characteristics.[48,49] However, even sister comparisons may overstate the deleterious consequences of teen childbearing because they may reflect differences between sisters that are unrelated to the age at first birth. For example, parents may favor, starting at an early age, the daughter they perceive to be the more able.

Comparisons of unmarried women who first gave birth to twins and unmarried women who first gave birth to singletons based on data from the 1970 and 1980 Censuses reveal large short-term effects of an unplanned birth on labor-force participation, poverty, and welfare receipt.[50] Consistent with the results from sister comparisons, these negative consequences are considerably smaller than those estimated in earlier studies. Most of the negative effects dissipate over time among whites but persist among blacks. Effects on poverty and welfare receipt were larger in 1980 than in

1970 and larger for blacks than whites. At the time of the 1980 Census, black but not white women who experienced an unplanned nonmarital birth were less likely to have completed high school and to be married.

STRATEGIES TO SOLVE THE PROBLEM

Many attempts have been made to reduce the incidence of teen pregnancy in the United States and to ease its health, social, educational, and economic consequences for mother and child. In this section we describe these approaches, with a special emphasis on what good evaluation research suggests about their effectiveness. In particular, we summarize what we know about the characteristics of programs that work. The limits of relying on programs alone to solve teen pregnancy are also discussed.

DEVELOPMENT OF INTERVENTION PROGRAMS: HISTORICAL PERSPECTIVE

Largely as a result of research findings described in the previous section on the negative consequences of teen pregnancy and parenthood, programs that provided care for pregnant teens, teen mothers, and their infants proliferated in the 1960s and 1970s. These programs generally provided comprehensive prenatal and postnatal health services for the young mother and her child. Many care programs also helped the teen mother stay in or return to school by offering special classes for these mothers and daycare for their children.

In the early 1980s, program planners began to look more to prevention as an effective way to address the problems of teen pregnancy and parenthood, in part because both research and common sense suggested that preventing adolescent pregnancy in the first place is far more cost-effective than trying to bolster the lives of young, largely unmarried mothers and their children after the fact. The prevention emphasis was also stimulated by the widespread availability and public acceptance of several forms of reversible contraception—oral contraceptives most importantly—which many believed would be especially effective in preventing teen pregnancy because they are coitus-independent. At the time, there also seemed to be adequate public tolerance for school-based sex education that discussed a wide range of reproductive health issues and for services that provided contraceptive care to teens without parental consent.

New programs aimed at preventing the occurrence of early pregnancy or birth began to emerge. Many different approaches were tried, based on the research literature as well as program planners' personal or ideologically based ideas about acceptable and effective means of preventing pregnancy. Several approaches were tried, sometimes simultaneously in a single program:

- **Abstinence education,** which teaches young people the benefits of refraining from sexual activity, the limits of contraception, and the skills to overcome temptation and/or refuse unwanted advances

- **Youth-friendly contraceptive services,** which ease access to contraception for sexually active young people (by, for example, establishing school-based contraceptive clinics)

- **Comprehensive sex education,** which focuses on teaching teens about human reproduction, contraception, and sexuality

- **Contraceptive negotiation skills,** which center on how to discuss and negotiate about sex and contraception with a romantic partner

- **Life option or youth development programs** that offer young people a variety of supports, such as academic assistance, job training, community service, and adult mentoring. This last approach is based partly on the premise that "hope is the best contraceptive"—that is, that having a compelling vision of a positive personal future or goal, and the skills to get there, are strong incentives to avoid teen pregnancy.

In the 1990s, three developments caused new intensity in the overall national effort to reduce teen pregnancy as well as new controversy. First, the deepening public understanding of the HIV/AIDs challenge (fueled in part by data that showed that heterosexual teens were not immune to this serious problem), and the heightened awareness of STIs generally led many teen programs to include a new emphasis on protecting against HIV and other STIs, not just unintended pregnancy. Second, the dramatic increase in both the teen pregnancy and birth rate in the late 1980s, which became apparent and widely recognized in the 1990s among demographers and policy leaders (see Figure 29-2) led to an outpouring of activities at the state and local level to reduce teen pregnancy. Many statewide coalitions were formed, governors' blue ribbon panels established, and private initiatives launched. For example, a survey of state-financed efforts to reduce teen pregnancy found dramatic increases in the last half of the decade in efforts to reduce teen pregnancy,[51] and in 1996, the National Campaign to Prevent Teen Pregnancy was established under the auspices of the White House and with the support of a diverse, bi-partisan group of national leaders from many social sectors.

And finally, in 1996, Congress passed and the President signed into law a complex revision of the nation's welfare system. Included in the legislation was a provision for $50 million in annual federal funding (which states must match on a 4:3 basis) for a narrowly defined set of abstinence education programs that some have called "abstinence-only" programs. This new money led to great controversy in the teen pregnancy prevention field; advocates of an exclusive message of abstinence for teens were pitted against those who asserted that a broader set of messages and services that included contraceptive information and care was the right path.

THE SEARCH FOR "WHAT WORKS"

Along with an increase in efforts to reduce teen pregnancy in the 1990s came more questions about the effectiveness of the many interventions being tried. Elected officials, foundation officers, and community leaders all began asking, "what works?" Unfortunately, the amount of high-quality data available at that time to answer this reasonable question was limited. Although by 1990, probably several thousand teen pregnancy prevention programs had been developed and put in place, few good evaluations existed. A variety of reasons underlay this dearth of scientifically valid program evaluations. First there were the tensions, some more real than others, between service and science. Service providers were often reluctant to direct dollars to scientific endeavors whose benefits were (perhaps erroneously) perceived as relatively remote rather than to services that help those in need. In addition, both funders and service providers were understandably wary about the possible fallout from negative evaluations. Beyond these reasons, some funders felt constrained, by fact or politics, from providing support for approaches not in line with their mission or their legislative mandate. As the national debate grew in the 1990s over issues such as abortion and the provision of contraception to minors, schools in particular became increasingly reluctant to ally themselves with controversial issues such as school-based clinics or contraceptive education and provision.

Tensions also existed between the requirements of science and the realities of program administration. For example, scientific evaluation encouraged the random assignment of subjects to treatment and control groups; administrators often replied it was unacceptable to withhold services from those in need, especially when the funds were available to provide services to all. Scientific rigor demanded that baseline and follow-up data be collected from identifiable individuals so these data could be linked; administrators often replied that, because of cost and confidentiality, this design could not be implemented. Moreover, when a good evaluation was designed and implemented, it was often discovered that members of the control or comparison group had been exposed to the influence of competing similar programs, often making the evaluation one of marginal effects of that program at best. Another problem was (and continues to be) the conflict between science and politics. There has been an unwillingness to use public funds (or allow public authorities) to ask adolescents about their sexual behavior, yet trends in sexual behavior cannot be monitored and programs cannot be evaluated without doing so.

Despite these obstacles, the field made laudable progress in the 1990s. Consciousness about the importance of evaluation was raised and evaluation methods advanced. Today, the field is more aware of the technical challenges of program evaluation, as well as the costs and benefits associated with various research designs. Moreover, the ways in which evaluation data may serve to improve prevention programs are now better appreciated and understood.

ASSESSING THE EVIDENCE

Reflecting the increasingly rigorous science of program evaluation, studies on the effectiveness of teen pregnancy prevention programs have increasingly asked whether the program in question actually changes behavior. Does it, for example, delay first sexual intercourse? Reduce the number of sexual partners? Reduce the frequency of intercourse? Increase the use of effective protection against pregnancy or STIs at first and subsequent episodes of sexual intercourse? This strong preference for examining changes in *behavior* rather than *knowledge* or *attitudes* reflects the growing understanding that knowledge gain, in particular, does not invariably lead to behavior change, so it is no longer enough for programs to show, for example, that they increase participants' understanding about how one gets pregnant, what contraceptive options are available to the sexually active, or where to go to obtain various contraceptive methods. They must actually show changes in behavior.

Over the last 10 years, at least 10 high quality reviews have been published that assess individual evaluations of programs to prevent teen pregnancy.[21,31,52-59] Each has used different criteria to decide which evaluations will be reviewed and which will be excluded. For example, some of these reviews have focused only on published, peer-reviewed evaluations, while others have broader inclusion criteria. Some include youth development programs while others are limited to more traditional teen pregnancy interventions that stress sex education and contraceptive services; some examine abstinence programs especially carefully, given their current political salience, while others pass them by. All, however, include the reviewers' insights about lessons learned from the programs and evaluations that were examined.

The most recent and comprehensive review (*Emerging Answers*) contains findings that are largely consistent with those of the previous nine reviews, but perhaps more importantly, concludes that after years of program innovation and rigorous research, there really are now some answers to the question, "What works? What should I put in place in my community?"[59]

One of this review's most important intellectual contributions is to point out that the risk factors—or "antecedents"—of teen pregnancy come in two broad categories: those that are *sexual* in nature (such as sexual attitudes, knowledge, beliefs, and skills) and those that are *non-sexual* (such as family composition, relationship to school, mental and emotional health, and several attributes of neighborhoods and communities), and that both sets of criteria can be used to design effective prevention programs. Indeed, evidence is now strong that there are effective models for reducing teen pregnancy that are based on trying to affect the sexual factors (which is the way most programs in this field have been conceptualized); but there are also effective models that reduce teen pregnancy by addressing the non-sexual factors. And, of course, some programs address both. This news is exceedingly good for the prevention field. Not only is the number of effective interventions increasing, but so also is the diversity; communities now have more opportunities to find programs that suit local values and preferences as well as budgets.

The 70+ programs included in *Emerging Answers* are divided into three categories, with several subcategories in each, as noted below. It is important to stress that effective programs were *not* identified in all categories; only those categories in **bold type** contain evaluated programs with very strong evidence that they are effective in changing behavior, although there is some hopeful news in virtually all categories:

Programs that focus on the *sexual antecedents* of teen pregnancy
- Curricula-based programs in schools
  1. abstinence-only programs
  2. **sex and HIV education programs**
- Sex and HIV education programs for parents and families
- Clinic or school-based programs to provide reproductive health care or to improve access to condoms or other contraceptives
  1. family planning clinics and services
  2. **clinic instructional programs with one-on-one consultation with a medical provider**
  3. **programs to change clinic protocols and policies**
  4. school-based and school-linked clinics
  5. school programs to make condoms available
- Community-wide initiatives with many components

Programs that focus on non-sexual antecedents
- Early childhood programs
- Youth development programs for adolescents
  1. **service learning programs**
  2. vocational education and employment programs
  3. selected other youth development programs

Programs that focus on both sexual and non-sexual antecedents
- **Programs with both sexuality and youth development components**

Abstinence-only

The "jury is still out" regarding the effectiveness of so-called "abstinence-only" programs, simply because very little rigorous evaluation of these programs has been completed. *Emerging Answers* also notes that the few studies that have been completed do not reflect the great diversity of the abstinence-only programs currently offered. For example, some of these programs adhere quite strictly to a strong "abstinence until marriage" message and do not address sexual activity and risk outside of marriage at all, while others are less clear cut about exactly when sexual activity is appropriate. Some include information about condoms and contraception (usually stressing the limitations of these methods), while others are silent on these issues altogether. All, however, unequivocally stress abstinence as the best choice for school-aged teens. The evidence available about the effectiveness of these programs is not encouraging, but all that can be conclusively said is that we still lack adequate information about the ability of these programs to increase abstinence among teens.

Sex and HIV Education

The overwhelming weight of evidence presented in *Emerging Answers* shows that sex and HIV education programs do not increase sexual activity—a concern that many parents and others have expressed from time to time. They do not hasten sexual debut, increase the frequency of sex, or increase the number of sexual partners. In fact, some sex and HIV education programs have just the opposite effect: they help to delay first intercourse, reduce the frequency of sex, or reduce the number of sexual partners. Among these curricula-based programs that have the strongest evidence of success are *Reducing the Risk*; *Safer Choices*; *Becoming a Responsible Teen*; *Making a Difference: An Abstinence Approach to STD, Teen Pregnancy, and HIV/AIDS Prevention*; and *Making a Difference: A Safer Sex Approach to STD, Teen Pregnancy, and HIV/AIDS Prevention*. Interestingly, it appears that these effective curricula share 10 common characteristics (see box).

Characteristics of Effective Sex and HIV Education Programs

1. Focus on reducing one or more sexual behaviors that lead to unintended pregnancy or HIV or other STIs.

2. Based on theoretical approaches demonstrated to influence other health-related behavior and identify specific important sexual antecedents to be targeted.

3. Deliver and consistently reinforce a clear message about abstaining from sexual activity and/or using condoms or other forms of contraception. This appears to be one of the most important characteristics that distinguishes effective from ineffective programs.

4. Provide basic, accurate information about the risks of teen sexual activity and about ways to avoid intercourse or use methods of protection against pregnancy and STIs.

5. Include activities that address social pressures that influence sexual behavior.

6. Provide examples of and practice with communication, negotiation, and refusal skills.

7. Employ teaching methods designed to involve participants and have them personalize the information.

8. Incorporate behavioral goals, teaching methods, and materials that are appropriate to the age, sexual experience, and culture of the students.

9. Last a sufficient length of time (i.e., more than a few hours).

10. Select teachers or peer leaders who believe in the program and then provide them with adequate training.

Family Planning Clinics

Family planning clinics are a very important part of this nation's effort to reduce unintended pregnancy, but their precise role in preventing teen pregnancy is not well understood, in part because they are rarely evaluated or even regarded as a discrete "program" intervention. It is clear that they provide many adolescents with contraceptive services, which presumably prevent pregnancies among the teens who present themselves at family planning clinics. Nonetheless, because the long-term impact of family planning services on whether teens choose to be sexually active or on the frequency of sexual activity is not known, the number of teen pregnancies prevented by family planning services is difficult to estimate.

However, the findings regarding particular clinic protocols or programs within health or family planning clinics present a much clearer picture. Studies have consistently shown that when clinics provide youth with quality information about abstinence and contraception, offer a clear message about sex and contraceptive use, engage youth in one-on-one discussions about their behavior, and provide contraceptives, they can increase contraceptive use among those who attend certain clinics (although not always for a prolonged period of time) without increasing sexual activity.

Service Learning Programs

Service learning programs—which may not focus on sexual issues at all—offer the strongest evidence to date that they reduce teen pregnancy rates while youth are engaged in the programs. Service learning programs offer youth opportunities to participate in community projects (such as tutoring or cleaning-up a park or river) while also providing them time to reflect on their experiences (through group discussions and journal writing, for example). The *Teen Outreach Program* and the *Reach for Health* program, in particular, have the best evidence of success. Research does not indicate why this type of intervention is successful, although *Emerging Answers* notes that several explanations seem plausible: "participants develop relationships with program facilitators, they gain a sense of autonomy and feel more competent in their relationships with peers and adults, and they feel empowered by the knowledge that they can make a difference in the lives of others. All such factors, in turn, may help increase teenagers' motivation to avoid pregnancy. In addition, participating in supervised activities—especially after school—may simply reduce the opportunities teens have to engage in risky behavior, including unprotected sex."[59]

Combined Sex Education and Youth Development

Finally, there is new research supporting the notion that programs which address both sexual and non-sexual risk factors for teen pregnancy may be highly effective. A recent, high-quality study found that the *Children's Aid Society-Carrera Program*—a long-term, intensive program that combines such things as tutoring, work, and sports-related activities, family life and sex education, and comprehensive medical care including mental health and reproductive health services—significantly delayed the onset of sex, increased the use of contraception, and reduced pregnancy and birth rates among girls.[60] The program did not reduce sexual risk-taking among boys. This is the first and only study to date that includes random assignment, multiple sites, and a large sample size and that found a positive impact on sexual and contraceptive behavior, pregnancy, and births among girls for as long as 3 years.

WHAT ELSE DO WE KNOW?

In addition to the specific findings noted in the previous section, there are also some more general points of consensus with special relevance to community-level programs to prevent teen pregnancy. These derive not only from the literature reviews already referenced, but also from public opinion polling, practical experience, and expert opinion:

Intervention intensity. The intensity of an intervention should match the level of risk among the teens one hopes to affect. Changing behavior (one's own or someone else's) is always difficult, but it may be especially so when many risk factors are present. Brief, superficial interactions will probably accomplish little when the odds are stacked in favor of early, unprotected sex and pregnancy. In addition, programs often make the mistake of starting too late. Given that the average age of first intercourse is now about 17 for girls and slightly younger for boys (see Figure 29-4), and that girls under 15 comprise the only group showing an increase in the proportion sexually active,[61] waiting to institute developmentally appropriate pregnancy prevention programs until high school is too late.

Abstinence and contraceptive use messages. There is a notable amount of national support for a strong message of abstinence to school-aged teens. For example, almost all adults (95%) and teens (93%) agree that "it is important for teens to be given a strong message from society that they should abstain from sex until they are at least out of high school."[62] At the same time, there is also strong support for these same young people to receive good reproductive health information and services. These are not inconsistent views: both abstinence and contraception can reduce teen pregnancy; both contributed to the decline in teen pregnancy and birth rates during the 1990s;[63] and the nation undoubtedly needs more of both among adolescents. Strident arguments over which strategy is better—sexual abstinence or contraceptive use—are a recipe for stalemate, and they obscure the more critical issue of motivation. Teens will do *neither* if they are not highly motivated to avoid pregnancy in the first place.

Partner involvement. Despite the accumulating evidence that decisions about sexual activity and contraception are affected by numerous factors within relationships, especially romantic relationships, few interventions try to work with couples or even to address couple interaction. Partners can be very influential in both choosing to use contraception and in continuing to use it effectively,[64] and programs need to find ways to build on this powerful reality.

Parental influence. Over two decades of research confirms that—whether they believe it or not—parents are an important influence on whether their children become pregnant or cause a pregnancy. Recent survey data confirm this view. Teens cited parents more than any other source as having the *most* influence over their sexual decision-making. For their part, *adults* believe that peers influence teens' sexual decision-making more than do parents.[62] Apparently, parents don't realize how influential they are in this area or how many opportunities they have to shape their children's behavior.

Peer norms. Peer pressure and teens' *perceptions* of the sexual behavior of others affect their own behavior. Teens report, common sense suggests, and research confirms that peer influence can play an important role in the sexual behavior of teens. Teens need accurate information about what their peers are doing (or not doing) because what they *think* other teens are doing has an impact on their behavior. A teen who believes his or her friends are sexually active is more likely to initiate sex, and is less likely to do so if he or she believe that peers are not sexually active. Peers can also have positive effects on teen behavior. A sexually active girl, for instance, is less likely to become pregnant if her peers are themselves at low risk of teen pregnancy. Conversely, after controlling for socioeconomic status, family characteristics, and popularity, a teen girl in a high-risk peer group is 3.5 times more likely to get pregnant within 18 months than a teen girl in a low-risk peer group.[65]

Directive expectations. Program messages must be clear and specific. It is not enough to give teens copious amounts of information about abstinence, sex, contraception, and related topics. If we want to reduce their risk of pregnancy, we also need to tell them what we expect them to actually do and why. Not have sex? Have sex only under certain conditions? Which ones? And why? In counseling theory, this approach is called "directive," and there is good reason to assert that in the sensitive, complex area of sexuality, teens benefit from clear guidance. Of course, taking a stand on what the desired sexual behavior is for teens involves value judgments as well as information, which is why these topics so often generate controversy (and why some object to having schools address these issues).

Community organizing. Putting programs into place at the community level is an arduous process, even when there is agreement on what needs to be done and for whom. Several groups have developed actual manuals for community organizers and activists to help them understand the sequence of steps that usually need to be taken. They cover everything from assessing needs, managing controversy, and finding needed money, to involving faith and business groups.[60,66,67]

Despite all these areas of consensus, there are many aspects of preventing teen pregnancy through community programs that remain obscure. For example, even with the proliferation of "male involvement" programs in reproductive health, no credible set of evaluation studies yet exists to suggest which approaches are more effective than others; and although it is well known that parents exert a strong influence on the sexual decision-making of their children, very little is known about what types of programs might harness these relationships to help reduce teen pregnancy. We also know virtually nothing about programs in faith settings that try to improve outcomes for youth, including reduced rates of teen pregnancy. Moreover, although some programs have been shown to be effective, as noted above, few have been assessed in more than a few populations, which means that we know less than we should about how teens from various racial/ethnic groups, income levels, or geographic areas might respond to particular interventions. We also do not know whether local- or state-level coalitions focused on preventing teen pregnancy are a useful way of achieving progress, despite the enduring popularity of this form of social organizing. In short, we know far more than we did even 5 years ago about programs to reduce teen pregnancy, but there are still important gaps.

THE LIMITS OF PROGRAMS

As this section makes clear, effective programs to reduce teen pregnancy exist and should be expanded, but it is unrealistic to assume that community programs alone will solve this problem. Not all teens are enrolled in programs, not all programs are well-run, and even those that ostensibly copy or "replicate" programs found to be effective do not always achieve the same result as the original model (in part because the original model is often not replicated faithfully). Many community-based programs are small, fragile, and poorly funded. And even the most effective programs may have only modest success. But there is another reason community programs cannot do it single-handedly: teen pregnancy is rooted partly (some would say mainly) in such broad social phenomena as popular culture, the images portrayed in the entertainment media, and the values articulated by parents and other adults. Community programs obviously cannot single-handedly counter or reshape these very powerful forces. Moreover, some organized programs are expensive; for example, the CAS-Carrera program estimates that it costs about $4,000 per participant per year.

Community programs are especially important for high-risk teens, but they need to be surrounded by *additional* activities best described as highly leveraged efforts to influence teen attitudes and cultural messages about sex, love, and relationships. Public and private funders and activists should continue looking for ways to influence broader social forces as a supplement to their more traditional focus on developing and funding local programs. For example, the National Campaign to Prevent Teen Pregnancy does so by working in partnership with the entertainment media to embed constructive messages and ideas into the television shows, internet sites, and magazines that are popular among teens and their parents. A message delivered by a favorite character on a soap opera, for instance, can make a lasting impression on a teen or an adult. There are undoubtedly other ways to influence the overall culture that should be developed as well. The simple point is that reducing teen pregnancy will likely require a combination of community programs *and* broader efforts to influence social norms, values, and popular culture.

PROGRAM PRIORITIES: AMELIORATING THE CONSEQUENCES OF CHILDBEARING

A final strategy commanding wide public support is ameliorating the negative consequences of adolescent childbearing. Demonstration projects have focused on several priorities for adolescent mothers:

- Ensuring a safe pregnancy and delivery
- Staying in school (particularly to increase employability)
- Avoiding additional pregnancies (secondary prevention)
- Increasing employment and earnings and decreasing welfare receipt
- Increasing parenting skills.

Health interventions are very effective. For young women in any socioeconomic category, adequate prenatal and obstetrical care greatly reduces the adverse health consequences to mother and child associated with pregnancy and childbirth at an early age.[68,69]

Prenatal Home Visits

Prenatal home-visitation programs for socially disadvantaged women have been designed to improve pregnancy outcomes, reduce dysfunctional care of children, and improve the maternal life course. Despite initial promising results, the effect of these programs on improving pregnancy outcomes has proved equivocal.[70,71] In contrast, the programs do have a beneficial impact on dysfunctional caregiving during the child's first 2 years of life and on some key maternal life-course outcomes (such as a reduction in the rate of subsequent pregnancies) among poor unmarried mothers. The more effective programs employ nurses who visit frequently enough during pregnancy and after delivery to establish a therapeutic alliance with the family and who address the material, social, psychological, and behavioral factors associated with maternal and child health. Results of randomized trials of home-visitation programs reveal that attempts to isolate only a few important aspects of such interventions are misguided. Social support during pregnancy is ineffective at improving pregnancy outcomes unless adverse maternal health behaviors are altered. Prenatal home visits alone, without continuing comprehensive postnatal visits, are insufficient to promote well-being past delivery. These programs benefit the neediest families (low income unmarried women) but provide little benefit for broader populations.

Comprehensive Services

The next priorities after ensuring a healthy delivery are to keep the mother in school, to prevent further pregnancies, to increase employment and income, and to increase parenting skills. The results of Project Redirection—a comprehensive program whose participants (who were extremely disadvantaged when compared not only with teenagers generally but also with other teen parents) were asked to organize and frequently reorient aspects of their lives while pursuing an education, training for a job, and learning about family planning—are sobering. When compared with control subjects not in the program, Redirection participants were more likely to be in school or have graduated, less likely to have become pregnant, and more likely to be practicing contraception at the time of the 1-year follow-up. After 2 years, however, the differentials had vanished.[72] This finding led the investigators to conclude that the impact of the intervention lasted no longer than the participants' stay in the program. Although Project Redirection was based on a research design substantially more rigorous than is typical for teenage parent programs, the comparison group had much wider access to local social service programs than had been anticipated. Thus, comparison of Redirection participants and controls does not reveal the difference in outcomes between "no treatment" and "comprehensive treatment" groups. A supplementary analysis compared four groups: Redirection participants in the program from 1 to 2 years, Redirection participants in the program for less than 1 year, controls who were ever in a similar program, and controls who were never in any program. The results, which must be interpreted with caution since the outcomes could reflect systematic variation in uncontrolled characteristics such as motivation, suggest that the more services a mother received, the better she performed. Nevertheless, the most reasonable conclusion is that short-term assistance does not have a long-term impact on educational attainment or subsequent pregnancy.

A 5-year follow-up of Project Redirection confirmed this conclusion: the experimental and control groups had equal educational attainment and equal numbers of subsequent pregnancies, on average. The experimental group actually had a greater average number of subsequent births (but fewer abortions) than the control group. In contrast, Redirection participants, when compared with controls, worked more hours and had higher weekly earnings from employment, were less likely to be receiving welfare, and scored higher on a widely used test of parenting ability. Moreover, participants' children showed better cognitive skills and exhibited fewer behavioral problems.[73] Although these results confirm that an intensive short-term program cannot eliminate the long-term disadvantages conferred by poverty, they do provide a basis for believing that the prospects for disadvantaged teenage mothers and their children can be improved by such an intervention.

Based in part on what was learned from Project Redirection, New Chance was a second test of whether providing comprehensive services could assist a disadvantaged group of families headed by young women who had first given birth as teenagers, who had dropped out of high school, and who were receiving welfare. Whereas Project Redirection was for pregnant teens and focused on education, New Chance was for teen mothers and their children and was more explicitly focused on preparation for work. As in Project Redirection, women were randomly assigned to the experimental group or the control group. The findings indicate that while those in both groups advanced in many ways, by the time of the 3½-year follow-up, those in the experimental group did not advance further than those in the control group in most respects.[74] When compared with those in the control group, women in the experimental group were more likely to have earned a GED but less likely to have graduated from high school, had similar rates of subsequent pregnancy, birth, and abortion, and similar rates of employment, earnings, and welfare receipt. Moreover, New Chance did not have an effect on children's cognitive development.

Project Redirection and New Chance are perhaps the best examples of comprehensive programs for pregnant teenagers and young mothers. Such programs have considerable appeal because they focus on the individual *after* she becomes pregnant, thereby avoiding the controversy surrounding the prevention of adolescent pregnancy and the seemingly insoluble problem of poverty. Moreover, focusing on local communities and the coordination of local programs appears to circumvent the need for additional resources. However, a review of the quality of such comprehensive programs has concluded that the comprehensive model is better suited to political compromise and rhetoric than to effective problem-solving.[75] The authors argue that many comprehensive programs are based on three faulty assumptions: that the requisite services are already locally available and need only be stitched together administratively, that this goal can be accomplished without a further infusion of state and federal financial assistance, and that the adolescent pregnancy problem can be best addressed by targeting services to those already pregnant.

Welfare Reform

The Teenage Parent Welfare Demonstration examined the potential of the institution of mandatory work-related activity, with case management and support services, to promote self-sufficiency and other positive outcomes for first-time teenage parents on welfare and their children. In 3 demonstration sites, young new mothers on welfare were randomly assigned to the prevailing welfare support policies or to the new regime requiring young mothers to work, attend school, or participate in job training for a minimum of 20 hours a week as a condition of receiving their full allotment of cash assistance. Case managers aided the young mothers in selecting their out-of-home activity, securing childcare and other required support services, and engaging in parenting and family management training. This demonstration program led to modest increases in employment and earnings, but did not change either economic well-being or welfare dependence. Moreover, the services to increase knowledge of and access to family planning services neither altered patterns of contraceptive use nor delayed subsequent pregnancies and births. The modest program investments—the parenting education together with the program-induced higher rates of non-maternal child care—did not alter significantly the developmental outcomes of the children of these teen mothers.[76,77]

Teen Family Home Visits

The Teenage Parent Home Visitor Services Demonstration was heavily influenced by both the highly favorable outcomes of the early demonstrations of the nurse home visitor services program in Elmira and Memphis and the mixed and disappointing findings from the Teenage Parent Welfare Demonstration. This demonstration tested the effectiveness of adding para-professional home visitor services to the type of mandatory work requirements and support services that formed the core of the Teenage Parent Welfare Demonstration and that were instituted as national policy in 1988. The appeal of this particular intervention model was in part its focus on a mechanism of intervention—home visitation—that had been demonstrated to reduce the rate of repeat pregnancies and births and improve parenting skills and child outcomes. However, it also was attractive for its relatively modest cost and potential to reach a majority of the welfare population. The results of the demonstration indicated that para-professional home visitor services can increase modestly the effectiveness of work-oriented programs for young mothers if the home visitors are well trained and supervised. They also can lead to higher rates of protection from STIs through higher rates of condom use and to lower exposure to unwanted pregnancies through higher rates of Norplant use. However, in order to achieve these impacts on condom use and choice of contraceptive methods, it was necessary to both provide substantial, highly directive training of the home visitors and closely supervise the home visitors.[78]

CONCLUSIONS

In summary, short-term interventions aimed at ensuring a safe pregnancy and delivery, reducing subsequent fertility, enhancing educational attainment, increasing parenting skills, enhancing employment, and reducing welfare dependency are expensive, and only those focused on prenatal care appear to be truly effective. The lesson to be learned is that no band-aid, quick-fix, inexpensive solutions exist for ameliorating the negative outcomes associated with adolescent childbearing.

A compelling question of public policy, therefore, is the relative effectiveness of fertility prevention versus ameliorative schemes for reducing poverty. Research suggests that preventing adolescent childbearing would be far more effective in reducing the proportion of young women who require public assistance than would increasing education, increasing marriage probabilities, or reducing subsequent fertility among adolescent mothers.[79] Such a finding is reassuring, because the public cost associated with teenage childbearing is substantial. The taxpayer cost of childbearing among women aged less than 18 is $6.9 billion, consisting of $2.2 billion for welfare and food stamps, $1.5 billion in medical care expenses, $1.0 billion to construct and maintain prisons to house the criminal teen sons who had been born to adolescent mothers, $0.9 billion for foster care, and $1.3 billion in lost tax revenue from the fathers. The total annual cost to society associated with childbearing by women under age 18 together with the other disadvantages faced by adolescent mothers is $29 billion.[80]

However, those who see lifelong economic and social disadvantage as the problem, and teenage childbearing as the consequence, warn that the conventional estimates such as those presented above overstate—perhaps substantially—the costs of teenage childbearing and therefore the benefits of reducing its incidence. The subtle danger is that research and analysis based on this perspective will. . .

. . . be used to argue that because teen pregnancy is not the linchpin that holds together myriad other social ills, it is not a problem at all. Concern about teen pregnancy has at least directed attention and resources to young, poor, and minority women. It has awakened many Americans to their diminished life chances. If measures aimed at reducing teen pregnancy are not the quick fix for much of what ails American society, there is the powerful temptation to forget these young women altogether and allow them to slip back to their traditional invisible place in American public debate. Teen pregnancy is less about young women and their sex lives than it is about restricted horizons and the boundaries of hope. It is about race and class and how those realities limit opportunities for young people. Most centrally, however, it is typically about being young, female, poor, and non-white and about how having a child seems to be one of the few avenues of satisfaction, fulfillment, and self-esteem. It would be a tragedy to stop worrying about these young women—and their partners—because their behavior is the measure rather than the cause of their blighted hopes.[81]

A sound rationale for supporting programs to reduce the incidence of adolescent pregnancy does not depend on resolving the current debate or on the accuracy of estimates about negative personal consequences or public costs. Few adolescents intentionally become pregnant. That adolescents want to avoid becoming pregnant is sufficient reason for helping them to do so.

TAILORING CLINIC SERVICES FOR THE NEEDS OF TEENS

The notion that many minors have the capacity and, indeed, the right to make important decisions about health care has been well established in federal and state policy. Many states explicitly authorize minors to consent to contraceptive services and testing and treatment for HIV and other STIs. Lawmakers have resisted attempts to impose parental notification or consent on minors' access to reproductive health care, with the exception of abortion (see Table 29-3).[82,83]

A review of more than 150 articles published since 1970 (with a focus on those published since 1980) has enriched our understanding of how clinics can best tailor their programs to meet the needs of sexually active teens.[84] Of these, 38 studies discussed aspects of adolescent behavior and sexual activity that could be related to the development of friendly and effective clinic practices, two studies on postponement of repeat teen pregnancies shed light on effective outreach and follow up practices, and six studies reported surveys of factors associated with improved services to teenagers. Three key features of effective and friendly clinics emerged: active outreach to attract clients, comprehensive services to meet individual needs, and thorough follow through to maintain clients in the program. In Table 29-4,[84] details of these features are classified under three acronyms: FIND, SERVE, and CARE. This model is an amalgam of characteristics of successful programs, presented within a theoretical context of adolescent growth and development. No program was identified that contains all the aspects of outreach, clinical services, and follow through in this model; thus, the overall impact of incorporating all programmatic aspects into one setting cannot yet be determined.

Table 29-3 Minor's right to consent to health care

MC = minor explicitly authorized to consent
NL = no law or policy found
PC = parental consent explicitly required
PN = parental notice explicitly required

State	Contraceptive Services	STD/HIV Services	Abortion Services
Alabama	NL	MC[1-3]	PC
Alaska	MC	MC	NL[4]
Arizona	MC	MC	NL
Arkansas	MC	MC[3,5]	PN[6]
California	MC	MC[1,7,8]	NL[4]
Colorado	MC[9,10]	MC[7]	NL[4]
Connecticut	NL	MC[7]	MC
Delaware	MC[1,3]	MC[1,3,5,7]	PN[11,12]
Dist. Of Colombia	MC	MC	MC
Florida	MC[9,10]	MC[2]	NL[4]
Georgia	MC	MC[2,3,5]	PN
Hawaii	MC[3,13,14]	MC[3,13,14]	NL
Idaho	MC	MC[2,13]	PC[6]
Illinois	MC[9,10]	MC[1-3]	NL[4]
Indiana	NL	MC	PC
Iowa	NL	MC[7,15]	PN[12]
Kansas	NL[16]	MC[3]	PN
Kentucky	MC[3]	MC[2,3]	PC
Louisiana	NL	MC[3]	PC
Maine	MC[9,10]	MC[3]	MC
Maryland	MC[3]	MC[3]	PN[12]
Massachusetts	NL[17]	MC	PC
Michigan	NL	MC[3,7]	PC
Minnesota	MC[3]	MC[3]	PN[6]
Mississippi	MC[9,10]	MC[2]	PC[6]
Missouri	NL	MC[3,5]	PC
Montana	MC[3]	MC[3,5,7]	NL[4]
Nebraska	NL	MC	PN
Nevada	NL	MC[2]	NL[4]
New Hampshire	NL	MC[13]	NL
New Jersey	NL	MC[3,5]	NL[4]
New Mexico	MC	MC[7,8]	NL[4]
New York	NL[17]	MC[7]	NL
North Carolina	MC	MC[2]	PC[12]
North Dakota	NL	MC[13,18]	PC[6]
Ohio	NL	MC[7,8]	PN[12,19]
Oklahoma	MC[3,20]	MC[2,3]	NL[4]
Oregon	MC[3]	MC[2,5]	NL
Pennsylvania	NL	MC[2]	PC
Rhode Island	NL	MC[7]	PC
South Carolina	MC[21]	MC[21]	PC[12,22]

(continued)

Table 29-3 Minor's right to consent to health care—(cont'd)

State	Contraceptive Services	STD/HIV Services	Abortion Services
South Dakota	NL	MC	PN
Tennessee	MC	MC^2	PC
Texas	NL^{23}	$MC^{2,3,5}$	PN
Utah	NL^{23}	MC	PN^{24}
Vermont	NL	$MC^{1,2}$	NL
Virginia	MC	MC^2	PN^{12}
Washington	NL^{25}	$MC^{2,5,13}$	NL
West Virginia	NL	MC	PN^{12}
Wisconsin	NL	MC	PC^{12}
Wyoming	MC	MC^2	PC
Total MC	26	51	3
Total PC/PN	0	0	31
Total NL/NA	25	0	17

Source: Boonstra and Nash (2000)[82] and AGI.[83]

Note: In all but 4 states, the age of majority is 18. In Alabama and Nebraska, it is 19, and in Pennsylvania and Mississippi, it is 21; however in Mississippi, 18 is the age of consent for health care.

1. Minor must be at least 12.
2. State officially classifies HIV/AIDS as an STI or infectious disease, for which minors may consent to testing and treatment.
3. Doctor may notify parents.
4. Law has been blocked by court action.
5. Includes surgery.
6. Involvement of both parents is required.
7. Law explicitly authorizes minor to consent to HIV testing and/or treatment.
8. Law does not apply to HIV treatment.
9. Minor may consent if a parent; also if married in DE, KY, ME, MD, MN, MS, MO and NV; also if married or pregnant in CO, FL, IL, MA, MT, NJ, NY and OK.
10. Minor may consent if she has a child or doctor believes minor would suffer "probable" health hazard if services not provided; in IL also if minor is referred by doctor, clergyman or Planned Parenthood clinic; in CO and MS also if minor is referred by a doctor, clergyman, family planning clinic, school of higher education or state agency.
11. Applies to minors younger than age 16.
12. Includes an alternative to parental involvement or judicial bypass. In MD the law provides for a physician bypass but does not have a judicial bypass.
13. Minor must be at least 14.
14. Excludes surgery.
15. Parent must be notified if HIV test is positive.
16. Any minor who is mature enough to understand the nature and consequences of the proposed medical or surgical treatment may consent.
17. The state funds a statewide program that gives minors access to confidential contraceptive care.
18. Parent must be shown the informed consent form for an HIV test before the minor signs it.
19. A revised law that requires parental consent is currently not in effect; meanwhile, the parental notification requirements remain in effect.
20. Minor may consent if she has ever been pregnant.
21. Any minor 16 or older may consent to any health service other than operations. Health services may be rendered to minors of any age without parental consent when the provider believes the services are necessary.
22. Applies to minors younger than age 17.
23. State funds may not be used to provide minors with confidential contraceptive services.
24. Law does not include a judicial bypass.
25. Providers rely on State v. Koome, which held that minors have the same constitutional rights as adults, to provide confidential contraceptive services and prenatal care to minors.

Table 29-4 Quick checklist for assessing whether contraceptive services to teens are optimal (FIND, SERVE, CARE Model)

FIND	
Are you maximizing the value of outreach? Specifically, are you:	**By:**
Providing a *Family-oriented* service?	• Recruiting clients through their mothers (who may have been teen mothers themselves) • Recruiting clients through their sister(s), who may have been teen mothers • Knowing what the teen's family has taught about sex • Knowing whether the teen is or has been sexually abused
Providing an *Integrated* service?	• Having an active, two-way referral system with schools • Having an active, two-way referral system with community-based organizations, clubs, etc. • Maximizing community interest in the clinic through advertisements, speeches, and community-based education programs

Providing a *Needed* service targeting teens who are more likely to have early or unprotected sex?	• Knowing which teens in the community are more likely to have sex at an early age; those who
	  — Are/were sexually abused
	  — Are substance abusers
	  — Are delinquents
	  — Lack adult supervision after school
	  — Live in poverty
	  — Live with one parent
	• Knowing which teens in the community are more likely to have unprotected sex; those who
	  — Initiated intercourse at an early age
	  — Are teen parents
	  — Are ambivalent about parenting
	  — Had a negative pregnancy test
	• Knowing where those teens are in the community
	• Getting into those areas and actively recruiting

Providing a *Determined* outreach effort?	• Having a sign on the clinic that is visible • Locating the clinic in a place accessible to teenagers • Encouraging clients to tell friends about the clinic and to bring friends with them • Including active outreach activities in the base budget • Evaluating the outreach efforts

(continued)

Table 29-4 Quick checklist for assessing whether contraceptive services to teens are optimal (FIND, SERVE, CARE Model)—*(cont'd)*

SERVE	
Are you maximizing the quality of your services? Specifically, are you:	**By:**
Making the services *Safe* for teen clients?	• Including a statement of confidentiality on advertising materials • Including a statement of confidentiality on clinic forms • Explaining the confidentiality policy to teens who visit the clinic
Making the services *Elastic* to fit individuals' needs?	• Providing services in late afternoons, evenings, weekends • Having few levels of hierarchy above the nursing level • Hiring female staff • Accepting governmental/state funding • Applying for external grants • Providing a mechanism to accept donations • Conducting community fund raisers • Accepting insurance coverage of services • Determining the dialects of the community • Determining literacy rates of the adolescent population • Hiring staff who speak the right languages at the right levels
Making the services *Related*?	• Working with parents in the community on ways to support teen contraceptive use • Counseling teens on ways they can involve their partners in contraceptive decision making • Encouraging teens to bring their partners and parents to clinic visits • Using peer counselors

Making the services *Varied*?	• Developing an intake screening tool that can be used to identify teens who may need additional attention which
	  — Identifies risks for early or unprotected sex (see *Needed*, under FIND)
	  — Assesses intention to use contraceptives (see *Assess*, under CARE)
	  — Contains a sexual and contraceptive history
	• Hiring staff with a background in recognizing sexual abuse and in counseling teens who have been abused
	• Through course work, workshops, and/or trainings, training current staff in recognizing and addressing sexual abuse

(continued)

Table 29-4 Quick checklist for assessing whether contraceptive services to teens are optimal (FIND, SERVE, CARE Model)—*(cont'd)*

SERVE	
Are you maximizing the quality of your services? Specifically, are you:	**By:**

Making the services *Varied?* (continued)	• Targeting materials and counseling to client's age
	• Administering medical protocols in an age-appropriate manner
	• Allowing clients to postpone the pelvic examination and blood work
	• Providing a broad range of contraceptive methods
	• Counseling on needed topics such as
	  — Sexual values
	  — Saying "no"
	  — Abstinence and alternate forms of intimacy
	  — Use, advantages, disadvantages, and effectiveness of various forms of birth control methods
	  — Signs and symptoms of STIs
	  — Family and peer relationships
	  — Decision making
	• Educating staff about the health and social services in the area available to teens
	• Discussing the personal goals of the client, including needs separate from family planning issues
	• Referring teen clients to health and social agencies in the area

Assuring that services are *Evaluated?*	• Obtaining ongoing feedback on service quality from clients • Establishing and periodically examining goals and objectives • Measuring progress towards goals achievement • Measuring impact of new program components

CARE	
Are you maximizing client continuation? Specifically, are you:	**By:**
Establishing and maintaining *Contact?*	• Getting the names and phone numbers of people the client says you may contact to help with return appointments • Getting mailing addresses that can be used • Creating a follow-up plan that does not compromise confidentiality

(continued)

Table 29-4 Quick checklist for assessing whether contraceptive services to teens are optimal (FIND, SERVE, CARE Model)—*(cont'd)*

Are you maximizing client continuation? Specifically, are you:	By:
Developing a means to *Assess* follow-up needs?	• Using a protocol to identify teens needing closer follow-up; those who — Are younger ages — Have a negative pregnancy test — Are ambivalent about using contraception — Are teen parents — Have experienced sexual abuse — Have a lower locus-of-control score — Have no articulated strong future goals
Assuring personal *Respect* for each client?	• Developing a system to collect information on the services used by each client and the outcome of her/his visits • Having teens see the same staff from visit to visit • Having teens see few staff at a given clinic visit • Training staff to apply developmental mileposts and longtudinal plans for contraceptive continuation
Doing what is required to *Encourage* continuation?	• Providing incentives for contraceptive continuation • Reviewing partner/parent involvement in ongoing contraceptive choices • Helping teens set goals and applauding their achievements

Source: Baden and Hogue (1997).[84]

This model can be used to conduct a program audit to determine which of these "best practices" are currently in place. Program managers in charge of more than one clinic could use the audit to determine whether differences in clinic performance are related to how closely each clinic reflects the ideal for teen friendly services. In setting priorities for program improvement, the director should involve teens from the community. They might jointly develop a "wish list" of components that might hold greater promise for improved clinic services within that community. Selected components can be added sequentially, with ongoing evaluation to determine their impact on the proportion of teens being served among those in need. Those additions that make an impact can be maintained, while those that do not can be replaced with other additions on the "wish list." In this systematic way, a program can be tailored to maximize its resources to meet the needs of its clientele. A related use of this model may be for the program administrator to justify additional financial support in order to add and evaluate a major new component (e.g., case management).

Adolescents with a negative pregnancy test result are an appropriate target group for contraceptive counseling and services. In one study, 62% of women aged 17 and younger seeking pregnancy tests in clinics tested negative. Many came for pregnancy tests even though they were certain they were not pregnant. Among those who had ever conceived, 1 in 4 had a prior negative test result at a clinic. Altogether almost 3 in 5 received a negative test result in a clinic prior to becoming pregnant.[85]

SUGGESTED READING

U.S. Department of Health and Human Services, Office of the Surgeon General. The Surgeon General's Call to Action to Promote Sexual Health and Responsible Sexual Behavior. Rockville MD: DHHS, 2001.

Luker K. Dubious conceptions: the politics of teenage pregnancy. Cambridge MA: Harvard University Press, 1996.

Brown SS, Eisenberg L. The best intentions: unintended pregnancy and the well-being of children and families. Washington DC: National Academy Press, 1995.

Kirby D. Emerging answers: research findings on programs to reduce teen pregnancy. Washington DC: The National Campaign to Prevent Teen Pregnancy, 2001.

REFERENCES

1. Henshaw SK. Personal communication to James Trussell, June 21, 2001.
2. Ventura SJ, Martin JA, Curtin SC, Mathews TJ. Births: final data for 1997. Nat Vital Stat Rep 1999;47(18).
3. Ventura SJ, Martin JA, Curtin SC, Menacker F, Hamilton BE. Births: final data for 1999. Nat Vital Stat Rep 2001;49(1).
4. Henshaw SK. Unintended pregnancy in the United States. Fam Plann Perspect 1998;30:24-29 & 46.
5. Abma JC, Chandra A, Mosher WD, Peterson LS, Piccinino LJ. Fertility, family planning, and women's health: new data from the 1995 National Survey of Family Growth. Vital Health Stat 1997;Series 23, Number 19.
6. Darroch JE, Landry DJ, Oslak S. Age differences between sexual partners in the United States. Fam Plann Perspect 1999;31:160-167.
7. Flanigan C. Personal communication to James Trussell, June 27, 2001.
8. Fields J. America's families and living arrangements: March 2000. Curr Popul Rep, Series P20-537. Washington DC: U.S. Census Bureau, 2001.
9. Abma JC, Sonenstein FL. Sexual activity and contraceptive practices among teenagers in the United States, 1988 and 1995. Vital Health Stat 2001;Series 23, Number 21.
10. Luker K. Dubious conceptions: the politics of teenage pregnancy. Cambridge MA: Harvard University Press, 1996.
11. Martin JA, Hamilton BE, Ventura SJ. Births: preliminary data for 2000. Nat Vital Stat Rep 2001;49(5).
12. Darroch JE, Singh S. Why is teenage pregnancy declining? The roles of abstinence, sexual activity and contraceptive use. New York NY: The Alan Guttmacher Institute, 1999.
13. Singh S, Darroch JE. Adolescent pregnancy and childbearing: levels and trends in developed countries. Fam Plann Perspect 2000;32:14-23.
14. Darroch JE, Frost JJ, Singh S. Can more progress be made? Teenage sexual and reproductive behavior in developed countries. New York NY: The Alan Guttmacher Institute, 2001.

15. Safer sex, condoms, and "the pill." Menlo Park CA: Henry J. Kaiser Family Foundation, November 2000.
16. David HP, Rademakers J. Lessons from the Dutch abortion experience. Stud Fam Plann 1996;27:341-343.
17. Furstenberg FF. When will teenage childbearing become a problem? The implications of western experience for developing countries. Stud Fam Plann 1998;29:246-253.
18. Gress-Wright J. The contraception paradox. Public Interest 1993;Number 113:15-25.
19. Dash L. When children want children: the urban crisis of teenage childbearing. New York NY: William Morrow, 1989. Reissued as: When children want children: an inside look at the crisis of teenage parenthood. New York NY: Penguin, 1990.
20. Forrest JD, Singh S. The sexual and reproductive behavior of American women, 1982-1988. Fam Plann Perspect 1990;22:206-214.
21. Brown SS, Eisenberg L. The best intentions: unintended pregnancy and the well-being of children and families. Washington DC: National Academy Press, 1995.
22. Zabin LS, Astone NM, Emerson MR. Do adolescents want babies? The relationship between attitudes and behavior. J Res Adolesc 1993;3:67-86.
23. Trussell J, Vaughan B. Selected results concerning sexual behavior and contraceptive use from the 1988 National Survey of Family Growth and the 1988 National Survey of Adolescent Males. Working Paper #91-12. Princeton NJ: Office of Population Research, Princeton University, 1991.
24. Harrison PF, Rosenfield A (eds). Contraceptive research and development: looking to the future. Washington DC: National Academy Press, 1996.
25. Mastroianni L, Donaldson PJ, Kane TT (eds). Developing new contraceptives: obstacles and opportunities. Washington DC: National Academy Press, 1990.
26. Trussell J, Stewart F, Guest F, Hatcher RA. Emergency contraceptive pills: a simple proposal to reduce unintended pregnancies. Fam Plann Perspect 1992;24:269-273.
27. Hoff T, Greene L, McIntosh M, Rawlings N, D'Amico J. Sex education in America: a view from inside the nation's classrooms. Menlo Park CA: Henry J. Kaiser Family Foundation, 2000.
28. Darroch JE, Landry DJ, Singh S. Changing emphases in sexuality education in U.S. public secondary schools, 1988-1999. Fam Plann Perspect 2000;32:204-211 & 265.
29. Landry DJ, Singh S, Darroch JE. Sexuality education in fifth and sixth grades in U.S. public schools, 1999. Fam Plann Perspect 2000;32:212-219.
30. Kirby D. Reducing adolescent pregnancy: approaches that work. Contemp Pediatr 1999;16:83-94.
31. Kirby D. Emerging answers: research findings on programs to reduce teen pregnancy. Washington DC: National Campaign to Prevent Teen Pregnancy, 2001.
32. Cates W, Berman SM, Darroch JE, Berkley S. Epidemiology of sexually transmitted diseases and STD sequelae. In: Hitchcock PJ, Boruch R, Flay B, Berkeley S, Kanouse D, Whitley R Darroch JE (eds). STDs in Adolescents: challenges for the 21st Century. New York NY: Oxford University Press, in press.
33. Centers for Disease Control and Prevention. Division of STD/HIV prevention annual report, 1993. Atlanta GA: Centers for Disease Control and Prevention, 1994.
34. Panchaud C, Singh S, Feivelson D, Darroch JE. Sexually transmitted diseases among adolescents in developed countries. Fam Plann Perspect 2000;32:24-32 & 45.
35. Division of STD Prevention, Centers for Disease Control and Prevention. Sexually transmitted disease surveillance 1999. Atlanta GA: Centers for Disease Control and Prevention, 2000.
36. Centers for Disease Control and Prevention. U.S. HIV and AIDS cases reported through June 2000. HIV/AIDS surveillance report. Atlanta GA: Centers for Disease Control and Prevention, 2000.
37. Kann L, Kinchen SA, Williams BI, Ross JG, Lowry R, Grunbaum JA, Kolbe LJ. Youth risk behavior surveillance—United States, 1999. MMWR 2000;49(SS-5).
38. Campbell AA. The role of family planning in the reduction of poverty. J Marriage Fam 1968;30:236-245.

39. Hayes CD (ed). Risking the future: adolescent sexuality, pregnancy and childbearing. Volume I. Washington DC: National Academy Press, 1987.
40. Clinton WJ. Address before a joint session of the Congress on the State of the Union. Washington DC, January 24, 1995. http://www.c-span.org/executive/stateofunion/sou95_trans.asp
41. Baldwin W, Cain VS. The children of teenage parents. Fam Plann Perspect 1980;12:34-43.
42. Fraser AM, Brockert JE, Ward RH. Association of young maternal age with adverse reproductive outcomes. N Engl J Med 1995;332:1113-1117.
43. Geronimus AT, Korenman S. Maternal youth or family background? On the health disadvantages of infants with teenage mothers. Am J Epidemiol 1993;137:213-225.
44. Rosenzweig MR, Wolpin KI. Sisters, siblings, and mothers: the effect of teen-age childbearing on birth outcomes in a dynamic family context. Econometrica 1995;63:303-326.
45. Speroff L, Glass RH, Kase NG. Clinical gynecologic endocrinology and infertility (Sixth Edition). Baltimore MD: Lippincott Williams and Wilkins, 1999.
46. Geronimus AT, Korenman S, Hillemeier MM. Does young maternal age adversely affect child development? Evidence from cousin comparisons in the United States. Popul Dev Rev 1994;20:585-609.
47. Moore KA, Snyder NO. Cognitive attainment among firstborn children of adolescent mothers. Am Sociol Rev 1991;56:612-624.
48. Geronimus AT, Korenman S. The socioeconomic consequences of teen childbearing reconsidered. Q J Econ 1992;107:1187-1214.
49. Hoffman SD, Foster EM, Furstenberg FF. Reevaluating the costs of teenage childbearing. Demography 1993;30:1-13.
50. Bronars SG, Grogger J. The economic consequences of unwed motherhood: using twin births as a natural experiment. Am Econ Rev 1994;84:1141-1156.
51. Wertheimer R, Jager J, Moore KA. State policy initiatives for reducing teen and adult non-marital childbearing. New Federalism: Issues and Options for States, No. A-43. Washington DC: Urban Institute, 2000.
52. Miller BC, Card JJ, Paikoff RL, Peterson, JL (eds). Preventing adolescent pregnancy: model programs and evaluations. Newbury Park CA: Sage Publications, 1992.
53. Kirby D, Short L, Collins J, Rugg D, Kolbe L, Howard M, Miller B, Sonenstein F, Zabin LS. School-based programs to reduce sexual risk behaviors: a review of effectiveness. Public Health Rep 1994;109:339-360.
54. Kirby D. A review of educational programs designed to reduce sexual risk-taking behaviors among school aged youth in the United States. Springfield VA: National Technical Information Service, 1995; #PB96108519.
55. Moore K, Sugland BW, Blumenthal C, Glei D, Snyder N. Adolescent pregnancy prevention programs: interventions and evaluations. Washington DC: Child Trends Inc., 1995.
56. Frost JJ, Forrest JD. Understanding the impact of effective teenage pregnancy prevention programs. Fam Plann Perspect 1995;27:188-195.
57. Philliber S, Namerow P. Trying to maximize the odds: using what we know to prevent teen pregnancy. Prepared for a technical assistance workshop to support the CDC Teen Pregnancy Prevention Program, 1995.
58. Card JJ, Niego S, Mallari A. Farrell WS. The program archive on sexuality, health & adolescence: promising "prevention programs-in-a-box." Fam Plann Perspect 1996;18:137-156.
59. Kirby D. Emerging answers: research findings on programs to reduce teen pregnancy. Washington DC: The National Campaign to Prevent Teen Pregnancy, 2001.
60. Philliber Research Associates (PRA). Creating and evaluating successful teen pregnancy prevention programs. Accord NY: PRA, 2001.
61. Terry E, Manlove J. Trends in sexual activity and contraceptive use among teens. Washington DC: The National Campaign to Prevent Teen Pregnancy, 2000.
62. With one voice: American adults and teens sound off about teen pregnancy. Washington DC: The National Campaign to Prevent Teen Pregnancy, 2001.

63. Flanigan C. What's behind the good news: the decline in teen pregnancy rates during the 1990s. Washington DC: The National Campaign to Prevent Teen Pregnancy, 2001.

64. Plichta SB, Weisman CS, Nathanson CA, Ensminger ME, Robinson JC. Partner-specific condom use among adolescent women clients of a family planning clinic. J Adol. Health 1992;13:506-11.

65. Bearman P, Bruckner H. Power in numbers: peer effects on adolescent girls' sexual debut and pregnancy. Washington DC: The National Campaign to Prevent Teen Pregnancy, 1999.

66. Brindis C, Davis L. Communities responding to the challenge of adolescent pregnancy prevention. Washington DC: Advocates for Youth, 1998.

67. Kreinin T, Kuhn S, Rodgers AB, Hutchins J (eds). Get organized: a guide to preventing teen pregnancy. Washington DC: The National Campaign to Prevent Teen Pregnancy, 1999.

68. Brown SS. Can low birth weight be prevented? Fam Plann Perspect 1985;17:112-118.

69. Makinson C. The health consequences of teenage fertility. Fam Plann Perspect 1985;17:132-139.

70. Olds DL, Kitzman H. Review of research on home visiting for pregnant women and parents of young children. Future Child 1993;3:53-92.

71. Olds DL, Henderson CR, Kitzman HJ, Eckenrode JJ, Cole RE, Tatelbaum RC. Prenatal and infancy home visitation by nurses: recent findings. Future Child 1999;9:44-65, 190-191.

72. Polit DF, Kahn JR. Project Redirection: evaluation of a comprehensive program for disadvantaged teenage mothers. Fam Plann Perspect 1985;17:150-155.

73. Polit DF. Effects of a comprehensive program for teenage parents: five years after Project Redirection. Fam Plann Perspect 1989;21:164-169, 187.

74. Quint JC, Bos JM, Polit DF. New Chance: final report on a comprehensive program for young mothers in poverty and their children. New York NY: Manpower Demonstration Research Corporation, 1997.

75. Weatherley RA, Perlman SB, Levine MH, Klerman LV. Comprehensive programs for pregnant teenagers and teenage parents: how successful have they been? Fam Plann Perspect 1986;18:73-78.

76. Maynard R, Rangarajan A. Prevalence and causes of repeat pregnancies among welfare-dependent teenage mothers. Fam Plann Perspect 1994;26:187-205.

77. Maynard R, Nicholson W, Rangarajan R. Breaking the cycle of poverty: the effectiveness of mandatory services for welfare dependent teenage parents. Princeton NJ: Mathematica Policy Research, Inc., 1993.

78. Kelsey M, Johnson A, Maynard R. The potential of home visitor services to strengthen welfare to work programs for teenage parents on cash assistance. Princeton NJ: Mathematica Policy Research, Inc., 2001.

79. Moore KA, Wertheimer RF. Teenage childbearing and welfare: preventive and ameliorative strategies. Fam Plann Perspect 1984;16:285-289.

80. Maynard RA (ed). Kids having kids: economic costs and social consequences of teen pregnancy. Washington DC: Urban Institute Press, 1996.

81. Luker K. Dubious conceptions: the controversy over teen pregnancy. Am Prospect 1991;5:73-83.

82. Boonstra H, Nash E. Minors and the right to consent to health care. Issues in Brief, 2000 Series, No. 2. New York NY: The Alan Guttmacher Institute, 2000.

83. AGI. State policies in brief: parental involvement in minors' abortions. New York NY: The Alan Guttmacher Institute, March 1, 2003.

84. Baden S, Hogue CJR. Family planning services for teens: a FIND, SERVE, CARE model. Unpublished manuscript. Atlanta GA: Rollins School of Public Health, Emory University, 1997.

85. Zabin LS, Emerson MR, Ringers PA, Sedivy V. Adolescents with negative pregnancy test results: an accessible at-risk group. JAMA 1996;275:113-117.

Dynamics of Reproductive Behavior and Population Change

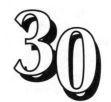

James Trussell, PhD

- Current population growth rates are very high by historical standards and cannot possibly persist indefinitely.
- Declining fertility inevitably leads to an aging of the population. Caring for an increasing proportion of elderly persons will be a significant problem in many countries.
- The impact of acquired immune deficiency syndrome (AIDS) on mortality rates and population growth could be dramatic and devastating in certain areas of the world, particularly in sub-Saharan Africa and Asia.
- Breastfeeding is an important contraceptive for a population even if an individual woman or couple cannot rely on it for very long.

In the United States, according to current experience, an average woman will bear 2.1 children in a lifetime that will last about 80 years. In Uganda, an average woman currently will produce 6.9 children; her life expectancy at birth is around 43 years. We will explore some of the reasons for these differences in the following sections. We will also examine the consequences of rapid population growth, the concepts of population momentum and population aging, and the results of governmental population policy.

Why should these issues be of concern to family planning practitioners? As firm believers in voluntary family planning, the authors of this book stress that we are dedicated to helping individuals achieve their reproductive life goals, whatever they may be. Nevertheless, individual reproductive choices do have aggregate consequences, because they determine the fertility of a population. It is only natural that those involved in family planning and reproductive health would be interested in understanding how the uses of contraception and its effectiveness, the prevalence of abortion, and the duration of lactation affect the aggregate level of fertility in a population. This chapter provides a framework of analysis for answering this question.

Fertility, however, is only one of the determinants of population change. The other two components—mortality and migration—are explored below in less detail. The final section describes several methodological tools for demographic analysis. We emphasize methodology for the sake of neither rigor nor completeness. Instead, such tools are necessary to avoid common pitfalls when thinking about reproductive issues that concern us all.

Determinants of Fertility

Why is fertility high in some populations and low in others? First, ages at menarche and menopause—which set biological limits on the start and end of childbearing—vary somewhat among populations. Second, proportions of females at each age who are sexually active and therefore exposed to the risk of pregnancy vary across populations. Third, populations vary in the spacing between initiation of sexual activity and the first live birth and in the spacing between one live birth and the next.

Menarche, Menopause, and Sterility

The average age of menarche normally varies only in a narrow range from about age 13 to about age 16.[1] The average age at menopause is much harder to measure; it is easy for a woman to know whether she has had a first period but hard to know if she has had her last. Ordinarily, menopause is assumed to have occurred if a specified period of time (e.g., 1 or 1.5 years) has passed since the last period. Menopause, too, appears to be largely confined to a rather narrow range, on average from about age 49 to age 52.[1]

The span between menarche and menopause could therefore be as short as 33 years or as long as 39 years. This difference of 6 years, all other factors being equal, could imply a difference in lifetime fertility of as much as 2 to 3 children, if, during the added 6 years, women experienced the maximum fertility rates that prevail in the primary childbearing years. For several reasons the difference is likely to be far smaller:

1. It is not possible to measure directly the age at which menopause occurs, so that 6 years may be an overestimate of the potential difference.

2. A difference of several years in estimated age at menopause between two populations, even if real, may mean only that in one population women have a longer period of subfecundity (reduced physiological capacity to produce a live birth) before becoming sterile. What we can observe directly is age at last birth, which seems to be on average near age 41 in populations not using contraception.[2,3]

3. Differences in age at menarche are unlikely to result in differences in fertility unless entry into a sexual union is tied closely to menarche. In most populations, women do not enter sexual unions until several years after menarche. Therefore, even though differences in the childbearing span could affect lifetime fertility, in practice the effect is likely to be small, at most a difference of 1 child over a lifetime and possibly much smaller.

AGE AT MARRIAGE AND PROPORTIONS MARRIED

A major determinant of fertility differences among populations is the age at which women begin sustained sexual activity.[4] In many populations, sexual intercourse is primarily confined to marriage, so that age at marriage, proportions ever marrying, and patterns of marital dissolution and remarriage are powerful determinants of fertility levels. One way to measure the impact of marriage on fertility is to compare the total fertility rates of married women with the total fertility rates of all women. Maximum fertility would be achieved if all women married at menarche and stayed married until menopause. This marriage pattern does not exist in any population. Estimates of the fertility-reducing effects of actual marriage patterns range from lows of 11% in Niger, 12% in Mali and Guinea, and 15% in Bangladesh to highs of 47% in Colombia, the Philippines, and Vietnam, and 50% in Kazakstan.[5]

While proportions of older women currently married do vary across populations, this variation is too small to account for a large portion of observed fertility differentials, particularly because marital fertility rates fall with age. In contrast, there is considerable variation in the proportions of young women who are married. For example, the fraction of 15 to 19 year-old women who are married varies from lows of 1% in a number of countries including Japan and Denmark, 2% in Hong Kong and 4% in China, to 38% in India, 48% in Bangladesh, and 58% in Sierra Leone.[6] Even if many developing countries adopted modern contraceptive practices, they are not likely to achieve growth rates lower than 1.5% per year unless age at marriage is also increased.[7] Increasing the age at which young women marry lowers total fertility by removing some young women from the risk of childbearing and raises the mean age at which women bear children, thereby lowering the annual population growth rate by lengthening the time between generations.[8]

Raising the age at which young women marry is almost certain to have effects other than the purely mechanically demographic. The most important is to enhance the status of women, allowing them to stay in school longer to acquire job-related skills, to work outside the home before marriage, and to enter marriage with more physical and emotional maturity and financial security. Such social changes are themselves likely to stimulate a demand for fertility control.[9,10] Because raising the age when women marry so profoundly alters the social fabric, governments may be unwilling or unable to use this potential instrument of public policy. In those populations with a high prevalence of consensual unions or premarital childbearing, a change in the legal minimum age for marriage may have little effect on fertility.

BIRTH INTERVAL LENGTH

Populations also differ widely in the length of time between one birth and the next, known as the birth interval. The shorter the average interval between births, the greater the number of births that can be squeezed into the childbearing span, and vice versa. The birth interval can be divided into three parts: the period of postpartum non-susceptibility during which a woman is not at risk of conception following a birth, the waiting time to a conception leading to the next live birth once she returns to risk, and the gestation period itself.[11] The last of these parts, the gestation period, does not vary from population to population. There is, however, considerable variation in the other two components.

Postpartum non-susceptibility. The period of postpartum non-susceptibility is primarily governed by the length of lactation. If women do not breastfeed, this period can be as short as 2 months. With prolonged breastfeeding, the period can be up to 1.5 years on average. For example, urban women in the Philippines breastfeed for an average of 5.6 months and do not resume menses for an average of 3.3 months.[12] In rural Nigeria, women breastfeed for 19.1 months and amenorrhea lasts for 14.3 months.[13] The contraceptive effect depends on the intensity (frequency and duration) of the infant's suckling, which in turn is heavily influenced by the extent of supplemental feeding, particularly by bottle.[14] (See Chapter 23 on Postpartum Contraception and Lactation.) In developing countries, particularly in sub-Saharan Africa, women may abstain from having intercourse during some or all of the period of breastfeeding.[15]

Waiting time to conceive. The length of time a sexually active woman must wait before conceiving a pregnancy that leads to a live birth is determined by the underlying fecundity (physiological capacity to produce a live birth) of the man and woman, the frequency and timing of intercourse, the prevalence and effectiveness of use of contraception, and the frequency of abortion (both spontaneous and induced). Of these four factors, the prevalence and effectiveness of contraceptive use and the frequency of induced abortion are the most important sources of fertility differences. Fetal wastage in the absence of induced abortion is certainly not constant across populations, but it is a relatively unimportant cause of differentials in fertility unless there is a high prevalence of syphilis. Likewise, fecundity, which declines with age within a given population, does not seem to vary much among populations unless there is a high prevalence of pelvic inflammatory disease (PID).

EFFECTS OF BREASTFEEDING AND CONTRACEPTION

Consider a typical developing country in which contraceptive use is low, but prolonged breastfeeding is nearly universal. Postpartum non-susceptibility lasts an average of 12 months. When not using contraception or breastfeeding, young women typically take about 6 months to become pregnant. Pregnancy lasts 9 months. Then the interval between one birth and the next (ignoring spontaneous abortions) is 12 + 6 + 9 = 27 months, or 2.25 years. The average fertility rate per year is therefore 1/2.25, or 444 births per 1,000 sexually active women.[a] A common effect of modernization is to decrease breastfeeding but increase contraceptive use. However, breastfeeding often decreases before contraceptive use increases.

If breastfeeding were completely abandoned in the population described above, the period of postpartum non-susceptibility would decrease to only 2 months. Thus the typical interval between births would also decrease: 2 + 6 + 9 = 17 months, or 1.42 years. The average fertility rate would rise from 444 to 706 births per 1,000 sexually active women—a rise of 59%. This simple calculation demonstrates the importance of lactation as a contraceptive to a population, even though it is not dependable enough for any individual woman to rely on it for very long to prevent pregnancy. (See Chapter 23.)

As contraceptive use increases, the waiting time to conception will rise and the birth interval will lengthen accordingly. If all women use contraception that reduces the monthly risk of pregnancy by 80% (say from .1667 to .0333), then the waiting time to conception would rise to about 30 months, since the waiting time can be shown to be the reciprocal (1/p) of the monthly probability (p) of conception. This rise would more than compensate for the decrease in the postpartum non-susceptible period, since the resulting birth interval would become 2 + 30 + 9 = 41 months. The fertility rate would fall by 59%, from 706 to 293 per 1,000.

The same reasoning leads to the conclusion that breastfeeding has little effect on fertility in the United States. Suppose women use contraception that reduces the monthly probability of conception to .01. The typical birth interval would be 111 months in the absence of breastfeeding (2 months of postpartum non-susceptibility, 100 months to conceive, and 9 months of gestation). Even if breastfeeding produced an average of 8 months of postpartum non-susceptibility, then the typical birth interval would increase by only 5%; both the proportion of infants breastfed and the average duration of breastfeeding would have to increase substantially in the United States to produce even this small effect.

EFFECT OF ABORTION

Many people mistakenly assume that 1 abortion will prevent 1 birth. Consider again the developing country with a birth interval among young women of 27 months (a period of postpartum non-susceptibility of 12

---

[a] We ignore here the effects of spontaneous abortion, which on average would add about two months to the average birth interval.

months, 6 months to get pregnant, and a pregnancy of 9 months). Imagine that every other pregnancy is aborted. Then the waiting time to conception would consist of the following parts: 6 months to get pregnant the first time, 3 months of pregnancy until the abortion, 1 month of postpartum non-susceptibility following the abortion, and 6 more months of waiting until the next pregnancy. Thus the total waiting time goes from 6 to 16 months, a rise of 167%. But the birth interval (12 + 16 + 9 months) would increase by only 37%, from 27 to 37 months. Hence, when every other pregnancy is aborted, the fertility rate would decline by only 27%, not 50% as might initially be expected. In summary, fertility is inversely related to the length of the total birth interval. Thus, a change in any component will have a less-than-proportional impact on the total, and hence on fertility. But, one might object, an abortion certainly prevents 1 birth. However, this way of thinking ignores the fact that the next birth occurs sooner when a pregnancy is aborted than when it results in a live birth. Therefore, while an abortion prevents a particular birth, it reduces the woman's lifetime births by fewer than 1 if her reproductive behavior does not otherwise change.

In contrast, an abortion in a population practicing highly effective contraception will prevent nearly 1 birth. Suppose that effective contraception reduces the monthly probability of conception to .01 and that breastfeeding is minimal. The average birth interval would be 111 months, as described earlier. If every other pregnancy is aborted, then the birth interval would rise to 215 months, an increase of 94%, and the fertility rate would fall by nearly half (48%). Hence, in the United States, some abortions (those occurring to women who use contraceptives effectively) will prevent nearly 1 birth while other abortions (those occurring to women who do not use contraceptives effectively) will prevent substantially less than 1 birth.

EFFECTS OF SEXUALLY TRANSMITTED INFECTIONS

Sexually transmitted infections (STIs) substantially reduce fertility in selected populations, although not in the United States.[16] Syphilis is an important cause of fetal loss among women with primary or secondary infections and may be an important factor contributing to low fertility among certain tribal groups in Burkina Faso and the Central African Republic.[17] Untreated PID caused by chlamydia and gonorrhea is a major cause of tubal infertility and sterility. The low fertility in Central Africa (a belt extending from the west coast of Cameroon and Gabon through northern Zaire into southwest Sudan) in the 1950s and 1960s[18] was attributed to a high prevalence of gonorrhea,[19] long before the additional role of chlamydia was recognized. In sub-Saharan Africa, gonorrhea and chlamydia are still common infections; yaws and pinta, while not sexually transmitted, are closely related to syphilis and are also treated with penicillin. Mass penicillin campaigns against gonorrhea (New Guinea), yaws

(Martinique), and yaws and pinta (Cameroon, Upper Volta, Zaire, and Zambia) were followed by pronounced increases in fertility.[17,19] It is possible that improved STI diagnostic and treatment services in sub-Saharan Africa as a component of AIDS prevention programs will also result in increased fertility.[20]

EFFECTS OF NUTRITION

A link between nutrition and fertility has been postulated as a relatively simple explanation for variations in marital fertility in populations that do not use contraception.[21] It is suggested that the lower the nutritional status of a population, the lower the fecundity and hence fertility. If nutrition is to have a demographically important impact on fertility, it must affect the waiting time to conception or the duration of postpartum non-susceptibility. The evidence suggests that chronic malnourishment may slightly increase the duration of postpartum non-susceptibility. But this effect will not amount to a difference of even 1 child in completed lifetime fertility. Nutrition does not appear to affect the waiting time to conception in chronically malnourished populations.[2,22,23] Chronic malnutrition probably does result in a delay in menarche, though, as argued above, the impact on fertility is likely to be very small. When food supplies are so short that there is outright famine and starvation, fecundity and hence fertility are reduced. But when malnourishment is chronic and food intake is above starvation levels, there does not appear to be an important nutrition-fertility link.

DETERMINANTS OF MORTALITY

As living conditions in a country improve, the causes of death shift quite dramatically.[24] In developing countries, infectious diseases are major causes of death. In developed countries such as the United States, degenerative diseases such as cancer and cardiovascular disease are the primary causes of death. This shift occurs primarily because infant and child mortality are much higher in developing countries. Poor nutrition makes children more susceptible to infection and less able to withstand illness that otherwise would not prove fatal. Improvement in living conditions implies better nutrition, sanitation, water supply, and access to public health measures such as vaccination against tetanus, measles, and other common diseases. With such improvements, children survive to adulthood, when degenerative diseases claim more lives.

Among Guatemalan women in 1964, for example, elimination of diarrheal, infectious, and parasitic diseases would have raised expectation of life at birth by 16.4 years, and elimination of cancer and heart disease would have added only 1.7 years. In contrast, elimination of the first three categories of diseases in the United States would have added 0.8 years, and the elimination of the two degenerative causes of death, 19.6 years.[25] The reason for the contrast between the United States and

Guatemala is quite simple. In the United States, virtually nobody died of the diarrheal, infectious, and parasitic diseases, while in Guatemala, a smaller fraction of women lived long enough to die of cancer or heart disease. An even more interesting contrast occurs in the United States itself. As stated above, elimination of heart disease and cancer would have added 19.6 years to the expectation of life. But the contributions of the two causes were very lopsided. Cancer accounted for only 2.6 years, whereas heart disease accounted for 17.1.

REPRODUCTIVE AND SEXUAL BEHAVIORS AFFECTING MORTALITY

Reproductive and sexual behavior significantly affect mortality in three major ways:

- The total number of children women bear, the ages at which they bear children, and length of intervals between births all affect maternal and infant health. Short intervals between births are associated with higher rates of infant, child, and maternal mortality. Reducing the number of children women bear would reduce maternal morbidity and mortality. These reductions would be greatest in populations with high fertility rates, poor health conditions, and high reproductive morbidity rates. Parents can minimize the risk of infant and child death by not bearing children at very young and very old ages, by averting high-parity births, and by lengthening the interval between births.[26]

- Breastfeeding significantly lowers the risk of infant and child death.[27]

- Unprotected sexual intercourse entails the risk of transmitting and acquiring STIs, including the human immunodeficiency virus (HIV), the virus that causes AIDS. STIs other than HIV are themselves associated with higher risks of transmitting and acquiring HIV. Pregnant women infected with HIV may transmit the infection to their infants in utero, during childbirth, or through breastmilk.

MATERNAL MORTALITY AND MORBIDITY

Each year an estimated 585,000 women worldwide die during pregnancy or childbirth. About 146,000 die from hemorrhage, 44,000 from obstructed labor, 74,000 from eclampsia (which causes convulsions and brain and kidney damage), and 87,000 from sepsis. About 20 million abortions are performed in unsafe conditions each year, resulting in the deaths of an additional 76,000 women and girls. Another 15 million women annually incur pregnancy-related or birth-related injuries, infections, or disabilities that are often left untreated. As a result, about 300 million women—more than a quarter of the adult female population in developing countries—live with debilitating health problems. The most obvious and distressing is fistula, which allows leakage of urine or feces into the vagina, bypassing muscles that normally control the flow; as many as 1 million women suffer from fistula. Several million women face increased risk during childbirth each year because of the traditional practice of female genital mutilation, experienced by more than 130 million women, nearly three-quarters of whom live in Nigeria, Egypt, Ethiopia, Sudan and Kenya.[28,29]

HIV AND AIDS

By the end of the century, an estimated 34.3 million people were living with human immunodeficiency virus (HIV). During 1999 alone, 5.4 million were infected and 18.8 million people had already died of AIDS, 3.8 million of them children. Over the course of the pandemic, 13.2 million children have been orphaned by acquired immune deficiency syndrome (AIDS). Joint United Nations Programme on HIV/AIDS (UNAIDS) estimates that 71% of people currently infected with HIV live in sub-Saharan Africa, 1.5% in East Asia and the Pacific, 16% in South and South-East Asia, 1.2% in Eastern Europe and Central Asia, 1.5% in Western Europe, 5% in Latin America and the Caribbean, 2.6% in North America, and 0.6% in North Africa and the Middle East.[30]

Despite a steady increase in the amount of international development assistance for HIV/AIDS, the funding per HIV-infected person was more than halved between 1988 and 1997.[31] Public health spending in 1997 for AIDS alone already exceeded 2% of gross domestic product (GDP) in 7 of 16 African countries sampled, countries where total health spending accounts for 3 to 5% of GDP.[30]

The impact on mortality rates and on population growth could be dramatic and devastating in certain areas of the world. In several sub-Saharan African countries, AIDS has already become the leading cause of adult mortality, doubling or tripling death rates that were already eight times those in developed countries. In countries like Botswana, where an estimated third of all adults are infected with HIV, there will be more adults in their 60s and 70s in 20 years time than there will be adults in their 40s and 50s. In practically any country where at this time at least 15% of adults are infected with HIV, at least 35% of boys currently aged 15 will die of AIDS, and the projections for women are just as sobering. Child mortality has risen sharply in such countries as well, rolling back important gains in child survival.[30] Population growth rates were estimated to be at least 1 percentage point lower in 2000 because of HIV/AIDS in Burundi, the Central African Republic, Malawi, Rwanda, Tanzania, Uganda, Zambia, and Zimbabwe.[32] The prognosis for several countries in Asia, particularly India, Indonesia, Myanmar, and Vietnam, is just as bleak.

DETERMINANTS OF MIGRATION

Compared with fertility and mortality, migration receives relatively less academic attention. It is also the process that is least linked to biology and most linked to economic, social, and political conditions. When assessing the determinants of migration, investigators have traditionally emphasized "push" and "pull" factors. Push factors include extraordinary events such as wars, floods, famines, political or religious persecution, and more ordinary conditions associated with depressed economic conditions: high unemployment, low wages, and little hope. Pull factors are those that attract people to a location. They are often those associated with economic opportunity: good jobs, high wages, and good public services such as education. They may also include an attractive environment, religious freedom, and proximity to family or large ethnic groups. These factors help to explain why people in the United States have been moving from the north and east to the south and west, from the frostbelt to the sunbelt. These factors also help explain rural-to-urban migration in developing and developed countries. Urban wages are typically higher, and public services are better.

The rapid growth of cities in developing countries is a matter of great concern to policymakers. However, careful examination of available data leads to several conclusions that do not support popular perceptions.[33] First, the rate of out-migration from rural to urban areas is higher in developed than in developing countries. Second, rates of urbanization in currently developing countries are not especially high if compared with currently developed countries when they were in a similar stage of development. Third, the primary determinant of the growth of urban areas in developing countries is the rate of natural increase, which accounts for about three-fifths of the growth while net in-migration explains the remaining two-fifths. However, the rate of growth of the absolute size of the urban population, as opposed to the rate of growth of the proportion urban in the total population, is very high by historical standards— precisely because the rate of natural increase is so high. This observation suggests that policies that slow the rate of natural increase, such as provision of family planning services, can have the added benefit of reducing urban growth.

POPULATION GROWTH AND AGE STRUCTURE

The age structure of a population is completely determined by its history of fertility, mortality, and migration. In Figure 30-1,[34,35] we see two examples of age pyramids, one for the United States and one for Mexico. We notice immediately that the profile for the United States is more nearly vertical (or steeper). Although one might think that the difference is due to mortality, it is, in fact, due almost entirely to fertility. This fact can be demonstrated by examining populations with different levels of fertility and mortality. If fertility and mortality remain constant for a long time, then the age distribution of the population will also become

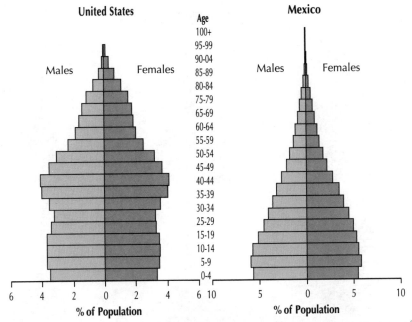

United States   Age   Mexico

Males   Females   Males   Females

100+
95-99
90-04
85-89
80-84
75-79
65-69
60-64
55-59
50-54
45-49
40-44
35-39
30-34
25-29
15-19
10-14
5-9
0-4

6   4   2   0   2   4   6   10   5   0   5   10

% of Population   % of Population

Source: INEGI (2001),[34] U.S. Census Bureau (2002).[35]

Figure 30-1 Age pyramids for the United States and Mexico

constant. The population itself may grow, shrink, or remain the same size, but the proportion of the population in each age group will remain the same. Such a population is known as a stable population; if its growth rate is zero, it is called stationary. The age distributions of the six stable populations resulting from combinations of three levels of fertility (total fertility rates of 2, 5, and 8 lifetime births per typical woman) and two levels of mortality (life expectations of 35 and 70) are shown in Figure 30-2.[36] Mortality plays the smaller role in determining the shape of the age profile; whether women have 2 or 8 children has a far greater impact on the age profile than whether they live 35 or 70 years.

POPULATION MOMENTUM

The age profile of a population contains momentum, just as a moving locomotive does. This momentum occurs because the number of persons already born implies much about future growth. The easiest way to understand the power of momentum is to ask how large the population would ultimately be if (1) the number of births in future years remains the same as the number this year, and (2) mortality remains constant. As is demonstrated in the last section of this chapter, a population with the same number of births each year and constant mortality will ultimately have the same age distribution as the underlying life table. Life expectancy (E) is the ratio of total person-years lived to the number of births

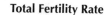

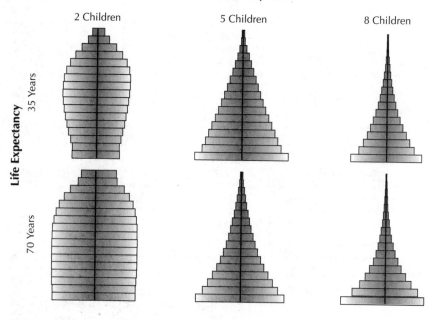

Source: Coale and Demeny (1966).[36]
For interpretation of population pyramids, see Figure 30-1.

Figure 30-2 Age pyramids for six stable populations

(B). Then the total person-years lived by the population, or equivalently the total size of the stationary population, is E times B. Consider again the case of the United States and Mexico. (See Figure 30-1.) The number of births in 2001 in Mexico was 2.4 million and the expectation of life was 75 years.[37] Hence the ultimate size of the stationary population would be 180 million or 81% larger than the 2001 population. In the United States, the number of births was about 4.3 million and the life expectancy about 77 years.[37] Hence, the ultimate size would be 331 million, about 16% larger than the 2001 population. We see that the Mexican population currently contains more momentum than does the U.S. population. The larger momentum results from its past high fertility, which has produced an age distribution with a very wide base (Figures 30-1 and 30-2).

These calculations are "quick and dirty" estimates. They give a precise answer to the question of what the size of the population would be if the number of births and mortality rates remained constant. But it is very unlikely that the number of births in Mexico will remain the same. From the age distribution shown in Figure 30-1, it is clear that the age-specific fertility rates would have to fall over time for the number of births to remain constant because the number of women of childbearing age will continue to increase for many years. Therefore, the size of the Mexican population is very likely to surpass 180 million in the future. In the United States, on the other hand, the number of births would decrease over time because the number of women currently of childbearing age is atypically large (the children of the baby boom). In fact, if the current age-specific mortality and fertility rates continued into the future, the size of the U.S. population (ignoring migration) would ultimately neither grow nor shrink in the distant future since the typical woman now bears almost exactly 1 daughter (see the section on Gross and Net Reproduction Rates at the end of this chapter).

SOCIETAL CONSEQUENCES OF IRREGULAR AGE DISTRIBUTIONS

Age distributions convey more than information about population momentum. Often they imply real problems for society. In the United States, the size of the population age 65 and over rose only from 17% of the size of the working age (18 to 64) population in 1960 to 20% in 2000.[35,38] If current trends continue, however, the fraction will rise to 32% by the year 2025 and to 36% by the year 2050.[35] Those projections also indicate that the size of the population age 85 and over will rise only from 2.5% of the size of the working age population in 2000 to 3.8% in 2025; however, it will increase rapidly thereafter, reaching 8.6% in 2050.[35] This rise in the fraction of old persons in the population is mostly the consequence of the rapid decline in fertility levels, from "baby boom" to "baby bust." The increase in population over age 65 has strained the social security system, which relies on the contributions of the current workers to finance benefits for the current retired population. The challenge of caring for the elderly is perhaps even more severe in Japan, where changes in the age structure will occur more rapidly than in the United States. For example, the elderly dependency ratio (population age 65+/population aged 15 to 64) in Japan will nearly double between 2000 and 2025, from 25% to 45%, and then rise to 58% by 2050.[39] Perhaps of greater importance for social and economic planning is the absolute increase in the number of elderly persons. Between 2000 and 2025, the size of the population age 65 and over is expected to nearly double in the United States, from 35 million people to 63 million, and to more than double in China, from 87 million to 195 million.[35,39] In the United States, the population age 85 and older is projected to grow rapidly, from 4.3 million in 2000, to 7.4 million in 2025, to 19.3 million in 2050 when it will comprise nearly 5% of the total population.[35]

In the United States, fertility fell as a consequence of decisions by millions of couples to limit childbearing. Government policy, especially after the 1973 Supreme Court decision legalizing abortion, did not attempt to limit individual control of reproductive behavior. Two more examples reveal the potential power of government action; they also highlight the value of demographic analysis before action is taken. In 1966 the government of Romania introduced pronatalist policies, including banning virtually all abortions and discontinuing importation of oral contraceptives and intrauterine devices (IUDs). The result was as instantaneous as it was stunning.[40,41] Within 8 months, the monthly birth rate doubled; within 11 months, it tripled. The birth cohorts of 1967 and 1968 were twice the size of the cohorts preceding them. What were the economic and social effects? Inadequate hospital care for the babies and their mothers caused infant and maternal mortality to rise sharply. As a consequence of unsafe illegal abortion, maternal mortality increased to a level 10 times that in any other European country. In the 23 years the policy was enforced, more than 10,000 women died from unsafe abortions. Many women who did not resort to unsafe abortion bore unwanted children, whom they placed in institutions. Such large-scale warehousing of children overwhelmed these institutions and severely degraded the quality of care. The educational system had to digest a giant bulge of students. Other problems, such as employment and housing, also arose as the large cohorts aged. The government took action because it was worried about low levels of fertility (fertility rates in 1965 implied that the typical woman who lived to age 50 would bear only 1.9 children). Its action certainly had the result of increasing fertility, but obviously the government had not thought clearly about the consequences. The ban on abortion was reversed immediately after the Ceaucescu regime was overthrown in December 1989.

Another example illustrates the problems caused by government attempts to lower fertility quickly. From 1979 through 1983, the government of China vigorously promoted the policy of one child per family.[b,42,43] What would be the consequences if the one-child policy were strictly adopted? By the year 2035, about a quarter of the population would be age 65 and over, versus only about 5% in 1975.[44] Only a tiny minority of Chinese are eligible for the state system of social security for the aged, so the state-financed system of old-age security would not be in danger of collapsing. Nevertheless, the traditional family structure would change radically in ways that would jeopardize the family's ability to care for the elderly and reduce its potential as a production unit; there would be no brothers, sisters, aunts, or uncles. The one-child policy may have already had the unintended side-effect of inducing female infanticide or female-specific abortion due to a cultural preference for sons.[42,45–47] Results of demographic analysis suggest that the Chinese could meet their aggregate population targets by replacing the one-child policy with a two-

---

[b] Since that time, the government has pursued a more flexible policy by allowing certain categories of couples to have 2 (but never 3) children. Furthermore, clear repudiation from the central government appears to have throttled the excessive zeal with which subordinate officials implemented the policy (mandatory insertion of IUDs for women with 1 child, abortion for unauthorized pregnancies, and sterilization for couples with 2 or more children).

child policy having a minimum age at first birth of 27 and a minimum birthspacing interval of 4 years.[48] While the two-child policy would not avoid the adverse age distribution effect, it would offer couples greater choice (they could have 1 child any time or 2 children subject to the rules) and reduce the adverse effects on the family.

DEMOGRAPHIC TRANSITION

Historically, the national populations of Western Europe tended to undergo first a fall in mortality and only later a fall in fertility. This observation led to a formal description of the process known as the demographic transition, which is shown in Figure 30-3. The paradigm is one of high birth and death rates in the pre-transition phase. Birth and death rates were not necessarily equal in every year. Fertility was the more stable. In good years, mortality was low. But the population was subject to chronic food shortage resulting from vagaries of the weather and limited storage and transport capacities, as well as periodic epidemics. Generally, mortality fluctuated widely and birth and death rates, on the average, balanced.

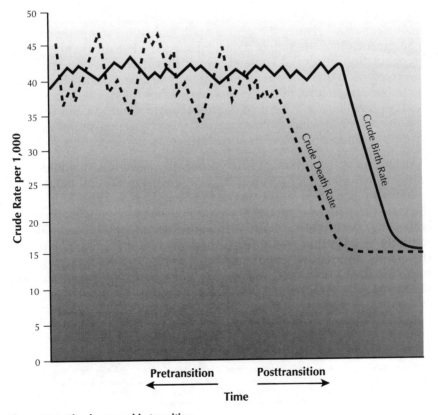

Figure 30-3 The demographic transition

At the time of the industrial revolution, mortality fell because of improvements in living conditions, such as better housing and food distribution networks, and public health measures, such as the provision of clean water. These changes required little or no individual action. Lowering fertility, however, requires that individuals make conscious decisions about postponing marriage or controlling fertility within marriage. These personal decisions were made only after standards of living had improved considerably. Several mechanisms have been suggested. As couples realized that mortality had fallen, they would need to have fewer births in order to attain the same number of surviving children. As the status of women changed, primarily through mass education, high fertility became less desirable to them.[49,50] Moreover, the changing economic value of children would motivate a desire to limit fertility. In traditional societies wealth flows upward, from the young to the old. In modern societies, wealth flows from the old to the young, as parents invest heavily in their children's education.

All developed countries have experienced a demographic transition. For some, however, the lag between the fall in mortality and the fall in fertility was short and for others, long. The strict interpretation of the classical paradigm has been shown to be incorrect. When the countries of Europe are examined on a provincial basis, the results indicate that fertility sometimes fell before mortality declined and before education became general.[51] Hence, the demographic transition is a more complicated process than the simple paradigm suggests. Exhaustive analysis of the population history of England reveals that it did not correspond to the prototypical high-pressure regime of high birth and death rates before the transition. Instead, mortality was, on average, moderate and fertility was kept moderate, not through control of marital fertility, but through controls on age at which women marry.[52] Other pre-transition societies have also been found to have moderate levels of marital fertility.[51,53]

Demographic transition theory is especially relevant if, in addition to telling us why fertility fell historically, it yields predictions about what would cause fertility to fall in currently developing countries. Appeal to the classical statement of the theory would suggest that development is the best contraceptive. Indeed, this was the position taken by many at the World Population Conference in Bucharest in 1974, a conference split between those who thought that family planning programs were the key to reducing fertility and hence population growth, and those who felt that policy makers should concentrate on development, and population would take care of itself.[c,54,55]

---

[c] The United States was the leader of the family planning approach in Bucharest but reversed its position at the 1984 International Conference on Population held in Mexico City due to intense political pressure from social conservatives, particularly anti-abortion groups. The U.S. position that rapid population growth does not hinder and even fosters economic development was supported only by the Vatican. Ironically, those developing countries that had been the most vocal critics of the U.S. position in Bucharest also switched sides in Mexico City. The 1994 International Conference on Population and Development held in Cairo resulted in a shift of focus away from demographic targets and toward reproductive health and the empowerment of women and sustainable development.

A careful reading of the evidence from the historical experience of current developed countries and the recent experience of developing countries suggests that (1) declines in marital fertility occurred in a wide variety of social and economic settings, (2) deliberate attempts to limit family size were not only largely absent but also probably unknown prior to the onset of the decline in fertility, even though a substantial fraction of births may have been unwanted, (3) the decline of marital fertility and the adoption of family limitation were essentially irreversible processes once under way, (4) cultural setting had an important and independent effect on the onset and spread of fertility decline, and (5) social interaction, through which people exchange and evaluate information and ideas and exert and receive social influence, plays a central role in fertility decline.[56,57] These considerations lead one to adopt a position midway between the two extremes adopted at Bucharest. Although the empirical record does confirm a relationship, albeit loose, between socioeconomic modernization and fertility decline, it also reveals important innovation-diffusion and social interaction aspects of the practice of fertility control. Emphasizing the right of couples to make an informed decision about the number of children they want to have, and providing them with information and technical assistance to give meaning to this right, particularly when coupled with advances in the status of women, and the educational power of mass media, can markedly reduce fertility.[58] Access to the broadest array of fertility-regulating technologies consistent with the principle of informed consent is essential.[59]

Considerable survey evidence suggests that large fractions of women in developing countries desire increased spacing between children or termination of childbearing.[60,61] Consequently, as three recent comprehensive reviews of and two international conferences on population and development have concluded, voluntary family planning could play an important role in aiding the development process.[62-66] While slower population growth would benefit development in most developing countries, it would not automatically make poor countries rich and is no substitute for the elimination of market imperfections.

China illustrates an alternative to voluntary family planning that is clearly effective in reducing fertility and the rate of population growth. However, it is unlikely that many other governments would have the authority to implement such compulsory policies, even if they had the desire. Human-rights issues aside, experience with mass sterilization campaigns in India suggests that coercive or compulsory attempts to bring down the birth rate are more likely to bring down the government instead.

Nevertheless, it is doubtful that further investments in voluntary family planning programs alone would halt rapid population growth. About 700 million people are projected to be added to the population of developing countries in each of the following two decades.[39] The population of the developing world is estimated to grow from 4.1 billion in 1990 to 10.2 billion in 2100. Of this increase of 5.7 billion, 1.9 billion can be attributed to unwanted fertility, 1.0 billion to high desired family size and 2.8 billion to population momentum. Therefore, if such growth is to be avoided, further policy options to reduce demand for large families and to limit population momentum are needed. These include enhancing the status of women, raising the average age at childbearing by increasing age at marriage, reducing adolescent childbearing, and increasing intervals between births.[67]

MEASURING FERTILITY, MORTALITY AND POPULATION GROWTH

The population of a state, county, city, or country can change in only three ways: through births, deaths, or migration. New persons can be added by birth or in-migration; persons can exit through death or out-migration. Total world population can change in only two ways: births and deaths.

The question of how to measure these processes immediately arises. For example, how should one compare mortality across populations? In 2001, there were an estimated 2.6 million deaths in the United States and only 456 thousand in Uganda.[37] Does the fact that there were more than five times as many deaths in the United States as in Uganda indicate that it is healthier to live in Uganda? A moment's reflection will convince one that it is not. There were 284.5 million people in the United States (and therefore at risk of dying) and only 24.0 million people in Uganda. If one divides the number of deaths by the population at risk, one obtains the *crude death rate* (CDR). The CDR provides a simple index of mortality conditions. These rates were 9 per 1,000 population (.009) in the United States and 19 per 1,000 (.019) in Uganda.

Many readers will immediately recognize the necessity of controlling for the size of the population at risk of dying when comparing the mortality conditions in different populations. But in other contexts, this same methodological principle is often overlooked. For example, in 1982 the Centers for Disease Control issued a report calling attention to its estimate that for the first time in the United States contraceptive-related deaths outnumbered pregnancy-related deaths.[68] This finding was widely (mis)interpreted by the press to mean that it is just as dangerous to prevent pregnancy as it is to become pregnant. But such reasoning ignores the fact that there are two different populations at risk in this comparison. Only women who become pregnant can die of pregnancy-related causes. A much larger number of women is at risk of death from contraception-related causes. Most of the contraceptive-related deaths were estimated to occur among women using the pill; even so, more than twice as many women used the pill as became pregnant. Hence the risk of death from prevention of pregnancy is far lower than the risk of death from pregnancy.[69]

CRUDE RATES

Rates are defined by demographers to be the number of events divided by the average number of persons exposed to the risk of the event in a year. The denominator of a rate can also be described as the number of *person-years* lived; the concept of person-years is a natural generalization of man-hours or person-hours. Using a rate, such as the CDR, avoids the severe problems in interpretation, as illustrated above, caused by examination of the numerator alone (e.g., deaths), without reference to the population at risk (the denominator). Another example of a rate is the *crude birth rate* (CBR), the number of births in a year divided by the total mid-year population. The difference between the crude birth rate and the crude death rate is known as the *crude rate of natural increase* (CRNI). If migration is negligible, the CRNI is also the *crude growth rate* (CGR), usually referred to more simply as the growth rate; otherwise, the CGR is the sum of the crude birth rate and the crude rate of in-migration minus the sum of the crude death rate and the crude rate of out-migration.

The population of the world in mid-2001 is estimated to have been 6.137 billion. It is currently growing at a rate of 1.3% per year.[37] In 2001 approximately 80 million people—a number comparable to the total population of Germany, the twelfth largest country in the world—were added; this growth results in the addition of 219 thousand people every day, or 9 thousand people every hour. Should this growth of 1.3% continue, in 50 years' time the population would be 11.7 billion, and in 100 years would be 22.3 billion. Of course, such growth could not continue indefinitely. Indeed, the growth rate has fallen after having reached a peak of 2.04% per year in the period 1965–70.[39]

DOUBLING TIME

The growth rate is a simple measure of the rapidity of population growth. It can be used to determine the length of time it would take a population to double, known as the *doubling time*. If a population is growing at a rate of r% per year, then it will double in approximately T = 69.3/r years (see Figure 30-4).[d,37,39,70]

The concept of geometric growth or doubling (1, 2, 4, 8, 16 . . .) originally led Malthus to the dismal conclusion that population would soon outstrip the food supply.[71] He reached this conclusion by arguing that if population growth continued unchecked, it would increase in a geometric sequence (1, 2, 4, 8, 16, 32, 64, 128 . . .), while food supply could grow only in an arithmetic sequence (1, 2, 3, 4, 5, 6, 7, 8 . . .). Under such conditions the ratio of food to population would diminish rapidly. Fortunately, as we all know, Malthus' prediction has thus far been incorrect. He did not foresee improvements in agricultural technology and the widespread acceptance of contraception in many societies.

---

[d] This formula is correct for all values of r if r is the continuously compounded (exponential) rate of growth. If r is derived from the formula r={P(2)/P(1)-1.0}×100 (i.e., the population this year is r% bigger than the population last year), then the doubling time formula is a very good approximation for values of r up to 10%. The exact formula in this case, used to derive the figures in the text, is $T = \ln(2)/\ln(1 + r/100)$, where ln is the natural logarithm.

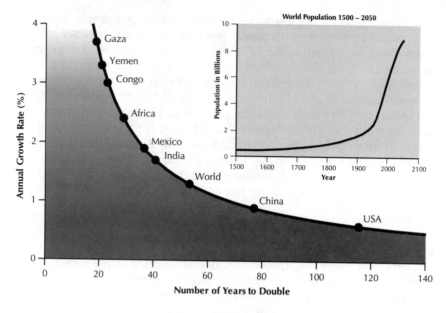

Sources: Haub and Cornelius (2001);[37] United Nations (1995,[65] 1999[39]).

Figure 30-4 Doubling time and world population growth curve

Nevertheless, geometric growth is still staggering. Many students who are first introduced to the concept are surprised to learn that the world population growth rate is 1.47%. After all, this number is small compared with inflation rates in excess of 10% and interest rates of 15% or more common in many countries. Still, at the current growth rate, the population of the world would double in 54 years and quadruple in 107 years. To see just how great the current growth rate is, let us compare it with the population growth rate in the past. Imagine that Adam and Eve lived about 100,000 years ago. What average growth rate would result in a population of 2 growing to a population of 6.137 billion in 100,000 years? The answer is a very small number, only .0218%. Another way of looking at this issue is to determine what the population of the earth would be if it had grown at 1.3% for 100,000 years. The answer is ridiculously large: approximately the number 176 followed by 559 zeroes! Finally, we might work backwards from the present by asking when Adam and Eve would have lived if the population growth rate had remained constant at 1.3% ever since. A population of 2 would grow to 6.137 billion in 1,691 years; hence Adam and Eve would have lived in the Garden of Eden in the year 310 A.D., in reality just 4 years after Constantine the Great became emperor of the Holy Roman Empire. We see from these three calculations that the current growth rate is very large by historical standards.

PROBLEMS WITH CRUDE RATES

All the rates discussed above are called crude rates because they make no allowance for the age distribution of the population. A simple example will demonstrate that they are indeed crude and that more refined measurement is needed. In 1980, the CDR in Mexico was 6.2 per 1,000 population, while in the United States it was 8.8.[72] One might be tempted to conclude that the United States provided a less healthy environment. In fact, the death rates in every age group (0-14, 15-44, 45-64, and 65+) were higher in Mexico. How could this anomaly arise? The answer is quite simple. The crude death rate in the United States was higher because its population was older (a much smaller fraction aged 0-14 and a much larger fraction over age 45) than Mexico's. If the United States' age-specific death rates had prevailed in Mexico, the CDR in Mexico would have been only 3.8 instead of 6.2. Similarly, if the Mexican death rates at all ages had prevailed in the United States, the CDR would have been 11.4 instead of 8.8.

Why does the age distribution of a population affect the CDR? It does so because death rates are not the same at every age. A typical example of death rates by age is shown in Figure 30-5.[36] Examination reveals that age-specific death rates after childhood rise with age; the probability of dying at age 60 is much higher than the probability of dying at age 40, which in turn is higher than the probability of dying at age 20. This example helps us to understand why the current CDR in the United States is higher than the CDR in Egypt, Indonesia, Iran, Libya, Malaysia, Mexico, Nicaragua, Syria, Thailand, and Vietnam, although mortality, when properly measured, is higher in these countries. The crude birth rate is less problematic because childbearing, unlike death, is confined to the middle of the age distribution.

PEARL INDEX: A PROBLEMATIC CRUDE RATE

There is a parallel between problems with crude death rates and a crude technique of determining contraceptive effectiveness called the Pearl index, which is calculated as the number of unintended pregnancies divided by the number of women-years of exposure to risk of pregnancy. Each woman contributes to the denominator the number of years of exposure from the beginning of use of a method until the end of the study, until the occurrence of an unintended pregnancy, or until she stops using the method for other reasons. The problem arises because contraceptive failure rates decline with duration of use, just as in the previous mortality example death rates in adulthood rise with age. Failure rates fall with duration of use because those women most prone to fail become pregnant early after starting use, so that over time the group of continuing users becomes increasingly composed of those least likely to fail. As a consequence, the longer the study runs, the more years of exposure each individual woman is allowed to contribute and the lower will be the failure rate.

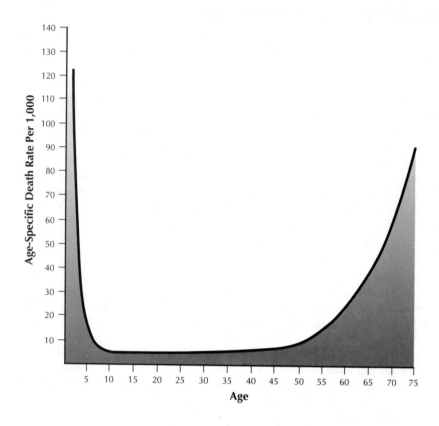

Source: Coale and Demeny (1966).[36]

Figure 30-5 Age-specific mortality rates for a typical population with expectation of life of 50 years

Hence, two investigators using data from a survey designed to yield estimates of contraceptive failure in the United States could obtain Pearl-index pregnancy rates of 7.5 and 4.4 per 100 women-years of exposure for the condom.[73] How could the two investigators get such different rates? One (who got 4.4) allowed each woman to contribute a maximum of 5 years of exposure while the other (who got 7.5) allowed each woman to contribute only 1 year. Which investigator is incorrect? Neither. The two rates are simply not comparable. The lesson is that when comparing the effectiveness of different contraceptive methods, one must be careful to ensure that failure is measured in the same way. We suggest, in fact, that the common measure be the probabilities of failure within the first, second, third, fourth and fifth years of use, calculated by life table techniques, which are discussed below.

AGE-SPECIFIC RATES

Crude rates can often hide more than they reveal because of the influence of the age structure of the population. Therefore, demographers prefer to calculate age-specific rates. These can be one-year rates calculated for every single age, but they are more commonly 5-year rates computed for standard 5-year age groups. Age-specific death rates are computed by dividing the number of persons alive in the age group into the number of deaths to persons in that group; they may, of course, be computed for each sex separately. Age-specific birth rates are normally computed in a different way. Only women enter the denominator, since only women bear children. Births to women in each age group are divided by the number of women in that group. The problem with age-specific rates is that there are many numbers. It is inconvenient to compare fertility in the United States and Mexico by looking at 35 single-year age-specific fertility rates, or even seven 5-year rates. Hence, there is a need to combine the age-specific rates into a single fertility or mortality index that is free of any age-distribution effect.

TOTAL FERTILITY RATE

Suppose we simply add all the age-specific fertility rates together. If we do so in the United States, we get 2.1. What does this number mean? Recall that the fertility rate at age 20, for example, is the number of births to women aged 20 divided by the number of women aged 20. Thus, the age-specific fertility rate is the number of babies produced by the typical woman of that age. If we add the fertility rates at ages 20 and 21 together, we get the number of babies produced by the typical woman during the 2-year period from her 20th birthday to her 22nd birthday. Therefore, if we add all the age-specific fertility rates together, we get the number of births that the typical woman would have if she experienced the fertility rates prevailing at every age and lived through the end of the childbearing ages. Hence, at current rates, the typical woman would produce 2.1 children by age 50. This index is known as total fertility, or the *total fertility rate* (TFR).

GROSS AND NET REPRODUCTION RATES

If we count just female births (we sum the age-specific female-birth rates), the measure is known as the *gross reproduction rate* (GRR). Since there are approximately 105 male births for every 100 female births in all populations (except among blacks, whose sex ratio at birth is about 103 males per 100 females), the fraction of female births is about .488. Thus we have the simple relationship that the GRR = .488 × TFR. Hence, the GRR in the United States is now about 1.02. This number directly tells us that women are barely reproducing themselves; 100 female babies would by age 50 produce only 102 daughters. Thus, over the long run (ignoring migration), the population of the United States would grow only very slowly if these age-specific birth rates remained constant. Actually, to reach this conclusion, we must also account for the fact that each girl baby does not necessarily live through the childbearing years. If the probability of survival is also factored in, the fertility index is known as the *net reproduction rate* (NRR). It is the number of daughters that the average girl baby will subsequently produce during her lifetime. Because not all girl babies survive to age 50, the NRR is always less than the GRR; the difference increases as mortality becomes higher. If the NRR is greater than 1.0, each woman will more than replace herself so that the population will in each succeeding generation grow (ignoring migration); and if the NRR is less than 1.0, it will decline. If the NRR equals 1.0, the population will ultimately neither shrink nor grow—it will become stationary, or constant.

LIFE TABLE AND EXPECTATION OF LIFE

A life table can best be imagined as a table showing how many people are still alive at each birthday out of the total number born at a particular time. Suppose that we observe 1,000 births in 2001. Then we simply record the number who have their first birthday in 2002, their second in 2003, and so forth. We can also record how many person-years were lived between birth and age 1, between age 1 and age 2, and so on. If we add up all the years lived and divide by the number who were born, we get the average number of years lived, or the expectation of life at birth. We could also find, for example, the expectation of life at age 40 by dividing the total years lived after age 40 by the number who survived to age 40. While this exercise is revealing, we usually do not want to wait the 100 or so years it would take to find the answer. It is possible, however, to take the current age-specific death rates and convert them into a life table. This life table would not, of course, represent the experience of an actual birth cohort. It tells us at what ages members of a cohort would die if current age-specific mortality rates persisted in the future. Life tables are not mere mathematical games; they affect our everyday lives, for they are used in setting insurance rates and in developing pension plans.

Life-table methodology is not restricted just to deaths. One can use the same techniques to measure contraceptive failure (where initiation of use of a method and accidental pregnancy, respectively, take the place of birth and death in the life table),[74,75] marital dissolution (marriage replacing birth and divorce or separation replacing death),[76] and other events of interest. In these other applications, the expectation of life is not always the most convenient measure; instead, one may be interested directly in the proportion failing within 6 or 12 or 24 months (e.g., contraceptive failure) or 5 years (e.g., marriage dissolution).

It is also very enlightening to realize that a life table can be thought of as a stationary population. If mortality is constant, and if there is the same number of births every year, then (ignoring migration) the number of persons at each age will be the same year after year. Furthermore, the number of person-years lived in the life table between ages 6 and 7 for example, will be the same as the number of 6-year-olds in the population.

SUGGESTED READING

Cohen JE. How many people can the earth support? New York NY: WW Norton & Company, 1995.

Tsui AO, Wasserheit J, Haaga JG (eds). Reproductive health in developing countries: expanding dimensions, building solutions. Washington DC: National Academy Press, 1997.

REFERENCES

1. Morabia A, Costanza MC. International variability in ages of menarche, first live birth, and menopause. Am J Epidemiol 1998;148:1195-1205.
2. Menken J, Trussell J, Watkins S. The nutrition fertility link: an evaluation of the evidence. J Interdisciplinary History 1981;11:425-441.
3. Desjardins B, Bideau A, Brunet G. Age of mother at last birth in two historical populations. J Biosoc Sci 1994;26:509-516.
4. Bongaarts J. A framework for analyzing the proximate determinants of fertility. Popul Dev Rev 1978;4:105-132.
5. Rutstein SO. Fertility levels, trends, and differentials: 1995-1999. Demographic and Health Surveys, Comparative Report No. 2. Calverton, Maryland: Macro International Inc., 2001.
6. Boyd A. The world's youth 2000. Washington, DC: Population Reference Bureau, 2001.
7. Lesthaeghe R. Nuptiality and population growth. Popul Stud 1971;25:415-432.
8. Trussell J. The impact of birthspacing on fertility. Int Fam Plann Perspect 1986;12:80-82.
9. Henry A, Piotrow PT. Age at marriage and fertility. Popul Rep 1979;7, Series M(4).
10. Mason KO. The impact of women's position on demographic change during the course of development. In: Federici N, Mason KO, Sogner S (eds). Women's position and demographic change. Oxford, UK: Clarendon Press, 1993:19-42.
11. Menken J, Bongaarts J. Reproductive models in the study of nutrition-fertility interrelationships. In: Mosley WH (ed). Nutrition and human reproduction. New York NY: Plenum Press, 1978:261-311.
12. Republic of the Philippines, national demographic and health survey 1998. Manila, Philippines: National Statistics Office and Department of Health, 1999.
13. Nigeria demographic and health survey 1999. Abuja, Nigeria: National Population Commission, 2000.
14. Campbell OMR, Gray RH. Characteristics and determinants of postpartum ovarian function in women in the United States. Am J Obstet Gynecol 1993;169:55-60.
15. Haggerty PA, Rutstein SO. Breastfeeding and complementary infant feeding, and the postpartum effects of breastfeeding. Demographic and Health Surveys, Comparative Studies No. 30. Calverton, Maryland: Macro International Inc., 1999.
16. Sherris JD, Fox G. Infertility and sexually transmitted disease: a public health challenge. Popul Rep 1983;11, Series L(4).
17. Gray RH. Biological factors other than nutrition and lactation which may influence natural fertility: a review. In: Leridon H, Menken J (eds). Natural fertility: patterns and determinants of natural fertility: proceedings of a seminar on natural fertility. Liege, Belgium: Ordina Editions, 1979:217-251.
18. Adegbola O. New estimates of fertility and child mortality in Africa, south of the Sahara. Popul Stud 1977;31:467-486.
19. Frank O. Infertility in sub-Saharan Africa: estimates and implications. Popul Dev Rev 1983;9:137-144.
20. Brunham RC, Cheang M, McMaster J, Garnett G, Anderson R. Chlamydia trachomatis, infertility and population growth in sub-Saharan Africa. Sex Transm Dis 1993;20:168-173.

21. Frisch RE. Demographic implications of the biological determinants of female fecundity. Soc Biol 1975;22:17-22.
22. Bongaarts J. Does malnutrition affect fecundity? A summary of evidence. Science 1980;208:564-569.
23. Ford K, Huffman SL, Chowdhury AKMA, Becker S, Allen H, Menken J. Birth-interval dynamics in rural Bangladesh and maternal weight. Demography 1989;26:425-437.
24. Preston SH. Mortality patterns in national populations. New York NY: Academic Press, 1976.
25. Preston SH, Keyfitz N, Schoen R. Causes of death: life tables for national populations. New York NY: Seminar Press, 1972.
26. National Research Council. Contraception and reproduction: health consequences for women and children in the developing world. Washington DC: National Academy Press, 1989.
27. VanLandingham M, Trussell J, Grummer-Strawn L. Contraceptive and health benefits of breastfeeding: a review of the recent evidence. Int Fam Plann Perspect 1991;17:131-136.
28. Adamson P (ed). The progress of nations 1996. New York NY: UNICEF, 1996.
29. United Nations. Reproductive rights and reproductive health: a concise report. New York NY: United Nations, 1996.
30. Report on the global HIV/AIDS epidemic, June 2000. Geneva, Switzerland: UNAIDS, 2000.
31. Ernberg G, Opuni M, Schwartländer B, Walker N, Tarantola D, Kieffer MP. Level and flow of national and international resources for the response to HIV/AIDS, 1996-1997. Geneva, Switzerland: UNAIDS, 1999.
32. Cohen B, Trussell J. Preventing and mitigating AIDS in sub-Saharan Africa. Washington DC: National Academy Press, 1996.
33. Preston SH. Urban growth in developing countries: a demographic reappraisal. Popul Dev Rev 1979;5:195-215.
34. INEGI (Instituto Nacional de Estadistica Geografia e Informatica). XII Censo General de Población y Vivienda, 2000. Tabulados Básicos y por Entidad Federativa. Bases de Datos y Tabulados de la Muestra Censal. México, 2001. http://www.inegi.gob.mx/estadistica/espanol/sociodem/sexo/sex_01.html.
35. U.S. Census Bureau. Statistical abstract of the United States: 2000. Washington DC: GPO, 2000. Table 14.
36. Coale AJ, Demeny P. Regional model life tables and stable populations. Princeton NJ: Princeton University Press, 1966.
37. Haub C, Cornelius D. 2001 World population data sheet. Washington DC: Population Reference Bureau, 2001.
38. Spencer G. Projections of the population of the United States, by age, sex, and race: 1988 to 2080. Curr Popul Rep, Series P25-1018. Washington DC: Government Printing Office, 1989.
39. United Nations. World population prospects: the 1998 revision. New York NY: United Nations, 1999.
40. Stephenson P, Wagner M, Badea M, Serbanescu F. Commentary: the public health consequences of restricted induced abortion—lessons from Romania. Am J Public Health 1992;82:1328-1331.
41. Teitelbaum MS. Fertility effects of the abolition of legal abortion in Romania. Popul Stud 1972;26:405-417.
42. Aird JS. Coercion in family planning: causes, methods, and consequences. Congressional Record-Senate 1985:S7776-S7788.
43. Greenhalgh S. Shifts in China's population policy, 1984-86: views from the central, provincial, and local levels. Popul Dev Rev 1986;12:491-515.
44. Coale AJ. Population trends, population policy, and population studies in China. Popul Dev Rev 1981;7:85-97.
45. Banister J. China's changing population. Stanford CA: Stanford University Press, 1987.

46. Coale AJ, Banister J. Five decades of missing females in China. Demography 1994;31:459-479.
47. Yi Z, Ping T, Baochang G, Yi X, Bohua L, Yongping L. Causes and implications of the recent increase in the reported sex ratio at birth in China. Popul Dev Rev 1993;19:283-302.
48. Bongaarts J, Greenhalgh S. An alternative to the one-child policy in China. Popul Dev Rev 1985;11:585-617.
49. Caldwell JC. A theory of fertility: from high plateau to destabilization. Popul Dev Rev 1978;4:553-577.
50. Caldwell JC. Mass education as a determinant of the timing of fertility decline. Popul Dev Rev 1980;6:225-255.
51. Coale AJ, Watkins SC. The decline of fertility in Europe: the revised proceedings of a conference on the Princeton European fertility project. Princeton NJ: Princeton University Press, 1986.
52. Wrigley EA, Schofield RS. The population history of England 1541-1871. Cambridge MA: Harvard University Press, 1981.
53. Barclay GW, Coale AJ, Stoto MA, Trussell TJ. A reassessment of the demography of traditional rural China. Popul Index 1976;42:606-635.
54. Demeny P. Bucharest, Mexico City, and beyond. Popul Dev Rev 1985;11:99-106.
55. McIntosh CA, Finkle JL. The Cairo conference on population and development: a new paradigm? Popul Dev Rev 1995;21:223-260.
56. Bongaarts J, Watkins SC. Social interactions and contemporary fertility transitions. Popul Dev Rev 1996;22:639-682.
57. Knodel J, van de Walle E. Lessons from the past: policy implications of historical fertility studies. Popul Dev Rev 1979;5:217-245.
58. Robey B, Rutstein SO, Morris L. The fertility decline in developing countries. Sci Am 1993;269:30-37.
59. Potts M. Sex and the birth rate: human biology, demographic change, and access to fertility-regulation methods. Popul Dev Rev 1997;23:1-39.
60. Westoff CF, Bankole A. Unmet need 1990-1994. Comparative Studies No. 16. Calverton MD: Macro International Inc, June 1995.
61. Westoff CF, Ochoa LH. Unmet need and the demand for family planning. Comparative Studies No. 5. Columbia MD: Institute for Resource Development, July, 1991.
62. Graham-Smith F (ed). Population—the complex reality: a report of the Population Summit of the world's scientific academies. Golden CO: North American Press, 1994.
63. Menken, J (ed). World population and U.S. policy: the choices ahead. New York NY: WW Norton, 1986.
64. National Research Council. Population growth and economic development: policy questions. Washington DC: National Academy Press, 1986.
65. United Nations. Population and development: programme of action adopted at the International Conference on Population and Development, Cairo, 5-13 September 1994. New York NY: United Nations, 1995.
66. World Bank. World development report, 1984. New York NY: Oxford University Press, 1984.
67. Bongaarts J. Population policy options in the developing world. Science 1994;263:771-776.
68. Sachs BP, Layde PM, Rubin GL, Rochat RW. Reproductive mortality in the United States. JAMA 1982;247:2789-2792.
69. Trussell J, Menken J. Comment: reproductive mortality. Fam Plann Perspect 1982;14:263.
70. United Nations. World population prospects: the 1994 revision. New York NY: United Nations, 1995: Table 43.
71. Malthus TR. An essay on the principle of population, as it affects the future improvement of society. London, England: J Johnson, 1798.

72. Smith DP. Formal Demography. New York NY: Plenum Press, 1992: Table 3.3.
73. Trussell J, Menken J. Life table analysis of contraceptive failure. In: Hermalin AI, Entwisle B (eds). The role of surveys in the analysis of family planning programs. Liege, Belgium: Ordina Editions, 1982:537-571.
74. Potter RG. Application of life table techniques to measurement of contraceptive effectiveness. Demography 1966;3:297-304.
75. Vaughan B, Trussell J, Menken J, Jones EF. Contraceptive failure among married women in the United States, 1970-1973. Fam Plann Perspect 1977;9:251-258.
76. Menken J, Trussell J, Stempel D, Babakol O. Proportional hazards life table models: an illustrative analysis of socio-demographic influences on marriage dissolution in the United States. Demography 1981;18:181-200.

Contraceptive Efficacy

James Trussell, PhD

- Pregnancy rates during *perfect use* reflect how effective methods can be in preventing pregnancy when used *consistently and correctly* according to instructions.

- Pregnancy rates during *typical use* reflect how effective methods are for the average person who does not always use methods correctly or consistently.

- Pregnancy rates during typical use of adherence-dependent methods generally vary widely for different groups using the same method, primarily due to differences in the propensity to use the method perfectly.

- Additional empirically-based estimates of pregnancy rates during perfect use are needed.

A general explanation of the sources of evidence and the logic underlying the summary table on contraceptive efficacy (Table 9-2) is provided in Chapter 9 on Essentials of Contraception. This chapter more completely explains the derivation of the estimates of the first-year probabilities of pregnancy during typical use (column 2) and perfect use (column 3) in Table 9-2, reproduced as Table 31-1.[1,2] The chapter also contains tables summarizing the literature on contraceptive efficacy for each method. These are arranged in the order in which they appear in summary Table 31-1. In these tables, all studies were conducted in the United States unless otherwise noted. In the epidemiology literature, the term *efficacy* refers to how well an intervention (in this case a contraceptive method) works in clinical trials and the term *effectiveness* refers to how well it works in actual practice. We use both sorts of evidence in this chapter, but in this chapter and in Chapter 9 and throughout the book, we use these terms interchangeably in the common everyday sense of how well a method works.

NO METHOD

Our estimate of the percentage of women becoming pregnant among those not using contraception is based on populations in which the use of contraception is rare and on couples who report that they stopped using contraceptives because they want to conceive. Based on this evidence, we conclude that 85 of 100 sexually active couples would experience an accidental pregnancy in the first year if they used no contraception. Available evidence in the United States suggests that only about 40% of married couples who do not use contraception (but who still wish to avoid pregnancy) become pregnant within 1 year.[3] However, such couples are almost certainly selected for low fecundity or low frequency of intercourse. They do not use contraception because, in part, they are aware that they are unlikely to conceive. The probability of pregnancy of 85%, therefore, is our best guess of the fraction of women now using reversible methods of contraception who would become pregnant within 1 year if they were to abandon their current method but not otherwise change their behavior. Couples who have unprotected intercourse for a year without achieving pregnancy are, by definition, infertile (but by no means are they necessarily sterile—see Chapter 9 and Chapter 27 on Impaired Fertility). Table 31-2 summarizes the studies of the risk of pregnancy among women who are neither using contraception nor breastfeeding.

TYPICAL USE OF SPERMICIDES, WITHDRAWAL, PERIODIC ABSTINENCE, DIAPHRAGM, MALE CONDOM, PILL, MINIPILL, AND DEPO-PROVERA

Our estimates of the probability of pregnancy during the first year of typical use for spermicides, withdrawal, periodic abstinence, the diaphragm, the male condom, the pill, and Depo-Provera are taken from the 1995 National Survey of Family Growth (NSFG) corrected for underreporting of abortion.[4] The characteristics of users of different methods, while reflecting the population actually using each method in the United States, vary greatly. For example, 63% of the number of intervals of use of the diaphragm were contributed by women aged 30 and older, compared with only 16% for Depo-Provera and 24% for the male condom. Therefore, the estimates are standardized to reflect the estimated probabilities of pregnancy that would be observed if users of each method had the same characteristics (for example, the same age distribution, marital/cohabiting status distribution, and the same fraction living in poverty).

The correction for underreporting of abortion may produce estimates that are too high because women in abortion clinics (surveys of whom provided the information for the correction) overreport use of a contraceptive method at the time they became pregnant. Moreover, women in personal interviews for the NSFG also might overreport use of a contraceptive method at the time of a conception leading to a live birth. Evidence for this suspicion is provided by uncorrected first-year probabilities of pregnancy of 3.7% for the IUD and 2.3% for Norplant (methods with little or no scope for user error) in the 1995 NSFG; these probabilities are much higher than rates observed in clinical trials of these methods, and for this reason we did not base the typical-use estimates for these two methods on the NSFG.[5] We would naturally expect overreporting of contraceptive use in both the NSFG and surveys conducted in abortion clinics, because the woman (couple) can then blame the pregnancy on contraceptive "failure."

Thus, biases in opposite directions affect these estimates. Pregnancy rates based on the NSFG alone would tend to be too low because induced abortions (and contraceptive failures leading to induced abortions) are underreported but would tend to be too high because contraceptive failures leading to live births are overreported. We reason that the former bias is the more important one.

The NSFG does not ask for brand of pill; thus combined and progestin-only pills cannot be distinguished; however, since use of the combined pill is far more common than use of the progestin-only pill, the results from the NSFG overwhelmingly reflect typical use of combined pills. The efficacy of progestin-only pills may be lower than that for combined pills since progestin-only pills are probably less forgiving of nonadherence to the dosing schedule.

PERFECT USE OF THE CERVICAL CAP, SPONGE, AND DIAPHRAGM

Our estimates of the probabilities of pregnancy during the first year of perfect use of the cervical cap and sponge correspond with results of a reanalysis of data from clinical trials in which women were randomly assigned to use the diaphragm or sponge or the diaphragm or cervical cap.[6] The results indicate that among parous women who use the sponge perfectly, 19.4% to 20.5% will experience a pregnancy within the first year. The corresponding range for nulliparous women is 9.0% to 9.5%. Among parous women who use the cervical cap perfectly, 25.7% to 27.0% will experience a pregnancy within the first year. The range for nulliparous women is 7.6% to 9.9%. In contrast, parous users of the diaphragm do not appear to have higher pregnancy rates during perfect use than do nulliparous users; 4.3% to 8.4% of all women experience an accidental pregnancy during the first year of perfect use of the diaphragm. Our revised estimates in the third column of Table 31-1 (and 9-2 in Chapter 9 on Essentials of Contraception) are obtained from the midpoints of these ranges.

TYPICAL USE OF THE CERVICAL CAP AND SPONGE

We next faced the problem of whether and how to revise the estimates for these methods during typical use (the second column). The proportions becoming pregnant during the first year of typical use for parous users of the sponge (27.4%) and cervical cap (30.3%) were about twice as high as for nulliparous users of these methods (14.0% and 15.2%, respectively). The evidence for the diaphragm is mixed. In the sponge-diaphragm trial, the proportion becoming pregnant in the first year of typical use for parous users of the diaphragm (12.4%) was marginally lower than that for nulliparous users (12.8%). In the cap-diaphragm trial, the proportion becoming pregnant among parous users (29.0%) is almost double that among nulliparous users (14.8%).[7] Faced with this information, we set the estimates for nulliparous users of the cervical cap and sponge equal to the estimate for all users of the diaphragm based on the NSFG (16%). We doubled the estimates for nulliparous users of the cervical cap and sponge to obtain the estimates for parous users.

FEMALE CONDOM

The typical-use estimate for the female condom is based on the results of a 6-month clinical trial of the Reality female condom; 12.4% of women in the United States experienced a pregnancy during the first 6 months of use.[7] The 12-month probability of pregnancy for users of Reality in the United States was projected from the relation between the pregnancy rates in the first 6 months and the pregnancy rates in the second 6 months for users of the diaphragm, sponge and cervical cap.[7] The probability of pregnancy during 6 months of perfect use of Reality by U.S. women who met the adherence criteria stipulated in the study protocol was 2.6%. Those who reported fewer than 4 acts of intercourse during the month prior to any follow-up visit, who did not use Reality at every act of intercourse, who ever reported not following the Reality instructions, or who used another method of contraception were censored at the beginning of the first interval where nonadherence was noted.[8] Under the assumption that the probability of pregnancy in the second six months of perfect use would be the same, the probability of pregnancy during a year of perfect use would be 5.1%.

PERFECT USE OF WITHDRAWAL AND SPERMICIDES

Our estimate of the proportion becoming pregnant during a year of perfect use of withdrawal is an educated guess based on the reasoning that pregnancy resulting from preejaculatory fluid is unlikely.[9,10]

Our estimate of the proportion becoming pregnant during a year of perfect use of spermicides is based on a recent NIH trial of 5 spermicides.[40] We assumed that the pregnancy rate per cycle during perfect use would be constant, extrapolated a one-year probability from the 6-cycle probability reported for each method, and took as our estimate the median (18%) of those 5 estimates. Our estimate is considerably higher than would be expected from the extensive literature on the contraceptive efficacy of spermicides.

Six studies outside the United States,[11-16] in addition to several U.S. studies reviewed earlier,[1] have yielded very low probabilities of pregnancy during the first year of typical use of spermicides, much lower than any estimates for barriers with spermicides. The efficacy literature on spermicides is dominated by studies of suppositories, foams, and film, and high spermicide efficacy is documented only in these studies. There are few studies of creams and gels used alone, and those with the lowest pregnancy rates are more than 30 years old (Table 31-3). We consider it likely that the spermicide studies suffer from flaws in analysis or design that are not apparent in the brief published descriptions. For example, an FDA advisory committee was openly skeptical of one German study[11]: "the way in which the survey was designed and the manner in which the various incentives were offered" (physicians reportedly received a fee for completing survey data forms) "would clearly make the data resulting from the survey unacceptable to any scientific group or regulatory agency."[17,18]

The first clinical trial of Emko vaginal foam is also one of the few studies to compute separate pregnancy rates for cycles in which the product was used at every act of intercourse and for cycles in which unprotected intercourse occurred.[19] The design of that trial was also quite sophisticated. Women were randomly assigned to six groups. Each group used three different spermicidal products for three cycles each. The six groups represented all possible permutations of orders of use of the three products. If the pregnancy rate for three cycles of consistent use of Emko vaginal foam is extrapolated, then the implied proportion becoming pregnant in the first year of consistent use is 8.9%.

A recent randomized clinical trial comparing the efficacy of a film and a foaming tablet—the first trial of spermicides conducted according to modern standards of design, execution, and analysis—supports the conclusion that the contraceptive efficacy of spermicides is considerably lower than was previously thought.[20] In that trial, 6-month probabilities of pregnancy during consistent use were 28% for the tablet and 24% for the film, probabilities that were nearly identical to the risks during typical use in that trial and that are about the same as the 12-month probability of pregnancy during typical use of spermicides in the 1995 NSFG.

PERFECT USE OF PERIODIC ABSTINENCE

The perfect-use estimates for periodic abstinence are based on an empirical estimate of 3.2% for the ovulation method.[21] Common sense dictates that the newer variants of periodic abstinence should be inherently efficacious because they demand abstinence during large portions of each cycle and particularly during times near estimated peak fecundity. They are relatively ineffective in actual use because perfect use is so difficult to achieve, and the consequence of imperfect use is a high risk of pregnancy. The post-ovulation variant of periodic abstinence requires the longest periods of abstinence, followed in order by the sympto-thermal, ovulation, and calendar variants. Consequently, we have assigned probabilities of pregnancy during perfect use that are consistent with that ordering with the realization that we can be confident only about the rate for the ovulation method. Given the dearth of evidence, higher or lower estimates for calendar rhythm would be as plausible and defensible.

PERFECT USE OF THE MALE CONDOM

Our estimate of the proportion becoming pregnant during a year of perfect use of the male condom is based on results from the only three studies of the male condom meeting modern standards of design, execution, and analysis.[22,41,42] In each study couples were randomly assigned to use either a latex condom or a polyurethane condom. All three studies reported efficacy during consistent use but only one reported efficacy during perfect use;[41] in that study the 6-cycle probability of pregnancy during perfect use (0.7%) was 70% of that (1%) during typical use. We assumed that in the other two studies the 6-cycle probability of pregnancy during perfect use would also be 70% of the 6-cycle probability during typical use, assumed that the pregnancy rate per cycle during perfect use would be constant, extrapolated a one-year probability from the 6-cycle probability reported for the latex condom in each trial, and took as our estimate the median (2%, also the mean) of those 3 estimates. This estimate is consistent with an estimate based on studies of condom breakage and slippage.[23] Under the assumption that 1.5% of condoms break or slip off the penis and that women have intercourse twice a week, then about 1.5% of women would experience condom breaks during the half-week that they are at risk of pregnancy during each cycle. The per-cycle probability of conception would be reduced by 98.5%, from 0.1358 to only 0.0020, if a condom failure results in no protection whatsoever against pregnancy, so that about 2.6% of women would become pregnant each year.[24] Unfortunately, breakage and slippage rates did not accurately predict pregnancy rates during consistent use in one clinical trial of the latex and polyurethane male condom,[22] and estimates of condom breakage and slippage during intercourse or withdrawal vary substantially across studies in developed countries,[23] from a low of 0.6% among commercial sex workers in Nevada's legal brothels[23] to a high of 7.2% among monogamous couples in North Carolina.[25]

PERFECT USE OF THE PILL, MINIPILL, DEPO-PROVERA, AND NORPLANT, AND TYPICAL USE OF NORPLANT

Although the lowest reported pregnancy rate for the combined pill during typical use is 0% (Table 31-11), recent studies indicate that pregnancies do occur, albeit rarely, during perfect use. Hence we set the perfect-use estimate for the pill at the very low level of 0.3%. The lowest reported pregnancy rate for the progestin-only pill (minipill) exceeds 1% (see Table 31-10). It is likely that the progestin-only pill is less effective than the combined pill during typical use, since the progestin-only pill is probably less forgiving of nonadherence to the dosing schedule. Whether the progestin-only pill is also less effective during perfect use is unknown.

The perfect-use estimate for Depo-Provera is the weighted average of the seven studies of the 150 mg dose shown in Table 31-12. These trials yield an estimate of efficacy during perfect rather than typical use because either women late for an injection were discontinued or all pregnancies reported occurred during actual use (after one injection but before the next was scheduled). The perfect-use estimate for Norplant (6 capsules) and Norplant-2 (2 rods) is the weighted average of the results from the four clinical trials reported in Table 31-14. Because there is no scope for user error, we set the typical use-estimate for Norplant equal to the perfect use estimate.

LUNELLE, EVRA, AND NUVARING

Clinical trials of Lunelle cannot yield an estimate of efficacy during typical use, because the design of those trials calls for removing from the study women who return late for their injections.[26,27] The estimate is therefore set equal to that for Depo-Provera. Although those clinical trials revealed no pregnancies, it is unlikely that Lunelle never fails; we therefore arbitrarily set the perfect-use estimate for Lunelle equal to that for Norplant and Norplant-2. The typical- and perfect-use estimates for the Evra patch and NuvaRing were set equal to those for the pill. It is possible that the patch and ring will prove to have better efficacy than the pill during typical use, because of better adherence with the dosing schedule. However, such superior efficacy has not been demonstrated in randomized trials. While in one trial the failure rate was lower among women randomly assigned to use the Evra patch (1.2%) than among those assigned to use the pill (2.2%), the difference was not statistically significant (P=0.6).[28] In a subsequent paper that argues that better adherence to the dosing schedule leads to better contraceptive efficacy of the patch than the pill during typical use, the authors acknowledge that it would require a trial with 24,143 subjects to demonstrate such superiority and conclude that "studies of this size to compare effectiveness may not be practical."[43] There are no published studies in which women were randomly assigned to the NuvaRing and the pill.

IUD

The estimate for typical use of the ParaGard (Copper T 380A) IUD is taken directly from the large study for that method shown in Table 31-13. The estimate for Mirena (LNG-IUS) is the weighted average of the results from the two studies shown in Table 31-13. The estimate for perfect use of the Copper T 380A was obtained by removing the pregnancies that resulted when the device was not known to be in situ,[29] on the perhaps-questionable assumption that these pregnancies should be classified as user failures and the empirically-based assumption that expulsions are so uncommon that the denominator of the perfect-use pregnancy rate is virtually the same as the denominator for the typical-use rate (Table 31-13). The perfect-use estimate for the LNG-IUS was derived analogously. No differences in the typical-use and perfect-use estimates for LNG-IUS are apparent due to the fact that only one significant digit is shown.

STERILIZATION

The weighted average of the results from the eight vasectomy studies in Table 31-16 analyzed with life-table procedures is 0.01% becoming pregnant in the year following the procedure. In these studies, pregnancies occurred after the ejaculate had been declared to be sperm-free. This perfect-use estimate of 0.01% is undoubtedly too low, because clinicians are understandably loath to publish articles describing their surgical failures and journals would be reluctant to publish an article documenting poor surgical technique. The difference between typical-use and perfect-use pregnancy rates for vasectomy would depend on the frequency of unprotected intercourse after the procedure had been performed but before the ejaculate had been certified to be sperm-free. We arbitrarily set the typical- and perfect-use estimates to 0.15% and 0.10%, respectively. For female sterilization, there is no scope for user error. The typical- and perfect-use estimates are the pooled results from the U.S. Collaborative Review of Sterilization, a prospective study of 10,685 women undergoing tubal sterilization.[30] We are less concerned about publication bias with female than with male sterilization because the largest studies of female sterilization are based on prospective, multicenter clinical trials, not retrospective reports from one investigator.

CONTRACEPTIVE CONTINUATION

Contraceptives will be effective at preventing unintended pregnancy only if women or couples continue to use them once they have initiated use. The proportions of women continuing use at the end of the first year for spermicides, withdrawal, periodic abstinence, the diaphragm, the male condom, the pill, Depo-Provera and Norplant were obtained from the 1995 NSFG.[5] Only method-related reasons for discontinuation (pregnancy, changing methods or termination of contraceptive use while still at risk for unintended pregnancy) were counted. Other reasons for discontinuing use of a method (such as attempting to get pregnant or not having intercourse) are not counted in the discontinuation rate because these reasons are unrelated to the method and do not apply to women seeking to avoid pregnancy and at risk of becoming pregnant. For nulliparous users of the sponge and cervical cap, we used the continuation rate for the diaphragm; for parous users, we adjusted the continuation rate for the diaphragm to reflect higher pregnancy rates. For the female condom, we adjusted the continuation rate for the male condom to reflect a higher pregnancy rate.

We set the continuation rate for Lunelle equal to that for Depo-Provera; we set the continuation rates for the Evra patch and NuvaRing equal to that for the pill.

Discontinuation rates of the two IUDs (for reasons related to the contraceptive) are based on clinical trials. The estimate for the Copper T 380A IUD was taken directly from the large study for that method shown in Table 31-13. The estimate for the LNG-IUS is the weighted average from the two studies shown in Table 31-13.

EMERGENCY CONTRACEPTION

Typically, if 100 women have unprotected intercourse once during the second or third week of their menstrual cycle, about 8 would become pregnant. If those same women used combined emergency contraceptive pills (ECPs), only 2 would become pregnant (a 75% reduction);[31] if they used the progestin-only ECP, only 1 would become pregnant (an 89% reduction).[32] Copper-T IUD insertion is extremely effective, reducing the risk of pregnancy following unprotected intercourse by more than 99%.[33] Moreover, a copper-T IUD can be left in place to provide continuous effective contraception for up to 10 years.

THE LACTATIONAL AMENORRHEA METHOD (LAM)

LAM is a highly effective, *temporary* method of contraception. If the infant is being fed only its mother's breastmilk (or is given supplemental non-breastmilk feeds only to a minor extent) and if the woman has not experienced her first postpartum menses, then breastfeeding provides more than 98% protection from pregnancy in the first 6 months following a birth.[34,35] Four prospective clinical studies of the contraceptive effect of this Lactational Amenorrhea Method (LAM) demonstrated cumulative 6-month life-table perfect-use pregnancy rates of 0.5%, 0.6%, 1.0%, and 1.5% among women who relied solely on LAM.[36–39]

TEXT REFERENCES

1. Trussell J, Kost K. Contraceptive failure in the United States: a critical review of the literature. Stud Fam Plann 1987;18:237-283.
2. Trussell J, Hatcher RA, Cates W, Stewart FH, Kost K. Contraceptive failure in the United States: an update. Stud Fam Plann 1990;21:51-54.
3. Grady WR, Hayward MD, Yagi J. Contraceptive failure in the United States: estimates from the 1982 National Survey of Family Growth. Fam Plann Perspect 1986;18:200-209.
4. Fu H, Darroch JE, Haas T, Ranjit N. Contraceptive failure rates: new estimates from the 1995 National Survey of Family Growth. Fam Plann Perspect 1999;31:56-63.
5. Trussell J, Vaughan B. Contraceptive failure, method-related discontinuation and resumption of use: results from the 1995 National Survey of Family Growth. Fam Plann Perspect 1999;31:64-72 & 93.
6. Trussell J, Strickler J, Vaughan B. Contraceptive efficacy of the diaphragm, the sponge and the cervical cap. Fam Plann Perspect 1993;25:100-105, 135.
7. Trussell J, Sturgen K, Strickler J, Dominik R. Comparative contraceptive efficacy of the female condom and other barrier methods. Fam Plann Perspect 1994;26:66-72.

8. Farr G, Gabelnick H, Sturgen K, Dorflinger L. Contraceptive efficacy and acceptability of the female condom. Am J Public Health 1994;84:1960-1964.
9. Ilaria G, Jacobs JL, Polsky B, Koll B, Baron P, MacLow C, Armstrong D, Schlegel PN. Detection of HIV-1 DNA sequences in pre-ejaculatory fluid. Lancet 1992;340:1469.
10. Pudney J, Oneta M, Mayer K, Seage G, Anderson D. Pre-ejaculatory fluid as potential vector for sexual transmission of HIV-1. Lancet 1992;340:1470.
11. Brehm H, Haase W. Die alternative zur hormonalen kontrazeption? Med Welt 1975;26:1610-1617.
12. Dimpfl J, Salomon W, Schicketanz KH. Die spermizide barriere. Sexualmedizin 1984;13:95-98.
13. Florence N. Das kontrazeptive vaginal-suppositorium: ergebnisse einer klinischen fünfjahresstudie. Sexualmedizin 1977;6:385-386.
14. Godts P. Klinische prüfung eines vaginalem antikonzipiens. Ars Medici 1973;2:589-593.
15. Iizuka R, Kobayashi T, Kawakami S, Nakamura Y, Ikeuchi M, Chin B, Mochimaru F, Sumi K, Sato H, Yamaguchi J, Ohno T, Shiina M, Maeda N, Tokoro H, Suzuki T, Hayashi K, Takahashi T, Akatsuka M, Kasuga Y, Kurokawa H. Clinical experience with the Vaginal Contraceptive Film containing the spermicide polyoxyethylene nonylphenyl ether (C-Film study group). Jpn J Fertil Steril 1980;25:64-68. (In Japanese; translation supplied by Apothecus Inc.)
16. Salomon W, Haase W. Intravaginale kontrazeption. Sexualmedizin 1977;6:198-202.
17. Over-the-Counter Contraceptives and Other Vaginal Drug Products Review Panel (Elizabeth B. Connell, Chairman). Encare Oval. Memorandum to Food and Drug Administration Commissioner Donald Kennedy, February 9, 1978.
18. Stewart FH, Stewart G, Guest FJ, Hatcher RA. My body, my health: the concerned woman's guide to gynecology. New York NY: John Wiley & Sons, 1979.
19. Mears E. Chemical contraceptive trial: II. J Reprod Fertil 1962;4:337-343.
20. Raymond E, Dominik R, the spermicide trial group. Contraceptive effectiveness of two spermicides: a randomized trial. Obstet Gynecol 1999;93:896-903.
21. Trussell J, Grummer-Strawn L. Contraceptive failure of the ovulation method of periodic abstinence. Fam Plann Perspect 1990;22:65-75.
22. Frezieres RG, Walsh TL, Nelson AL, Clark VA, Coulson AH. Evaluation of the efficacy of a polyurethane condom: results from a randomized controlled clinical trial. Fam Plann Perspect 1999;31:81-87.
23. Albert AE, Warner DL, Hatcher RA, Trussell J, Bennett C. Condom use among female commercial sex workers in Nevada's legal brothels. Am J Public Health 1995;85:1514-1520.
24. Kestelman P, Trussell J. Efficacy of the simultaneous use of condoms and spermicides. Fam Plann Perspect 1991;23:226-227, 232.
25. Steiner M, Piedrahita C, Glover L, Joanis C. Can condom users likely to experience condom failure be identified? Fam Plann Perspect 1993;25:220-223, 226.
26. Hall P, Bahamondes L, Diaz J, Petta C. Introductory study of the once-a-month, injectable contraceptive Cyclofem in Brazil, Chile, Colombia, and Peru. Contraception 1997;56:353-359.
27. Kaunitz AM, Garceau RJ, Cromie MA, Lunelle Study Group. Comparative safety, efficacy, and cycle control of Lunelle monthly contraceptive injection (medroxyprogesterone acetate and estradiol cypionate injectable suspension) and Ortho-Novum 7/7/7 oral contraceptive (norethindrone/eithinyl estradiol triphasic). Contraception 1999;60:179-187.
28. Audet MC, Moreau M, Koltun WD, Waldbaum AS, Shangold G, Fisher AC, Creasy GW. Evaluation of contraceptive efficacy and cycle control of a transdermal contraceptive patch vs an oral contraceptive. JAMA 2001;285:2347-2354.
29. Sivin I. Personal communication to James Trussell, August 13, 1992.
30. Peterson HB, Xia Z, Hughes JM, Wilcox LS, Tylor LR, Trussell J. The risk of pregnancy after tubal sterilization: findings from the U.S. Collaborative Review of Sterilization. Am J Obstet Gynecol 1996;174:1161-1170.
31. Trussell J, Rodríguez G, Ellertson C. Updated estimates of the effectiveness of the Yuzpe regimen of emergency contraception. Contraception 1999;59:147-151.

32. Task Force on Postovulatory Methods of Fertility Regulation. Randomised controlled trial of levonorgestrel versus the Yuzpe regimen of combined oral contraceptives for emergency contraception. *Lancet* 1998;352:428-433.
33. Trussell J, Ellertson C. Efficacy of emergency contraception. Fertil Control Rev 1995;4:8-11.
34. Kennedy KI, Rivera R, McNeilly AS. Consensus statement on the use of breastfeeding as a family planning method. Contraception 1989;39:477-496.
35. Kennedy KI, Labbok MH, Van Look PFA. Lactational amenorrhea method for family planning. Int J Gynaecol Obstet. 1996;54:55-57.
36. Kazi A, Kennedy KI, Visness CM, Khan T. Effectiveness of the lactational amenorrhea method in Pakistan. Fertil Steril 1995;64:717-723.
37. Labbok MH, Hight-Laukaran V, Peterson AE, Fletcher V, von Hertzen H, Van Look PFA. Multicenter study of the Lactational Amenorrhea Method (LAM): I. Efficacy, duration, and implications for clinical application. Contraception 1997;55:327-336.
38. Pérez A, Labbok MH, Queenan JT. Clinical study of the lactational amenorrhoea method for family planning. Lancet 1992;339:968-970.
39. Ramos R, Kennedy KI, Visness CM. Effectiveness of lactational amenorrhea in prevention of pregnancy in Manila, the Philippines: non-comparative prospective trial. Br Med J 1996;313:909-912.

LATE REFERENCES

40. Raymond EG, Chen PL, Luoto J. Contraceptive effectiveness and safety of five nonoxynol-9 spermicides: a randomized trial. Obstet Gynecol 2004;103:430-439.
41. Walsh TL, Frezieres RG, Peacock K, Nelson AL, Clark VA, Bernstein L. Evaluation of the efficacy of a nonlatex condom: results from a randomized, controlled clinical trial. Perspect Sex Reprod Health 2003;35:79-86.
42. Steiner MJ, Dominik R, Rountree RW, Nanda K, Dorflinger LJ. Contraceptive effectiveness of a polyurethane condom and a latex condom: a randomized controlled trial. Obstet Gynecol 2003;101:539-547.
43. Archer DF, Cullins V, Creasy GW, Fisher AC. The impact of improved compliance with a weekly contraceptive transdermal system (Ortho Evra®) on contraceptive efficacy. Contraception 2004;69:189-195.

TABLE REFERENCES

Åkerlund M, Røde A, Westergaard J. Comparative profiles of reliability, cycle control and side effects of two oral contraceptive formulations containing 150 µg desogestrel and either 30 µg or 20 µg ethinyl oestradiol. Brit J Obstet Gynaecol 1993;100:832-838.

Alderman PM. The lurking sperm: a review of failures in 8879 vasectomies performed by one physician. JAMA 1988;259:3142-3144.

Anderson FD, Hait H, the Seasonale-301 Study Group. A multicenter, randomized study of an extended cycle oral contraceptive. Contraception 2003;68:89-96.

Apothecus Pharmaceutical Corporation. VCF®: Vaginal Contraceptive Film™. East Norwich NY: Apothecus Inc, 1992.

Archer DF, Maheux R, DelConte A, O'Brien FB. North American levonorgestrel study group (NALSG). Efficacy and safety of a low-dose monophasic combination oral contraceptive containing 100 µg levonorgestrel and 20 µg ethinyl estradiol (Alesse). Am J Obstet Gynecol 1999;181:S39-S44.

Arévalo M Jennings V, Sinai I. Efficacy of a new method of family planning: the Standard Days Method. Contraception 2002;65:333-338.

Audet MC, Moreau M, Koltun WD, Waldbaum AS, Shangold G, Fisher AC, Creasy GW. Evaluation of contraceptive efficacy and cycle control of a transdermal contraceptive patch vs an oral contraceptive. JAMA 2001;285:2347-2354.

Ball M. A prospective field trial of the ovulation method of avoiding conception. Eur J Obstet Gynecol Reprod Biol 1976;6:63-66.

Bannemerschult R, Hanker JP, Wunsch C, Fox P, Albring M, Brill K. A multicenter, uncontrolled clinical investigation of the contraceptive efficacy, cycle control, and safety of a new low dose oral contraceptive containing 20 μg ethinyl estradiol and 100 μg levonorgestrel over six treatment cycles. Contraception 1997;56:285-90.

Bartzen PJ. Effectiveness of the temperature rhythm system of contraception. Fertil Steril 1967;18:694-706.

Belhadj H, Sivin I, Diaz S, Pavez M, Tejada AS, Brache V, Alvarez F, Shoupe D, Breaux H, Mishell DR, McCarthy T, Yo V. Recovery of fertility after use of the levonorgestrel 20 mcg/d or copper T 380 Ag intrauterine device. Contraception 1986;34:261-267.

Bernstein GS. Clinical effectiveness of an aerosol contraceptive foam. Contraception 1971;3:37-43.

Bernstein GS, Clark V, Coulson AH, Frezieres RG, Kilzer L, Moyer D, Nakamura RM, Walsh T. Use effectiveness study of cervical caps. Final report. Washington DC: National Institute of Child Health and Human Development, Contract No. 1-HD-1-2804, July, 1986.

Bhiwandiwala PP, Mumford SD, Feldblum PJ. A comparison of different laparoscopic sterilization occlusion techniques in 24,439 procedures. Am J Obstet Gynecol 1982;144:319-331.

Board JA. Continuous norethindrone, 0.35 mg, as an oral contraceptive agent. Am J Obstet Gynecol 1971;109:531-535.

Boehm D. The cervical cap: effectiveness as a contraceptive. J Nurse Midwifery 1983;28:3-6.

Bounds W, Guillebaud J. Randomised comparison of the use-effectiveness and patient acceptability of the Collatex (Today) contraceptive sponge and the diaphragm. Br J Fam Plann 1984;10:69-75.

Bounds W, Guillebaud J, Dominik R, Dalberth BT. The diaphragm with and without spermicide: a randomized, comparative efficacy trial. J Reprod Med 1995;40:764-774.

Bounds W, Vessey M, Wiggins P. A randomized double-blind trial of two low dose combined oral contraceptives. Brit J Obstet Gynaecol 1979;86:325-329.

Bracher M, Santow G. Premature discontinuation of contraception in Australia. Fam Plann Perspect 1992;24:58-65.

Brehm H, Haase W. Die alternative zur hormonalen kontrazeption? Med Welt 1975;26:1610-1617.

Brigato G, Pisano G, Bergamasco A, Pasqualini M, Cutugno G, Luppari T. Vaginal topical chemical contraception with C-Film. Ginecol Clinica 1982;3:77-80. (In Italian; translation supplied by Apothecus Inc.)

Bushnell LF. Aerosol foam: a practical and effective method of contraception. Pac Med Surg 1965;73:353-355.

Cagen R. The cervical cap as a barrier contraceptive. Contraception 1986;33:487-496.

Carpenter G, Martin JB. Clinical evaluation of a vaginal contraceptive foam. Adv Plann Parent 1970;5:170-175.

Chi IC, Laufe LE, Gardner SD, Tolbert MA. An epidemiologic study of risk factors associated with pregnancy following female sterilization. Am J Obstet Gynecol 1980;136:768-773.

Chi IC, Mumford SD, Gardner SD. Pregnancy risks following laparoscopic sterilization in nongravid and gravid women. J Reprod Med 1981;26:289-294.

Chi IC, Siemens AJ, Champion CB, Gates D, Cilenti D. Pregnancy following minilaparotomy tubal sterilization: an update of an international data set. Contraception 1987;35:171-178.

Cliquet RL, Schoenmaeckers R, Klinkenborg L. Effectiveness of contraception in Belgium: results of the second national fertility survey, 1971 (NEGO II). J Biosoc Sci 1977;9:403-416.

Cox M, Blacksell S. Clinical performance of the levonorgestrel intra-uterine system in routine use by the UK Family Planning and Reproductive Health Research Network: 12-month report. Br J Fam Plann 2000;26:143-147.

Debusschere R. Effectiviteit van de anticonceptie in Vlaanderen: resultaten van het NEGO-III-onderzoek 1975-1976. Bevolking en Gezin 1980;1:5-28.

Denniston GC, Putney D. The cavity rim cervical cap. Adv Plann Parent 1981;16:77-80.

Dieben TOM, Roumen JME, Apter D. Efficacy, cycle control and user acceptability of a novel combined contraceptive vaginal ring. Obstet Gynecol 2002;100:585-93.

Dimpfl J, Salomon W, Schicketanz KH. Die spermizide barriere. Sexualmedizin 1984;13:95-98.

Dingle JT, Tietze C. Comparative study of three contraceptive methods: vaginal foam tablets, jelly alone, and diaphragm with jelly or cream. Am J Obstet Gynecol 1963;85:1012-1022.

Dolack L. Study confirms values of ovulation method. Hospital Progress 1978;59: 64-66,72-73.

Dominik R, Gates D, Sokal D, Cordero M, Lasso de la Vega J, Remes Ruiz A, Thambu J, Lim D, Louissaint S, Galvez RS, Uribe L, Zighelboim I. Two randomized controlled trials comparing the Hulka and Filshie Clips for tubal sterilization. Contraception 2000;62:169-175.

Dubrow H, Kuder K. Combined postpartum and family-planning clinic. Obstet Gynecol 1958;11:586-590.

Edelman DA. Nonprescription vaginal contraception. Int J Gynecol Obstet 1980;18:340-344.

Edelman DA, McIntyre SL, Harper J. A comparative trial of the Today contraceptive sponge and diaphragm. Am J Obstet Gynecol 1984;150:869-876.

Ellis JW. Multiphasic oral contraceptives: efficacy and metabolic impact. J Reprod Med 1987;32:28-36.

Ellsworth HS. Focus on triphasil. J Reprod Med 1986;31:559-564.

Endrikat J, Jaques MA, Mayerhofer M, Pelissier C, Müller U, Düsterberg B. A twelve-month comparative clinical investigation of two low-dose oral contraceptives containing 20 µg ethinylestradiol/75 µg gestodene and 20 µg ethinylestradiol/150 µg desogestrel, with respect to efficacy, cycle control and tolerance. Contraception 1995;52:229-235.

Engel T. Laparoscopic sterilization: electrosurgery or clip application? J Reprod Med 1978;21:107-110.

Florence N. Das kontrazeptive vaginal-suppositorium: ergebnisse einer klinischen fünfjahresstudie. Sexualmedizin 1977;6:385-386.

Frank R. Clinical evaluation of a simple jelly-alone method of contraception. Fertil Steril 1962;13:458-464.

Frankman O, Raabe N, Ingemansson CA. Clinical evaluation of C-Film, a vaginal contraceptive. J Int Med Res 1975;3:292-296.

Frezieres RG, Walsh TL, Nelson AL, Clark VA, Coulson AH. Evaluation of the efficacy of a polyurethane condom: results from a randomized controlled clinical trial. Fam Plann Perspect 1999;31:81-87.

Fu H, Darroch JE, Haas T, Ranjit N. Contraceptive failure rates: new estimates from the 1995 National Survey of Family Growth. Fam Plann Perspect 1999; 31:56-63.

Gibor Y, Mitchell C. Selected events following insertion of the Progestasert system. Contraception 1980;21:491-503.

Glass R, Vessey M, Wiggins P. Use-effectiveness of the condom in a selected family planning clinic population in the United Kingdom. Contraception 1974;10:591-598.

Godts P. Klinische prüfung eines vaginalem antikonzipiens. Ars Medici 1973;28: 584-593.

Grady WR, Hayward MD, Yagi J. Contraceptive failure in the United States: estimates from the 1982 National Survey of Family Growth. Fam Plann Perspect 1986;18:200-209.

Grady WR, Hirsch MB, Keen N, Vaughan B. Contraceptive failure and continuation among married women in the United States, 1970-75. Stud Fam Plann 1983;14:9-19.

Hall P, Bahamondes L, Diaz J, Petta C. Introductory study of the once-a-month, injectable contraceptive Cyclofem in Brazil, Chile, Colombia, and Peru. Contraception 1997;56:353-359.

Hall RE. Continuation and pregnancy rates with four contraceptive methods. Am J Obstet Gynecol 1973;116:671-681.

Hawkins DF, Benster B. A comparative study of three low dose progestogens, chlormadinone acetate, megestrol acetate and norethisterone, as oral contraceptives. Br J Obstet Gynaecol 1977;84:708-713.

Howard G, Blair M, Chen JK, Fotherby K, Muggeridge J, Elder MG, Bye PG. A clinical trial of norethisterone oenanthate (Norigest) injected every two months. Contraception 1982;25:333-343.

Hughes I. An open assessment of a new low dose estrogen combined oral contraceptive. J Int Med Res 1978;6:41-45.

Hulka JF, Mercer JP, Fishburne JI, Kumarasamy T, Omran KF, Phillips JM, Lefler HT, Lieberman B, Lean TH, Pai DN, Koetsawang S, Castro VM. Spring clip sterilization: one-year follow-up of 1,079 cases. Am J Obstet Gynecol 1976;125:1039-1043.

Iizuka R, Kobayashi T, Kawakami S, Nakamura Y, Ikeuchi M, Chin B, Mochimaru F, Sumi K, Sato H, Yamaguchi J, Ohno T, Shiina M, Maeda N, Tokoro H, Suzuki T, Hayashi K, Takahashi T, Akatsuka M, Kasuga Y, Kurokawa H. Clinical experience with the Vaginal Contraceptive Film containing the spermicide polyoxyethylene nonylphenyl ether (C-Film study group). Jpn J Fertil Steril 1980;25:64-68. (In Japanese; translation supplied by Apothecus Inc.)

John APK. Contraception in a practice community. J R Coll Gen Pract 1973;23: 665-675.

Johnston JA, Roberts DB, Spencer RB. A survey evaluation of the efficacy and efficiency of natural family planning services and methods in Australia: report of a research project. Sydney, Australia: St. Vincent's Hospital, 1978.

Jones EF, Forrest JD. Contraceptive failure rates based on the 1988 NSFG. Fam Plann Perspect 1992;24:12-19.

Jubhari S, Lane ME, Sobrero AJ. Continuous microdose (0.3 mg) quingestanol acetate as an oral contraceptive agent. Contraception 1974;9:213-219.

Kambic R, Kambic M, Brixius AM, Miller S. A thirty-month clinical experience in natural family planning. Am J Public Health 1981;71:1255-1258. Erratum. Am J Public Health 1982;72:538.

Kasabach HY. Clinical evaluation of vaginal jelly alone in the management of fertility. Clin Med 1962;69:894-897.

Kase S, Goldfarb M. Office vasectomy review of 500 cases. Urology 1973;1:60-62.

Kassell NC, McElroy MP. Emma Goldman Clinic for Women study. In: King L (ed). The cervical cap handbook for users and fitters. Iowa City IA: Emma Goldman Clinic for Women, 1981:11-19.

Kaunitz AM. Efficacy, cycle control, and safety of two triphasic oral contraceptives: Cyclessa (desogestrel/ethinyl estradiol) and Ortho-Novum 7/7/7 (norethindrone/ethinyl estradiol): a randomized clinical trial. Contraception 2000;61:295-302.

Kaunitz AM, Garceau RJ, Cromie MA, Lunelle Study Group. Comparative safety, efficacy, and cycle control of Lunelle monthly contraceptive injection (medroxyprogesterone acetate and estradiol cypionate injectable suspension) and Ortho-Novum 7/7/7 oral contraceptive (norethindrone/eithinyl estradiol triphasic). Contraception 1999;60:179-187.

Keifer W. A clinical evaluation of continuous Norethindrone (0.35 mg). In: Ortho Pharmaceutical Corporation. A clinical symposium on 0.35 mg. Norethindrone: continuous regimen low-dose oral contraceptive. Proceedings of a symposium, New York City, February 22, 1971. Raritan NJ: Ortho Pharmaceutical Corporation, 1973:9-14.

Klapproth HJ, Young IS. Vasectomy, vas ligation and vas occlusion. Urology 1973;1:292-300.

Klaus H, Goebel JM, Muraski B, Egizio MT, Weitzel D, Taylor, RS, Fagan MU, Ek K, Hobday K. Use-effectiveness and client satisfaction in six centers teaching the Billings ovulation method. Contraception 1979;19:613-629.

Kleppinger RK. A vaginal contraceptive foam. Penn Med J 1965;68:31-34.

Koch JP. The Prentif contraceptive cervical cap: a contemporary study of its clinical safety and effectiveness. Contraception 1982;25:135-159.

Korba VD, Heil CG. Eight years of fertility control with norgestrel-ethinyl estradiol (Ovral): an updated clinical review. Fertil Steril 1975;26:973-981.

Korba VD, Paulson SR. Five years of fertility control with microdose norgestrel: an updated clinical review. J Reprod Med 1974;13:71-75.

Kovacs GT, Jarman H, Dunn K, Westcott M, Baker HWG. The contraceptive diaphragm: is it an acceptable method in the 1980s? Aust NZ J Obstet Gynaecol 1986;26:76-79.

Lane ME, Arceo R, Sobrero AJ. Successful use of the diaphragm and jelly by a young population: report of a clinical study. Fam Plann Perspect 1976;8:81-86.

Ledger WJ. Ortho 1557-O: a new oral contraceptive. Int J Fertil 1970;15:88-92.

Lehfeldt H, Sivin I. Use effectiveness of the Prentif cervical cap in private practice: a prospective study. Contraception 1984;30:331-338.

Loffer FD, Pent D. Risks of laparoscopic fulguration and transection of the fallopian tube. Obstet Gynecol 1977;49:218-222.

Loudon NB, Barden ME, Hepburn WB, Prescott RJ. A comparative study of the effectiveness and acceptability of the diaphragm used with spermicide in the form of C-film or a cream or jelly. Br J Fam Plann 1991;17:41-44.

Luukkainen T, Allonen H, Haukkamaa M, Holma P, Pyörälä T, Terho J, Toivonen J, Batar I, Lampe L, Andersson K, Atterfeldt P, Johansson EDB, Nilsson S, Nygren KG, Odlind V, Olsson SE, Rybo G, Sikström B, Nielsen NC, Buch A, Osler M, Steier A, Ulstein M. Effective contraception with the levonorgestrel-releasing intrauterine device: 12-month report of a European multicenter study. Contraception 1987;36:169-179.

Margaret Pyke Centre. One thousand vasectomies. Br Med J 1973;4:216-221.

Marshall J. Cervical-mucus and basal body-temperature method of regulating births: field trial. Lancet 1976;2:282-283.

Marshall S, Lyon RP. Variability of sperm disappearance from the ejaculate after vasectomy. J Urol 1972;107:815-817.

Mauck C, Callahan M, Weiner DH, Dominik R, FemCap investigators' group. A comparative study of the safety and efficacy of FemCap, a new vaginal barrier contraceptive, and the Ortho All-Flex diaphragm. Contraception 1999;60:71-80.

Mauck C, Glover LH, Miller E, Allen S, Archer DF, Blumenthal P, Rosenzweig BA, Dominik R, Sturgen K, Cooper J, Fingerhut F, Peacock L, Gabelnick HL. Lea's Shield®: a study of the safety and efficacy of a new vaginal barrier contraceptive used with and without spermicide. Contraception 1996;53:329-335.

McIntyre SL, Higgins JE. Parity and use-effectiveness with the contraceptive sponge. Am J Obstet Gynecol 1986;155:796-801.

McQuarrie HG, Harris JW, Ellsworth HS, Stone RA, Anderson AE. The clinical evaluation of norethindrone in cyclic and continuous regimens. Adv Plann Parent 1972;7:124-130.

Mears E. Chemical contraceptive trial: II. J Reprod Fertil 1962;4:337-343.

Mears E, Please NW. Chemical contraceptive trial. J Reprod Fertil 1962;3:138-147.

The Mircette Study Group. An open-label, multicenter, noncomparative safety and efficacy study of Mircette, a low-dose estrogen-progestin oral contraceptive. Am J Obstet Gynecol 1998;179:S2-S8.

Mishell DR, El-Habashy MA, Good RG, Moyer DL. Contraception with an injectable progestin. Am J Obstet Gynecol 1968;101:1046-1053.

Morigi EM, Pasquale SA. Clinical experience with a low dose oral contraceptive containing norethisterone and ethinyl oestradiol. Curr Med Res Opin 1978;5: 655-662.

Moss WM. A comparison of open-end versus closed-end vasectomies: a report on 6220 cases. Contraception 1992;46:521-525.

Mumford SD, Bhiwandiwala PP, Chi IC. Laparoscopic and minilaparotomy female sterilisation compared in 15,167 cases. Lancet 1980;2:1066-1070.

Nelson JH. The use of the mini pill in private practice. J Reprod Med 1973;10: 139-143.

Parsey KS, Pong A. An open-label, multicenter study to evaluate Yasmin, a low-dose combination oral contraceptive containing drospirenone, a new progestogen. Contraception 2000;61:105-111.

Peel J. The Hull family survey: II. Family planning in the first five years of marriage. J Biosoc Sci 1972;4:333-346.

Peterson HB, Xia Z, Hughes JM, Wilcox LS, Tylor LR, Trussell J. The risk of pregnancy after tubal sterilization: findings from the U.S. Collaborative Review of Sterilization. Am J Obstet Gynecol 1996;174:1161-1170.

Philp T, Guillebaud J, Budd D. Complications of vasectomy: Review of 16,000 patients. Br J Urol 1984;56:745-748.

Postlethwaite DL. Pregnancy rate of a progestogen oral contraceptive. Practitioner 1979;222:272-275.

Potts M, McDevitt J. A use-effectiveness trial of spermicidally lubricated condoms. Contraception 1975;11:701-710.

Powell MG, Mears BJ, Deber RB, Ferguson D. Contraception with the cervical cap: effectiveness, safety, continuity of use, and user satisfaction. Contraception 1986;33:215-232.

Preston SN. A report of a collaborative dose-response clinical study using decreasing doses of combination oral contraceptives. Contraception 1972;6:17-35.

Preston SN. A report of the correlation between the pregnancy rates of low estrogen formulations and pill-taking habits of females studied. J Reprod Med 1974;13: 75-77.

Raymond EG, Chen PL, Luoto J. Contraceptive effectiveness and safety of five nonoxynol-9 spermicides: a randomized trial. Obstet Gynecol 2004;103:430-439.

Raymond E, Dominik R, the spermicide trial group. Contraceptive effectiveness of two spermicides: a randomized trial. Obstet Gynecol 1999;93:896-903.

Rice FJ, Lanctôt CA, Garcia-Devesa C. Effectiveness of the sympto-thermal method of natural family planning: an international study. Int J Fertil 1981;26:222-230.

Richwald GA, Greenland S, Gerber MM, Potik R, Kersey L, Comas MA. Effectiveness of the cavity-rim cervical cap: results of a large clinical study. Obstet Gynecol 1989;74:143-148.

Roumen FJME, Apter D, Mulders TMT, Dieben TOM. Efficacy, tolerability and acceptability of a novel contraceptive vaginal ring releasing etonogestrel and ethinyl oestradiol. Hum Reprod 2001;16:469-475.

Rovinsky JJ. Clinical effectiveness of a contraceptive cream. Obstet Gynecol 1964;23:125-131.

Royal College of General Practitioners. Oral contraceptives and health. New York NY: Pitman Publishing Corp., 1974.

Salomon W, Haase W. Intravaginale kontrazeption. Sexualmedizin 1977;6:198-202.

Sangi-Haghpeykar H, Poindexter AN, Bateman L, Ditmore JR. Experiences of injectable contraceptive users in an urban setting. Obstet Gynecol 1996;88:227-233.

Schirm AL, Trussell J, Menken J, Grady WR. Contraceptive failure in the United States: the impact of social, economic, and demographic factors. Fam Plann Perspect 1982;14:68-75.

Schmidt SS. Vasectomy. JAMA 1988;259:3176.

Schwallie PC, Assenzo JR. Contraceptive use-efficacy study utilizing Depo-Provera administered as an injection once every six months. Contraception 1972;6:315-327.

Schwallie PC, Assenzo JR. Contraceptive use-efficacy study utilizing medroxyprogesterone acetate administered as an intramuscular injection once every 90 days. Fertil Steril 1973;24:331-339.

Scutchfield FD, Long WN, Corey B, Tyler CW. Medroxyprogesterone acetate as an injectable female contraceptive. Contraception 1971;3:21-35.

Sheps MC. An analysis of reproductive patterns in an American isolate. Popul Stud 1965;19:65-80.

Sheth A, Jain U, Sharma S, Adatia A, Patankar S, Andolsek L, Pretnar-Darovec A, Belsey MA, Hall PE, Parker RA, Ayeni S, Pinol A, Foo CLH. A randomized, double-blind study of two combined and two progestogen-only oral contraceptives. Contraception 1982;25:243-252.

Shihata AA, Trussell J. New female intravaginal barrier contraceptive device: preliminary clinical trial. Contraception 1991;44:11-19.

Shroff NE, Pearce MY, Stratford ME, Wilkinson PD. Clinical experience with ethynodiol diacetate 0.5 mg daily as an oral contraceptive. Contraception 1987;35:121-134.

Sivin I, Alvarez F, Mishell DR Jr, Darney P, Wan L, Brache V, Lacarra M, Klaisle C, Stern J. Contraception with two levonorgestrel rod implants: a 5-year study in the United States and Dominican Republic. Contraception 1998a;58:275-282.

Sivin I, Campodonico I, Kiriwat O, Holma P, Diaz S, Wan L, Biswas A, Viegas O, el din Abdalla K, Anant MP, Pavez M, Stern J. The performance of levonorgestrel rod and Norplant contraceptive implants: a 5 year randomized study. Hum Reprod 1998b;13:3371-3378.

Sivin I, El Mahgoub S, McCarthy T, Mishell DR, Shoupe D, Alvarez F, Brache V, Jimenez E, Diaz J, Faundes A, Diaz MM, Coutinho E, Mattos CER, Diaz S, Pavez M, Stern J. Long-term contraception with the Levonorgestrel 20 mcg/day (LNG-IUS) and the Copper T 380Ag intrauterine devices: a five-year randomized study. Contraception 1990;42:361-378.

Sivin I, Lähteenmäki P, Ranta S, Darney P, Klaisle C, Wan L, Mishell DR, Lacarra M, Viegas OAC, Bilhareus P, Koetsawang S, Piya-Anant M, Diaz S, Pavez M, Alvarez F, Brache V, LaGuardia K, Nash H, Stern J. Levonorgestrel concentrations during use of levonorgestrel rod (LNG ROD) implants. Contraception 1997;55:81-85.

Sivin I, Mishell DR Jr, Diaz S, Biswas A, Alvarez F, Darney P, Holma P, Wan L, Brache V, Kiriwat O, Abdalla K, Campodonico I, Pasquale S, Pavez M, Schechter J. Prolonged effectiveness of Norplant capsule implants: a 7-year study. Contraception 2000;61:187-194.

Sivin I, Shaaban M, Odlind V, Olsson SE, Diaz S, Pavez M, Alvarez F, Brache V, Diaz J. A randomized trial of the Gyne T 380 and Gyne T 380 Slimline intrauterine copper devices. Contraception 1990;42:379-389.

Sivin I, Stern J. Long-acting, more effective copper T IUDs: a summary of U.S. experience, 1970-1975. Stud Fam Plann 1979;10:263-281.

Smith C, Farr G, Feldblum PJ, Spence A. Effectiveness of the non-spermicidal fit-free diaphragm. Contraception 1995;51:289-291.

Smith GG, Lee RJ. The use of cervical caps at the University of California, Berkeley: a survey. Contraception 1984;30:115-123.

Smith M, Vessey MP, Bounds W, Warren J. C-Film as a contraceptive. Br Med J 1974;4:291.

Sokal D, Gates D, Amatya R, Dominik R, Clinical investigator team. Two randomized controlled trials comparing the tubal ring and Filshie Clip for tubal sterilization. Fertil Steril. 2000;74:525-533.

Steiner MJ, Dominik R, Rountree RW, Nanda K, Dorflinger LJ. Contraceptive effectiveness of a polyurethane condom and a latex condom: a randomized controlled trial. Obstet Gynecol 2003;101:539-547.

Stim EM. The nonspermicidal fit-free diaphragm: a new contraceptive method. Adv Plann Parenthood 1980;15:88-98.

Squire JJ, Berger GS, Keith L. A retrospective clinical study of a vaginal contraceptive suppository. J Reprod Med 1979;22:319-323.

Tatum HJ. Comparative experience with newer models of the copper T in the United States. In: Hefnawi F, Segal SJ (eds). Analysis of intrauterine contraception. Amsterdam, Netherlands: North Holland, 1975:155-163.

Tietze C, Lewit S. Comparison of three contraceptive methods: diaphragm with jelly or cream, vaginal foam, and jelly/cream alone. J Sex Res 1967;3:295-311.

Tietze C, Lewit S. Evaluation of intrauterine devices: ninth progress report of the cooperative statistical program. Stud Fam Plann 1970;1:1-40.

Tietze C, Poliakoff SR, Rock J. The clinical effectiveness of the rhythm method of contraception. Fertil Steril 1951;2:444-450.

Trussell J, Grummer-Strawn L. Contraceptive failure of the ovulation method of periodic abstinence. Fam Plann Perspect 1990;22:65-75.

Trussell J, Hatcher RA, Cates W, Stewart FH, Kost K. Contraceptive failure in the United States: an update. Stud Fam Plann 1990;21:51-54.

Trussell J, Kost K. Contraceptive failure in the United States: a critical review of the literature. Stud Fam Plann 1987;18:237-283.

Trussell J, Vaughan B. Contraceptive failure, method-related discontinuation and resumption of use: results from the 1995 National Survey of Family Growth. Fam Plann Perspect 1999;31:64-72, 93.

Tyler ET. Current developments in systemic contraception. Pac Med Surg 1965;93: 79-85.

Valle RF, Battifora HA. A new approach to tubal sterilization by laparoscopy. Fertil Steril 1978;30:415-422.

Vaughan B, Trussell J, Menken J, Jones EF. Contraceptive failure among married women in the United States, 1970-1973. Fam Plann Perspect 1977;9:251-258.

Vessey M, Huggins G, Lawless M, McPherson K, Yeates D. Tubal sterilization: findings in a large prospective study. Br J Obstet Gynaecol 1983;90:203-209.

Vessey M, Lawless M, Yeates D. Efficacy of different contraceptive methods. Lancet 1982;1:841-842.

Vessey MP, Lawless M, Yeates D, McPherson K. Progestogen-only oral contraception. Findings in a large prospective study with special reference to effectiveness. Br J Fam Plann 1985;10:117-121.

Vessey MP, Villard-Mackintosh L, McPherson K, Yeates D. Factors influencing use-effectiveness of the condom. Br J Fam Plann 1988;14:40-43.

Vessey M, Wiggins P. Use-effectiveness of the diaphragm in a selected family planning clinic population in the United Kingdom. Contraception 1974;9:15-21.

Vessey MP, Wright NH, McPherson K, Wiggins P. Fertility after stopping different methods of contraception. Br Med J 1978;1:265-267.

Wade ME, McCarthy P, Braunstein GD, Abernathy JR, Suchindran CM, Harris GS, Danzer HC, Uricchio WA. A randomized prospective study of the use-effectiveness of two methods of natural family planning. Am J Obstet Gynecol 1981;141:368-376.

Walsh TL, Frezieres RG, Peacock K, Nelson AL, Clark VA, Bernstein L. Evaluation of the efficacy of a nonlatex condom: results from a randomized, controlled clinical trial. Perspect Sex Reprod Health 2003;35:79-86.

Westoff CF, Potter RG, Sagi PC, Mishler EG. Family growth in metropolitan America. Princeton NJ: Princeton University Press, 1961.

Wolf L, Olson HJ, Tyler ET. Observations on the clinical use of cream-alone and gel-alone methods of contraception. Obstet Gynecol 1957;10:316-321.

World Health Organization. A multicentered phase III comparative clinical trial of depot-medroxyprogesterone acetate given three-monthly at doses of 100 mg or 150 mg: I. Contraceptive efficacy and side effects. Contraception 1986;34:223-235.

World Health Organization. A multicentered phase III comparative study of two hormonal contraceptive preparations given once-a-month by intramuscular injection: I. Contraceptive efficacy and side effects. Contraception 1988;37:1-20.

World Health Organization. A prospective multicentre trial of the ovulation method of natural family planning. II. The effectiveness phase. Fertil Steril 1981;36:591-598.

World Health Organization. Multinational comparative clinical evaluation of two long-acting injectable contraceptive steroids: norethisterone oenanthate and medroxyprogesterone acetate. Contraception 1977;15:513-533.

World Health Organization. Multinational comparative clinical trial of long-acting injectable contraceptives: norethisterone enanthate given in two dosage regimens and depot-medroxyprogesterone acetate. Final report. Contraception 1983;28:1-20.

Woutersz TB. A low-dose combination oral contraceptive: experience with 1,700 women treated for 22,489 cycles. J Reprod Med 1981;26:615-620.

Woutersz TB. A new ultra-low-dose combination oral contraceptive. J Reprod Med 1983;28:81-84.

Wyeth Laboratories. NORPLANT® SYSTEM Prescribing Information. Philadelphia PA: Wyeth Laboratories, December 10, 1990.

Yoon IB, King TM, Parmley TH. A two-year experience with the Falope ring sterilization procedure. Am J Obstet Gynecol 1977;127:109-112.

Table 31-1 Percentage of women experiencing an unintended pregnancy during the first year of typical use and the first year of perfect use of contraception and the percentage continuing use at the end of the first year. United States.

Method (1)	% of Women Experiencing an Unintended Pregnancy within the First Year of Use		% of Women Continuing Use at One Year[3] (4)
	Typical Use[1] (2)	Perfect Use[2] (3)	
No method[4]	85	85	
Spermicides[5]	29	18	42
Withdrawal	27	4	43
Periodic abstinence	25		51
Calendar		9	
Ovulation method		3	
Sympto-thermal[6]		2	
Post-ovulation		1	
Cap[7]			
Parous women	32	26	46
Nulliparous women	16	9	57
Sponge			
Parous women	32	20	46
Nulliparous women	16	9	57
Diaphragm[7]	16	6	57
Condom[8]			
Female (Reality)	21	5	49
Male	15	2	53
Combined pill and minipill	8	0.3	68
Evra patch	8	0.3	68
NuvaRing	8	0.3	68
Depo-Provera	3	0.3	56
Lunelle	3	0.05	56
IUD			
ParaGard (copper T)	0.8	0.6	78
Mirena (LNG-IUS)	0.1	0.1	81
Norplant and Norplant-2	0.05	0.05	84
Female sterilization	0.5	0.5	100
Male sterilization	0.15	0.10	100

Emergency Contraceptive Pills: Treatment initiated within 72 hours after unprotected intercourse reduces the risk of pregnancy by at least 75%.[9]

Lactational Amenorrhea Method: LAM is a highly effective, *temporary* method of contraception.[10]

Source: See text.

1 Among *typical* couples who initiate use of a method (not necessarily for the first time), the percentage who experience an accidental pregnancy during the first year if they do not stop use for any other reason. Estimates of the probability of pregnancy during the first year of typical use for spermicides, withdrawal, periodic abstinence, the diaphragm, the male condom, the pill, and Depo-Provera are taken from the 1995 National Survey of Family Growth corrected for underreporting of abortion; see the text for the derivation of estimates for the other methods.

2 Among couples who initiate use of a method (not necessarily for the first time) and who use it *perfectly* (both consistently and correctly), the percentage who experience an accidental pregnancy during the first year if they do not stop use for any other reason. See the text for the derivation of the estimate for each method.

3 Among couples attempting to avoid pregnancy, the percentage who continue to use a method for 1 year.

4 The percentages becoming pregnant in columns (2) and (3) are based on data from populations where contraception is not used and from women who cease using contraception in order to become pregnant. Among such populations, about 89% become pregnant within 1 year. This estimate was lowered slightly (to 85%) to represent the percentage who would become pregnant within 1 year among women now relying on reversible methods of contraception if they abandoned contraception altogether.

5 Foams, creams, gels, vaginal suppositories, and vaginal film.

6 Cervical mucus (ovulation) method supplemented by calendar in the pre-ovulatory and basal body temperature in the post-ovulatory phases.

7 With spermicidal cream or jelly.

8 Without spermicides.

9 The treatment schedule is one dose within 120 hours after unprotected intercourse, and a second dose 12 hours after the first dose. Both doses of Plan B can be taken at the same time. Plan B (1 dose is 1 white pill) is the only dedicated product specifically marketed for emergency contraception. The Food and Drug Administration has in addition declared the following 18 brands of oral contraceptives to be safe and effective for emergency contraception: Ogestrel or Ovral (1 dose is 2 white pills), Alesse, Lessina, or Levlite, (1 dose is 5 pink pills), Levlen or Nordette (1 dose is 4 light-orange pills), Cryselle, Levora, Low-Ogestrel, or Lo/Ovral (1 dose is 4 white pills), Tri-Levlen or Triphasil (1 dose is 4 yellow pills), Portia, Seasonale, or Trivora (1 dose is 4 pink pills), Aviane (one dose is 5 orange pills), and Empresse (one dose is 4 orange pills).

10 However, to maintain effective protection against pregnancy, another method of contraception must be used as soon as menstruation resumes, the frequency or duration of breastfeeds is reduced, bottle feeds are introduced, or the baby reaches 6 months of age.

Table 31-2 Summary of studies of pregnancy rates among women neither contracepting nor breastfeeding[a]

Reference	N for Analysis	Life-Table 12-Month % Pregnant	Characteristics of the Sample	LFU (%)[g]	Comments
Grady et al., 1986	1,028	43.1	All married	20.6[f]	1982 NSFG; estimate far too low; see text
Sivin and Stern, 1979	420	78.1	48% nulliparous	?	Following removal of copper–medicated IUD for planned pregnancy
Vessey et al., 1978	779	82	All nulligravid	?	Britain; Oxford/FPA study following cessation of method use for planned pregnancy; conceptions leading to a live birth
Tatum, 1975	553	84.6		17.2	Following removal of copper–medicated IUD for planned pregnancy
Sivin, 1987	96	87	All parous	?	Chile, Dominican Republic, Finland, Sweden, United States; following removal of Norplant for planned pregnancy
Tietze and Lewit, 1970	378	88.2	89% aged 15–29	19.0	Following removal of nonmedicated IUD for planned pregnancy
Sheps, 1965	397	88.8	All married Hutterites	?	Conceptions leading to the first live birth following marriage among women reporting no fetal losses before the first conception
Vessey et al., 1978	1,343	89	All parous	?	Britain; Oxford/FPA study following cessation of method use for planned pregnancy; conceptions leading to a live birth
Belhadj et al., 1986	110	94.0[c]	All parous; aged 18–36	9.1	Brazil, Chile, Dominican Republic, Singapore, United States; following removal of medicated IUD for planned pregnancy

Notes:

[a] Updated from Trussell and Kost (1987), Table 1.

[c] Calculated by James Trussell from data in the article.

[g] Most of these studies incorrectly report the loss to follow-up probability as the number of women lost at any time during the study divided by the total number of women entering the study. Thus, these are the probabilities presented in the table. However, the correct measure of LFU would be a gross life-table probability. When available, gross 12-month probabilities are denoted by the letter "g."

[f] Nonresponse rate for entire survey.

For table references, see reference section.

Table 31-3 Summary of studies of contraceptive failure: spermicides[a]

Reference	Method Brand	N for Analysis	Life-Table 12-Month % Pregnant	Pearl Index Pregnancy Rate			Characteristics of the Sample	LFU (%)[g]	Comments
				Index	Total Exposure	Maximum Exposure			
Edelman, 1980	S'positive	200		0.0	2,682 Mo.	?		?	Study conducted by Jordan-Simmer, Inc., as reported by Edelman
Squire et al., 1979	Semicid Suppository	326	0.3				69% aged 20–34; 55% married; "well educated"; "highly motivated"; 24% prior use of oral contraceptives	0.0[c]	89% reported exclusive use of foam
Soloman and Haase, 1977	Patentex (Encare) Oval	1,652		0.3[c]	34,506 Cy.	54 Mo.	13% aged 15–20, 48% aged 21–30, 33% aged 31–40, 6% aged 41–45, 42% nulliparous	?	Subjects who used for less than one year excluded? Germany
Iizuka et al., 1980	Vaginal Contraceptive Film (C-Film)	168		0.6	2,161 Mo.	?	All women had been pregnant before; 20% aged <25, 64% aged 25–34,17% aged 35+	?	Japan
Brehm and Haase, 1975	Patentex (Encare) Oval	10,017		0.9[c]	63,759 Cy.	?	18% aged <21, 20% aged >35; 46% parity 0	?	Germany; FDA rejected this study because of flawed design (see text)
Florence,1977	a-gen 53	103		1.2[c]	2,255 Cy.	61 Mo.	17% aged 17–20, 51% aged 21–30, 20% aged 31–40,12% aged 41+	?	Belgium
Dimpfl et al., 1984	Pantentex (Encare) Oval	482	1.5				22% aged <21,25% aged >31; 44% parity 0; 60% married	?	Denmark, Germany, Poland, Switzerland
Bushnell, 1965	Emko Vaginal Foam	130		1.8	2,737 Mo.	57 Mo.	Aged 17–51; 76% aged 20–35	?	

(continued)

Table 31-3 Summary of studies of contraceptive failure: spermicides[a]—(cont'd)

Reference	Method Brand	N for Analysis	Life-Table 12-Month % Pregnant	Pearl Index Pregnancy Rate — Index	Pearl Index Pregnancy Rate — Total Exposure	Pearl Index Pregnancy Rate — Maximum Exposure	Characteristics of the Sample	LFU (%)[g]	Comments
Godts, 1973	a-gen 53	56		1.9[c]	1,344 Cy.	32 Mo.	21% aged 18–20, 46% aged 21–30, 18% aged 31–40, 14% aged 41+; all gravid	?	
Carpenter and Martin, 1970	Emko Pre-fil Vaginal Foam	1,778		3.4[c]	17,200 Cy.	18 Cy.	69% aged 21–35; 24% ≥12 years education; 44% no previous contraceptive experience	14.2[c]	All women agreed to exclusive use of foam
Brigato et al., 1982	Vaginal Contraceptive Film (C-Film)	37		3.9[c]	924 Mo.	?		?	Italy
Wolf et al., 1957	Preceptin Vaginal Gel	112		4.2[c]	1,145 Mo.	29 Mo.	All aged 13–40; mean age = 25[f]; all married	8.9[c]	
Bernstein, 1971	Emko Pre-fil Vaginal Foam	2,932		4.3[c]	28,332 Cy.	20 Cy.	70% aged 21–35; 39% ≥12 years education	16.1[c]	All women agreed to exclusive use of foam
Tyler, 1965	Delfen Vaginal Foam	672		6.0	9,486 Cy.	>16 Mo.	Rates for full applicator doses and half doses combined	?	
Apothecus, 1992	Vaginal Contraceptive Film (C-Film)	761		6.5	6,501 Mo.	?			Belgium, Netherlands, Britain, Germany, Switzerland, Denmark, Sweden, Israel, Egypt; results never published; quality of study unknown
Kleppinger, 1965	Delfen Vaginal Foam	138		7.5	1,116 Mo.	19 Mo.	53% aged 21–30; 27% postpartum	0.0[c,g]	

(continued)

CONTRACEPTIVE TECHNOLOGY

Table 31-3 Summary of studies of contraceptive failure: spermicides[a]—(cont'd)

Reference	Method Brand	N for Analysis	Risk of Pregnancy				Characteristics of the Sample	LFU (%)[g]	Comments
			Life-Table 12-Month % Pregnant	Pearl Index Pregnancy Rate					
				Index	Total Exposure	Maximum Exposure			
Dubrow and Kuder, 1958	Delfen Vaginal Cream	338		7.6	633 Mo.	12 Mo.	Mean age = 25; 93% ≤12 years education; 39% black; 45% Puerto Rican[t]	59.5[c]	
Dubrow and Kuder, 1958	Preceptin Vaginal Gel	835		8.1	3,728 Mo.	23 Mo.	Mean age = 25; 93% ≤12 years education; 39% black; 45% Puerto Rican[t]	45.1[c]	
Wolf et al., 1957	Delfen Vaginal Cream	875		8.9[c]	5,232 Mo.	30 Mo.	All aged 13–40; mean age = 25[t]; all married	13.0[c]	
Frankman et al., 1975	Vaginal Contraceptive Film (C-Film)	237		9.0	1,866 Mo.	23 Mo.		?	Sweden; data included in Apothecus (1992)
Rovinsky, 1964	Delfen Vaginal Cream	251		9.1	2,915 Mo.	67 Mo.	70% aged 20–34; 55% Puerto Rican; 10% ≥13 years education	28.0[c]	
Raymond et al., 2004	100 mg suppository (Encare)	299	10.0[d]				44% aged 18–25	22	Random assignment to 100 mg suppository, 52.5 mg gel, 100 mg gel, 150 mg gel or 100 mg film
Raymond et al., 2004	100 mg film (Ortho Options Contraceptive Film)	295	11.9[d]				43% aged 18–25	24	Random assignment to 100 mg film, 52.5 mg gel, 100 mg gel, 150 mg gel or 100 mg suppository
Vessey et al., 1982		?		11.9	303 Yr.	?	All white; at recruitment aged 25–39 and married; at enrollment, all women had been using the diaphragm, IUD, or pill successfully for at least 5 months	0.3[t,v]	Britain; Oxford/FPA study

(continued)

Table 31-3 Summary of studies of contraceptive failure: spermicides[a]—(cont'd)

Reference	Method Brand	N for Analysis	Life-Table 12-Month % Pregnant	Risk of Pregnancy — Pearl Index Pregnancy Rate			Characteristics of the Sample	LFU (%)[g]	Comments
				Index	Total Exposure	Maximum Exposure			
Jones and Forrest, 1992		267	13.4				Aged 15–44[t]	21[r]	NSFG 1988; probablity when standardized and corrected for estimated underreporting of abortion = 30.2[s]
Raymond et al., 2004	150 mg gel (Ortho Options Conceptrol)	300	14.0[d]				43% aged 18–25	21	Random assignment to 150 mg gel, 52.5 mg gel, 100 mg gel, 100 mg film or 100 mg suppository
Vaughan et al., 1977		596	14.9[s]				Aged 15–44; all married[t]	19.0[r]	NSFG 1973
Trussell and Vaughan, 1999		164	15.3				Aged 15–44[t]	21[r]	NSFG 1995
Raymond et al., 2004	100 mg gel (Ortho Options Conceptrol)	295	15.5[d]				46% aged 18–25	25	Random assignment to 100 mg gel, 52.5 mg gel, 150 mg gel, 100 mg film or 100 mg suppository
Fu et al., 1999		?	16.6					21[r]	NSFG 1995; probablity when standardized and corrected for estimated underreporting of abortion = 29.0[s]
Grady et al., 1983		1,106	17.5[s,c]				Aged 15–44; all married[t]	18.2[r]	NSFG 1973 and 1976
Schirm et al., 1982		1,106	17.9[s]				Aged 15–44; all married[t]	18.2[r]	NSFG 1973 and 1976

(continued)

Table 31-3 Summary of studies of contraceptive failure: spermicides[a]—(cont'd)

Reference	Method Brand	N for Analysis	Risk of Pregnancy				Characteristics of the Sample	LFU (%)g	Comments
			Life-Table 12-Month % Pregnant	Pearl Index Pregnancy Rate					
				Index	Total Exposure	Maximum Exposure			
Mears, 1962	Emko Aerosol Foam (nonoxynol 10-11)	425		18.0c	722 Cy.	3 Cy.	Pearl index of 9.3 among consistent and 48.4 among inconsistent users	>20c,t	Britain; postal trial; random assignment to foam, foaming tablet, or pessary with crossover design
Kasabach, 1962	Koromex A Jelly	242		21.0c	2,058 Mo.	24 Mo.	36% aged 25–35; all married; 68% "had a high school education"; all parous	19.3c	
Bracher and Santow, 1992		89	21.5				27% aged <20, 56% aged 20–29, 17% aged 30+; 49% parity 0; 87% married or cohabiting	25r	Australian Family Survey; first use of method
Grady et al., 1986		284	21.8s				Aged 15–44; all married[t]	20.6r	NSFG 1982
Raymond et al., 2004	52.5 mg gel (Advantage S)	296	22.2d				43% aged 18–25	20	Random assignment to 52.5 mg gel, 100 mg gel, 100 mg gel, 150 mg gel, 100 mg film or 100 mg suppository
Frank, 1962	Koromex A Jelly	824		24.8c	5,767 Mo.	12 Mo.	72% aged 21–35	17.0c	
Dingle and Tietze, 1963	Lactikol	170		23.5	1,789 Mo.	36 Mo.	Median age = 24.5	3.2t	
Raymond et al., 1999	Vaginal Contraceptive Film	369	24.9d				Aged 18–35; 17% nulligravid	5.8	Mexico, Ecuador, Guatemala, Ghana, United States; random assignment to Vaginal Contraceptive Film or Conceptrol foaming tablets

(continued)

Table 31-3 Summary of studies of contraceptive failure: spermicides[a]—(cont'd)

Reference	Method Brand	N for Analysis	Risk of Pregnancy				Characteristics of the Sample	LFU (%)[g]	Comments
			Life-Table 12-Month % Pregnant	Pearl Index Pregnancy Rate					
				Index	Total Exposure	Maximum Exposure			
Raymond et al., 1999	Conceptrol foaming tablets	365	28.0[d]				Aged 18–35; 16% nulligravid	7.3	Mexico, Ecuador, Guatemala, Ghana, United States; random assignment to Conceptrol foaming tablets or Vaginal Contraceptive Film
Tietze and Lewit, 1967	Emko Vaginal Foam	779	28.3				86% < age 30; all married; 47% ≥ high school completion; 75% nonwhite	6.9[g]	
Dingle and Tietze, 1963	Durafoam	421		28.5	2,985 Mo.	36 Mo.	Median age = 26.1	3.2[t]	
Mears, 1962	Genexol Pessary (nonoxynol 10-11)	425		30.3	730 Cy.	3 Cy.		>20[c,t]	Britain; postal trial; random assingment to foam, foaming tablets, or pessary with crossover design
Tietze and Lewit, 1967	Cooper Creme and Creme Jel, Koromex A, Lactikol Creme and Jelly, Lanesta Gel	806	36.8				79% < age 30; all married; 53% ≥ high school completion; 75% nonwhite	3.4[g]	
Mears, 1962	Volpar Foaming Tablets (phenyl mercuric acetate)	425		48.2[c]	728 Cy.	3 Cy.	Pearl index of 44.4 among consistent and 64.1 among inconsistent users	>20[c,t]	Britain; postal trial; random assignment to foam, foaming tablet, or pessary with crossover design
Mears and Please, 1962	Staycept Cream (hexyl resorcinol)	678		49.6[c]	707 Cy.	3 Cy.	Pearl index of 31.4 among consistent and 132.0 among inconsistent users	>41[c,t]	Britain; postal trial; random assignment to cream, foaming tablet, or pessary with crossover design

(continued)

Table 31-3 Summary of studies of contraceptive failure: spermicides[a] —(cont'd)

Reference	Method Brand	N for Analysis	Life-Table 12-Month % Pregnant	Risk of Pregnancy Pearl Index Pregnancy Rate			Characteristics of the Sample	LFU (%)[g]	Comments
				Index	Total Exposure	Maximum Exposure			
Mears and Please, 1962	Genexol Pessary (quinine)	678		52.2	647 Cy.	3 Cy.		>41[c,t]	Britain; postal trial; random assignment to cream, foaming tablet, or pessary with crossover design
Smith et al., 1974	Vaginal Contraceptive Film (C-Film)	63[c]		55.7[c]	194[c] Mo.	<15[c] Mo.	Aged 16-35	9.5[c]	Britain; trial terminated for ethical reasons
Mears and Please, 1962	Volpar Foaming Tablets (phenyl mercuric acetate)	678		59.0[c]	705 Cy.	3 Cy.	Pearl index of 47.8 among consistent and 106.7 among inconsistent users	>41[c,t]	Britain; postal trial; random assignment to cream, foaming tablet, or pessary with crossover design

Notes:

a Updated from Trussell and Kost (1987), Table 2.

c Calculated by James Trussell from data in the article.

d 6-month probability; 12-month probability not available.

g Most of these studies incorrectly report the loss to follow-up probability (LFU) as the number of women lost at any time during the study divided by the total number of women entering the study. Thus, these are the probabilities presented in the table. However, the correct measure of LFU would be a gross life-table probability. When available, gross 12-month probabilities are denoted by the letter "g."

r Nonresponse rate for entire survey.

s Standardized: Vaughan et al., (1977) (1973 NSFG)—intention (the average of probabilities for preventers and delayers); Grady et al., (1983) (1973 and 1976 NSFG)—intention. Our calculation (the average of probabilities for preventers and delayers); Schirm et al., (1982) (1973 and 1976 NSFG)—intention, age, and income; Grady et al., (1986) (1982 NSFG)—intention, age, poverty status, and parity; Jones and Forrest, (1992) (1988 NSFG)—age, marital status, and poverty status; Fu et al., (1999) (1995 NSFG)—age, union status, poverty status.

t Total for all methods in the study.

v The authors report that LFU for "relevant reasons (withdrawal of cooperation or loss of contact)" was 0.3% per year in the 1982 study. In the 1982 study, women had been followed for 9.5 years on average; if 0.3% are LFU per year, then 2.8% would be LFU in 9.5 years. LFU including death and emigration is about twice as high as LFU for "relevant reasons."

For table references, see reference section.

Table 31-4 Summary of studies of contraceptive failure: withdrawal

Reference	N for Analysis	Life-Table 12-Month % Pregnant	Pearl Index Pregnancy Rate			Characteristics of the Sample[w]	LFU (%)[g]	Comments
			Index	Total Exposure	Maximum Exposure			
Vessey et al., 1982	?		6.7	674 Yr.	?	All white; at recruitment aged 25–39 and married; at enrollment, all women had been using the diaphragm, IUD, or pill successfully for at least 5 months	0.3[t,v]	Britain; Oxford/FPA study
Bracher and Santow, 1992	94	14.2				25% aged <20, 66% aged 20–29, 9% aged 30+; 57% parity 0; 92% married or cohabiting	25[r]	Australian Family Survey; first use of method
Westoff et al., 1961	~74		16.7	1,287 Mo.	?	All married; all white	5.7[r]	FGMA study
Cliquet et al., 1977	2,316	17.3				All aged 30–34 living in Belgium; 93% living as married[t]	22[r]	Belgium; 1971 National Survey on Family Development (NEGO II)
Trussell and Vaughan, 1999	440	18.8				Aged 15–44[t]	21[r]	NSFG 1995
Fu et al., 1999	?	20.1					21[r]	NSFG 1995; probability when standardized and corrected for estimated underreporting of abortion = 27.1[s]

(continued)

Table 31-4 Summary of studies of contraceptive failure: withdrawal—(cont'd)

Reference	N for Analysis	Risk of Pregnancy					Characteristics of the Sample[w]	LFU (%)[g]	Comments
		Life-Table 12-Month % Pregnant	Pearl Index Pregnancy Rate						
			Index	Total Exposure	Maximum Exposure				
Debusschere, 1980	3,561	20.8				Aged 16–44 living in Flanders; 85% married[t]	40[r]	Belgium; 1975–1976 National Survey on Family Development (NEGO III)
Peel, 1972	62		21.9	1,640 Mo.	60 Mo.	All married	2.9[t]	Britain; Hull Family Survey

Notes:

a Updated from Trussell and Kost (1987), Table 1.

c Calculated by James Trussell from data in the article.

g Most of these studies incorrectly report the loss to follow-up probability (LFU) as the number of women lost at any time during the study divided by the total number of women entering the study. Thus, these are the probabilities presented in the table. However, the correct measure of LFU would be a gross life-table probability. When available, gross 12-month probabilities are denoted by the letter "g."

r Nonresponse rate for entire survey.

s Fu et al., (1999) (1995 NSFG) — age, union status, poverty status.

t Total for all methods in the study.

v The authors report that LFU for "relevant reasons" (withdrawal of cooperation or loss of contact)" was 0.3% per year in the 1982 study. In the 1982 study, women had been followed for 9.5 years on average; if 0.3% are LFU per year, then 2.8% would be LFU in 9.5 years. LFU including death and emigration is about twice as high as LFU for "relevant reasons."

w Unless otherwise noted, characteristics refer to females.

For table references, see reference section.

Table 31-5 Summary of studies of contraceptive failure: periodic abstinence[a]

Reference	Method	N for Analysis	Life-Table 12-Month % Pregnant	Pearl Index Pregnancy Rate			Characteristics of the Sample	LFU (%)[g]	Comments
				Index	Total Exposure	Maximum Exposure			
Trussell and Grummer-Strawn, 1990	Ovulation	725	3.2				Mean age = 30; proven fertility; agreed to use OM alone; cohabiting; 765 of 869 learned OM to satisfaction of teachers; 725 entered effectiveness study	?	Reanalysis of W.H.O. (1981) trial; probability based on 13 cycles of *perfect* use
Rice et al., 1981	Calendar + BBT	723	8.2				Aged 19–44; 9% aged 19–24, 54% aged 25–34, 37% aged 35–44; all parity 1+	3.4[c]	United States, France, Colombia, Canada, Mauritius
Dolack, 1978	Ovulation	329		10.5[c]	3,354 Cy.	?	Aged 19–48; mean age = 28; 40% had used oral contraceptives prior to study	18.0[c]	
Arévalo et al., 2002	Standard Days	478	12.0					7.1	Bolivia, Peru, Phillipines
Johnston et al., 1978	Cervical Mucus + BBT + Other Signs	268	13.3[c]				73% aged 22–32; all married or de facto married; 48% ≥12 years education (n = 460)	33.9[c,t]	Australia; probability based on 13 cycles
Wade et al., 1981	Cervical Mucus + BBT + Calendar	239	13.9[c]				Aged 20–39; 78% married	11.4[c,g]	Random assignment to OM or CM + BBT + Cal
Johnston et al., 1978	Calendar + BBT + Other Signs	192	14.3				73% aged 22–32; all married or de facto married; 48% ≥ 12 years education (n = 460)	33.9[c,t]	Australia; probability based on 13 cycles
Tietze et al., 1951	Calendar	409		14.4	7,267 Mo.	>60 Mo.	57% aged 25–34	13.4[c,t]	

(continued)

Table 31-5 Summary of studies of contraceptive failure: periodic abstinence[a]—(cont'd)

				Risk of Pregnancy					
					Pearl Index Pregnancy Rate				
			Life-Table						
Reference	Method	N for Analysis	12-Month % Pregnant	Index	Total Exposure	Maximum Exposure	Characteristics of the Sample	LFU (%)[g]	Comments
Vessey et al., 1982	Rhythm	?		15.5	161 Yr.	?	All white; at recruitment aged 25–39 and married; at enrollment, all women had been using the diaphragm, IUD, or pill successfully for at least 5 months	0.3[t,v]	Britain; Oxford/FPA study
Klaus et al., 1979	Ovulation	?	15.8[n]				67% aged 18–34; 52% ≥13 years education; some use of concurrent methods	2.9[n]	Probability based on only 12 cycles
Johnston et al., 1978	Cervical Mucus + BBT + Other Signs + Other Methods	94	16.0				78% aged 22–32; all married or de facto married; 53% ≥12 years education ("other" not limited to rhythm)	33.9[c,t]	Australia; probability based on 13 cycles
Grady et al., 1986	Rhythm	167	16.1[s]	16.8[c]	1,626 Cy.	22 Cy.	Aged 15–44; all married[t]	20.6[f]	NSFG 1982
Ball, 1976	Ovulation	124					Aged 20–39	1.6[c]	Australia
Bracher and Santow, 1992	Rhythm	137	17.9				14% aged <20, 75% aged 20–29, 11% aged 30+; 46% parity 0; 92% married or cohabiting	25[r]	Australian Family Survey; first use of method
Kambic et al., 1981, 1982	Ovulation or Cervical Mucus + BBT	235	18.2[n]				81% aged 20–34; 83% married; approx. 30% used barrier methods concurrently[t]	6.5[n]	
Grady et al., 1983	Rhythm	412	18.3[s,c]				Aged 15–44; all married[t]	18.2[r]	NSFG 1973 and 1976

(continued)

Table 31-5 Summary of studies of contraceptive failure: periodic abstinence[a]—(cont'd)

Reference	Method	N for Analysis	Life-Table 12-Month % Pregnant	Pearl Index Pregnancy Rate — Index	Pearl Index Pregnancy Rate — Total Exposure	Pearl Index Pregnancy Rate — Maximum Exposure	Characteristics of the Sample	LFU (%)[g]	Comments
Johnston et al., 1978	Ovulation + Other Methods	71	18.8				80% aged 22–32; all married or de facto married; 49% ≥12 years education ("other" not limited to rhythm)	33.9[c,t]	Australia; probability based on 13 cycles
Vaughan et al., 1977	Rhythm	220	19.1[s]				Aged 15–44; all married[t]	19.0[r]	NSFG 1973
W.H.O., 1981	Ovulation	725	19.6				Mean age about 30; proven fertility; agreed to use OM alone; 54% desired no more children; 765 of 869 learned OM to satisfaction of teachers; 725 entered effectiveness study	?	New Zealand, India, Ireland, Philippines, El Salvador; probability based on 13 cycles
Trussell and Vaughan, 1999		250	19.8				Aged 15–44[t]	21[r]	NSFG 1995
Fu et al., 1999		?	20.2					21[r]	NSFG 1995; probability when standardized and corrected for estimated underreporting of abortion = 25.3[s]

(continued)

Table 31-5 Summary of studies of contraceptive failure: periodic abstinence[a]—(cont'd)

				Risk of Pregnancy					
					Pearl Index Pregnancy Rate				
			Life-Table 12-Month						
Reference	Method	N for Analysis	% Pregnant	Index	Total Exposure	Maximum Exposure	Characteristics of the Sample	LFU (%)[g]	Comments
Jones and Forrest, 1992	Rhythm	289	20.9				Aged 15–44[t]	21[r]	NSFG 1988; probability when standardized and corrected for estimated underreporting of abortion = 31.4[s]
Bartzen, 1967	BBT	335		21.3[c]	4,824 Cy.	58 Mo.	Aged 19–45; mean age = 28	11.6[c]	
Schirm et al., 1982	Rhythm	412	23.7[s]				Aged 15–44; all married[t]	18.2[r]	NSFG 1973 and 1976
Marshall, 1976	Ovulation + BBT	84		23.9[c]	1,195 Cy.	32 Mo.	67% aged 20–34	1.2[c]	Britain
Johnston et al., 1978	Ovulation	586	26.4				69% aged 22–32; all married or de facto married; 44% ≥12 years education	33.9[c,t]	Australia; probability based on 13 cycles

(continued)

Table 31-5 Summary of studies of contraceptive failure: periodic abstinence[a]—*(cont'd)*

Reference	Method	N for Analysis	Risk of Pregnancy Life-Table 12-Month % Pregnant	Pearl Index Pregnancy Rate Index	Pearl Index Pregnancy Rate Total Exposure	Pearl Index Pregnancy Rate Maximum Exposure	Characteristics of the Sample	LFU (%)[g]	Comments
Wade et al., 1981	Ovulation	191	37.2[c]				Aged 20–39; 74% married	13.8[c,g]	Random assignment to OM or CM + BBT + Cal

Notes:

[a] Updated from Trussell and Kost (1987), Table 3.

[c] Calculated by James Trussell from data in the article.

[g] Most of these studies incorrectly report the loss to follow-up probability (LFU) as the number of women lost at any time during the study divided by the total number of women entering the study. Thus, these are the probabilities presented in the table. However, the correct measure of LFU would be a gross life-table probability. When available, gross 12-month probabilities are denoted by the letter "g."

[n] Only net probabilities for this study.

[r] Nonresponse rate for entire survey.

[s] Standardized: Vaughan et al., (1977) (1973 NSFG)—intention (the average of probabilities for preventers and delayers); Grady et al., (1983) (1973 and 1976 NSFG)—intention. Our calculation (the average of probabilities for preventers and delayers); Schirm et al., (1982) (1973 and 1976 NSFG)—intention, age, and income; Grady et al., (1986) (1982 NSFG)—intention, age, poverty status, and parity; Jones and Forrest, (1992) (1988 NSFG)—age, marital status, and poverty status; Fu et al., (1999) (1995 NSFG)—age, union status, poverty status.

[t] Total for all methods in the study.

[v] The authors report that LFU for "relevant reasons (withdrawal of cooperation or loss of contact)" was 0.3% per year in the 1982 study. In the 1982 study, women had been followed for 9.5 years on average; if 0.3% are LFU per year, then 2.8% would be LFU in 9.5 years. LFU including death and emigration is about twice as high as LFU for "relevant reasons."

For table references, see reference section.

Table 31-6 Summary of studies of contraceptive failure: cervical cap and other female barrier methods with spermicide[a]

Reference	Method Brand	N for Analysis	Life-Table 12-Month % Pregnant	Risk of Pregnancy Pearl Index Pregnancy Rate — Index	Total Exposure	Maximum Exposure	Characteristics of the Sample	LFU (%)[g]	Comments
Shihata and Trussell, 1991	Fem Cap	106	4.8					0.0[g]	Probability based on 13 cycles
Denniston and Putney, 1981	Prentif Cavity-rim	110	8.0 [b,n]				98% aged 20–35; 70% nulliparous	20.9[c]	
Cagen, 1986	Prentif Cavity-rim	620	8.1[n]				87% aged 20–34; 80% always used spermicide and 14% never did	38.5[c]	LFU = "no response"
Koch, 1982	Prentif Cavity-rim	372	8.4				76% aged 20–29; 65% college graduates	8.0[c]	Women advised also to use condom for the first several cap uses
Mauck et al., 1996	Lea's Shield	79	8.7[b]				Mean age = 29.6; mean education = 14.2 years; 19% nulliparous	6.4[b,g]	
Richwald et al., 1989	Prentif Cavity-rim	3,433	11.3				Mean age 29.0; 91% white non-Hispanic; 80% unmarried; almost 60% college graduates; 64% one or more previous pregnancies; 6.1% failure rate among perfect users, 11.9% among imperfect users	18[g]	Women advised to use extra spermicide or use condoms during first 2 months of use; 15 sites; 14 in Los Angeles, 1 in Santa Fe
Mauck et al., 1999	FemCap	355	13.5[d]				Mean age = 29.1; 23% nulligravid	3.7[c]	Random assignment to FemCap or Ortho All-Flex diaphragm

(continued)

Table 31-6 Summary of studies of contraceptive failure: cervical cap and other female barrier methods with spermicide[a]—(cont'd)

| | | | | Risk of Pregnancy | | | | | |
| | | | Life-Table 12-Month | Pearl Index Pregnancy Rate | | | | | |
Reference	Method Brand	N for Analysis	% Pregnant	Index	Total Exposure	Maximum Exposure	Characteristics of the Sample	LFU (%)[g]	Comments
Powell et al., 1986	Prentif Cavity-rim and Vimule	477	16.6				67% aged 25–34 "about half" unmarried; 97% high school graduates; 17% using the pill when fitted for cap	43.8[c]	Canada; back-up methods encouraged (including the emergency contraceptive pills used by 23 women in cases of cap dislodgement)
Bernstein et al., 1986	Prentif Cavity-rim	687[c]	17.4				95% aged ≤35, 16% married, 96% ≥ high school completion	26.3[c,g]	Random assignment to the diaphragm or cervical cap
Kassell and McElroy, 1981	Prentif Cavity-rim	90		18.1[c]	731 Mo.	12 Mo.	Mean age = 23.6; mean education = 14.7 years	10.0[c]	
Boehm, 1983	Prentif Cavity-rim	47		18.1[c]	397 Mo.	12 Mo.		31.6	All women reported exclusive use of cap
Lehfeldt and Sivin, 1984	Prentif Cavity-rim	130	19.1				37% aged 16–25; 72% college graduates; 91% nulliparous	7.2[c]	All women agreed to exclusive use of cap

(continued)

CONTRACEPTIVE TECHNOLOGY

Table 31-6 Summary of studies of contraceptive failure: cervical cap and other female barrier methods with spermicide[a]—(cont'd)

Reference	Method Brand	N for Analysis	Life-Table 12-Month % Pregnant	Index	Total Exposure	Maximum Exposure	Characteristics of the Sample	LFU (%)[g]	Comments
				Risk of Pregnancy					
				Pearl Index Pregnancy Rate					
Smith and Lee, 1984	Prentif Cavity-rim and Vimule	33	27.0				80% aged 20–29; clients at university student health service	1.5–4.6[c]	Regular users for whom the cap (with spermicide) was the sole method used "during the fertile portion of the cycle"

Notes:

[a] Updated from Trussell and Kost (1987), Table 4.

[b] 6-month probability; 12-month probability not available.

[c] Calculated by James Trussell from data in the article.

[g] Most of these studies incorrectly report the loss to follow-up (LFU) probability as the number of women lost at any time during the study divided by the total number of women entering the study. Thus, these are the probabilities presented in the table. However, the correct measure of LFU would be a gross life-table probability. When available, gross 12-month probabilities are denoted by the letter "g."

[n] Only net probabilities available for this study.

For table references, see reference section.

Table 31-7 Summary of studies of contraceptive failure: sponge[a]

Reference	N for Analysis	Life-Table 12-Month % Pregnant	Characteristics of the Sample	LFU (%)[g]	Comments
Jones and Forrest, 1992	227	14.5	Aged 15–44[t]	21[r]	NSFG 1988
Edelman et al., 1984	722	17.0	89% aged 20–34, 28% married; 77% ≥13 years education; 94% white, 49% never-married; 38% used oral contraceptives prior to entering study	33.2[c,g]	Random assignment to the diaphragm or sponge
McIntyre and Higgins, 1986	723	17.4	89% aged 20–34, 28% married; 77% ≥13 years education; 94% white, 49% never-married; 38% used oral contraceptives prior to entering the study	33.2[c,g]	A reanalysis of data used by Edelman et al. (1984); random assignment to the diaphragm or sponge; much higher probability for parous women
Trussell and Vaughan, 1999	111	18.4	Aged 15–44[t]	21[r]	NSFG 1995
Bounds and Guillebaud, 1984	126	24.5	92% aged 20–34; all married/consensual union; "most" ≥13 years education; 99% white	1.7[g]	Britain; random assignment to the diaphragm or sponge

Notes:

[a] Updated from Trussell and Kost (1987), Table 4.

[c] Calculated by James Trussell from data in the article.

[g] Most of these studies incorrectly report the loss to follow-up (LFU) probability as the number of women lost at any time during the study divided by the total number of women entering the study. Thus, these are the probabilities presented in the table. However, the correct measure of LFU would be a gross life-table probability. When available, gross 12-month probabilities are denoted by the letter "g."

[r] Nonresponse rate for entire survey.

[t] Total for all methods in the study.

For table references, see reference section.

Table 31-8 Summary of studies of contraceptive failure: diaphragm with spermicide[a]

Reference	N for Analysis	Life-Table 12-Month % Pregnant	Pearl Index Pregnancy Rate			Characteristics of the Sample	LFU (%)[g]	Comments
			Index	**Total Exposure**	**Maximum Exposure**			
Stim, 1980	1,238		1.1[c]	911 Yr.	4 Yr.	Median age = 24	19.5	Fit-free diaphragm without spermicides; continuous wearing with brief daily removal for cleaning but not within 6 hours after intercourse; 1,238 women given device, with follow-up of 997
Lane et al., 1976	2,168	2.1[c]				61% aged 21–34; 71% unmarried; 92% white	1.2[c,g]	Probability downward biased due to improper exposure allocated to women LFU
Vessey and Wiggins, 1974	4,052		2.4	5,909 Mo.	>60 Mo.	All white; at recruitment aged 25–39 and married; all had been using the diaphragm for at least 5 months at enrollment; no previous pill use	1.0[v]	Britain; Oxford/FPA study
Vessey et al., 1982	?		5.5	2,582 Yr.	24 Mo.	All white and aged 25–34; all married at recruitment; at enrollment, all women had been using the diaphragm, IUD, or pill successfully for at least 5 months	0.3[t,v]	Britain; Oxford/FPA study
Mauck et al., 1999	403	7.9[d]				Mean age = 28.8; 25% nulligravid	4.2[c]	Ortho All-Flex diaphragm; random assignment to Ortho All-Flex diaphragm or FemCap

(continued)

Table 31-8 Summary of studies of contraceptive failure: diaphragm with spermicide[a]—(cont'd)

Reference	N for Analysis	Life-Table 12-Month % Pregnant	Pearl Index Pregnancy Rate — Index	Pearl Index Pregnancy Rate — Total Exposure	Pearl Index Pregnancy Rate — Maximum Exposure	Characteristics of the Sample	LFU (%)[g]	Comments
Trussell and Vaughan, 1999	166	8.1				Aged 15–44[t]	21[r]	NSFG 1995
Loudon et al., 1991	269		8.7	2,350 Mo.	12 Mo.	Mean age = 28.6; 57% gravidity 0; 68% married or cohabiting; 54% already using the diaphragm at start of trial	>3.7	Britain; random assignment of spermicide: either C-Film or jelly
Fu et al., 1999	?	9.2					21[r]	NSFG 1995; probability when standardized and corrected for estimated underreporting of abortion = 15.9[s]
Dubrow and Kuder, 1958	873		9.3	5,814 Mo.	48 Mo.	Mean age = 25; 39% black; 45% Puerto Rican; 93% ≤12 years education[t]	38.0[c]	
Jones and Forrest, 1992	472	10.4				Aged 15–44[t]	21[r]	NSFG 1988; probability when standardized and corrected for estimated underreporting of abortion = 22.0[s]
Hall, 1973	347	10.6				Approximately 75% aged 20–24; 47% black; 38% Hispanic; all postpartum	16.0	
Bounds and Guillebaud, 1984	123	10.9				90% aged 20–34; all married/consensual union; "most" ≥13 years education; 96% white	0.0	Britain; random assignment to the diaphragm or sponge

(continued)

Table 31-8 Summary of studies of contraceptive failure: diaphragm with spermicide[a]—(cont'd)

| Reference | N for Analysis | Life-Table 12-Month % Pregnant | Risk of Pregnancy — Pearl Index Pregnancy Rate | | | Characteristics of the Sample | LFU (%)[g] | Comments |
			Index	Total Exposure	Maximum Exposure			
Edelman et al., 1984	717	12.5				88% aged 20–34; 55% never married; 76% ≥13 years education; 94% white; 39% used oral contraceptives prior to entering study	37.8[c,g]	Random assignment to the diaphragm or sponge
McIntyre and Higgins, 1986	717	12.9				88% aged 20–34; 55% never married; 76% ≥13 years education; 94% white; 39% used oral contraceptives prior to entering study	37.8[c,g]	A reanalysis of data used by Edelman et al. (1984); random assignment to the diaphragm or sponge
Vaughan et al., 1977	166	13.1[s]				Aged 15–44; all married[t]	19.0[r]	NSFG 1973
Dingle and Tietze, 1963	189		14.3	2,012 Mo.	36 Mo.	Median age = 22.8	3.2[t]	
Grady et al., 1983	349	14.3[c,s]				Aged 15–44; all married[t]	18.2[r]	NSFG 1973 and 1976
Bernstein et al., 1986	707[c]	16.7				96% aged ≤35; 17% married; 97% ≥ high school completion	33.5[c,g]	Random assignment to the diaphragm or cervical cap
Grady et al., 1986	257	17.0[s]				Aged 15–44; all married[t]	20.6[r]	NSFG 1982
Tietze and Lewit, 1967	1,197	17.9				86% aged <30; all married; 60% ≥ high school completion; 50% white	7.2[g]	

(continued)

Table 31-8 Summary of studies of contraceptive failure: diaphragm with spermicide[a]—(cont'd)

| | | | Risk of Pregnancy | | | | | |
| | | Life-Table 12-Month % Pregnant | Pearl Index Pregnancy Rate | | | Characteristics of the Sample | LFU (%)[g] | Comments |
Reference	N for Analysis		Index	Total Exposure	Maximum Exposure			
Schirm et al., 1982	349	18.6[s]				Aged 15–44; all married[t]	18.2[r]	NSFG 1973 and 1976
Kovacs et al., 1986	324	20.9[t]				28% aged 24–26	52.2	Australia
Bracher and Santow, 1992	219	21.0				12% aged <20; 77% aged 20–29, 11% aged 30+; 56% parity 0; 87% married or cohabiting	25[r]	Australian Family Survey; first use of method
Bounds et al., 1995	80	21.2				Mean age = 29.6; 60% nulliparous	1.3	Britain; probability during consistent use = 12.3; random assignment to diaphragm with spermicide or diaphragm only
Smith et al., 1995	110	24.1				Mean age = 28.8	26.0	Britain; fit-free diaphragm without spermicide; continuous wearing with brief daily removal for cleaning but not within 6 hours after intercourse

(continued)

Table 31-8 Summary of studies of contraceptive failure: diaphragm with spermicide[a]—(cont'd)

Reference	N for Analysis	Risk of Pregnancy — Life-Table 12-Month % Pregnant	Pearl Index Pregnancy Rate — Index	Pearl Index Pregnancy Rate — Total Exposure	Pearl Index Pregnancy Rate — Maximum Exposure	Characteristics of the Sample	LFU (%)g	Comments
Bounds et al., 1995	84	28.6				Mean age = 29.5; 55% nulliparous	0.08	Britain; diaphragm without spermicide; probability during consistent use = 19.3; random assignment to diaphragm only or diaphragm with spermicide

Notes:

[a] Updated from Trussell and Kost (1987), Table 5.

[c] Calculated by James Trussell from data in the article.

[d] 6-month probability; 12-month probability not available.

[g] Most of these studies incorrectly report the loss to follow-up (LFU) probability as the number of women lost at any time during the study divided by the total number of women entering the study. Thus, these are the probabilities presented in the table. However, the correct measure of LFU would be a gross life-table probability. When available, gross 12-month probabilities are denoted by the letter "g."

[r] Nonresponse rate for entire survey.

[s] Standardized: Vaughan et al., (1977) (1973 NSFG)—intention (the average of probabilities for preventers and delayers); Grady et al., (1983) (1973 and 1976 NSFG)—intention. Our calculation (the average of probabilities for preventers and delayers); Schirm et al., (1982) (1973 and 1976 NSFG)—intention, age, and income; Grady et al., (1986) (1982 NSFG)—intention, age, poverty status, and parity; Jones and Forrest, (1992) (1988 NSFG)—age, marital status, and poverty status; Fu et al., (1999) (1995 NSFG)—age, union status, poverty status.

[t] Total for all methods in the study.

[v] The authors report that LFU for "relevant reasons (withdrawal of cooperation or loss of contact)" was 0.3% per year in the 1982 study and "about 10 per 1,000" per year in the 1974 study. In the 1982 study, women had been followed for 9.5 years on average; if 0.3% are LFU per year, then 2.8% would be LFU in 9.5 years. LFU including death and emigration is about twice as high as LFU for "relevant reasons."

For table references, see reference section.

Table 31-9 Summary of studies of contraceptive failure: male condom[a]

| Reference | N for Analysis | Life-Table 12-Month % Pregnant | Risk of Pregnancy — Pearl Index Pregnancy Rate | | | Characteristics of the Sample[w] | LFU (%)[g] | Comments |
			Index	Total Exposure	Maximum Exposure			
Potts and McDevitt, 1975	397	2.1[b]				77% males ≥ age 40; all married	4.8[c]	Britain; postal trial of spermicidally lubricated condom
Steiner et al., 2003	436	3.3[d]				72% living with partner	5.8	Kimono Select latex condom; random assignment to Kimono Select latex or eZ-on plastic condom
Frezieres et al., 1999	383	4.1[d]				Mean age of male and female subjects = 27	3.9[c]	Avanti plastic condom; random assignment to Avanti plastic or Ramses latex condom
Peel, 1972	96		3.9	3,689 Mo.	60 Mo.	All married	2.9[t]	Britain; Hull Family Survey
Glass et al., 1974	2,057	4.2				All white; at recruitment aged 25–39 and married; at enrollment, all women had been using the diaphragm, IUD, or pill successfully for at least 5 months	<1.0[v]	Britain; Oxford/FPA study
Vessey et al., 1988	?		4.4	10,000[c] Yr.	24 Mo.	All white; at recruitment aged 25–39 and married; at enrollment, all women had been using the diaphragm, IUD, or pill successfully for at least 5 months	?	Britain; Oxford/FPA study
John, 1973	85		5.7[c]	261 Yr.	>7 Yr.	?	?	Britain; retrospective study
Vessey et al., 1982	?		6.0	4,317 Yr.	24 Mo.	All white and aged 25–34; all married at recruitment all women were using the diaphragm, IUD, or pill successfully for at least 5 months	0.3[t,v]	Britain; Oxford/FPA study

(continued)

Table 31-9 Summary of studies of contraceptive failure: male condom[a]—(cont'd)

		Risk of Pregnancy						
			Pearl Index Pregnancy Rate					
Reference	N for Analysis	Life-Table 12-Month % Pregnant	Index	Total Exposure	Maximum Exposure	Characteristics of the Sample[w]	LFU (%)[g]	Comments
Frezieres et al., 1999	384	6.2[d]				Mean age of male and female subjects = 27	2.9[c]	Ramses latex condom; random assignment to Ramses latex or Avanti plastic condom
Jones and Forrest, 1992	1,728	7.2				Aged 15–44[t]	21[r]	NSFG 1988; probability when standardized and corrected for estimated underreporting of abortion = 15.8[s]
Walsh et al., 2003	415	7.9[d]				74% > high school education[t]	0.7	Trojan-Enz or LifeStyles latex condom; random assignment to Trojan-Enz latex or LifeStyles latex condom or Tactylon plastic condom
Bracher and Santow, 1992	262	8.1				16% aged <20, 65% aged 20–29, 19% aged 30+; 48% parity 0; 83% married or cohabiting	25[r]	Australian Family Survey; first use of method
Trussell and Vaughan, 1999	2,925	8.7				Aged 15–44[t]	21[r]	NSFG 1995
Steiner et al., 2003	442	9.2[d]				73% living with partner	5.1	eZ-on plastic condom; random assignment to eZ-on plastic or Kimono Select latex condom
Schirm et al., 1982	1,223	9.6[s]				Aged 15–44; all married[t]	18.2[r]	NSFG 1973 and 1976
Grady et al., 1983	1,223	9.7[s,c]				Aged 15–44; all married[t]	18.2[r]	NSFG 1973 and 1976
Fu et al., 1999	?	9.7					21[r]	NSFG 1995; probability when standardized and corrected for estimated underreporting of abortion = 14.7[s]

(continued)

Table 31-9 Summary of studies of contraceptive failure: male condom[a]—(cont'd)

Reference	N for Analysis	Life-Table 12-Month % Pregnant	Pearl Index Pregnancy Rate — Index	Pearl Index Pregnancy Rate — Total Exposure	Pearl Index Pregnancy Rate — Maximum Exposure	Characteristics of the Sample[w]	LFU (%)[g]	Comments
Vaughan et al., 1977	696	10.1[s]				Aged 15–44; all married[t]	19.0[r]	NSFG 1973
Walsh et al., 2003	415	10.8[d]				74% > high school education[t]	0.7	Tactylon plastic condom; random assignment to Tactylon plastic or Trojan-Enz latex or LifeStyles latex condom
Grady et al., 1986	526	13.8[s]				Aged 15–44; all married[t]	20.6[r]	NSFG 1982
Westoff et al., 1961	~212		13.8[c]	10,062 Mo.	?	All married	5.7[r]	FGMA study

Notes:

[a] Updated from Trussell and Kost (1987), Table 6.

[b] 24-month probability; 12-month probability not published.

[c] Calculated by James Trussell from data in the article.

[d] 6-month probability; 12-month probability not available.

[g] Most of these studies incorrectly report the loss to follow-up probability (LFU) as the number of women lost at any time during the study divided by the total number of women entering the study. Thus, these are the probabilities presented in the table. However, the correct measure of LFU would be a gross life-table probability. When available, gross 12-month probabilities are denoted by the letter "g."

[r] Nonresponse rate for entire survey.

[s] Standardized: Vaughan et al., (1977) (1973 NSFG)—intention (the average of probabilities for preventers and delayers); Grady et al., (1983) (1973 and 1976 NSFG)—intention. Our calculation (the average of probabilities for preventers and delayers); Schirm et al., (1982) (1973 and 1976 NSFG)—intention, age, and income; Grady et al., (1986) (1982 NSFG)—intention, age, poverty status, and parity; Jones and Forrest, (1992) (1988 NSFG)—age, marital status, and poverty status; Fu et al., (1999) (1995 NSFG)—age, union status, poverty status.

[t] Total for all methods in the study.

[v] The authors report that LFU for "relevant reasons (withdrawal of cooperation or loss of contact)" was 0.3% per year in 1982 study. In the 1982 study, women had been followed for 9.5 years on average; if 0.3% are LFU per year, then 2.8% would be LFU in 9.5 years. LFU including death and emigration is about twice as high as LFU for "relevant reasons."

[w] Unless otherwise noted, characteristics refer to females.

For table references, see reference section.

Table 31-10 Summary of studies of contraceptive failure: minipill[a]

Reference	Method Brand	N for Analysis	Risk of Pregnancy				Characteristics of the Sample	LFU (%)[g]	Comments
			Life-Table 12-Month % Pregnant	Pearl Index Pregnancy Rate					
				Index	Total Exposure	Maximum Exposure			
Postlethwaite, 1979	Femulen (Ethynodiol diacetate 0.5 mg)	309	1.1[c]				Aged 17–48	21.0[c]	Britain
Shroff et al., 1987	Femulen (Ethynodiol diacetate 0.5 mg)	425	1.1[n]				72% aged 16–34; 25% nulligravid	12.7[c]	Britain; authors employed by manufacturer
Board, 1971	Micronor (Norethindrone 0.35 mg)	154		1.3	1,882 Mo.	19 Mo.		?	
Keifer, 1973	Micronor (Norethindrone 0.35 mg)	151		1.68	2,141 Mo.	26 Mo.	Aged 18–45; 84% aged 21–35; 74% previous oral contraceptive users; at least 32% current users at start	4.6[c]	
Vessey et al., 1985		?		1.98[c]	404 Yr.	12 Mo.	All white and aged 25–34; all married at recruitment; at enrollment, all women had been using the diaphragm, IUD, or pill successfully for at least 5 months	0.3[t,v]	Britain; Oxford/FPA study
Korba and Paulson, 1974	Ovrette (Norgestrel 0.075 mg)	2,202		2.19[c]	29,006 Mo.	67 Mo.		?	Authors employed by manufacturer

(continued)

Table 31-10 Summary of studies of contraceptive failure: minipill[a]—(cont'd)

Reference	Method Brand	N for Analysis	Life-Table 12-Month % Pregnant	Risk of Pregnancy — Pearl Index Pregnancy Rate			Characteristics of the Sample	LFU (%)[g]	Comments
				Index	Total Exposure	Maximum Exposure			
McQuarrie et al., 1972	Micronor (Norethindrone 0.35 mg)	318		2.64[c]	3,453 Cy.	27 Mo.	Aged 16–42; mean age = 26; all white	2.2[c]	
Nelson, 1973	Megestrol acetate (0.5 mg)	342		2.7	3,552 Mo.	41 Mo.		14.6[c]	
Jubhari et al., 1974	Quingestanol acetate (0.3 mg)	382	2.9[n]				Mean age = 23; "predominantly white, single and nulliparous"	14.0	
Hawkins and Benster, 1977	Norethisterone (0.35 mg)	200	6.8				Mean age = 25; postpartum women, 71% within 3 months of delivery[t]	5.2[c]	Britain
Hawkins and Benster, 1977	Megestrol acetate (0.5 mg)	174	8.7				Mean age = 25; postpartum women, 71% within 3 months of delivery[t]	8.4[c]	Britain
Sheth et al., 1982	Levonorgestrel (0.30 mg)	128	9.5[n]				Mean age = 25.7	2.1[t]	Yugoslavia, India
Hawkins and Benster, 1977	Chlormadinone acetate (0.5 mg)	182	9.6				Mean age = 26; postpartum women, 71% within 3 months of delivery[t]	3.3[c]	Britain

(continued)

Table 31-10 Summary of studies of contraceptive failure: minipill[a]—(cont'd)

Reference	Method Brand	N for Analysis	Risk of Pregnancy				Characteristics of the Sample	LFU (%)[g]	Comments
			Life-Table 12-Month % Pregnant	Pearl Index Pregnancy Rate					
				Index	Total Exposure	Maximum Exposure			
Sheth et al., 1982	Norethisterone (0.35 mg)	130	13.2[n]				Mean age = 25.6	2.1[t]	Yugoslavia, India

Notes:

[a] Updated from Trussell and Kost (1987), Table 8.

[c] Calculated by James Trussell from data in the article.

[g] Most of these studies incorrectly report the loss to follow-up (LFU) probability as the number of women lost at any time during the study divided by the total number of women entering the study. Thus, these are the probabilities presented in the table. However, the correct measure of LFU would be a gross life-table probability. When available, gross 12-month probabilities are denoted by the letter "g."

[n] Only net probabilities available for this study.

[t] Total for all methods in the study.

[v] The authors report that LFU for "relevant reasons (withdrawal of cooperation or loss of contact)" was 0.3% per year in the 1982 study. In the 1985 study, women had probably been followed for 12.5 years on average; if 0.3% are LFU per year, then 3.7% would be LFU in 12.5 years. LFU including death and emigration is about twice as high as LFU for "relevant reasons."

For table references, see reference section.

Table 31-11 Summary of studies of contraceptive failure: combined oral contraceptives, vaginal rings, and patches[a]

Reference	Method Brand	N for Analysis	Life-Table 12-Month % Pregnant	Risk of Pregnancy Pearl Index Pregnancy Rate			Characteristics of the Sample	LFU (%)g	Comments
				Index	Total Exposure	Maximum Exposure			
Preston, 1972	Norlestrin 2.5 (80%)	378	0.0c				Aged 15–46; 46% aged 25–34; 36% white; 64% on pill at start	9.5	Author employed by manufacturer; pill not marketed
Ledger, 1970	Ortho-Novum 1/80	144	0.0c				All aged 14–43; mean age = 24; mostly graduate students or wives of students	14.0c	
Woutersz, 1981	Lo/Ovral	1,700		0.12	22,489 Cy.	53 Cy.	65% aged 20–29; 55% on pill at start	23.8	Author employed by manufacturer
Korba and Heil, 1975	Ovral	6,806		0.19	127,872 Cy.	110 Cy.	Mean age = 25; 26% white; approximately 80% had not used other oral contraceptives within 3 months	?	Mexico, Puerto Rico, United States; author employed by manufacturer
Lammers and op ten Berg, 1991	Mercilon	1,684		0.20	25,970 Cy.	36 Cy.	23% aged <20, 51% aged 20–29, 14% aged 30–34; 12% aged 35+	?	Authors employed by manufacturer; Belgium, Denmark, Finland, France, Hungary, Netherlands, Norway, Poland, Sweden, Switzerland, West Germany, Yugoslavia
Ellis, 1987	Ortho-Novum 7/7/7	619		0.22	909c Yr.	?	Mean age = 24.5; 40.5% nulligravid	?	United States, Canada, France

(continued)

Table 31-11 Summary of studies of contraceptive failure: combined oral contraceptives, vaginal rings, and patches[a]—(cont'd)

Reference	Method Brand	N for Analysis	Life-Table 12-Month % Pregnant	Pearl Index Pregnancy Rate			Characteristics of the Sample	LFU (%)[g]	Comments
				Index	Total Exposure	Maximum Exposure			
Morigi and Pasquale, 1978	Modicon	1,168		0.24[c]	16,345 Cy.	53 Cy.	Aged 13–54; 85% aged 19–36; 61% previous use of oral contraceptives	?	Mexico, Puerto Rico, Canada, United States; author employed by manufacturer
Hughes, 1978	Ovamin	453	0.24[c]				Aged 16–40; % new users not stated	11.9[c]	Britain
Vessey et al., 1982	50 µg estrogen	?		0.25	10,400 Yr.	24 Mo.	All white and aged 25–34; all married at recruitment; at enrollment, all women had been using the diaphragm, IUD, or pill successfully for at least 5 months	0.3[t,v]	Britain; Oxford/FPA study
Runnebaum et al., 1992	Ortho-Cyclen	59,701		0.27[c]	342,348 Cy.	6 Cy.	Mean age = 24.0; 32% parous	?	Germany
Kaunitz et al., 1999	Ortho-Novum 7/7/7	321	0.30				Mean age = 27.8; 65% used hormonal contraception in prior month	6.9[c]	Trial design discontinued subjects who did not adhere to dosing schedule
Bannemerschult et al., 1997	Alesse	805		0.30	4,400 Cy.	6 Cy.	Mean age = 25.6	0.6[c]	Germany; some women who did not return for follow-up visits were excluded

(continued)

Table 31-11 Summary of studies of contraceptive failure: combined oral contraceptives, vaginal rings, and patches[a]—(cont'd)

Reference	Method Brand	N for Analysis	Risk of Pregnancy — Life-Table 12-Month % Pregnant	Risk of Pregnancy — Pearl Index Pregnancy Rate — Index	Total Exposure	Maximum Exposure	Characteristics of the Sample	LFU (%)[g]	Comments
Royal College, 1974		23,611		0.34	?	48 Mo.	75% aged 20–34; all married/living as married; 62% on pill at start (20% new users)	32.0[c]	Britain
Woutersz, 1983	Nordette	1,130		0.35	11,064 Cy.	31 Cy.	71% aged 20–30; 48% no use of hormones and not pregnant within 60 days of start	8.1[c]	Author employed by manufacturer
Vessey et al., 1982	<50 µg estrogen	?		0.38	3,158 Yr.	24 Mo.	All white and aged 25–34; all married at recruitment; at enrollment, all women had been using the diaphragm, IUD, or pill successfully for at least 5 months	0.3[t,v]	Britain; Oxford/FPA study
Kaunitz, 2000	Ortho-Novum 7/7/7	2,675	0.39[d]				Mean age = 28.5[t]	6.0[c]	Random assignment to Ortho-Novum 7/7/7 or Cyclessa; 2.5% of subjects discontinued for noncompliance
Parsey and Pong, 2000	Yasmin	326		0.41	3,201 Cy.	13 Cy.	Mean age = 26.4	?	
Kaunitz, 2000	Cyclessa	2,643	0.51[d]				Mean age = 28.5[t]	5.8[c]	Random assignment to Cyclessa or Ortho-Novum 7/7/7; 2.4% of subjects discontinued for non-compliance
Gauthier et al., 1992	Ortho Tri-Cyclen	661	0.57[b]				Mean age = 27.9; 24% nulligravid	?	France; 2 authors employed by manufacturer

(continued)

Table 31-11 Summary of studies of contraceptive failure: combined oral contraceptives, vaginal rings, and patches[a]—(cont'd)

			Risk of Pregnancy					
			Life-Table 12-Month % Pregnant	Pearl Index Pregnancy Rate				
Reference	Method Brand	N for Analysis		Index	Total Exposure	Maximum Exposure	Characteristics of the Sample	LFU (%)[g]	Comments
Åkerlund et al., 1993	Mercilon	485		0.57[c]	4,543 Cy.	12 Mo.	Mean age = 23.8	?	Denmark, Norway, Sweden; random assignment to Mercilon or Marvelon; cycles excluded if the pill-taking period was less than 18 or more than 33 days or if the pill-free period was less than 5 or more than 9 days
Preston, 1974 and 1972	Norlestrin 2.5 (60%)	1,192		0.63[c]	14,536 Cy.	>18 Cy.	Aged 14–47; 35% aged 25–34; 47% white; 56% on pill at start	13.7	Author employed by manufacturer; pill not marketed
Roumen et al., 2001	NuvaRing	1,145		0.64[c]	12,109 Cy.	13 Cy.	Mean age = 28.2	?	Austria, Belgium, Denmark, Finland, France, Germany, Israel, Netherlands, Norway, Spain, Sweden, United Kingdom

(continued)

Table 31-11 Summary of studies of contraceptive failure: combined oral contraceptives, vaginal rings, and patches[a]—(cont'd)

Reference	Method Brand	N for Analysis	Risk of Pregnancy				Characteristics of the Sample	LFU (%)[g]	Comments
			Life-Table 12-Month % Pregnant	Pearl Index Pregnancy Rate					
				Index	Total Exposure	Maximum Exposure			
Archer et al., 1999	Alesse	1,708	0.69[b]				Mean age = 27.2	12.1	Cycles in which 3 or more consecutive active pills were missed and all subsequent cycles from that subject were excluded from the analysis
London et al., 1992	Triphasil (Tri-Levlen)	2,124		0.80	11,306 Cy.	6 Cy.	Mean age = 25.5	?	Random assignment to Triphasil or Ortho Tri-Cyclen
Åkerlund et al., 1993	Marvelon (Ortho-Cept, Desogen)	497		0.83[c]	4,688 Cy.	12 Mo.	Mean age = 23.1	?	Denmark, Norway, Sweden; random assignment to Marvelon or Mercilon; cycles excluded if the pill-taking period was less than 18 or more than 33 days or if the pill-free period was less than 5 or more than 9 days
Anderson et al., 2003	Seasonale	456	0.9					8.6	Random assignment to Seasonale or Nordette; noncompliant patients excluded
Corson, 1990	Lo/Ovral	737		0.94[c]	9,727 Cy.	24 Cy.	Mean age = 24.3	?	Random assignment to Lo/Ovral or Ortho-Cyclen

(continued)

Table 31-11 Summary of studies of contraceptive failure: combined oral contraceptives, vaginal rings, and patches[a]—*(cont'd)*

		Life-Table 12-Month % Pregnant	Risk of Pregnancy Pearl Index Pregnancy Rate					
Reference	Method Brand	N for Analysis		Index	Total Exposure	Maximum Exposure	Characteristics of the Sample	LFU (%)[g]	Comments
London et al., 1992	Ortho Tri-Cyclen	2,110		0.94	11,006 Cy.	6 Cy.	Mean age = 25.6	?	Random assignment to Ortho Tri-Cyclen or Triphasil
Preston, 1974 and 1972	Norlestrin 2.5 (40%)	1,393		0.94[c]	15,265 Cy.	>18 Cy.	Aged 13–42; 27% aged 25–34; 39% white; 49% on pill at start	16.3	Author employed by manufacturer; pill not marketed
The Mircette Study Group, 1998	Mircette	1,226		1.02	14,050 Cy.	13 Cy.	Mean age = 28.3	6.8[c]	
Endrikat et al., 1995	Mercilon	219		1.04[c]	2,496 Cy.	12 Cy.	Mean age = 25.0	?	Austria, France; random assignment to Mercilon or Meliane; cycles excluded if more than two pills were missed or pill-taking was irregular
Ellsworth, 1986	Triphasil	1,264		1.09	8,349 Cy.	34 Cy.	All < age 38	?	17 U.S. centers
Corson, 1990	Ortho-Cyclen	736		1.11[c]	9,351 Cy.	24 Cy.	Mean age = 24.6	?	Random assignment to Ortho-Cyclen or Lo/Ovral
Dieben et al., 2002	NuvaRing	2,322		1.18	23,298 Cy.	13 Cy.	Mean age = 28.2	?	United States, Canada, Europe; Pearl index for United States = 1.75; European results published separately by Roumen et al. (2001)

(continued)

Table 31-11 Summary of studies of contraceptive failure: combined oral contraceptives, vaginal rings, and patches[a]—*(cont'd)*

			Risk of Pregnancy						
			Life-Table	Pearl Index Pregnancy Rate					
Reference	Method Brand	N for Analysis	12-Month % Pregnant	Index	Total Exposure	Maximum Exposure	Characteristics of the Sample	LFU (%)[g]	Comments
Anderson et al., 2003	Nordette	226	1.3					9.3	Random assignment to Nordette or Seasonale; noncompliant patients excluded
Audet et al., 2001	Evra patch	811	1.3				Mean age = 28.0	3.9[c]	Random assignment to Evra patch or Triphasil
Preston, 1974 and 1972	Norlestrin 1.0 (60%)	1,872		1.47[c]	20,341 Cy.	>18 Cy.	Aged 14–44; 30% aged 25–34; 42% white; 55% on pill at start	13.1	Author employed by manufacturer; pill not marketed
Preston, 1974	Norlestrin 1.0 (20%)	276		1.59[c]	2,449 Cy.	?		?	Author employed by manufacturer; pill not marketed
Audet et al., 2001	Triphasil	605	1.8				Mean age = 27.8	7.9[c]	Random assignment to Triphasil or Evra patch
Vaughan et al., 1977		2,434	2.0[s]				Aged 15–44; all married[t]	19.0[r]	NSFG 1973
Bracher and Santow, 1992		1,830	2.2				42% aged <20, 49% aged 20–29, 9% aged 30+; 67% parity 0; 45% married or cohabiting	25[r]	Australian Family Survey, first use of method
Schirm et al., 1982		4,487	2.4[s]				Aged 15–44; all married[t]	18.2[r]	NSFG 1973 and 1976
Grady et al., 1983		4,487	2.5[c,s]				Aged 15–44; all married[t]	18.2[r]	NSFG 1973 and 1976

(continued)

Table 31-11 Summary of studies of contraceptive failure: combined oral contraceptives, vaginal rings, and patches[a]—(cont'd)

Reference	Method Brand	N for Analysis	Risk of Pregnancy				Characteristics of the Sample	LFU (%)[g]	Comments
			Life-Table 12-Month % Pregnant	Pearl Index Pregnancy Rate					
				Index	Total Exposure	Maximum Exposure			
Bounds et al., 1979	Microgynon-30	55	2.6[c]				Aged 16–39; mean age = 26; 62% used oral contraceptives as last contraceptive before study	5.5[c]	Britain; probability based on only 12 cycles
Grady et al., 1986		856	2.9[s]				Aged 15–44; all married[t]	20.6[r]	NSFG 1982
Jones and Forrest, 1992		3,041	5.1				Aged 15–44; all married[t]	21[r]	NSFG 1988; probability when standardized and corrected for estimated under-reporting of abortion = 7.3[s]
Preston, 1974	Norlestrin 1.0 (40%)	313		5.80[c]	1,570 Cy.	?		?	Author employed by manufacturer; pill not marketed
Bounds et al., 1979	Loestrin-20	55	5.9[c]				Aged 16–39; mean age = 26; 65% used oral contraceptives as last contraceptive before study	5.5[c]	Britain; probability based on only 12 cycles
Trussell and Vaughan, 1999		2,130	6.9				Aged 15–44[t]	21[r]	NSFG 1995
Fu et al., 1999		?	7.3					21[r]	NSFG 1995; probability when standardized and corrected for estimated underreporting of abortion = 8.1[s]

(continued)

Table 31-11 Summary of studies of contraceptive failure: combined oral contraceptives, vaginal rings, and patches[a] — *(cont'd)*

			Risk of Pregnancy					
			Life-Table 12-Month	Pearl Index Pregnancy Rate				
Reference	Method Brand	N for Analysis	% Pregnant	Index	Total Exposure	Maximum Exposure	Characteristics of the Sample	LFU (%)[g]	Comments
Preston, 1974	Norlestrin 2.5 (20%)	178		10.45[c]	871 Cy.	?		?	Author employed by manufacturer; pill not marketed

Notes:

[a] Updated from Trussell and Kost (1987), Table 8.

[b] 12-cycle probability; 12-month probability not available.

[c] Calculated by James Trussell from data in the article.

[d] 6-cycle probability.

[g] Most of these studies incorrectly report the loss to follow-up (LFU) probability as the number of women lost at any time during the study divided by the total number of women entering the study. Thus, these are the probabilities presented in the table. However, the correct measure of LFU would be a gross life-table probability. When available, gross 12-month probabilities are denoted by the letter "g."

[r] Nonresponse rate for entire survey.

[s] Standardized: Vaughan et al., (1977) (1973 NSFG)—intention (the average of probabilities for preventers and delayers); Grady et al., (1983) (1973 and 1976 NSFG)—intention. Our calculation (the average of probabilities for preventers and delayers); Schirm et al., (1982) (1973 and 1976 NSFG)—intention, age, and income; Grady et al., (1986) (1982 NSFG)—intention, age, poverty status, and parity; Jones and Forrest, (1992) (1988 NSFG)—age, marital status, and poverty status; Fu et al., (1999) (1995 NSFG)—age, union status, poverty status.

[t] Total for all methods in the study.

[v] The authors report that LFU for "relevant reasons (withdrawal of cooperation or loss of contact)" was 0.3% per year in the 1982 study. In the 1982 study, women had probably been followed for 9.5 years on average; if 0.3% are LFU per year, then 2.8% would be LFU in 9.5 years. LFU including death and emigration is about twice as high as LFU for "relevant reasons."

For table references, see reference section.

Table 31-12 Summary of studies of contraceptive failure: injectables[a]

Reference	Method Brand	N for Analysis	Life-Table 12-Month % Pregnant	Characteristics of the Sample	LFU (%)[g]	Comments
W.H.O., 1988	Depo-Provera 25 mg + Estradiol Cypionate 5 mg (30-Day)	1,168	0.0	Aged 18–35; mean age = 26; proven fertility	11.4[g]	Egypt, Thailand, Mexico, Guatemala, Cuba, Indonesia, Pakistan, U.S.S.R., Philippines, Italy, Hungary, Chile
W.H.O., 1986	Depo-Provera 150 mg (90-Day)	607	0.0	Mean age = 27.7[t]	8.6[g]	7 developing countries
Mishell et al., 1968	Depo-Provera 150 mg (90-Day)	100	0.0[c]	59% aged 21–30	24.0[c]	Injection immediately postpartum
Howard et al., 1982	Norigest 200 mg (56-Day)	383	0.0[c]		6.5[n]	Britain
Kaunitz et al., 1999	Lunelle	782	0.0	Mean age = 27.3; 44% used hormonal contraception in prior month	8.6[c]	Trial design discontinued subjects who did not adhere to dosing schedule
Hall et al., 1997	Cyclofem (Lunelle)	3,183	0.0		12.9[c]	Brazil, Chile, Colombia, Peru. Perfect use analysis since trial design discontinued women who were late for injections
W.H.O., 1983	Depo-Provera 150 mg (90-Day)	1,587	0.1	Mean age = 27.4[t]	8.1	87% of women from 9 developing countries
W.H.O., 1988	Norigest 50 mg + Estradiol Valerate 5 mg (30-Day)	1,152	0.18	Aged 18–35; mean age = 26.7; proven fertility	10.5[g]	Egypt, Thailand, Mexico, Guatemala, Cuba, Indonesia, Pakistan, U.S.S.R., Philippines, Italy, Hungary, Chile

(continued)

Table 31-12 Summary of studies of contraceptive failure: injectables[a]—*(cont'd)*

Reference	Method Brand	N for Analysis	Life-Table 12-Month % Pregnant	Characteristics of the Sample	LFU (%)[g]	Comments
Sangi-Haghpeykar et al., 1996	Depo-Provera 150 mg (3-Month)	536	0.2	25% nulligravid; mean age = 24.4; primarily low income	5.4[c]	
Scutchfield et al., 1971	Depo-Provera 150 mg (90-Day)	650	0.2[c]	66% aged 20–34; 50% married	6.8[n]	
Schwallie and Assenzo, 1973	Depo-Provera 150 mg (90-Day)	3,857	0.3	86% aged 20–39	18.6	Primarily United States; also Chile, Jamaica, Mexico; authors employed by manufacturer
W.H.O., 1983	Norigest 200 mg (60-Day)	789	0.4	Mean age = 27.4[t]	7.1	87% of women from 9 developing countries
W.H.O., 1986	Depo-Provera 100 mg (90-Day)	609	0.4	Mean age = 27.7[t]	8.2[g]	7 developing countries
W.H.O., 1983	Norigest 200 mg (84-Day)	796	0.6	Mean age = 27.4[t]	7.4	87% of women from 9 developing countries
W.H.O., 1977	Depo-Provera 150 mg (84-Day)	846	0.7	87% aged 20–34	6.2	10 developing countries
Schwallie and Assenzo, 1972	Depo-Provera 300 mg (180-Day)	991	2.3[n]	88% aged 20–39	28.9	United States, Chile; authors employed by manufacturer
Fu et al., 1999	Depo-Provera 150 mg	?	2.8		21[r]	NSFG 1995; probability when standardized and corrected for estimated underreporting of abortion = 2.6[s]

(continued)

Table 31-12 Summary of studies of contraceptive failure: injectables[a] —(cont'd)

Reference	Method Brand	N for Analysis	Life-Table 12-Month % Pregnant	Characteristics of the Sample	LFU (%)[g]	Comments
Trussell and Vaughan, 1999	Depo-Provera 150 mg	209	3.2	Aged 15–44[t]	21[r]	NSFG 1995
W.H.O., 1977	Norigest 200 mg (84-Day)	832	3.6	84% aged 20–34	5.8	10 developing countries

Notes:

[a] Updated from Trussell and Kost (1987), Table 9.

[c] Calculated by James Trussell from data in the article.

[g] Most of these studies incorrectly report the loss to follow-up (LFU) probability as the number of women lost at any time during the study divided by the total number of women entering the study. Thus, these are the probabilities presented in the table. However, the correct measure of LFU would be a gross life-table probability. When available, gross 12-month probabilities are denoted by the letter "g."

[n] Only net probabilities available for this study.

[r] Nonresponse rate for entire survey.

[s] Fu et al., (1995 NSFG)—age, union status, poverty status.

[t] Total for all methods in the study.

For table references, see reference section.

Table 31-13 Summary of studies of contraceptive failure: IUD[a]

Reference	Method Brand	N for Analysis	Life-Table 12-Month % Pregnant	Characteristics of the Sample	LFU (%)[g]	Comments
Luukkainen et al., 1987	LNG20	1,821	0.1	15% aged 17–25, 60% aged 26–35, 25% aged 36–40; 7% parity 0, 27% parity 1, 50% parity 2, 16% parity 3+	5.7[c]	Denmark, Finland, Hungary, Norway, Sweden
Sivin et al., 1990	LNG20	1,124	0.2	Mean age 26.6; mean parity = 2.4	5.7[g,x]	Brazil, Chile, Dominican Republic, Egypt, Singapore, United States
Sivin et al., 1990	TCu380A Slimline	698	0.3	Mean age = 28.5; mean parity = 2.7; 47.4% prior IUD use	6.0	Randomized trial of TCu380A and TCu380A Slimline. Egypt, Chile, Sweden, Dominican Republic, Brazil
Sivin et al., 1990	TCu380A	298	0.4	Mean age = 28.1; mean parity = 2.6; 49.0% prior IUD use	9.7	Randomized trial of TCu380A and TCu380A Slimline. Egypt, Chile, Sweden, Dominican Republic, Brazil
Cox and Blacksell, 2000	LNG20	692	0.6	All parous	0?	United Kingdom
Sivin and Stern, 1979	TCu380A	3,536	0.8	72% aged 20–29; 64% nulliparous	18.3[n]	
Gibor and Mitchell, 1980	Progestasert	6,261	2.0[n]		?	Authors employed by manufacturer; United States (51%), Canada (5%), and at least 11 other countries
Trussell and Vaughan, 1999		59	3.7	Aged 15–44[t]	21[r]	NSFG 1995
Bracher and Santow, 1992		408	3.9	10% aged <20, 68% aged 20–29, 22% aged 30+; 25% parity 0; 87% married or cohabiting	25[r]	Australian Family Survey, first use of method
Vaughan et al., 1977		576	4.2[s]	Aged 15–44; all married[t]	19.0[r]	NSFG 1973

(continued)

Table 31-13 Summary of studies of contraceptive failure: IUD[a]—(cont'd)

Reference	Method Brand	N for Analysis	Life-Table 12-Month % Pregnant	Characteristics of the Sample	LFU (%)[g]	Comments
Schirm et al., 1982		1,070	4.6[s]	Aged 15–44; all married[t]	18.2[r]	NSFG 1973 and 1976
Grady et al., 1983		1,070	4.8[c,s]	Aged 15–44; all married[t]	18.2[r]	NSFG 1973 and 1976
Grady et al., 1986		235	5.9[s]	Aged 15–44; all married[t]	20.6[r]	NSFG 1982

Notes:

[a] Updated from Trussell and Kost (1987), Table 7.

[c] Calculated by James Trussell from data in the article.

[g] Most of these studies incorrectly report the loss to follow-up (LFU) probability as the number of women lost at any time during the study divided by the total number of women entering the study. Thus, these are the probabilities presented in the table. However, the correct measure of LFU would be a gross life-table probability. When available, gross 12-month probabilities are denoted by the letter "g."

[n] Only net probabilities available for this study.

[r] Nonresponse rate for entire survey.

[s] Standardized: Vaughan et al., (1977) (1973 NSFG)—intention (the average of probabilities for preventers and delayers); Grady et al., (1983) (1973 and 1976 NSFG)—intention. Our calculation (the average of probabilities for preventers and delayers); Schirm et al., (1982) (1973 and 1976 NSFG)—intention, age, and income; Grady et al., (1986) (1982 NSFG)—intention, age, poverty status, and parity.

[t] Total for all methods in the study.

[x] Irving Sivin, personal communication to James Trussell, August 13, 1992.

For table references, see reference section.

Table 31-14 Summary of studies of contraceptive failure: Implants[a]

Reference	Method Brand	N for Analysis	Life-Table 12-Month % Pregnant	Characteristics of the Sample	LFU (%)[g]	Comments
Sivin et al., 1997	Norplant-2 (2 Rods)	199	0.0		2.0	Chile, Dominican Republic, Singapore, Thailand, United States; current version with core of rods made of new elastomer; random assignment to new or old version of Norplant-2
Sivin et al., 2000	Norplant (6 capsules)	1,210	0.0	Mean age = 27.4; 13% nulliparous	1.2	Chile, Dominican Republic, Egypt, Finland, Singapore, Thailand, United States; current version with capsules made of new elastomer
Sivin et al., 1998b	Norplant (2 Rods)	600	0.0	Mean age = 28.3; 2% nulliparous	0.3[c]	Chile, Egypt, Finland, Singapore, Thailand, United States; current version with core of rods made of new elastomer
Sivin et al., 1998a	Norplant (2 Rods)	594	0.2	Mean age = 25.5; 17% nulliparous	2.2	Dominican Republic, United States; current version with core of rods made of new elastomer
Fu et al., 1999		?	1.8		21[r]	NSFG 1995; probability when standardized and corrected for estimated under-reporting of abortion = 1.4[s]
Trussell and Vaughan, 1999		146	2.3	Aged 15–44[t]	21[r]	NSFG 1995

Notes:

[a] Updated from Trussell and Kost (1987), Table 9.

[c] Calculated by James Trussell from data provided by Sivin (1992).

[g] Proportion LFU in the first year (number of women LFU in the first year divided by the number entering the study); gross 12-month life-table probabilities denoted by the letter "g."

[r] Nonresponse rate for entire survey.

[s] Fu et al., (1999) (1995 NSFG)—age, union status, poverty status.

[t] Total for all methods in the study.

For table references, see reference section.

Table 31-15 Summary of studies of contraceptive failure: female sterilization[a]

Reference	Procedure	N for Analysis	Life-Table 12-Month % Pregnant	Pearl Index Pregnancy Rate — Index	Pearl Index Pregnancy Rate — Total Exposure	Pearl Index Pregnancy Rate — Maximum Exposure	Characteristics of the Sample	LFU (%)[g]	Comments
Engel, 1978	Laparoscopy	182	0.0[c]				"No failures" presumably some women followed for at least 12 months	?	
Valle and Battifora, 1978	Laparoscopy	165	0.0[c]				"Failure rate after 2 years follow-up is zero" all aged 22–38; 80% had at least 12 months follow-up	?	
Vessey et al., 1983	Procedures other than laparotomy and laparoscopy	345		0.0	331 Yr.	12 Mo.	All white; at recruitment aged 25–39 and married; at enrollment, all women had been using the diaphragm, IUD, or pill successfully for at least 5 months	0.3[v]	Britain; Oxford/FPA study
Chi et al., 1980	Culdoscopy: Pomeroy	392	0.0				Mean age = 32[t]	?	IFRP (19 countries)
Loffer and Pent, 1977	Laparoscopy	1,717		0.0[c]		≥6 Mo.	Duration of follow-up not reported	?	
Chi et al., 1987	Minilaparotomy: Pomeroy	445	0.0[c]				Median age = 32	31.6	IFRP (19 countries)
Peterson et al., 1996	Postpartum partial salpingectomy	1,637	0.06				43% aged 18–27, 38% aged 28–33, 18% aged 34+	8.8	U.S. Collaborative Review of Sterilization

(continued)

Table 31-15 Summary of studies of contraceptive failure: female sterilization[a]—(cont'd)

Reference	Procedure	N for Analysis	Risk of Pregnancy — Life-Table 12-Month % Pregnant	Pearl Index Pregnancy Rate — Index	Pearl Index Pregnancy Rate — Total Exposure	Pearl Index Pregnancy Rate — Maximum Exposure	Characteristics of the Sample	LFU (%)[g]	Comments
Peterson et al., 1996	Unipolar coagulation	1,432	0.07				20% aged 18–27, 39% aged 28–33, 42% aged 34+	5.0	U.S. Collaborative Review of Sterilization
Dominik et al., 2000	Filshie Clip	1,063	0.11					31.3[c]	Dominican Republic, Guatemala, Haiti, Malaysia, Mexico, Panama, Venezuela
Sokal et al., 2000	Filshie Clip	1,378	0.17				Mean age = 31	18.1[c]	Brazil, Dominican Republic, Indonesia, Kenya, Mexico, Panama, Peru, Thailand
Sokal et al., 2000	Tubal Ring	1,355	0.17				Mean age = 31	17.6[c]	Brazil, Dominican Republic, Indonesia, Kenya, Mexico, Panama, Peru, Thailand
Bhiwandiwala et al., 1982	Rocket Clip	630	0.18[u]					42.1[c,t]	IFRP (27 countries)
Peterson et al., 1996	Bipolar coagulation	2,267	0.23				31% aged 18–27, 35% aged 28–33, 35% aged 34+	10.5	U.S. Collaborative Review of Sterilization
Chi et al., 1980	Minilaparotomy	3,988	0.24				Mean age = 32[t]	?	IFRP (19 countries)

(continued)

Table 31-15 Summary of studies of contraceptive failure: female sterilization[a]—*(cont'd)*

Reference	Procedure	N for Analysis	Life-Table 12-Month % Pregnant	Risk of Pregnancy			Characteristics of the Sample	LFU (%)[g]	Comments
				Pearl Index Pregnancy Rate					
				Index	Total Exposure	Maximum Exposure			
Bhiwandiwala et al., 1982	Electro-coagulation	6,542	0.26[u]					42.1[c,t]	IFRP (27 countries)
Vessey et al., 1983	Laparotomy: all procedures	743		0.28	716 Yr.	12 Mo.	All white; at recruitment aged 25–39 and married; at enrollment, all women had been using the diaphragm, IUD, or pill successfully for at least 5 months	0.3[t,v]	Britain; Oxford/FPA study
Mumford et al., 1980	Minilaparoscopy: Pomeroy	2,022	0.3[u]					?	IFRP (23 countries)
Chi et al., 1980	Electro-coagulation	3,594	0.32[c]					?	IFRP (19 countries)
Bhiwandiwala et al., 1982	Tubal Ring	5,046	0.47[u]					42.1[c,t]	IFRP (27 countries)
Mumford et al., 1980	Minilaparoscopy: Ring	1,324	0.51[u]					?	IFRP (23 countries)
Vessey et al., 1983	Laparoscopy: Tubal Diathermy	776		0.53	755 Yr.	12 Mo.	All white; at recruitment aged 25–39 and married; at enrollment, all women had been using the diaphragm, IUD, or pill successfully for at least 5 months	0.3[t,v]	Britain: Oxford/FPA study

(continued)

Table 31-15 Summary of studies of contraceptive failure: female sterilization[a] —(cont'd)

Reference	Procedure	N for Analysis	Life-Table 12-Month % Pregnant	Risk of Pregnancy — Pearl Index Pregnancy Rate Index	Risk of Pregnancy — Pearl Index Pregnancy Rate Total Exposure	Risk of Pregnancy — Pearl Index Pregnancy Rate Maximum Exposure	Characteristics of the Sample	LFU (%)[g]	Comments
Chi et al., 1981	Tubal Ring	4,106	0.54[c]					?	IFRP (19 countries)
Peterson et al., 1996	All methods combined	10,685	0.55				33% aged 18–27, 35% aged 28–33, 32% aged 34+	10.8	U.S. Collaborative Review of Sterilization
Chi et al., 1980	Laparoscopy: Rocket Clip	457	0.59				Mean age = 32[t]	?	IFRP (19 countries)
Peterson et al., 1996	Rubber band	3,329	0.59				30% aged 18–27, 36% aged 28–33, 34% aged 34+	12.1	U.S. Collaborative Review of Sterilization
Mumford et al., 1980	Laparoscopy: Rings	4,262	0.60[u]					?	IFRP (23 countries)
Vessey et al., 1983	Laparoscopy: Rings, Clips, etc.	379		0.60	334 Yr.	12 Mo.	All white; at recruitment aged 25–39 and married; at enrollment, all women had been using the diaphragm, IUD, or pill successfully for at least 5 months	0.3[t,v]	Britain; Oxford/FPA study
Dominik et al., 2000	Hulka Clip	1,062	0.69				Dominican Republic, Guatemala, Haiti, Malaysia, Mexico, Panama, Venezuela	33.1[c]	
Peterson et al., 1996	Interval partial salpingectomy	425	0.73				28% aged 18–27, 32% aged 28–33, 40% aged 34+	7.3	U.S. Collaborative Review of Sterilization
Chi et al., 1987	Minilaparotomy: Rings and Clips	1,146		0.79	1,143 Yr.	12 Mo.	Median age = 32 years	13.5	IFRP (19 countries)
Yoon et al., 1977	Falope Ring	902		1.33[c]	3,617[c] Mo.	12 Mo.		21.0[c]	
Peterson et al., 1996	Spring Clip	1,595	1.82				44% aged 18–27, 30% aged 28–33, 26% aged 34+	16.4	U.S. Collaborative Review of Sterilization

(continued)

Table 31-15 Summary of studies of contraceptive failure: female sterilization[a]—(cont'd)

Reference	Procedure	N for Analysis	Risk of Pregnancy					Characteristics of the Sample	LFU (%)[g]	Comments
			Life-Table 12-Month % Pregnant	Pearl Index Pregnancy Rate						
				Index	Total Exposure	Maximum Exposure				
Hulka et al., 1976	Spring Clip	1,079	2.3[c]						9.5[c]	United States, UK, Jamaica, Thailand, Singapore, El Salvador (defective clips)
Chi et al., 1981	Spring Clip	1,699	4.19[c]						?	IFRP (19 countries) (defective clips)
Chi et al., 1980	Culdoscopy; Tantalum Clip	498	8.19					Mean age = 32[t]	?	IFRP (19 countries)

Notes:

[a] Updated from Trussell and Kost (1987), Table 10.

[c] Calculated by James Trussell from data in the article.

[g] Most of these studies incorrectly report the loss to follow-up (LFU) probability as the number of women lost at any time during the study divided by the total number of women entering the study. Thus, these are the probabilities presented in the table. However, the correct measure of LFU would be a gross life-table probability. When available, gross 12-month probabilities are denoted by the letter "g."

[t] Total for all methods in the study.

[u] Study did not report whether the cumulative life-table probability was net or gross.

[v] The authors report that LFU for "relevant reasons (withdrawal of cooperation or loss of contact)" was 0.3% per year in the 1983 study. In the 1983 study, women had probably been followed for 10 years on average; if 0.3% are LFU per year, then 3.0% would be LFU in 10 years. LFU including death and emigration is about twice as high as LFU for "relevant reasons."

For table references, see reference section.

Table 31-16 Summary of studies of contraceptive failure: vasectomy[a]

Reference	N for Analysis	Life-Table 12-Month % Pregnant	Pearl Index Pregnancy Rate			Characteristics of the Sample	LFU (%)[g]	Comments
			Index	Total Exposure	Maximum Exposure			
Moss, 1992	6,220	0.0[c]					?	1 pregnancy 10 years after vasectomy
Schmidt, 1988	5,000	0.0[c]					?	Presumably 0 pregnancies
Alderman, 1988	5,331	0.0[c]				5,331 of 8,879 had at least 2 post-op semen tests	?	Canada; 4 pregnancies, 4.5–8.6 years after vasectomy
Philip et al., 1984	16,039	0.0[c]				16,039 of 16,796 provided requested post-op semen samples	?	Britain; 6 pregnancies, 1.3–3 years after vasectomy; 3 pregnancies in first year among 757 men who did not supply post-op semen samples
Kase and Goldfarb, 1973	500	0.0[c]				2% ≥ aged 41	?	1 pregnancy 15 months after vasectomy
Vessey et al., 1982	?		0.08	2,500 Yr.	24 Mo.	Females all white; females at recruitment aged 25–39 and married; at enrollment, all women had been using the diaphragm, IUD, or pill successfully for at least 5 months	0.3[t,v]	Britain; Oxford/FPA study
Margaret Pyke Center, 1973	1,000	0.1[c]				24% ≥ age 41	?	Britain; 1 pregnancy in first year
Klapproth and Young, 1973	1,000	0.2[c]				35% ≥ age 41	10.0?	2 pregnancies, 3 and 4 months after vasectomy

(continued)

Table 31-16 Summary of studies of contraceptive failure: vasectomy[a]—*(cont'd)*

Reference	N for Analysis	Risk of Pregnancy				Characteristics of the Sample	LFU (%)[g]	Comments
		Life-Table 12-Month % Pregnant	Pearl Index Pregnancy Rate					
			Index	Total Exposure	Maximum Exposure			
Marshall and Lyon, 1972	200	0.5[c]				Age 25–60; "majority" aged 35–39	?	1 pregnancy 3 months after vasectomy

Notes:

[a] Updated from Trussell and Kost (1987), Table 10.

[c] Calculated by James Trussell from data in the article.

[g] Most of these studies incorrectly report the loss to follow-up (LFU) probability as the number of women lost at any time during the study divided by the total number of women entering the study. Thus, these are the probabilities presented in the table. However, the correct measure of LFU would be a gross life-table probability. When available, gross 12-month probabilities are denoted by the letter "g."

[t] Total for all methods in the study.

[v] The authors report that LFU for "relevant reasons (withdrawal of cooperation or loss of contact)" was 0.3% per year in the 1982 study. In the 1982 study, women had probably been followed for 9.5 years on average; if 0.3% are LFU per year, then 2.8% would be LFU in 9.5 years. LFU including death and emigration is about twice as high as LFU for "relevant reasons."

For table references, see reference section.

Index

A

Abortion
- adjunctive techniques, 688–689
- adolescent pregnancy, 703–704
- aspiration, 681–682
- cautions, 689–690
- clinical management, 687
- complications, 686(t), 690–696
- contraception after, 696–697
- decisions regarding, 676–677
- first trimester, **681–687**, 691–692
- follow-up care, 696–697
- legal status of, 674–675
- levels/trends in, 704–705, 706(f), 707(f)
- medication, **682–687**, 691–692
- method of, selecting, 677–678, 678(f), 678(t)
- ongoing pregnancy after, 693–694
- osmotic dilators, 688–689
- overview, 673–674
- population change and, 749–750
- precautions, 689–690
- procedures, pre-abortion, 679–681
- public health impact of, 675
- second trimester, **687–689**
- statistics, 702(t)
- sterilization after, 548, 549
- warning signs, 686(t), 690–696
- women seeking, characteristics of, 675–676, 677(t)

Abortion, incomplete, 693

Abortion, spontaneous, 642, 644(t), 646

Abstinence
- as contraceptive choice, 237, **305–309**, 703, 720, 723–724, 726
- defined, 305–306
- efficacy/effectiveness, **774–775, 777–778**, 792(t), **804(t)–808(t)**
- indications for, 307–308
- natural family planning and, 317
- sexuality and, 23–24

Accutane, 468

Acne, 401, 428–429

Acquired Immune Deficiency Syndrome (AIDS)—*See* HIV/AIDS

Actinomyces spp., 48–49, 502

Acute urethral syndrome, **201–202**

Acyclovir, 178

Adenomyosis, 141, 142, 499

Adnexal pelvic masses, benign, 140–141

Adolescent pregnancy
- comparisons, other countries, 705, 708(f), 709–710
- consequences of, 716–719, 729–734
- determinants of, 711–714
- FIND, SERVE, CARE programs, 734, 737(t)–740(t)
- home visits, 729–730, 732
- intervention programs, 719–720, 737(t)–740(t)
- levels/trends in, 704–705, 706(f), 707(f)
- prevention, 257, 703, **719–741**
- service learning programs, 725
- socioeconomic aspects, 704, 718–719, 732
- support services, 703–704
- welfare reform, 732

Adolescents
- abstinence and, 23, 703, 720, 723–724, 726
- clinic services for, 734, 737(t)–740(t), 740–741
- contraceptive use, 710, 713–714, 720, 726, 737(t)–740(t)
- counseling/education and, 254–259
- HBV vaccinations, 211
- HIV/AIDS prevention and, 164–165, 724
- informed consent and, 734, 735(t)–736(t)
- male condom use, promoting, 344–345
- oral contraceptives and, 424
- RTIs/STIs among, 192, 715–716
- sexual behavior, 12–13, 701–704, 711, 712(f), 713

Adoption, 668–669

Age and aging—*See also* Menopause; Population change; Reproductive life
- contraceptive choice and, 231–232, 468
- counseling/education and, 254–259
- menstrual cycle and, 71

Agglutination inhibition slide tests, 638–639

AIDS—*See* HIV/AIDS

Alcohol abuse—*See* Substance abuse

Alesse-28 Tablets, *(A), (B), (H),* 280(t), 394(f), 825(t), 828(t)

Allergies, 336, 358, 359, 470, 481—*See also* Latex allergy

Alzheimer's disease, 90

Amenorrhea
· lactational, 579–581
· "post-pill," 398
· primary, 113–115
· progestin-only contraceptives and, 467
· secondary, 115–118

Anal intercourse, 14, 337

Anatomy—*See* Sexual anatomy

Androgen—*See also* Combined hormonal contraceptives
· indications, 401
· menopause, use in, 83, 99–100
· menstrual cycle and, 64, 66, 70

Anemia, 401–402, 680—*See also* Sickle cell anemia

Anogenital intercourse—*See* Anal intercourse

Anovulation, 70–71, 73, 657

Anovulatory bleeding, 399

Anti-HIV protease inhibitors, 436

Anti-tuberculosis drugs—*See* Tuberculosis

Antibiotics
· IUDs and, 500
· oral contraceptives and, 436–437
· post-abortion use, 691, 692
· RTIs, use in, 196, 201

Anticonvulsants, 436

Antifungal agents, 436

Antiprogestins, 281

Anxiety, premenstrual syndrome and, 132

Arousal disorders, 30–32

Aspiration abortion, 681–682

Assisted reproductive technologies, 666–667

Atrophy—*See* Genitourinary atrophy

Aviane, *(B), (H),* 280(t)

Azospermia, 667

B

Bacterial vaginosis, 48, **202–203**, 359

Barrier methods—*See also* Caps; Diaphragms; Female condoms; Male condoms; Sponges
· advantages/indications, 372–373
· cost, 372
· dental dams/oral dams, 337

Barrier methods—*continued*
· disadvantages/cautions, 373–375
· efficacy/effectiveness, 370–371, **774–776**, 778, **809(t)–811(t)**
· FAB methods and, 317
· follow-up, 382–383
· future fertility and, 237
· history, 365–366
· lubricants and, 377
· mechanism of action, 366–370
· perimenopause, use in, 77
· postpartum use, 586
· problems, managing, 382–383
· providing, 375–382
· research/development, 609–610
· risk factors, 237
· sexuality and, 21–22
· using, guidelines for, 376, 383–388

Basal body temperature (BBT), 67, 69(f), 318, 319, **325–326**, 327(f), 659

Bellergal-S, 82

Benign pelvic mass(es), 140–142

Bethesda System Classification, PAP smears, 45, 45(t), 46, 47(t)

Biphasic oral contraceptives, 397, 422

Birth defects, 321, 359, 374, 621, 626(t)

Black cohosh, 84

Bleeding—*See* Uterine bleeding; Vaginal bleeding

Bone disorders—*See* Osteopenia/osteoporosis

Bone mineral density (BMD)
· medications, 89(t)
· menopause and, 86, 87
· progestin-only contraceptives and, 470, 478–479
· screening guidelines, 88(t)

Breakthrough spotting—*See* Vaginal bleeding

Breast cancer
· abortion and, 696
· contraceptive choice and, 237
· menopause and, 76, 78
· oral contraceptives and, 443–444
· progestin-only contraceptives and, 478
· risk factors for, 57(t), 92–94, 410
· screening for, 56–59
· sterilization and, 539

Breast self-examination (BSE), 56

Breastfeeding
· contraception, emergency, and, 291
· contraceptive benefits of, 579–581, 794(t)

Breastfeeding—*continued*
· contraceptive methods with, 585–590
· contraceptives, hormonal, and, 589–590
· contraceptives, oral, and, 426
· contraceptives, progestin-only, and, 468, 478, 481
· HIV transmission and, 182, 183, 590–591, 594
· infant, advantages to, 590
· instructions/information, 592–594
· lactational infertility, 575–579
· management guidelines, 577(f)
· mother, effects on, 592
· population change and, 748–749
Breast(s)
· amenorrhea and, 114–115
· benign conditions, 400–401
· tenderness, 469
Brevicon® 28-Day Tablets, *(D)*, 394(f)

C

CA-125 blood test, 55, 142–143
Calcium intake, 87
Calendar rhythm method, of fertility awareness, 318, 319, 322
Cancer—*See also* Breast cancer; Cervical cancer; Ovarian cancer; Uterine cancer
· colorectal, 90
· contraceptive choice, risks and, 235
· endometrial, 400, 498–499
· hormone therapy and, 95
· liver, 408
· prostate, 539
· screening, in females, **37–59**
Candidiasis *(Candida)* spp., 47(t), 48, 135, 178, **203**, 359
Caps, cervical—*See also* FemCap; Prentif Cavity-Rim cervical caps
· efficacy/effectiveness, **775–776**, 792(t), **809(t)–811(t)**
· fitting/disinfecting, 380–381
· HIV/AIDS transmission and, 162, 181(t)
· instructions for using, 383, 384, 385, 386, 387
· mechanism of action, 368–369
· sexuality and, 21
· spermicides and, 355
Cardiovascular disease—*See* Heart disease

Cervical cancer—*See also* PAP smears
· contraceptive choice and, 237, 373
· HIV infection and, 41–42
· human papilloma virus (HPV) and, 178
· incidence, 142
· pathophysiology, 39–40
· risk factors for, 40–42, 409–410
· screening for, **38–54**
Cervical dysplasia, 373, 409–410, 427
Cervical mucous/secretions
· FAB methods and, 318, 323–325, 325(t), 328
· menstrual cycle and, 65, 66, 69(f), 70
Cervicitis, **213–214**
Cervix, 49, 65–66
Cesarean section, 549
Chancroid, 135, **204–205**
Chasteberry, 84
Chastity—*See* Abstinence
Childbearing—*See also* Pregnancy
· birth rates, trends in, 704–705, 706(f), 707(f), 708(f)
· maternal mortality/morbidity, 752–753
· statistics, 702(t)
Children
· herpes transmission in, 206–207
· HIV/AIDS and, 182
· sexual assault and, 16
· STI transmission in, 200
Chlamydia, 140, 196, 197, **205**, 214, 504
Chloasma, 433
Cholestatic jaundice, 408
Cholesterol—*See* Hyperlipidemia
Cialis, 31
Cigarette smoking—*See* Smoking
CIN classification, PAP smears, 45, 45(t)
Circumcision, 162
Clomiphene citrate, 664–665, 667, 668
Clonidine, 82
Clot formation—*See* Thrombosis
Cocaine use—*See* Substance abuse
Cognition, 90–91
Coitus interruptus (withdrawal)
· advantages/indications, 313
· disadvantages/cautions, 313–314
· efficacy/effectiveness, 312, 312(t), **774–777**, 792(t), **802(t)–803(t)**
· instructions for using, 314–315
· mechanism of action, 311–312
· sexuality and, 23

Color photos, of contraceptive pills, (A–H)

Colorectal cancer, 90, 403

Colposcopy, 42, 50–51, 52(t), 134

Combined hormonal contraceptives—*See also* Oral contraceptives; Transdermal contraceptive patches; Vaginal contraceptive rings
· advantages/indications, 398–404
· color photos, *(A–H)*
· cost, 397–398
· disadvantages, 404–410
· efficacy/effectiveness, 395–396
· estrogens in, 392, **393**, 394(t)
· follow-up, 419–420
· history, 391–392
· instructions for use, **438–451**
· mechanism of action, 392
· patient selection, 410–411
· postpartum use, 588–589
· progestins in, 392, 393, **393**, 394(t)
· side effects, managing, 427–438
· special populations, 424–427

Competence, issues of, 264

Conception, 70

Condoms—*See* Female condoms; Male condoms

Condyloma acuminata—*See* Warts, genital

Consent—*See* Informed consent

Contact lenses, 432

Contraceptive choice—*See also* Abstinence; Barrier methods; Coitus interruptus; Emergency contraception; Hormonal contraceptives; Intrauterine devices; Postpartum contraception; Spermicides; Sterilization
· abortion, after, 696–697
· adolescents and, 710, 713–714, 720
· benefits, noncontraceptive, 240, 241(t)
· breastfeeding and, 585–590
· comfort/confidence scale, 244(t)
· cost, 243, 245(t), 246(f), 246–247
· counseling for, 234, 248–249
· efficacy/effectiveness, **224–234**, 773–774, 780–781, **792(t)–794(t)**
· failures in a lifetime, 229–230
· future fertility and, 237–238
· HIV/AIDS transmission and, 160–162, 181(t)
· perimenopause and, **75–77**

Contraceptive choice—*continued*
· personal considerations, **221–224**, 223(t), **240–248**
· population change and, 748–749
· postpartum, 585–590
· risks, major health, 235–237, 236(t)
· safety concerns, 235–239, 241(t)
· sexuality and, 20(t), **20–25**, 21–25
· side effects, 238, 241(t)
· simultaneous use of methods, 228–229, 234
· STIs and, 194

Contraceptive research
· barrier methods, 609–610
· current, 607–615
· future, 615
· history, 603–606
· men, methods for, 611–613
· microbicides, 607–609
· need(s) for, 601–603, 606–607
· systemic methods, 610–613
· women, methods for, 610–611

Convulsions, 436, 467

Copper T 380A (ParaGard) IUDs
· availability in US, 495
· efficacy/effectiveness, **779–780**, 781, 792(t), **836(t)**
· emergency contraception and, 281, 285–286, 290
· insertion, 519–520, 520(f)–521(f)
· mechanism of action, 462
· menopause, use in, 76
· postpartum use, 582–583, 586

Corpus luteum, 63, 67

Counseling/education—*See also* Sexual counseling/education
· abstinence, 308–309
· coitus interruptus, 314–315
· contraceptive choice, 248–249
· contraceptive effectiveness, 234
· contraceptive safety, 239
· early pregnancy, 646–647
· emergency contraception, 292–294, 298–299
· FAB methods, 322–327
· infertility, 669
· informed consent and, 263–265
· IUDs, about, 504, 505
· key points, 262(t)
· male condom use, 338–341, 342–348
· resources for, **267–277**, 298
· sexuality and, 10

Creams, spermicidal, 355, 356, 361

Cultural values—*See* Sociocultural values

Cunnilingus—*See* Oral intercourse

Cycle beads™, 323, 324(f)
Cyclessa, *(E)*, 393, 826(t)
Cystitis, 22, 195, 201
Cytological screening—*See* PAP smears
Cytotec—*See* Misoprostol (Cytotec)

D

Danazol, 111, 138, 282
D&E—*See* Dilation & evacuation (D&E)
Dehydroepiandrosterone (DHEA), 100
Dementia—*See* Cognition
Demulen® 1/35-28, *(D)*, 394(f)
Demulen® 1/50-28, *(G)*
Dental dams (oral dams), 337
Depo-Provera (DMPA)
· advantages, 467
· bone density and, 478–479
· breastfeeding and, 478
· cancer and, 478, 479(t)
· cost, 465
· disadvantages, 470
· efficacy/effectiveness, 464,
    774–775, 778–779, 792(t),
    833(t)–835(t)
· endometriosis, use in, 138
· follow-up, 480–481
· formulation, 461
· HIV-infected women, use in, 181(t)
· instructions for using, 481–484
· mechanism of action, 461–462
· menopause, use in, 75, 77, 82
· menstrual problems, treatment for,
    111
· perimenopause, use in, 71
· postpartum use, 585, 587, 588, 590
· problems, managing, 480–481
· providing, 479–480
· warning signs, 484
Depot medroxyprogesterone acetate
    (DMPA)—*See* Depo-Provera (DMPA)
Depression, 132, 433, 470
DES (Diethylstilbestrol), 282
Desire disorders, 29
Desogen® 28 Tablets, *(C)*, 828(t)
DHEA (Dehydroepiandrosterone), 100
Diabetes, 407–408, 426, 503, 504, 626
Diaphragms
· efficacy/effectiveness, **774–775**,
    792(t), **813(t)–817(t)**
· fitting/disinfecting, 379–380
· HIV/AIDS transmission and, 162,
    181(t)
· instructions for using, 383, 384,
    385, 386, 387

Diaphragms—*continued*
· mechanism of action, 367–368
· postpartum use, 582
· RTI risks and, 194
· sexuality and, 21, 22
· spermicides and, 355, 356
· styles, 378–380
Diarrhea, 440
Diet—*See* Nutrition
Diethylstilbestrol (DES), 282
Dilapan, 688–689
Dilation & evacuation (D&E), 687–689
DMPA—*See* Depo-Provera (DMPA)
Dong Quai, 84
Douching, 194–195, 357, 362
Down's syndrome—*See* Birth defects
Drospirenone, 393, 410, 427, 437–438
Drug abuse—*See* Substance abuse
Dual-method contraception, 234, 339
Dysfunctional uterine bleeding (DUB),
    123, 124, 125(t)
Dysmenorrhea, **110–113**, 399
Dyspareunia, 31, 33, 85, 143–145
Dysuria, 209

E

Eating disorders, 70, 118
ECPs—*See* Emergency contraception
Ectopic pregnancy
· emergency contraception and, 290
· managing, 643–645, 644(t)
· as pelvic mass, 139–140
· risk factors for, 357, 399, 466–467,
    692
· sterilization and, 560
· treatment, 682–683
Education—*See* Counseling/education
Emergency contraception
· advantages/indications, 288–289
· color photos, *(H)*
· costs, 246–247
· counseling for, 234, 292–294
· disadvantages/cautions, 289–291
· efficacy/effectiveness, 286–288, 781,
    792(t)
· follow-up care, 296(t), 297
· future potential for, 282–284
· history, 281–282
· hormonal methods, 279–282,
    284–285, 289–290, 298–299
· instructions for using, 298–299
· IUDs, 285–286, 290, 297, 298
· mechanism of action, 284–286

Follicular ovarian cysts, 140
Follicular phase, of menstrual cycle, 63, 66
Fractures, 86–89, 91, 402
FSH—*See* Follicle stimulating hormone (FSH)
Fungal infections, 436

G

Gabapentin, 83
Gallbladder disease, 94, 408, 426
Gamete intrafallopian transfer (GIFT), 664, 666
Gastrointestinal problems, 429
Gels, spermicidal, 355, 356, 360, 361
Gender—*See* Female(s); Male(s)
Genetic disorders, 621
Genital herpes—*See* Herpes simplex virus
Genital warts—*See* Warts, genital
Genitourinary atrophy, 85–86, 96—*See also* Vaginal atrophy
GIFT—*See* Gamete intrafallopian transfer (GIFT)
Ginseng, 84
Glandular cells, atypical, 47(t), 53
Glucose/glucose tolerance—*See* Diabetes
Gonadotropin-releasing hormone (GnRH), 64, 66, 68(f), 111, 114, 665–666
Gonorrhea, 140, **209–210**, 401, 504
Grafenberg (G) spot, 17
Granuloma inguinale, 135, **210–211**
Gynecological problems—*See also* Menstrual problems
· abstinence and, 308
· endometriosis, 136–138
· HIV/AIDS, management of, 175, 176(t)–177(t), 178–179
· pelvic mass, 139–143
· sexual dysfunction, 143–146
· vulvar lesions, 133–136

H

HAART—*See* Highly Active Antiretroviral Therapy (HAART)
hCG—*See* Human chorionic gonadotropin (hCG)
Headaches, 429–430, 431(f)
Health—*See also* Medical problems; Reproductive health
· contraceptive choice, risks and, 235–237, 236(t)

Health—*continued*
· menopause and, 78–79
· mortality in women, leading causes of, 2(t)
· preventative, 2–4
· screening recommendations, periodic, 3(t)–4(t)
· women's, 3(t)–4(t), 4–6
Health care providers—*See also* Counseling/education
· access to, contraceptive choice and, 248
· HIV/AIDS and, 183–185
· professional education, 268–271
Heart disease
· contraceptive choice and, 235
· hormone treatment and, 92
· IUD use and, 503–504
· menopause and, 76, 77, 78, 79
· risk factors for, 6
Hepatic neoplasms, 408
Hepatitis B virus (HBV), 5, 183, **211–212**
Hermaphrodites, 113
Herpes simplex virus (HSV), **205–207**
· cervical changes with, 47(t), 49
· HIV/AIDS and, 178
· reporting, 197
· symptoms, 135
Highly Active Antiretroviral Therapy (HAART), 174–175, 182
Hirsutism, 428–429
HIV/AIDS
· breastfeeding and, 590–591, 594
· cervical cancer and, 41–42
· coitus interruptus and, 313–314
· condom use and, 195
· contraceptive choice and, 313–314, 321
· contraceptives, oral, and, 408–409
· counseling/education and, **165–174, 168(t)–171(t)**, 260, 724
· in women, **174–183**
· incidence, 153–154
· IUD use and, 503
· male condom use and, 331–332, 336–337
· partner selection/assessment skills, 159
· population change and, 753
· post-exposure prophylaxis, 159
· prevention, 155–165, 163–165
· psychological support/care, 174, 179
· risk factors for, 15, 155–157, 156(t)
· safe sex skills, 157–158, 158(t)

Levonorgestrel intrauterine (LNG IUS)—*See* Mirena (LNG IUS) IUDs

Levora Tablets, *(C), (H)*, 280(t)

Libido, decreased, 80, 145, 403, 432

Lichen sclerosis, 134

Lipids—*See* Hyperlipidemia

Liver disease, 408

LNG IUS—*See* Mirena (LNG IUS) IUDs

Lo/Ovral®-28 Tablets, *(C), (H)*, 280(t), 394(f), 824(t), 828(t)

LoEstrin® 21 1.5/30, *(C)*, 394(f)

LoEstrin® FE 1/20, *(A), (B)*, 394(f)

Low-Ogestrel-28, *(C), (H)*, 280(t)

Lubricant products, 30, 85, 344, 347, 377

Lunelle (Cyclofem) injection, 393, 582, 611, 779, 792(t), 833(t)

Luteal ovarian cysts, 140

Luteal phase, of menstrual cycle, 63, 67

Luteinizing hormone (LH)
- infertility and, 665
- menopause and, 78
- menstrual cycle and, 64, 66, 68(f)
- menstrual problems and, 114

M

Male condoms
- adolescents, promoting use among, 344–345
- advantages/indications, 335–337
- anal intercourse, use during, 337
- cost, 335
- disadvantages/cautions, 338
- dual method use, 339
- efficacy/effectiveness, **333–335**, 774–775, 778, 792(t), **818(t)–820(t)**
- follow-up, 345–346
- HIV/AIDS prevention and, 157, 160, 161, 181(t), 336–337
- incidence of use, 331–332
- instructions for using, 346–348
- mechanism of action, 332–333
- options, 332–333, 333(t)
- oral intercourse, use during, 337
- partner negotiation, 340
- preferences, 341–342
- problems, managing, 345–346
- providing, 338–346
- RTI/STI prevention and, 194, 336–337
- sexuality and, 22–23
- spermicidal, 333, 356
- user error, minimizing, 342–344

Male(s)—*See also* Infertility
- contraceptive research/development for, 611–613
- erectile disorders, 30–32
- orgasmic disorders, 32–33
- sexual anatomy, 16
- sexual attitudes of, 10–12, 13

Mammography, **58–59**, 93–94

Marijuana, 5

Mastalgia, 432–433

Masters and Johnson, 18, 27, 28, 31

Masturbation, 32

Medical problems
- abstinence and, 308
- adolescent pregnancy and, 717–718
- infertility and, 657
- IUD use and, 503–504
- menopause and, 77
- menstruation and, 126–127
- oral contraceptives and, **404–411**, **412(t)–419(t)**, 426–427, 436–438
- preconception care and, 625–626
- sexual arousal disorders and, 30, 31

Medication abortion, 682–687, 691–692

Medications—*See also* Over-the-counter medications
- bone mineralization, 88(t), 88–89, 89(t)
- dysmenorrhea, 111–112
- fetal development, effect on, 626(t)
- HIV/AIDS post-exposure prophylaxis, 159
- hormone therapy (HT), **97(t)–99(t)**
- interactions, drug, 31, 291, 377, 410, **436–438**, 443, 467, 471
- libido, effect on, 145–146
- menopausal symptoms, 82–84
- preconception care and, 626
- premenstrual syndrome, 130–133
- RTIs, presumptive treatment for, 200

Medroxyprogesterone acetate, 116, 124, 660

Megestrol acetate, 82, 822(t)

Melanoma, 409

Melasma, 433

Memory loss, 90–91

Men—*See* Male(s)

Menometrorrhagia, 121

Menopause—*See also* Hormone therapy (HT); Perimenopause
- aging and, stages of, 74(t), 77
- bones, impact on, 86–89, 91
- diagnosis of, 78
- genitourinary atrophy, 85–86
- health risks in, 78–79

Mucopurulent cervicitis, **213–214**
Mulluscum contagiosum, 135, **213**
Multiphasic oral contraceptives, 397
Myocardial infarction, 404–405, 692

N

Naltrexone, 118
Natural family planning (NFP) method, 317, 321, 322
Natural membrane condoms, 332, 333
Nausea and vomiting, 289, 295(t), 440
Necon 1/35-28, *(E)*
Neural tube defects, 6
NFP—*See* Natural family planning (NFP) method
Nongonococcal urethritis, **214–215**
Nonoxynol-9 (N-9) products, 161, 333, 355, 358
Nor-QD® Tablets, *(A)*, *(B)*, 394(f), 462
Nordette®-28 Tablets, *(C)*, *(H)*, 280(t), 394(f), 826(t), 830(t)
Norethin 1/35E-28, *(E)*
Norethindrone, 393, 462, 589
Norgestrel, 393, 462, 589
Norinyl® 1+35 28-Day Tablets, *(E)*, 394(f)
Norplant
  · advantages, 467–468
  · availability in US, 461
  · contraceptive research, 610
  · cost, 466
  · disadvantages, 470–471
  · efficacy/effectiveness, 464, **778–779**, 792(t), **838(t)**
  · postpartum use, 582, 585, 587
  · removal, 484–487
Nutrition
  · as health risk factor, 6
  · population change and, 751
  · preconception care and, 624–625
  · premenstrual syndrome and, 130
NuvaRing, 21, **448–451**, 779, 792(t), 827(t), 829(t)

O

Obesity, 6, 75, 657, 667
Occupationally acquired HIV/AIDS, 183–185
Ogestrel, *(G)*, *(H)*, 280(t)
Oligomenorrhea, 119–121
Oocytes, 63, 65

Oral contraceptives—*See also* Emergency contraception
  · adolescents and, 424
  · advantages/indications, 398–404
  · breast cancer, 410, 431, 433–434
  · cautions, 441–444
  · color photos, *(A–H)*
  · cost, 397–398
  · diabetes and, 407–408, 418, 426
  · disadvantages, 404–410
  · dysmenorrhea, 111
  · efficacy/effectiveness, 395–396, 774–775, 778–779, 792(t), 824(t)–832(t)
  · extended use, 422
  · follow-up, 419–420
  · formulation, choosing a, 422, 423(f)
  · headaches, 407, 415, 420, 422–423, **429–430**, 431(f)
  · initiation, choices for, 420–423, 438–439
  · instructions for using, 421–422, 438–444
  · interactions, drug, 436–438, 443
  · menstrual cycle and, 71
  · missed pills, 439–440
  · ovarian cancer and, 54
  · patient selection/precautions, 410–411, 412(t), 413(t)–419(t)
  · perimenopausal women and, 424–425
  · postpartum women and, 426
  · pregnancy and, 433–434
  · providing, 411–412
  · risk factors, 237
  · RTI risks and, 194
  · sexuality and, 21
  · side effects, 427–438, 428(t), 441–444
  · switching from other methods, 421
  · warning signs, 441–444
  · WHO medical eligibility criteria, 413–419
Oral intercourse, 14, 337
Organizations, reproductive health—*See* Reproductive health resources
Orgasm(s), 17, 32–33
Orogenital intercourse—*See* Oral intercourse
Ortho-Cept® Tablets 28-Day Regimen, *(C)*, 828(t)
Ortho-Cyclen® 28 Tablets, *(D)*, 393, 825(t), 829(t)

PMS—*See* Premenstrual syndrome (PMS)
Podophyllin/Podofilox 0.5%, 208
Polycystic ovary syndrome (PCOS), **119–121**
- infertility treatment and, 665, 667–668
- menstrual cycle and, 71
- ovarian cancer and, 54
Polymenorrhea, 121
POPs—*See* Minipills (progestin-only pills, POPs)
Population change
- abortion and, 749–750
- age distributions, 754–759
- age-specific rates, 767
- birth interval length and, 748
- breastfeeding and, 748–749
- contraception and, 748–749
- crude rates, 762–768
- demographic transition, 759–762
- doubling time, 763–764
- fertility determinants and, 746–751, 762–768
- gross reproduction rates, 767–768
- HIV/AIDS and, 753
- life table/expectation of life, 768
- marriage age/proportions and, 747–748
- measuring, 762–768
- menarche/menopause and, 746–747
- migration, determinants of, 753–754
- momentum, 755–757
- mortality, determinants of, 751–753, 762–768
- net reproduction rates, 767–768
- nutrition and, 751
- Pearl index, 765–766
- reproductive behavior and, 745–746
- STIs and, 750–751
- total fertility rates, 767
Post-exposure HIV prophylaxis, 159
Post-menopause—*See* Menopause
"Post-pill amenorrhea," 398
Postabortal syndrome, 693
Postcoital contraception—*See* Emergency contraception
Postpartum contraception
- breastfeeding woman, 585–590
- infertile period, 575–579
- initiating, 582–585
- lactational infertility, 575–579
- nonbreastfeeding woman, 585
- oral contraceptives and, 426
- sexuality and, 581–582
- sterilization, 548–549, 556–557

Poverty, 6, 710
Preconception care
- health precautions, 619(t)
- immunizations, 623
- importance of, 617
- information, essential, 618
- male partner's risk factors, 627
- prenatal care, 627
- visit services, 620–627
Preejaculatory fluid, 314, 776
Pregnancy—*See also* Adolescent pregnancy; Unintended pregnancy
- clinical evaluation, 630–631, 679–681
- contraceptive choice and, 21, 773–774, 792(t)–794(t)
- counseling objectives, 646–647
- early, problem management in, 642–646, 644(t)
- hCG levels, during/after, 631–635
- HIV/AIDS and, 173–174, 179–183
- IUDs and, 526
- maternal mortality/morbidity, 752–753
- oral contraceptives and, 433–434, 441
- preconception care, **617–627**
- probability of, 652–653
- RTIs and, 197, 198(t)–199(t)
- sex selection, FAB methods and, 322
- sexual disinterest and, 146
- spermicidal exposure during, 359–360
- statistics, 702(t)
Pregnancy testing
- agglutination inhibition slide, 638–639
- biology of, 631–635
- hCG levels, 631–635
- home, 635, 636(t)–637(t), 638, 639–642
- hormone structure, test design and, 635
- immunometric, 635, 636, 636(t)–637(t), 637–638
- importance of, 629–630
- interpretation errors, avoiding, 640–642
- options, 635, 636(t)–637(t), 638–642
- quantitative beta hCG RIA, 638
Premarin, 97(t), 98(t)
Premature ejaculation, 33
Premenstrual dysphoric disorder (PMDD), 127, 128(t)
Premenstrual syndrome (PMS), 110, **127–133**, 399

Prenatal care, importance of, 627
Prentif Cavity-Rim cervical caps, 380,
  809(t), 810(t), 811(t)
Presumptive treatment, sexual assault
  and, 200
Preventative health services, 2–4
Previn, 280, 295
Primary amenorrhea, 113–115
Primary dysmenorrhea, 110–112
Primary infertility, 652
Progestasert (Progesterone T) IUDs
  · availability in US, 496
  · efficacy/effectiveness, 779–780, 781,
    792(t)
  · mechanism of action, 71
  · postpartum use, 587, 588
Progesterone
  · menopause and, 96, 99(t)
  · menstrual cycle and, 64, 65, 66, 67,
    68(f)
  · menstrual problems and, 110
  · mid-luteal phase serum, 660
Progestin—See also Combined
  hormonal contraceptives
  · menstrual cycle and, 65, 66
  · postmenopausal use, 95–99,
    97(t)–99(t)
Progestin challenge test, 116, 117(f),
  660, 667
Progestin-only contraceptives—See also
  Depo-Provera; Implants; Minipills;
  Mirena (LNG IUS) IUDs
  · advantages/indications, 466–468
  · color pictures, (A), (B), (H)
  · costs, 465–466
  · delivery methods, 461–462, 463(t)
  · disadvantages/cautions, 469–471,
    472(t)–477(t)
  · efficacy/effectiveness, 462, 464–465
  · mechanism of action, 462
  · menstrual cycle and, 71
  · perimenopause, use in, 77
  · postpartum use, 587–588
  · providing, 478–491
Prolactin, 116
Prolapse, uterine, 85–86
Prostaglandins, 110, 111, 112
Prostate cancer, 539–540
Pseudogestational sac, 645
Psychiatric problems, abortion and,
  695–696
Public health, 1

Q

Quantitative beta hCG
  radioimmunoassay (RIA), 638,
  643–644
Quick Start methods, OC pills, 420, 438

R

Rape—See Sexual assault
Reading level, SMOG formula for, 259
Red clover/red clover isoflavones, 83, 84
Red vulvar lesions, 135–136
"Redo" syndrome, 693
Reed, David M., 18–19, 29
Religious values—See Sociocultural
  values
Reproductive health
  · abortion and, 695
  · perspectives on, 1–6
  · preventative services, 2–4
  · screening recommendations,
    periodic, 3(t)–4(t)
  · sexuality and, 9–10
Reproductive health resources
  · emergency contraception, 298
  · multimedia materials, **268–272**
  · organizations, 267(t), 268(t)
  · pharmaceutical houses, 272(t)
  · print materials, **268–272**
  · telephone numbers/hotlines,
    273(t)–277(t), 298
Reproductive life, stages of—See also
  Menopause
  · contraceptive choices and, 242(t),
    243(f)
  · counseling/education and, 254–259
  · pelvic masses in women, 139–140
Reproductive tract infections (RTIs),
  201–218— See also Sexually
  transmitted diseases (STIs)
  · assessment, 195–200
  · diagnosis, 195–200
  · incidence, 191–192
  · IUD use and, 500–502, 504, 526
  · PAP smear results, 48–49
  · partner notification, 197
  · preconception care and, 622–623
  · pregnancy and, 197, 198(t)–199(t)
  · prevention, 193–195
  · reporting, 197
  · risks of, 192–193, 193(t)
  · treatment, 195–200
Rh sensitization, 642

Rheumatoid arthritis, 402
Roe v. Wade, 674–675
RTIs—*See* Reproductive tract Infections (RTIs)
RU 486—*See* Mifepristone (Mifeprex)
Rupture, of the uterus, 694

S

Safer sex skills, 157–158, 158(t), 193, 239
Seasonale, *(C),* 280(t), 398, 422, 435, 828(t)
Second-trimester abortion, 687–689
Secondary amenorrhea, 115–118
Secondary dysmenorrhea, 112–113
Secondary infertility, 652
Seizures—*See* Convulsions
Selective serotonin reuptake inhibitors (SSRIs), 30, 82, 130–132, 131(t)
Semen analysis, 656, 661—*See also* Infertility
Sexual abuse, 15–16, 146, 200, 340
Sexual anatomy, 16–17
Sexual assault—*See also* Emergency contraception
· as health risk factor, 5
· HIV prophylaxis postexposure, 159
· incidence of, 15–16
· presumptive treatment, 200
· RTI transmission and, 200
Sexual behavior
· adolescents, 12–13, **701–704**, 711, 712(f), 713
· contraceptive choice and, 231–232, 247–248
· counseling/education and, 260–263
· fertility awareness-based methods and, 322
· history, taking a, 25(t)
· mortality, affecting, 752
· partner, choosing a, 255(t)
· questions, commonly asked, 26–27
· RTI prevention and, 193–195
· same gender, 13
· United States, in the, **10–16**, 11(t)
Sexual counseling/education
· abstinence, regarding, 305–309
· adolescents, 254–259, 714, 720, 724, 725–729
· age, development and, 254–259
· behavior change, to support, 260–263
· emotional state and, 259–260
· factors influencing, **253–260**

Sexual counseling/education—*continued*
· introduction to, 25–27
· literacy level and, 258–259
· questions, commonly asked, 26, 28
· resources for, 267–277, 298
· values, personal/cultural and, 258
Sexual dysfunction(s)
· arousal disorders, 30–32
· common, introduction to, **27–33**
· desire disorders, 29, 145–146
· disinterest, 80, 145–146
· dyspareunia, 143–145
· etiology, 28–29
· orgasmic disorders, 32–33
· pain disorders, 33, 143–145
Sexual response, 17–19, 18(f)
Sexuality
· abstinence and, 305–309
· contraceptive choice and, 20(t), **20–25**
· postpartum, 581–582
· reproductive health and, 9–10
· sterilization and, 561
Sexually transmitted diseases (STIs)—*See also* HIV/AIDS
· in adolescents, 715–716
· contraceptive choice and, 20, 240, 313, 372–373, 469
· health risk factor, 5
· male condom use and, 336–337, 339
· partner notification, 196
· population change and, 750–751
· reporting, 196, 197
· risk factors for, 15
· vaginal barriers/spermicides and, 358, 372–373
Sickle cell anemia, 426, 467
Simple observation method, of fertility awareness, 328
Sleep disorders, 75, 80, 84
SMOG formula, for reading level, 259
Smoking
· breastfeeding and, 593
· as health risk factor, 5
· menopause and, 77, 78, 87
· oral contraceptives and, 410–411, 425, 443
· preconception care, 623
Sociocultural values
· adolescent pregnancy and, 709–710
· sexual counseling and, 258
· sexual dysfunction and, 29
Sonohysterography, 661

Tension headaches, 430
Teratomas, 140–141
Testosterone, 30, 64, 99, 115
"Third-generation" pills, 393
Thrombosis, 405–406, 468
Thyroid dysfunction, 657
Thyroid stimulating hormone (TSH), 78, 116
Tibolone, 83
Tinea, 135
Tobacco use—*See* Smoking
Toxic shock syndrome (TSS), 367, 369, 374, 376, 383, 388
Transdermal contraceptive patches—*See also* Ortho Evra patch
· advantages/indications, 391, 444–445
· disadvantages/cautions, 445–446
· efficacy/effectiveness, 396, 824(t)–832(t)
· follow-up, 446–447
· instructions for using, 447–448
· mechanism of action, 393
· postpartum use, 582, 585
· problems, managing, 446–447
· providing, 446
· side effects, 445
· switching from other methods, 446
Tri-Levlen® 28 Tablets, *(E)*, 280(t), 394(f)
Tri-Norinyl® 28-Day Tablets, *(F)*, 394(f)
Trichloroacetic acid (TCA), 208
Trichomonas vaginalis, 47(t), 48, **218**
Triphasic model, of sexual response, 18
Triphasic oral contraceptives, *(A)*, *(E–F)*, 397, 422
Triphasil®-28 Tablets, *(E)*, *(H)*, 280(t), 324(f), 828(t), 829(t)
Trivora®, *(E)*, *(H)*, 280(t)
TSH—*See* Thyroid stimulating hormone
TSS—*See* Toxic shock syndrome (TSS)
Tubal ligation—*See* Sterilization, female
Tuberculosis, 291, 436
Tumors—*See* Pelvic mass(es)

U

Ultrasound, use of, 644–645, 660
Unintended pregnancy—*See also* Emergency contraception
· contraceptive choice and, **225–234**, 226(t)–227(t)
· health risk factor, 4–5
· RTIs and, 193(t)

United States
· adolescent pregnancy, 706(f), 707(f), 708(f)
· contraceptives available in, 461, 484, 495–496, 674–675
· sexual behavior in, **10–16**, 11(t)
Urethral syndrome, acute, 201
Urethritis, nongonococcal, **214–215**
Urinary tract atrophy, 85–86
Urinary tract infections (UTIs), 85, 201, 333, 359, 374
Uterine bleeding—*See also* Menstruation
· excessive/irregular, 121–126, 122(t)
· post-abortion, 694
· side effect of HT, 94
Uterine cancer, 92, 142
Uterine pelvic masses, benign, 141–142
Uterine perforation, 500, 525, 694

V

Vacuum curettage—*See* Aspiration abortion
Vaginal atrophy, 50, 85
Vaginal barriers—*See* Barrier methods
Vaginal bleeding
· breakthrough, 434–435
· oral contraceptives and, 440
· withdrawal, managing, 427–428
Vaginal contraceptive rings—*See also* NuvaRing
· advantages, 391, 449
· disadvantages/cautions, 449
· efficacy/effectiveness, 396, 824(t)–832(t)
· follow-up, 450
· mechanism of action, 393
· menopause, use in, 96
· postpartum use, 582, 585
· problems, managing, 450
· providing, 450
· side effects, 449
· using, 448, 450–451
Vaginal discharge, 434
Vaginal spermicides—*See* Spermicides, vaginal
Vaginismus, 33, 144
Vaginosis—*See* Bacterial vaginosis
Vasectomy
· advantages/indications, 531–532, 534–535
· cost, 534
· counseling, 555–557
· disadvantages/cautions, 538

Vasectomy—*continued*
- efficacy/effectiveness, 533–534, 780, 792(t), **844(t)–845(t)**
- follow-up, 561–562
- HIV/AIDS transmission in, 162
- informed consent, 264
- instructions for, 566–567
- mechanism of action, 532
- methods/techniques, 551–554
- postpartum, 584
- problems, managing, 561–562
- providing, 551–554
- research/development, 614
- reversal of, 562–564
- sexuality and, 24
- special issues, 539–540

Vasopressin, 689

Venereal diseases—*See* Sexually transmitted diseases (STIs)

Venous thromboembolism (VTE), 405–406

Viagra, 30, 31

Vibrators, 32

Violence, against women, 5–6, 248—*See also* Sexual assault

Vitamin therapy, 84, 87, 130, 403

Voluntary surgical contraception—*See* Sterilization

Vomiting—*See* Nausea and vomiting

Vulvar lesions, 133–136

Vulvodynia, 33, 136

Vulvovaginitis, candida, 135, 178

W

Warts, genital
- condyloma acuminata, 20, 41, 53, 134–135, 178, **207–209**
- lymphogranuloma venereum, 135, 212

Water retention, 133

Websites, 272(t), **273(t)–277(t)**, 298

Weight/weight change, 435–436, 469, 481, 483—*See also* Eating disorders; Obesity

Wellbutrin, 30

Western blot testing, 167

White vulvar lesions, 134–135

Withdrawal—*See* Coitus interruptus (withdrawal)

Women—*See* Female(s)

World Health Organization (WHO) Medical Eligibility Criteria, for IUDs, 502–503, 507(t)–518(t)

Y

Yasmin 28 Tablets, *(C)*, 410, 429, 826(t)

Yeast vaginitis—*See* Candidiasis *(Candida)* spp.

Yohimbine, 31

Yuzpe regimen, 281, 282

Z

Zidovudine (AZT), 182

ZIFT—*See* Zygote intra-fallopian transfer (ZIFT)

Zovia® 1/35E-28, *(D)*

Zygote intra-fallopian transfer (ZIFT), 664, 666

Network

The organizations listed here play key roles in family planning, reproductive health, and population activities.

Advocates for Youth
2000 M Street NW, Suite 750
Washington, DC 20036
202-419-3420
202-419-1448 FAX
email: questions@advocatesforyouth.org
http://www.advocatesforyouth.org

AIDS Clinical Trials Information Service (ACTIS)
P.O. Box 6303
Rockville, MD 20849
1-800-448-0440
1-301-519-6616 FAX
email: ContactUs@aidsinfo.nih.gov
http://www.aidsinfo.nih.gov

Alan Guttmacher Institute (AGI)
120 Wall Street, 21st Floor
New York, NY 10005
212-248-1111
212-248-1951 FAX
email: info@guttmacher.org
http://www.guttmacher.org

Alliance for Microbicide Development
8484 Georgia Ave., Suite 940
Silver Spring, MD 20910
301-587-9690
301-588-8390 FAX
email: info@microbicide.org
http://www.microbicide.com

American Association of Sex Educators, Counselors, and Therapists
P.O. Box 5488
Richmond, VA 23220
804-644-3288
email: aasect@aasect.org
http://www.aasect.org

American College Health Association
P.O. Box 28937
Baltimore, MD 21240
410-859-1500
410-859-1510 FAX
email: contact@acha.org
http://www.acha.org

American College of Obstetricians and Gynecologists (ACOG)
409 12th Street, SW
P.O. Box 96920
Washington, DC 20090
202-863-2518
202-484-1595 FAX
email: resources@acog.org
http://www.acog.org

American Public Health Association (APHA)
800 I Street NW
Washington, DC 20001
202-777-2742 (APHA)
202-777-2534 FAX
email: comments@apha.org
http://www.apha.org

American Social Health Association (ASHA)
P.O. Box 13827
Research Triangle Park, NC 27709
919-361-8400
919-361-8425 FAX
http://www.ashastd.org

American Society for Reproductive Medicine (ASRM)
1209 Montgomery Highway
Birmingham, AL 35216
205-978-5000
205-978-5005 FAX
email: asrm@asrm.org
http://www.asrm.org

Association of Reproductive Health Professionals (ARHP)
2401 Pennsylvania Avenue NW, Suite 350
Washington, DC 20037
202-466-3825
202-466-3826 FAX
http://www.arhp.org

California Family Health Council
3600 Wilshire Boulevard, Suite 600
Los Angeles, CA 90010
213-386-5614
213-368-4410 FAX
http://www.cfhc.org

Catholics for a Free Choice
1436 U Street NW, Suite 301
Washington, DC 20009
202-986-6093
202-332-7995 FAX
email: cffc@catholicsforchoice.org
http://www.cath4choice.org

Centre for Development and Population Activities (CEDPA)
1400 16th Street NW Suite 100
Washington, DC 20036
202-667-1142
202-332-4496 FAX
email: cmail@cedpa.org
http://www.cedpa.org

Centers for Disease Control and Prevention (CDC)
Public Inquiries/MASO
Mailstop F-07
1600 Clifton Road NE
Atlanta, GA 30333
404-639-3353
800-311-3435
http://www.cdc.gov/netinfo.htm
CDC Division of HIV/AIDS Prevention
Mailstop E-49
Atlanta, GA 30333
800-458-5231
404-639-2007 FAX
http://www.cdc.gov/hiv/contactus.htm

Columbia University
The Harriet and Robert Heibrunn
Department of Population and Family Health
Mailman School of Public Health
60 Haven Avenue, B-2
New York, NY 10032
212-304-5200
http://cpmcnet.columbia.edu/dept/sph/popfam

Committee on Population, National Research Council
500 5th Street, NW, TNA 1133
Washington, DC 20001
202-334-3167
202-334-3768 FAX
http://www7.nationalacademies.org/cpop

Contraceptive Research and Development Program (CONRAD)
Eastern Virginia Medical School
1611 North Kent Street, Suite 806
Arlington, VA 22209
703-524-4744
703-524-4770 FAX
email: info@conrad.org
http://www.conrad.org

Contraceptive Technology
Contraceptive Technology
Communications, Inc.
P.O. Box 49007
Atlanta, GA 30359
email: authors@contraceptivetechnology.org
http://www.contraceptivetechnology.org

East-West Center Program on Population
1601 East-West Road
Honolulu, HI 96848
808-944-7111
808-944-7376 FAX
http://www.eastwestcenter.org/res-ph.asp

Education Program Associates (EPA)
492 Division St.
Campbell, CA 95008
408-374-3720
408-374-7385 FAX
email: epa@cfhc.org
http://epa.cfhc.org

Education and Training Resource Associates (ETR)
4 Carbonero Way
Scotts Valley, CA 95066
408-438-4060
http://www.etr.org

Emory University Family Planning Program
Department of Gynecology and Obstetrics
69 Jesse Hill Jr. Dr.
Atlanta, GA 30303
404-616-3709
404-521-3589 FAX

Engender Health
440 9th Ave.
New York, NY 10001
212-561-8000
212-561-8067 FAX
email: info@engenderhealth.org
www.engenderhealth.org

Family Health International (FHI)
P.O. Box 13950
Research Triangle Park, NC 27709
919-544-7040
919-544-7261 FAX
http://www.fhi.org

Family Violence Prevention Fund
383 Rhode Island St., Suite 304
San Francisco, CA 94103-5133
415-252-8000
415-252-8991 FAX
email: info@endabuse.org
http://www.endabuse.org

868

Ford Foundation
320 East 43rd Street
New York, NY 10017
212-573-5000
212-351-3677 FAX
http://www.fordfound.org

Hewlett Foundation
2121 Sand Hill Rd.
Menlo Park, CA 94025
650-234-4500
650-234-4501 FAX
http://www.hewlett.org

Ibis Reproductive Health
2 Brattle Square
Cambridge, MA 02138-3742
617-349-0040
617-349-0041 FAX
http://www.ibisreproductivehealth.org

Institute for Reproductive Health
4301 Connecticut Ave., NW, Suite 310
Washington, DC 2008
202-687-1392
email: irhinfo@georgetown.edu
http://www.irh.org

International Partnership for Microbicides
1010 Wayne Ave, Suite 510
Silver Spring, MD 20910
301-608-2221
301-608-2241 FAX
http://www.ipm-microbicides.org

International Planned Parenthood Federation (IPPF)
120 Wall Street, 9th Floor
New York, NY 10005
212-248-6400
212-248-4221 FAX
email: info@ippfwhr.org
http://www.ippfwhr.org

International Union for the Scientific Study of Population (IUSSP)
3-5, rue Nicolas
F-75980
Paris Cedex 20, France
331-56-06-2173
331-56-06-2204 FAX
email: iussp@iussp.org
http://www.iussp.org

IPAS
300 Market St., Suite 200
Chapel Hill, NC 27516
919-967-7052
919-929-0258 FAX
email: ipas@ipas.org
http://www.ipas.org

John Snow, Inc.
44 Farnsworth Street
Boston, MA 02111
617-482-9485
617-482-0617 FAX
email: jsinfo@jsi.com
http://www.jsi.com

Johns Hopkins University
Center for Communication Programs
111 Market Place, Suite 310
Baltimore, MD 21202
410-659-6300
410-659-6266 FAX
email: webadmin@jhuccp.org
http://www.jhuccp.org

Kaiser Family Foundation
2400 Sand Hill Road
Menlo Park, CA 94025
650-854-9400
650-854-4800 FAX
http://www.kff.org

National Abortion Federation (NAF)
1755 Massachussetts Ave., NW
Washington, DC 20036
202-667-5881
202-667-5890 FAX
email: naf@prochoice.org
http://www.prochoice.org

National Abortion and Reproductive Rights Action League (NARAL)
1156 15th Street NW, Suite 700
Washington, DC 20005
202-973-3000
202-973-3030 FAX
http://www.prochoiceamerica.org

National Association of Nurse Practitioners Women's Health (NPWH)
1090 Vermont Avenue NW, Suite 800
Washington, DC 20005
202-543-9693
202-408-0902 FAX
http://www.npwh.org

National Family Planning and Reproductive Health Association (NFPRHA)
1627 K St., NW, 12th Floor
Washington, DC 20006
202-293-3114
202-293-1990 FAX
email: info@nfprha.org
http://www.nfprha.org

National Institute of Child Health and Human Development (NICHD)
Center for Population Research
6100 Executive Blvd, Room 8B07-NIH
Bethesda, MD 20892
301-496-1101
301-496-0962 FAX
http://www.nichd.nih.gov/about/cpr/cpr.htm

Office on Women's Health
Department of Health and Human Services
8550 Arlington Blvd., Suite 300
Fairfax, VA 22031
800-994-woman
http://www.4woman.gov/healthpro
.index.htm

Pathfinder International
9 Galen Street, Suite 217
Watertown, MA 02172
617-924-7200
617-924-3833 FAX
email: information@pathfind.org
http://www.pathfind.org

Planned Parenthood Federation of America (PPFA)
434 West 33rd St.
New York, NY 10001
212-541-7800
800-230-PLAN (Smart Number)
212-245-1845 FAX
email: communications@ppfa.org
http://www.plannedparenthood.org

Population Action International (PAI)
1300 19th Street NW, 2nd Floor
Washington, DC 20036
202-557-3400
202-728-4177 FAX
email: pai@popact.org
http://www.populationaction.org

Population Association of America (PAA)
8630 Fenton St., Suite 722
Silver Spring, MD 20910
301-565-6710
301-565-7850 FAX
email: info@popassoc.org
http://www.popassoc.org

Population Council
1 Dag Hammarskjold Plaza
New York, NY 10017
212-339-0500
212-755-6052 FAX
email: pubinfo@popcouncil.org
http://www.popcouncil.org

Population Institute
107 2nd Street NE
Washington, DC 20002
202-544-3300
202-544-0068 FAX
email: web@populationinstitute.org
http://www.populationinstitute.org

Population Reference Bureau (PRB)
1875 Connecticut Avenue NW, Suite 520
Washington, DC 20009
202-483-1100
202-328-3937 FAX
email: popref@prb.org
http://www.prb.org

Princeton University
Office of Population Research
Wallace Hall, 2nd Floor
Princeton, NJ 08544
609-258-4870
609-258-1039 FAX
http://opr.princeton.edu

Program for Appropriate Technology in Health (PATH)
1455 NW Leary Way
Seattle, WA 98107-5136
206-285-3500
206-285-6619 FAX
email: info@path.org
http://www.path.org

Program for International Training and Health (INTRAH)
University of North Carolina
1700 Airport Rd., Suite 300
Chapel Hill, NC 27599-8100
919-966-5636
919-962-7178 FAX
email: intrah@intrahealth.org
http://www.intrahealth.org

Religious Institute on Sexual Morality, Justice, and Healing
304 Main Avenue, #335
Norwalk, CT 06851
203-840-1148
email: info@religiousinstitute.org
http://www.religiousinstitute.org

Reproductive Health Technologies Project (RHTP)
1300 19th St., 2nd Floor
Washington, DC 20036
202-557-3417
202-728-4177 FAX
email:rhtp@rhtp.org
http://www.rhtp.org

Rockefeller Foundation
420 Fifth Avenue
New York, NY 10018
212-869-8500
212-764-3468 FAX
http://www.rockfound.org

Sexuality Information and Education Council of the United States (SIECUS)
130 West 42nd Street, Suite 350
New York, NY 10036
212-819-9770
212-819-9776 FAX
email: siecus@siecus.org
http://www.siecus.org

United Nations Population Division
Department of Economics and Social Affairs
2 United Nations Plaza
DC 2-1950
New York, NY 10017
212-963-3179
212-963-2147 FAX
http://www.un.org/popin

United Nations Population Fund (UNFPA)
220 East 42nd Street
New York, NY 10017
212-297-5211
212-297-4915 FAX
email: ryanw@unfpa.org
http://www.unfpa.org/

University of Michigan
Population Studies Center
1225 South University Avenue
Ann Arbor, MI 48109
734-763-1414
http://www.psc.lsa.umich.edu/

University of North Carolina
Carolina Population Center
123 West Franklin Street
Chapel Hill, NC 27516
919-966-2157
919-966-6638 FAX
email: cpcweb@unc.edu
http://www.cpc.unc.edu

U.S. Agency for International Development (USAID)
Office of Population
Bureau for Research and Development
GH/PRH
Washington, DC 20523
202-712-0869
202-216-3485 FAX
email: jshelton@usaid.gov
http://www.maqweb.org

World Bank
Health, Nutrition and Population Department
1818 H Street NW
Washington, DC 20433
202-473-1000
202-477-6391 FAX
http://www.worldbank.org

World Health Organization
Special Programme of Research, Development, and Research Training in Human Reproduction
Avenia Appia 20
1211 Geneva 27
Switzerland
41-22-791-2111
41-22-791-3111 FAX
email: info@who.int
http://www.who.int

ARDENT MEDIA, INC.

AN INVITATION TO YOU FROM ARDENT MEDIA

Ardent Media seeks to expand its offerings in the health field, including mental and psychological health. As our name implies, we are open to publishing and distributing information in electronic form as well as print.

We are seeking material in formats such as internet web sites, video, audio and CD-ROM in addition to book and booklet material.

If you or your organization has produced material and is seeking distribution, or is planning to write or produce such material, please contact us.

We prefer that you fax or write us a description of your material prior to sending it. Please write us at Box 286, Cooper Station P.O. New York, N.Y., 10276-0286 or Fax us at (212) 861-0998. Thank You.

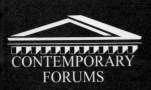

Forthcoming 2005

by the authors of *Contraceptive Technology*
from ARDENT MEDIA INC.

SAFELY SEXUAL

Written for the general public. Safely Sexual is the
practical guide to planning a safer sexual lifestyle,
preventing unplanned pregnancy, and protecting against HIV
and other sexually transmitted infections. It is perfect for distribution
to clients of family planning clinics and practitioners.

— 250 pages —
5.5" x 8.25"

ISBN 0-9664902-8-2 (*Safely Sexual* Paper) $16.95
ISBN 0-9664902-9-0 (*Safely Sexual* Cloth) $29.95

Visit our new website
Opening Fall 2004 for further information.
ardentmediainc.com

NOW AVAILABLE

A POCKET GUIDE TO

MANAGING CONTRACEPTION
2004-2005 Edition

by Robert A. Hatcher, MD et al.

$10.00 ISBN 0-9638875-4-8
— 160 pages —
3.5" x 5.5"

See order form in back of *Contraceptive Technology*
or visit our new website
Opening Fall 2004 for further information
ardentmediainc.com

Contracteptive Technology
❏ CD-ROM ❏ PDA Registration Form

Registration is required so we can send your access code to activate your CD-ROM and/or PDA. Mail your receipt or proof of purchase.
(See bottom of page for address.)

or

❏ New Media Survey

ABOUT YOU

1. Educational degree:_____
   Note: If you're a student, list degree you're studying for and expected date of graduation.

2. Describe your current position: _____

3. Circle your most important site of work:
   Managed care organization   Private practice   Health department
   Family planning clinic   Hospital   Other _____

4. Circle the number of women you have provided personal contraceptive or STI services in the past year:
   None   1-10   11-100   101-500   501-5000   More than 5000

5. I use a ❏ PDA or ❏ laptop while counseling patients.
   (please check one or both)

6. Name and address:

   Name _____

   Organization/Institution _____

   Address _____

   _____

   City _____ State _____ Zip _____

   Fax _____

   Email _____

   Website URL _____

   ❏ I am interested in linking my health related website to yours.

   (Please complete the Form found on the back of this page.)

Thank you for taking the time to help us serve you better!

Please photocopy or clip out both pages of this form and mail to:

Ardent Media Inc.
Box 286 Cooper Station P.O.
New York, New York 10276-0286

You may mail it along with your order.

PLEASE PHOTOCOPY THIS FORM OR CUT OUT AND MAIL TO ARDENT MEDIA, INC. BOX 286, COOPER STATION P.O., NEW YORK, NY 10276-0286

Contraceptive Technology
❏ CD-ROM ❏PDA Registration Form

Registration is required so we can send your access code to activate your CD-ROM and/or PDA. Mail your receipt or proof of purchase.
(See other side of this form for address.)

or

❏ New Media Survey

As our thank you for completing this form and the ABOUT YOU form on the adjoining page, you will receive a special prepublication discount on future new media published by us.

In addition, the most helpful surveys will receive a free copy of *Safety Sexual* upon publication.

1. Would you be interested in having access to an electronic version of *Safely Sexual* or *Contraceptive Technology* if it were offered on the Internet, PDA or on a CD-ROM?
    ❏ CT ❏ Safely Sexual ❏ CD-ROM ❏ PDA ❏ Internet

2. Would you be interested in receiving electronic updates of *Contraceptive Technology* and/or *Safely Sexual*?
    ❏ CT ❏ Safely Sexual ❏ Both

3. How often would you like to receive electronic updates?
    ❏ Every 3 months   ❏ Every 6 months   ❏ Other_____

4. What would you consider a fair price for an update as often as you specified above of a chapter or the entire *CT* book?
    Chapter $_____   Book $_____

5. Would you be interested primarily in receiving electronic updates of specific chapters of *CT*? If yes, please specify your top 5 choices in order of preference by chapter number. 1____ 2____ 3____ 4____ 5____

6. Let us know if you are interested in a *CT* and *Safely Sexual* CD-ROM or PDA:

    ❏ I am interested in a CD-ROM of ❏ *CT* ❏ *Safely Sexual* to printout information for patients.

    ❏ I am interested in a CD-ROM of ❏ *CT* ❏ *Safely Sexual* with additional information.
       Such as: ❏ audio ❏ video ❏ color graphics
                ❏ selected readings or source material

    ❏ I am interested in approximately ____ copies of a ❏ CD-ROM ❏ PDA for ❏ *CT* ❏ *Safely Sexual*.

    ❏ I am part of a network of _____ users and would like information on a network license or bulk purchase of ____ copies of ❏ *CT* ❏ *SS* on ❏ CD-ROM ❏ PDA.

    ❏ I am interested in a ❏ CD-ROM ❏ PDA with high-end capabilities such as searching with Boolean logic, word proximity, and key words or phrases for ❏ *CT* ❏ *SS*.

7. What could we do to improve the book and electronic media to make it more useful to you?

Please use additional sheet re: above questions 1-7 with your specific suggestions.

Please complete the other side of this form.

PLEASE PHOTOCOPY THIS FORM OR CUT OUT AND MAIL TO ARDENT MEDIA, INC. BOX 286, COOPER STATION P.O., NEW YORK, NY 10276-0286

ARDENT MEDIA INC
Box 286 Cooper Station P.O.
New York, New York 10276-0286

Please Print Clearly

Name _____

Address _____

_____

City _____

State _____ Zip _____

Telephone _____

Fax _____

E-mail _____

Method of Payment: ☐ Purchase Order enclosed (Institutions only)
☐ Check ☐ Money Order ☐ MasterCard ☐ Visa

Credit Card #: _____

Expiration Date _____

Name on Card _____
(Please Print Above)

Signature _____

Contact Ardent Media for discount information on bulk orders (*Contraceptive Technology*: 25 copies or more) at our fax (212) 861-0998, phone (212) 861-1501 or write to our New York address listed on this page. Please see reverse side for more information on bulk discounts.

Prices are subject to change without notice. All sales final. No returns. Our standard returns policy applies for bookstores.

Order Form

Ardent Media Inc Federal ID # 13-3984679

Description	Unit Price	Quantity	Total
Contraceptive Technology **New 18th Edition** • *New Hormonal Methods* • *New Contraceptive Efficacy Rates*			
Hardback with CD-ROM sewn binding for durability ISBN 0-9664902-3-1	$99.95		
Hardback sewn binding for durability ISBN 0-9664902-5-8	$79.95		
Paperback with CD-ROM ISBN 0-9664902-2-3	$79.95		
Paperback ISBN 0-9664902-6-6	$59.95		
CD-ROM ISBN 0-9664902-7-4	$59.95		
PDA (Personal Digital Assistant) ISBN 1-59708-000-4	$59.95		
Contraceptive Technology 17th Edition—Includes detailed information on Depo-Provera and Norplant Paperback (published 1998) ISBN 0-9664902-0-7	$39.95		
Managing Contraception 2004-2005: A Pocket Guide (paperback 3.5" x 5.5") ISBN 0-9638875-4-8	$10.00		

Subtotal	
10% Postage and handling (minimum $2.50) *International shipping additional (minimum $10.00)*	
NY residents add sales tax (NYC 8.625%)	
TOTAL DUE (US funds only)	

Note: When ordering CD-ROM or PDA format, please mail the Registration Form on next page. PDA format sent on CD-ROM or we will e-mail to you instructions to download from the web.

ARDENT MEDIA INC
Ordering Information
1-800-218-1535

Credit card orders (VISA or MasterCard) or institutional purchase orders may be placed toll-free 9 AM–5 PM EST weekdays at the above telephone number.

Credit card orders (VISA or MasterCard) or institutional purchase orders may be faxed *toll free* 24 hours to **1-800-711-3724.**

or

Please photocopy or clip the Order Form on the opposite side and mail with your check, money order, credit card information, or purchase order to:
ARDENT MEDIA INC Box 286, Cooper Station P.O., New York, NY 10276-0286

or

**Visit the website of ARDENT MEDIA INC
Scheduled opening October 2004**
www.ardentmediainc.com

This 18th edition of *Contraceptive Technology* is current until publication of the 19th edition, scheduled for release in 2007. Please write or fax ARDENT MEDIA to be notified of the publication of the 19th edition and receive a prepublication discount offer. Please state if you are a nonprofit organization and the number of copies you are interested in purchasing. Also check our website listed above for further information, sign up for e-mail notification and prepublication discount offer.

Bulk Purchase Discounts: Contraceptive Technology. For discounts on orders of 25 copies or more please call (212) 861-1501, fax (212) 861-0998 or write the address above. Please state if you are a nonprofit organization and the number of copies you are interested in purchasing. Bulk discount orders are nonreturnable. *Note:* Any of the ISBNs listed for *Contraceptive Technology,* including the electronic formats, may be combined to qualify for the 25 copy minimum: for example, 10 paperbacks, 10 hardbacks, and 5 PDAs.

Bulk Purchase Discounts: Managing Contraception. Minimum quantity for bulk discount is 100 copies. Please contact Special Sales Department at (212) 861-1501, fax (212) 861-0998 or write the address above.

Note to Book Sellers:
All returns require written permission and label from the publisher. CD-ROMs returnable only if packaging is unopened. Write to the address above or fax to the number above for permission.

ARDENT MEDIA INC
Box 286 Cooper Station P.O.
New York, New York 10276-0286

Order Form

Ardent Media Inc Federal ID # 13-3984679

Description	Unit Price	Quantity	Total
Contraceptive Technology **New 18th Edition** • New Hormonal Methods • New Contraceptive Efficacy Rates			
Hardback with CD-ROM sewn binding for durability ISBN 0-9664902-3-1	$99.95		
Hardback sewn binding for durability ISBN 0-9664902-5-8	$79.95		
Paperback with CD-ROM ISBN 0-9664902-2-3	$79.95		
Paperback ISBN 0-9664902-6-6	$59.95		
CD-ROM ISBN 0-9664902-7-4	$59.95		
PDA (Personal Digital Assistant) ISBN 1-59708-000-4	$59.95		
Contraceptive Technology 17th Edition—Includes detailed information on Depo-Provera and Norplant Paperback (published 1998) ISBN 0-9664902-0-7	$39.95		
Managing Contraception 2004-2005: A Pocket Guide (paperback 3.5" x 5.5") ISBN 0-9638875-4-8	$10.00		

Note: When ordering CD-ROM or PDA format, please mail the Registration Form on next page. PDA format sent on CD-ROM or we will e-mail to you instructions to download from the web.

Please Print Clearly

Name _____

Address _____

City _____

State _____ Zip _____

Telephone _____

Fax _____

E-mail _____

Method of Payment: ☐ Purchase Order enclosed (Institutions only)
☐ Check ☐ Money Order ☐ MasterCard ☐ Visa

Credit Card #: _____

Expiration Date _____

Name on Card _____
(Please Print Above)

Signature _____

Contact Ardent Media for discount information on bulk orders (Contraceptive Technology: 25 copies or more) at our fax (212) 861-0998, phone (212) 861-1501 or write to our New York address listed on this page. Please see reverse side for more information on bulk discounts.

Prices are subject to change without notice. All sales final. No returns. Our standard returns policy applies for bookstores.

Subtotal _____

10% Postage and handling (minimum $2.50)
International shipping additional (minimum $10.00)
NY residents add sales tax (NYC 8.625%)

TOTAL DUE (US funds only) _____

ARDENT MEDIA INC
Ordering Information
1-800-218-1535

Credit card orders (VISA or MasterCard) or institutional purchase orders may be placed toll-free 9 AM–5 PM EST weekdays at the above telephone number.

Credit card orders (VISA or MasterCard) or institutional purchase orders may be faxed *toll free* 24 hours to **1-800-711-3724**.

or

Please photocopy or clip the Order Form on the opposite side and mail with your check, money order, credit card information, or purchase order to:
ARDENT MEDIA INC Box 286, Cooper Station P.O., New York, NY 10276-0286

or

Visit the website of ARDENT MEDIA INC
Scheduled opening October 2004

www.ardentmediainc.com

This 18th edition of *Contraceptive Technology* is current until publication of the 19th edition, scheduled for release in 2007. Please write or fax ARDENT MEDIA to be notified of the publication of the 19th edition and receive a prepublication discount offer. Please state if you are a nonprofit organization and the number of copies you are interested in purchasing. Also check our website listed above for further information, sign up for e-mail notification and prepublication discount offer.

Bulk Purchase Discounts: Contraceptive Technology. For discounts on orders of 25 copies or more please call (212) 861-1501, fax (212) 861-0998 or write the address above. Please state if you are a nonprofit organization and the number of copies you are interested in purchasing. Bulk discount orders are nonreturnable. *Note:* Any of the ISBNs listed for *Contraceptive Technology,* including the electronic formats, may be combined to qualify for the 25 copy minimum: for example, 10 paperbacks, 10 hardbacks, and 5 PDAs.

Bulk Purchase Discounts: Managing Contraception. Minimum quantity for bulk discount is 100 copies. Please contact Special Sales Department at (212) 861-1501, fax (212) 861-0998 or write the address above.

Note to Book Sellers:
All returns require written permission and label from the publisher. CD-ROMs returnable only if packaging is unopened. Write to the address above or fax to the number above for permission.